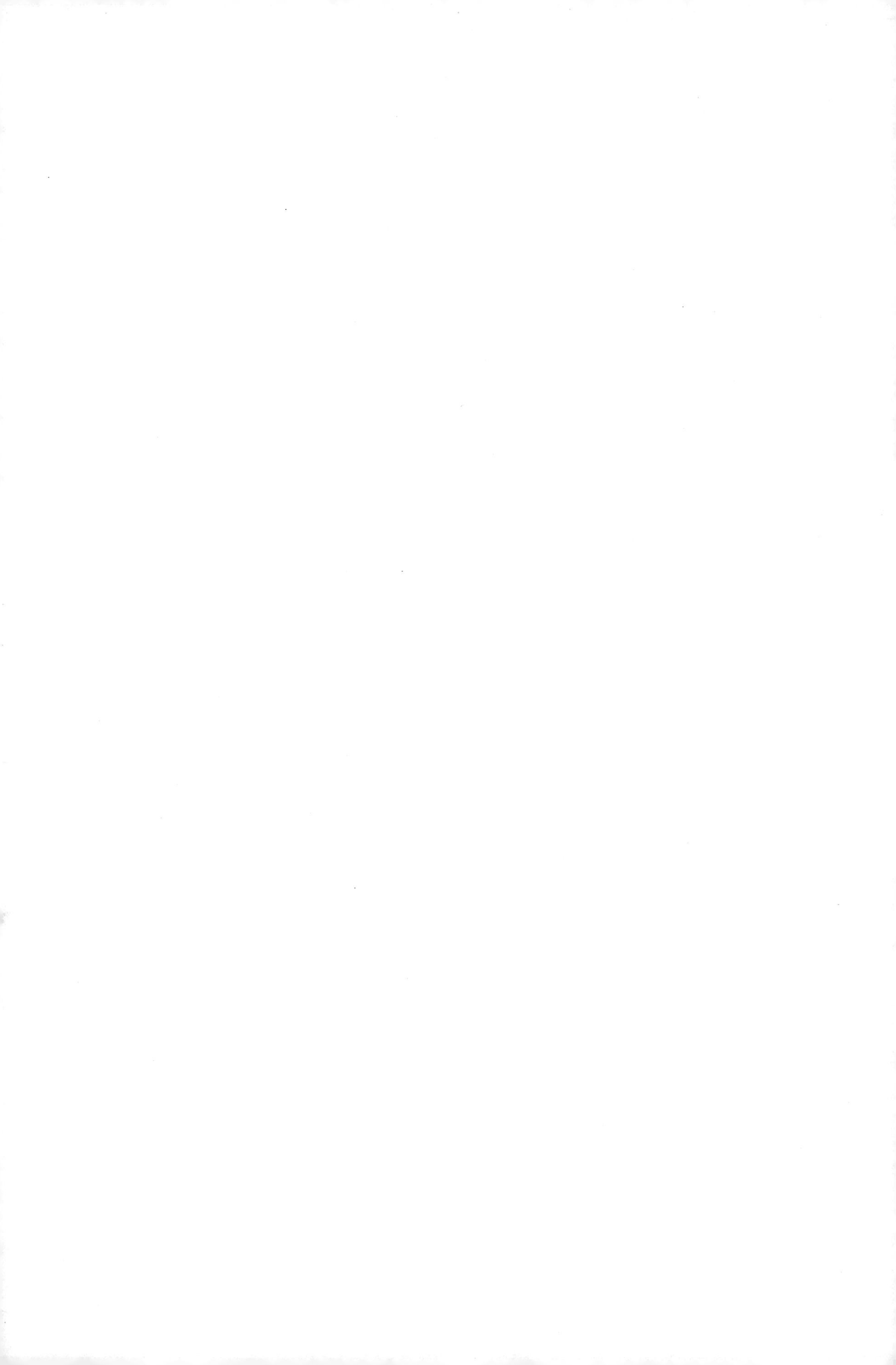

Aeromedical Evacuation

William W. Hurd • William Beninati
Editors

Aeromedical Evacuation

Management of Acute and Stabilized Patients

Second Edition

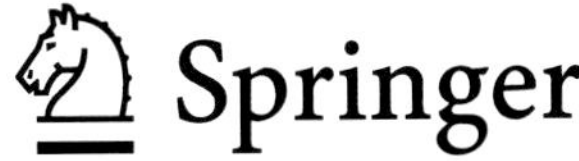

Editors
William W. Hurd, MD, MPH, FACOG, FACS
Col, USAF, MC, SFS (ret.)
Chief Medical Officer
American Society for Reproductive Medicine
Professor Emeritus
Department of Obstetrics and Gynecology
Duke University Medical Center
Durham, NC
USA

William Beninati, MD, FCCM
Col, USAF, MC, CFS (ret.)
Senior Medical Director
Intermountain Life Flight and Virtual Hospital
University of Utah School of Medicine
Salt Lake City, UT
USA

Clinical Associate Professor (Affiliated)
Stanford University School of Medicine
Stanford, CA
USA

ISBN 978-3-030-15902-3 ISBN 978-3-030-15903-0 (eBook)
https://doi.org/10.1007/978-3-030-15903-0

This Springer imprint is published by the registered company Springer Nature Switzerland AG
The registered company address is: Gewerbestrasse 11, 6330 Cham, Switzerland

Foreword

Killed in action (KIA), died of wounds (DOW), and case fatality (CF) rates among US service members are at their lowest points in the history of warfare. Directly attributable to this striking rise in survivability are numerous factors, which include highly effective body armor, widespread use of Tactical Combat Casualty Care at the point of injury (POI), rapid casualty evacuation/ tactical critical care evacuation from POI to higher levels of medical care, forward resuscitative surgery, a standardized trauma network that is integrated across all theaters of operation, and aeromedical evacuation (AE) bolstered by Critical Care Air Transport Teams (CCATT). Clearly, all of the aforementioned capabilities have saved thousands of lives and mitigated incalculable suffering. The en route care system (a series of clinical and mobility processes bridged by a command and control system, along with a network of organizations composed of highly trained, multidisciplinary personnel; machines, technology, and information systems) has been the keystone for the dramatic reduction in the footprint of medical personnel and infrastructure within the theater of operations. As a result, logistics support is freed up for other purposes while further advancing the quality of care for our injured and/or ailing service members. Moreover, whether supporting combat or humanitarian/disaster relief operations, the en route care system represents a national capability essential to the security of the United States.

Undoubtedly, America's national security is based on the appropriate application of the instruments of national power (diplomacy, information, military, and economic). However, without the patriotic, courageous, dedicated, and self-sacrificing men and women serving in our nation's armed forces, the instruments of national power would be fatally weakened. It is, therefore, critical for America's political and military leaders to heed the advice of Major (Dr.) Jonathan Letterman, Medical Director, Army of the Potomac, whose innovations still form the backbone of the US military's standardized battlefield trauma system, as well as its en route care casualty evacuation system: "It is the interest of the Government, aside from all the motives of humanity, to bestow the greatest possible care upon its wounded and sick, and to use every means to preserve the health of those who are well, since the greater the labor given to the preservation of health, the greater will be the number for duty, and the more attention bestowed upon the sick and wounded, the more speedily will they perform the duties for which they were employed." In other words, regardless of the cost, it is incumbent upon the US Government to provide all the resources required to optimize care for its armed service members, and it is incumbent upon the leadership of the Military Health System to ensure all military medical personnel are resourced, trained, experienced, and *always* ready to deliver increasingly sophisticated healthcare. This must encompass the total spectrum of care required to support the nation's defenders of freedom, whether it be at home garrison, the battlefield, and all points in-between. It is to this end this essential textbook lies. Its contents have been updated by a distinguished panel of experts in disciplines who collectively and synergistically compose the US military's unrivaled en route care system.

Bart O. Iddins, MD, DVM, SM
Maj Gen, USAF, MC, CFS (ret.)
Medical Director, Oak Ridge National Laboratory
Oak Ridge, TN, USA

Preface

Aeromedical evacuation (AE), the long-distance air transportation of patients, has advanced dramatically since the first edition of this book was published almost two decades ago. At that time, forward-deployed medical units have become lighter and more rapidly deployable, and thus have little patient-holding capacity. This evolution has made AE an essential element of contingency medical care throughout the world. The reach of AE is global, and it spans contingencies from humanitarian operations and disaster relief to support for combat operations and the response to terrorism. The second edition of this book is an update that summarizes much of what has been learned about important issues that should be considered in planning and executing long-distance AE.

We asked our expert authors to concentrate on two primary objectives as they rewrote their chapters. The first objective is to describe the problems and limitations of medical care in-flight. Ground-based medical teams manage patients before AE and determine the timing of when to request AE. Their clinical and operational decisions can have a major impact on how their patients will tolerate the stresses and limitations of the AE environment. The goal is to increase non-flying clinicians' appreciation of the medical flight environment so that they can better select and prepare their patients for AE.

The second objective is to examine the unique challenges that AE presents for patients with specific medical conditions. This applies to both elective and urgent AE. It is especially important for urgent AE, since recently stabilized patients have less physiologic reserve, and are often more sensitive to the stresses of flight. To minimize patient risks during flight, we have asked experts in their fields to provide criteria that patients with specific conditions should fulfill prior to AE. These experts have also outlined patient preparation and equipment required for safe air transportation and management of the most likely complications that can occur during flight.

Years of AE experience transporting stabilized patients who are critically ill or injured has greatly improved our understanding of the stresses of flight and the risks to specific patients during long-distance AE. We hope that the updated information in this edition will help guide medical planners and serve as a useful reference for the military and civilian clinicians who prepare patients for AE, and especially the medical flight crews who take care of them in the air.

William W. Hurd, MD, MPH, FACOG, FACS
Col, USAF, MC, SFS (ret.)
Durham, NC, USA

William Beninati, MD, FCCM
Col, USAF, MC, CFS (ret.)
Salt Lake City, UT, USA

Disclaimer

The views expressed herein are those of the authors and do not necessarily reflect the official policies or positions of any agency of the US Government, including the US Air Force, the US Army, the US Navy, the Department of Defense, the Department of Veterans Affairs, and the Federal Aviation Administration.

Contents

Contributors

Tamara A. Averett-Brauer, MN, BSN Col, USAF, NC. CFN, En Route Care and Expeditionary Medicine, Human Performance Wing, Aeromedical Research Department, USAF School of Aerospace Medicine, Wright Patterson AFB, Dayton, OH, USA

David J. Barillo, MD, FACS, FCCM COL, MC, USA (ret.), Former, Clinical Division/Director US Army Burn Center, Former, US Army Burn Flight Team, U.S. Army Institute of Surgical Research, Joint Base San Antonio-Fort Sam Houston, San Antonio, TX, USA

Disaster Response/Critical Care Consultants, LLC, Mount Pleasant, SC, USA

William Beninati, MD, FCCM Col, USAF, MC, CFS (ret.), Senior Medical Director, Intermountain Life Flight and Virtual Hospital, University of Utah School of Medicine, Salt Lake City, UT, USA

Clinical Associate Professor (Affiliated), Stanford University School of Medicine, Stanford, CA, USA

John R. Bennett, MD, FAAO-HNS, FAAFPRS Ear Nose & Throat Center of Utah, Salt Lake City, UT, USA

Matthew A. Borgman, MD, FCCM, CHSE LTC, MC, USA, Pediatric Critical Care Services, Brook Army Medical Center Simulation Center, Joint Base San Antonio - Fort Sam Houston, San Antonio, TX, USA

Department of Pediatrics, F. Edward Hebert School of Medicine - Uniformed Services University, Bethesda, MD, USA

Richard D. Branson, MS, RRT, FAARC, FCCM Department of Surgery, Division of Trauma/Critical Care, University of Cincinnati, Cincinnati, OH, USA

School of Aerospace Medicine, Wright Patterson Air Force Base, Dayton, OH, USA

Joseph A. Brennan, MD, FACS Col, USAF, MC (ret.), Clinical Operations, Department of Surgery, Uniformed Services University of the Health Sciences, Annapolis, MD, USA

Elizabeth Bridges, PhD, RN, CCNS Col, USAF, NC (ret.), Biobehavioral Nursing and Health Informatics, University of Washington School of Nursing, University of Washington Medical Center, Seattle, WA, USA

Kristine P. Broger, DNP, RN, MHA, CCRN, NE-BC LTC, NC, USA, US Army Burn Flight Team, Nursing, US Army Medical Department, Guthrie MEDDAC, Fort Drum, NY, USA

Melissa A. Buzbee-Stiles, MSN, RN, CEN Maj, USAF, NC, En Route Medical Care Division, Office of the Command Surgeon, Headquarters Air Mobility Command, Scott Air Force Base, IL, USA

Jeremy W. Cannon, MD, MS, FACS Col, USAFR, MC, Department of Surgery, Penn Presbyterian Medical Center, Perelman School of Medicine at the University of Pennsylvania, Philadelphia, PA, USA

Uniformed Services University of the Health Sciences, Bethesda, MD, USA

George W. Christopher, MD Col, USAF, MC (ret.), Medical Countermeasure Systems, Joint Program Executive Office for Chemical and Biological Defense, Fort Belvoir, VA, USA

Nicholas G. Conger, MD Col, USAF, MC, Wright Patterson Air Force Base, Dayton, OH, USA

Division of Infectious Disease, Department of Internal Medicine, Wright State University School of Medicine, Dayton, OH, USA

Cord W. Cunningham, MD, MPH, FACEP, FAEMS LTC (P), MC, FS, DMO, USA, Critical Care Flight Paramedic Program, Center for Prehospital Medicine, Army Medical Department Center and School Health Readiness Center of Excellence, Joint Trauma System Committee on En Route Combat Casualty Care, DoD EMS & Disaster Medicine Fellowship SAUSHEC, Joint Base San Antonio-Fort Sam Houston, San Antonio, TX, USA

Robert A. De Lorenzo, MD, MSM, MSCI, FACEP LTC, MC, FS, USA (ret.), Faculty Development, Department of Emergency Medicine, University of Texas Health Science Center at San Antonio, San Antonio, TX, USA

Lisa Diane DeDecker, MS, RN Lt Col, USAF, NC, CFN (ret.), En Route Critical Care Program, Division of En Route Medical Care, Headquarters Air Mobility Command, Command Surgeon's Office, Scott Air Force Base, IL, USA

Daniel J. Donovan, MD, MBA, MHCM COL, MC, USAR, 1252nd Medical Detachment, Tripler Army Medical Center, Department of Surgery, University of Hawaii John A. Burns School of Medicine, Honolulu, HI, USA

Gina R. Dorlac, MD Col, USAF, MC (ret.), Critical Care Medicine and Pulmonary Disease, University of Colorado Health, Fort Collins, CO, USA

Warren C. Dorlac, MD, FACS Col, USAF, MC, FS (ret.), Trauma and Acute Care Surgery, Department of Surgery, Medical Center of the Rockies and the University of Colorado School of Medicine, University of Colorado Health, Trauma Services, Loveland, CO, USA

Ryan E. Earnest, MD, FACS LtCol, USAF, MC, Surgical Critical Care, Department of Trauma and General Surgery, University of Cincinnati Medical Center, Cincinnati, OH, USA

Jo Ann Egan, BSN, MS Department of Ophthalmology, Madigan Army Medical Center, Tacoma, WA, USA

DoD-VA Vision Center of Excellence, Bethesda, MD, USA

Michael J. Eppinger, MD Col, USAF (ret.), Cardiothoracic Surgery, Department of Surgery, South Texas Veterans Health Care System, San Antonio, TX, USA

Angela M. Fagiana, MD, FAAP Maj, USAF, MC, Neonatal Transport, Department of Neonatology, Brooke Army Medical Center, Fort Sam Houston, TX, USA

Department of Pediatrics, F. Edward Hebert School of Medicine – Uniformed Services University, Bethesda, MD, USA

William F. Fallon Jr, MD, MBA LTC, MC, USA (ret.), Trauma Surgery & Surgical Critical Care, Summa Health System, Akron, OH, USA

Department of Surgery, Case West Reserve University School of Medicine, Cleveland, OH, USA

Raymond Fang, MD, FACS Col, USAF, MC (ret.), Department of Surgery, Johns Hopkins Bayview Medical Center, Baltimore, MD, USA

J. Christopher Farmer, MD, FACP, FCCP, FCCM Col, USAF, MC, FS (ret.), Department of Critical Care Medicine, Mayo Clinic Hospital, Phoenix, AZ, USA

Kathleen M. Flarity, DNP, PhD, CEN, CFRN, FAEN Col, USAF, NC, CFN, Air Mobility Command, Scott Air Force Base, IL, USA

Emergency Medicine, University of Colorado School of Medicine, UC Health, Aurora, CO, USA

Brian T. Garibaldi, MD Department of Medicine and Physiology, Division of Pulmonary and Critical Care Medicine, Johns Hopkins Biocontainment Unit, Johns Hopkins University School of Medicine, Baltimore, MD, USA

Thomas E. Grissom, MD, MSIS, FCCM Col, USAF, MC (ret.), Department of Anesthesiology, R Adams Cowley Shock Trauma Center, University of Maryland School of Medicine, Catonsville, MD, USA

Jose J. Gutierrez-Nunez, MD Col, USAF, MC (ret.), University of Puerto Rico School of Medicine, Department of Medicine, San Juan Veterans Administration Medical Center, San Juan, PR, USA

Steven J. Hatfill, MD, MSc, MSc, M.Med Department of Clinical Research and Leadership, Department of Microbiology, Immunology, and Tropical Medicine, George Washington University Medical School, Washington, DC, USA

Jennifer J. Hatzfeld, PhD, RN, APHN-BC Lt Col, USAF, NC, TriService Nursing Research Program, Uniformed Services University of Health Sciences, Bethesda, MD, USA

Anthony J. Hayes, BS, MD LT, MC, USN, Department of General Surgery, Navy Medical Center Camp Lejeune, Camp Lejeune, NC, USA

Howard S. Heiman, MD, FAAP COL, MC, USA (ret.), Neonatal Transport, Department of Pediatrics, Neonatal-Perinatal Division, Cohen Children's Medical Center of Greater New York, Northwell Health, New Hyde Park, NY, USA

William W. Hurd, MD, MPH, FACOG, FACS Col, USAF, MC, SFS (ret.), Chief Medical Officer, American Society for Reproductive Medicine, Professor Emeritus Department of Obstetrics and Gynecology, Duke University Medical Center, Durham, NC, USA

Formerly, CCATT physician and Commander, 445th ASTS, Wright-Patterson Air Force Base, Dayton, OH, USA

Bart O. Iddins, MD, DVM, SM Maj Gen, USAF, MC, CFS (ret.), Formerly, Command Surgeon, Air Mobility Command & Air Force Special Operations Command, Director, Health Services Division, Oak Ridge National Laboratory, Oak Ridge, TN, USA

T. Jacob Lee Jr, MD, FAAP Maj, USAF, MC, Pediatric Critical Care, Critical Care Air Transport, Department of Pediatrics, Brooke Army Medical Center, Joint Base San Antonio-Fort Sam Houston, San Antonio, TX, USA

John G. Jernigan, MPH, MD Brig Gen, USAF, CFS (ret.), Formerly Commander, Human Systems Center, Brooks Air Force Base, Texas, San Antonio, TX, USA

Nathan A. Jordan, MD MAJ, MC, USA, Department of Surgery, Tripler Army Medical Center, Uniformed Services University of the Health Sciences, Honolulu, HI, USA

Donald E. Keen, MD, MPH, EMTP MAJ, MC, FS, USA, Army Critical Care Flight Paramedic Program, Center for Pre-Hospital Medicine, U.S Army Medical Department Center and School, Joint Base San Antonio-Fort Sam Houston, San Antonio, TX, USA

Chetan U. Kharod, MD, MPH Col, USAF, MC, SFS (ret.), SAUSHEC Military EMS & Disaster Medicine Fellowship, Emergency Medicine, Uniformed Services University, Bethesda, MD, USA

Department of Emergency Medicine, San Antonio Military Medical Center, Joint Base San Antonio-Fort Sam Houston, San Antonio, TX, USA

Robert A. Klocke, MD, FACP Department of Medicine, Jacobs School of Medicine and Biomedical Education, State University of New York at Buffalo, Buffalo, NY, USA

Jose M. Lara-Ruiz, MA Department of Psychiatry, University of Texas Health Science Center, San Antonio, TX, USA

Rose M. Leary-Wojcik, DMD, MD Col, USAF, MC (ret.), Oral & Maxillofacial Surgery, Good Samaritan Clinic, DeLand, FL, USA

Amy T. Makley, MD Department of Surgery, University of Cincinnati, Cincinnati, OH, USA

Phillip E. Mason, MD, FACEP Lt Col, USAF, MC, Department of Surgery, San Antonio Military Medical Center, Fort Sam Houston, TX, USA

Robert A. Mazzoli, MD, FACS COL, MC, USA (ret.), Department of Ophthalmology, Ophthalmic Plastic, Reconstructive, and Orbital Surgery, Madigan Army Medical Center, Tacoma, WA, USA

Uniformed Services University of the Health Sciences, Bethesda, MD, USA

Former Consultant to the US Army Surgeon General, DoD-VA Vision Center of Excellence, Bethesda, MD, USA

Thomas J. McLaughlin, DO, FACEP Colonel, USAF, MC, SFS (ret.), Department of Emergency Medicine, Texas A&M University College of Medicine, Bryan, TX, USA

Department of Emergency Medicine, CHRISTUS Health/Texas A&M Spahn Emergency Medicine Residency, Corpus Christi, TX, USA

Skyler W. Nielsen, BS, DO Capt, USAF USARMY MEDCOM BAMC, Department of Otolaryngology, San Antonio Military Medical Center, Fort Sam Houston, TX, USA

Steven L. Oreck, SB, MA, MD CAPT, MC, USN (FMF) (ret.), Department of History, University of Wisconsin-Madison, Madison, WI, USA

Mick J. Perez-Cruet, MD, MS Department of Neurosurgery, Oakland University William Beaumont School of Medicine, Royal Oak, MI, USA

Alan L. Peterson, PhD, ABPP Col, USAF (ret.), Department of Psychiatry, Division of Behavioral Medicine, The Military Health Institute, University of Texas Health Science Center, San Antonio, TX, USA

Christopher J. Pickard-Gabriel, MD Maj, USAF, MC, Anesthesia Critical Care, Perelman School of Medicine at the University of Pennsylvania, Philadelphia, PA, USA

J. D. Polk, DO, MS, MMM, FACOEP, FAsMA LtCol, USAF, MC, CFS (ret.), National Aeronautics and Space Administration, Washington, DC, USA

Department of Policy, George Mason University, Fairfax County, VA, USA

Edward Via College of Osteopathic Medicine, Blacksburg, VA, USA

Bryan Propes, MD CDR, MC, USN, Department of Ophthalmology, Naval Medical Center San Diego, San Diego, CA, USA

Elspeth Cameron Ritchie, MD, MPH COL, MC, USA (ret.), Department of Psychiatry, Washington Hospital Center, Washington, DC, USA

Julie A. Rizzo, MD, FACS MAJ, MC, USA, Burn Unit, United States Army Institute of Surgical Research, Fort Sam Houston, TX, USA

Dario Rodriquez Jr, MSc, RRT, FAARC CMS, USAF (ret.), Research Health Science, CSTARS, Cincinnati, OH, USA

Department of Aeromedical Research, En Route Care Research Division, USAF School of Aerospace Medicine, University of Cincinnati, Cincinnati, OH, USA

Robert E. Rogers, MD, FACOG COL, MC, USA (ret.), Department of Obstetrics and Gynecology, Indiana University School of Medicine, Indianapolis, IN, USA

Jeffrey M. Rothenberg, MD, FACOG Obstetrics-Gynecology, St. Vincent Hospitals, Indianapolis, IN, USA

David G. Schall, MD, MPH, FACS Col, USAF, MC, CFS (ret.), Formerly Otolaryngology Head & Neck Surgery Consultant to the USAF Surgeon General, Regional Flight Surgery/Aerospace Neurology, Office of Aerospace Medicine, Federal Aviation Administration, Des Plaines, IL, USA

Steven G. Schauer, DO, MS MAJ, MC, USA, US Army Institute of Surgical Research, San Antonio Military Medical Center, Joint Base San Antonio-Fort Sam Houston, San Antonio, TX, USA

Dhiya V. Shah, PsyD Department of Psychiatry and Primary Care Center, Division of Behavioral Medicine, University of Texas Health Science Center, San Antonio, TX, USA

Kenton E. Stephens Jr, MD Cardiothoracic Surgery, Denali Cardiac & Thoracic Surgical Group, Anchorage, AK, USA

Russell K. Stewart, BA Wake Forest School of Medicine, Winston-Salem, NC, USA

Lucas Teske, MD Department of Orthopedic Surgery, Wake Forest Baptist Health, Winston Salem, NC, USA

Brian R. Waterman, MD Department of Orthopaedic Surgery, Wake Forest Baptist Health, Winston Salem, NC, USA

Robert J. Wells, MD Col, USAF, MC, CFS (ret.), Formerly, Department of Pediatrics, University Of Texas MD Anderson Cancer Center, Houston, TX, USA

Formerly Commander, 445th ASTS, Wright-Patterson AFB, Dayton, OH, USA

Mark R. Withers, MD COL, MC, USA (ret.), Office of Medical Support & Oversight, U.S. Army Research Institute of Environmental Medicine, Natick, MA, USA

Abbreviations

AFB	Air Force Base
APHN-BC	Advanced Public Health Nurse, Board Certified
Brig Gen	Brigadier General
BS	Bachelor of Science
BSN	Bachelor of Science in Nursing
CAPT	Captain (USN)
Capt	Captain (USAF)
CEN	Certified Emergency Nurse
CFN	Chief Flight Nurse
CFRN	Certified Flight Registered Nurse
CFS	Chief Flight Surgeon
CHSE	Certified Healthcare Simulation Educator
CNA	Certified Nursing Administrator
CNS	Clinical Nurse Specialist
COL	Colonel (USA)
Col	Colonel (USAF)
CPE	Certified Physician Executive
CPT	Captain (USA)
DC	District of Columbia
DNP	Doctor of Nursing Practice
DO	Doctor of Osteopathic Medicine
FAAFPRS	Fellow of the American Academy of Facial Plastic and Reconstructive Surgery
FAAO-HNS	Fellow of the American Academy of Otolaryngology-Head and Neck Surgery
FAAP	Fellow, American Academy of Pediatrics
FAARC	Fellow, American Association for Respiratory Care
FACOEP	Fellow, American College of Osteopathic Emergency Physicians
FACOG	Fellow, American College of Obstetricians and Gynecologists
FACP	Fellow, American College of Physicians
FAsMA	Fellow, Aerospace Medical Association
FACEP	Fellow, American College of Emergency Physicians
FACS	Fellow, American College of Surgeons
FACEM	Fellow, Australasian College for Emergency Medicine
FAEN	Fellow, Academy of Emergency Nursing
FCCP	Fellow, American College of Chest Physicians

FCCM	Fellow, American College of Critical Care Medicine
FS	Flight Surgeon
LT	Lieutenant (USN)
LTC	Lieutenant Colonel (USA)
LtCol	Lieutenant Colonel (USAF)
LTC(P)	Lieutenant Colonel, Promotable (USA)
MAJ	Major (USA)
Maj	Major (USAF)
Maj Gen	Major General (USAF)
MBA	Master of Business Administration
MC	Medical Corps
MD	Doctor of Medicine
MHA	Master of Health Administration
MMM	Master of Medical Management
MPH	Master of Public Health
MS	Master of Science
MSCI	Master of Science in Clinical Investigation
MSIS	Master of Science in Information Systems
MSM	Master of Science in Management
MSN	Master of Science in Nursing
NASA	National Aeronautics and Space Administration
NC	Nurse Corps
PhD	Doctor of Philosophy
RN	Registered Nurse
ret.	Retired
RRT	Registered Respiratory Therapist
SFS	Senior Flight Surgeon
USA	United States Army
USAR	United States Army Reserve
USAF	United States Air Force
USAFR	United States Air Force Reserve
USN	United States Navy
USNR	United States Navy Reserve

Part I

The Need

Introduction

1

William W. Hurd and William Beninati

Aeromedical evacuation (AE), the long-distance air transportation of patients, has seen dramatic advancements over the last two decades. As a result, AE has become an essential linchpin of contingency medical care throughout the world. Transportation of casualties from the site of injury to the highest levels of care has undergone two key technological revolutions in the last 60 years. During the Korean and Vietnam conflicts, battlefield and tactical medical evacuation (MEDEVAC) was greatly improved by the use of helicopters to augment ground transportation. The ability to transport seriously wounded soldiers quickly from the injury site to field hospitals for definitive surgical care dramatically reduced battlefield mortality. More recently, during the wars in Iraq and Afghanistan, the military medical system has been transformed by the earlier use of AE for the transport of both stable and stabilized patients as soon as possible after definitive therapy. Years of practical experience has dramatically improved our ability to maximize in-flight care and minimized the risk of adverse sequelae that can be associated with transporting these patients.

The majority of military AE remains elective, where air transportation is reserved for stable or convalescing patients who will be only minimally affected by the stresses of air transportation. Highly trained flight nurses and medical technicians monitor patients in-flight to minimize the chance that they will experience difficulty during AE. Elective AE continues to be performed using a variety of military and civilian aircraft with an assorted level of medical equipment and personnel required to deal with the uncommon medical emergencies that occur in-flight.

The last decade has seen the rapid development of a robust Urgent AE system as a result of increased training for AE flight crews and the total integration of specially trained and equipped Critical Care Air Transport Teams (CCATT). These highly trained Operational Support teams are comprised of physicians, critical care nurses, and cardiorespiratory therapists and their specialized equipment and remain on standby alert to transport stabilized patients to higher echelons of care whenever the need arises. This integrated system for transporting patients requiring ongoing intensive care greatly

W. W. Hurd (✉)
Col, USAF, MC, SFS (ret.), Chief Medical Officer, American Society for Reproductive Medicine, Professor Emeritus Department of Obstetrics and Gynecology, Duke University Medical Center, Durham, NC, USA

Formerly, CCATT physician and Commander, 445th ASTS, Wright-Patterson Air Force Base, Dayton, OH, USA
e-mail: whurd@asrm.org

W. Beninati
Col, USAF, MC, CFS (ret.), Senior Medical Director, Intermountain Life Flight and Virtual Hospital, University of Utah School of Medicine, Salt Lake City, UT, USA

Clinical Associate Professor (Affiliated), Stanford University School of Medicine, Stanford, CA, USA

W. W. Hurd, W. Beninati (eds.), *Aeromedical Evacuation*,
https://doi.org/10.1007/978-3-030-15903-0_1

enhances the US Air Force (USAF) capability to provide AE to stabilized critically ill or injured personnel anywhere in the world.

The original impetus for enhancing medical care capability of AE was to minimize the in-theater medical footprint, since quality postoperative care and large patient-holding facilities are difficult to maintain in a contingency environment. This contemporary AE paradigm has resulted in continued improvements in the survival of critically ill and severely injured patients throughout the world—particularly during armed conflicts, natural disasters, or other catastrophic events.

A great deal has been learned over the last decade about the optimal preparation for AE of patients with a broad spectrum of medical and surgical conditions, both in terms of patient preparation and AE crew preparation. However, not all of this new information has been well documented, primarily because the clinicians who have become experts in this type of Operational Support medicine are not always in environments conducive to such reporting.

The second edition of this book is an update that summarizes much of what has been learned over the last two decades about important issues that should be considered prior to and during long-distance AE. Since AE is a complex process with many steps, we have two primary objectives. The first is to describe the problems and limitations of medical care in-flight. The goal is to increase nonflying clinicians' appreciation of the medical flight environment when considering AE for their patients.

Our second objective is to examine the unique AE problems and risks for patients with specific conditions when considering either Elective or Urgent AE. This is especially important for Urgent AE, since it is well appreciated that recently treated patients are often more sensitive to the stresses of flight and at higher risk for decompensation. To minimize patient risks during flight, we have asked experts in their fields to provide criteria that patients with specific conditions should fulfill prior to AE. These experts have also outlined patient preparation and equipment required for safe air transportation and the most likely complications that can occur during flight.

Years of AE experience transporting critically ill patients has greatly improved our understanding of the stresses of flight and the risks to specific patients during long-distance AE. We hope that this updated information will serve as a useful reference source for both the military and civilian clinicians who prepare patients for AE and the medical flight crews who take care of them in the air.

2 Aeromedical Evacuation: A Historical Perspective

Kathleen M. Flarity, Tamara A. Averett-Brauer, and Jennifer J. Hatzfeld

Introduction

The origin of aeromedical evacuation (AE), the transport of the sick and wounded by aircraft, has a proud heritage that spans more than 100 years. The current AE system has been instrumental in saving thousands of lives in peace, war, contingencies, conflicts other than war, and during humanitarian missions. The resolute progress of AE, which parallels the advances in human flight, has been the result of humankind's desire to avoid the ultimate sacrifice of death while bravely defending their country's vital interests. Although early development of AE progressed slowly, its many champions steadfastly believed that air transport of the wounded could significantly decrease the morbidity and mortality of those injured in battle. The history of AE began in the early part of the twentieth century as an important part of military medicine. In the modern era, AE has risen to new heights with the implementation of technological advances in both flight and medicine [1–3].

K. M. Flarity (✉)
Col, USAF, NC, CFN, Air Mobility Command, Scott Air Force Base, IL, USA

Emergency Medicine, University of Colorado School of Medicine, UC Health, Aurora, CO, USA
e-mail: Kathleen.flarity@uchealth.org

T. A. Averett-Brauer
Col, USAF, NC. CFN, En Route Care and Expeditionary Medicine, Human Performance Wing, Aeromedical Research Department, USAF School of Aerospace Medicine, Wright Patterson AFB, Dayton, OH, USA

J. J. Hatzfeld
Lt Col, USAF, NC, TriService Nursing Research Program, Uniformed Services University of Health Sciences, Bethesda, MD, USA

Before World War I

The concept of moving the wounded by air began almost simultaneously with the concept of fixed-wing aircraft flight. Shortly after the Wright brothers successfully flew their first airplane, two US Army medical officers, Captain George H. R. Gosman and Lieutenant A. L. Rhodes, designed an airplane built to transport patients [1–3]. Using their own money, they built and flew the world's first air ambulance at Fort Barrancas, FL, in 1910. Unfortunately, on its first test flight, it only flew 500 yards at an altitude of 100 feet before crashing. This flight, followed by Captain Gosman's unsuccessful attempt to obtain official backing for the project, proved to be only the beginning of many challenges for this new concept [2, 3].

World War I Era

World War I will not be remembered for the extent that AE was used, but as a time when air ambulance design made significant progress by

W. W. Hurd, W. Beninati (eds.), *Aeromedical Evacuation*,
https://doi.org/10.1007/978-3-030-15903-0_2

trial and error. A French medical officer, Eugene Chassaing, first adapted French military planes for use as air ambulances [1, 2]. Two patients were inserted side-by-side into the fuselage behind the pilot's cockpit. Modified Dorand II aircraft were used on the battlefield in April 1918 in what was the first actual AE of the wounded in airplanes specifically equipped for patient movement [1, 2].

The United States also used airplanes for evacuating the injured from the battlefield in World War I, but found it difficult to use planes not suited for patient airlift [1]. Specifically, the fuselages were too small to accommodate stretchers and the open cockpit exposed patients to the elements. The US Army Medical Corps used airplanes primarily to transport flight surgeons to the site of airplane accidents to assist in the ground transportation of casualties [1–3].

By the end of the War, the US Army recognized the emerging requirement to transport the wounded by air. In 1918, Major Nelson E. Driver and Captain William C. Ocker converted a Curtiss JN-4 Jenny biplane into an airplane ambulance by modifying the rear cockpit to accommodate a standard Army stretcher (Fig. 2.1). This allowed the US Army to transport patients by airplane for the first time [1, 2].

Between the World Wars

The success of the Curtis JN-4 Jenny air ambulances during World War I paved the way for the further development of AE [1]. In 1920, the De Havilland DH-4 aircraft was modified to carry a medical attendant in addition to two side-by-side patients in the fuselage. Shortly thereafter, the Cox-Klemmin aircraft became the first aircraft built specifically as an air ambulance. This airplane carried two patients and a medical attendant enclosed within the aircraft. In 1921, the Curtis Eagle aircraft was built to transport four patients on litters and six ambulatory patients. Unfortunately, in its first year in service, a Curtis Eagle crashed during an electrical storm, killing seven people. Despite this apparent setback, aeromedical transportation continued to progress. In 1922, the US Army converted the largest single-engine airplane built at the time, the Fokker F-IV, into an air ambulance designated as the A-2. In the same year, a US Army physician,

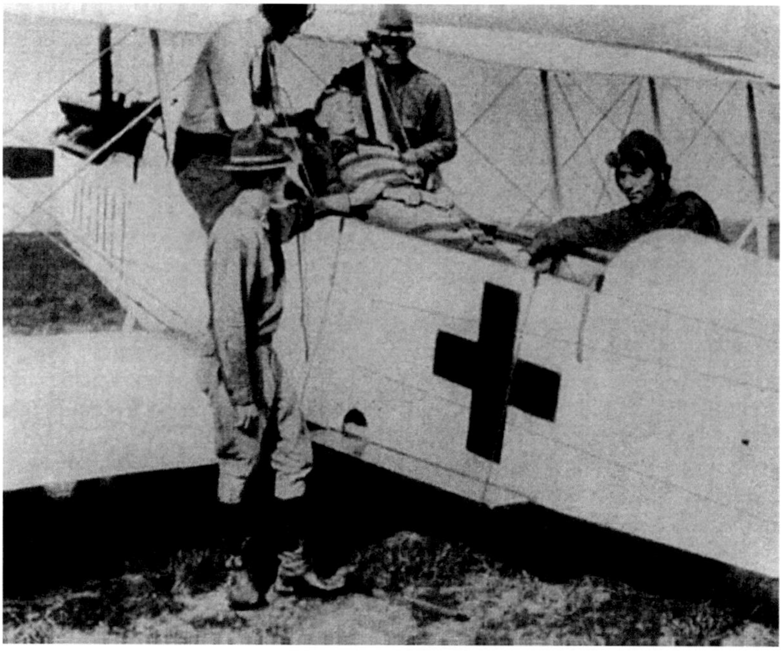

Fig. 2.1 The Curtiss JN-4 Jenny was converted to an air ambulance by removing the rear cockpit seat. (USAF photo, 311th Human Systems Wing Archives, Brooks AFB, TX)

Colonel Albert E. Truby, enumerated the potential uses of the airplane ambulances [3]:

- Transportation of medical officers to the site of aircraft crashes and evacuation of casualties from the crash back to hospitals
- Transportation of patients from isolated stations to larger hospitals where they could receive more definitive care
- In time of war, transportation of seriously wounded from the front to rear hospitals.
- Transportation of medical supplies in emergencies

Transportation of patients by air began to take on operational importance as well. In 1922, in the Riffian War in Morocco, the French Army transported more than 1200 patients by air with a fleet of 6 airplanes [3]. In 1928, a Ford Trimotor was converted to an air ambulance capable of carrying six litter patients, a crew of two pilots, a flight surgeon, and a medical technician [1]. Also in 1928, the US Marines in Nicaragua established that aircraft used to transport supplies into the jungle would then be used to evacuate sick and wounded patients to the rear on the return flight. This concept proved to be an essential part of modern AE doctrine.

In the 1930s, a registered nurse and visionary, Lauretta M. Schimmoler, believed that 1 day there would be a need to evacuate the wounded by air, and for 15 years was a proponent for establishing the Aerial Nurse Corps of America. However, not everyone supported this premise. Mary Beard, RN, the Director of the Red Cross Nursing Service in 1930, stated, "No one of our nursing organizations, no leading school of nursing, nor any other professional group, has taken up this subject seriously and definitely tried to promote the organization of a group of nurses who understand conditions surrounding patients when they are traveling by air" [2, 3]. In 1940, the Acting Superintendent of the Army Nurse Corps stated, "The present mobilization plan does not contemplate the extensive use of airplane ambulances. For this reason, it is believed that a special corps of nurses with qualifications for such assignment will not be required" [3].

The Surgeon General at the time, Major General C. R. Reynolds, added, "If commercial aviation companies require special nurses in any way, which at present I can't visualize, this is a matter which has nothing to do with the Medical Department of the Army" [3]. AE and flight nursing were yet to prove themselves in the quest to save lives through air transport.

World War II

At the beginning of World War II, it was commonly believed that air evacuation of the sick and wounded was dangerous, medically unsound, and militarily impossible [3]. The Army Medical Department did not believe that the airplane was a substitute for field ambulances, even when it was necessary to evacuate casualties over long distances. The Surgeon for the Army Air Force Combat Command, Major I. B. March, was concerned that field ambulances would not be sufficient to cover the aerial paths of the Air Forces. In response, the Surgeon of the Third Air Force, Lieutenant Colonel Malcolm C. Grow, stated that the "chief stumbling block in the way of air ambulances has been the lack of interest on the part of the Army Surgeon General. ...Until he accepts the airplane as a vehicle for casualty transportation, I doubt if very much can be done about it" [3].

The war soon demonstrated the necessity of AE. Large numbers of casualties needed to be transported back from distant theaters of war. Because designated AE aircraft did not exist, the Army Air Force made it their policy to use transport planes for AE flights as their secondary mission (Fig. 2.2). Regular transport aircraft were reconfigured for AE using removable litter supports (Fig. 2.3) [3]. In this way, aircraft that had transported troops and supplies to the theaters of operation could be utilized as AE aircraft for the return trip. By January 1942, Army Air Force C-47 aircraft had transported more than 10,000 casualties back from Burma, New Guinea, and Guadalcanal. In 1941, the first Air Surgeon of the Army Air Force, Colonel David N. Grant, advocated AE with airborne competent medical care as a way to increase the speed

MEDICAL - Air Evacuation
Rec'd 5 Dec. 1944 from Hq. Ferrying Division, Air Transport Command, Cincinnati, Ohio. Copied 6/9/45. Released 6/15/45.
(over)

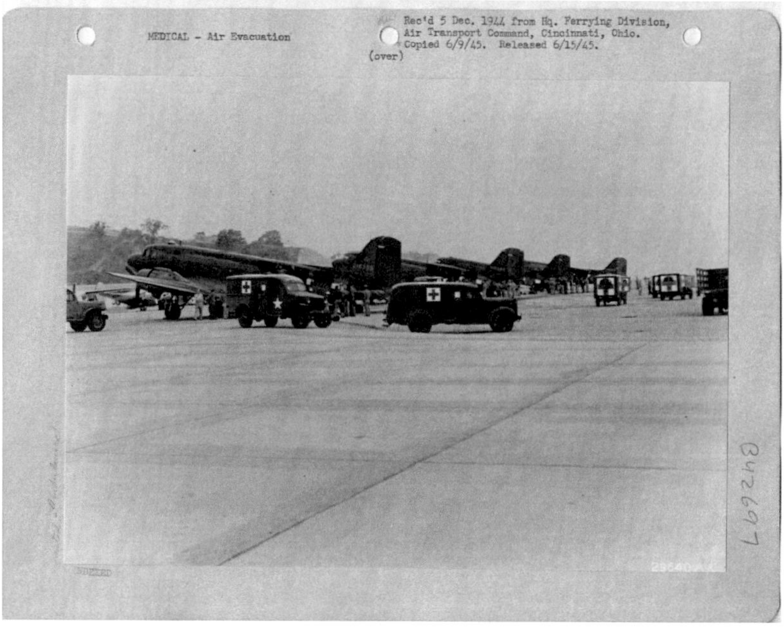

Fig. 2.2 World War II photo titled "MEDICAL – Air Evacuation" with multiple aircraft and vehicles used to transport patients in 1944. (AFMS History Office)

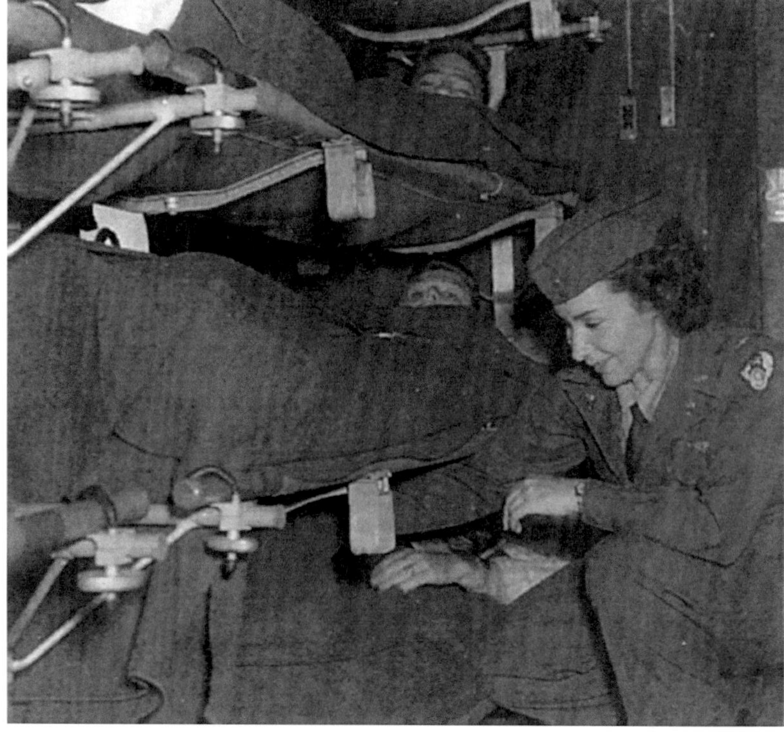

Fig. 2.3 A US Army Air Force flight nurse attends a wounded soldier being evacuated by air in 1944. (Department of the Army photo)

and caliber of casualty transportation and pointed out that AE would be available when other means of transportation were not [4]. The first Medical Air Ambulance Squadron was established in 1942 [1–3].

As AE evolved, it became clear that specially trained personnel were needed to optimize casualty care during air transport. Because there were not enough physicians to put on every AE flight, Grant proposed the establishment of a flight nurse corps [3]. Despite opposition from the Army Surgeon General, the designation of "Flight Nurse" was created for specially trained members of the Army Nurse Corps assigned to the Army Air Forces Evacuation Service. In February 1943, the first class of flight nurses graduated from Bowman Field, KY, after a 4-week course that included aeromedical physiology, aircraft loading procedures, and survival skills.

Soon regular AE routes were established and hospitals were built along airstrips to care for the wounded who needed to remain overnight along the route [5]. In early 1943, AE aircraft began transatlantic flights from Prestwick, Scotland, to the United States. By the end of the same year, the transpacific AE flights transported patients back to the continental United States via Hawaii. In 1944, a southern Atlantic route to the United States was added, originating in North Africa with stopovers in the Azores and Bermuda. Aircraft used for AE during the war included the C-54 Skymaster, C-46 Commando, C-47 Skytrain, C-64 Norseman, and C-87 Liberator Express. Bombers and tankers were sometimes used for tactical AE to move patients from forward battle zones [2, 3].

The number of patients transported reflects the importance of AE during World War II, with the number increasing by 500% from 1943 to 1945 [2, 5]. At its peak, the Army Air Force evacuated the sick and wounded at a rate of almost 100,000 per month. In 1945, a 1-day AE record was set at 4707 patients [5]. The risk of AE to the patient had been a concern since the beginning of the war. As the aeromedical crews gained experience, the risk of death during AE had dropped in 1943 to 6 of every 100,000 patients [1, 3]. By the end of the war, the risk of death during AE was only 1.5 of every 100,000 patients [3]. In fact, AE was listed along with antibiotics and blood products as among the most important medical advances in decreasing the mortality rate associated with warfare during World War II. In 1945, General Dwight D. Eisenhower stated, "We evacuated almost everyone from our forward hospitals by air, and it has unquestionably saved hundreds of lives, thousands of lives" [1, 3].

Postwar Period and a New Service

The postwar drawdown changed the face of the US military AE system. By 1946, the system consisted of 12 aircraft at the School of Aviation Medicine and one C-47 at each of 12 regional US hospitals. In 1947, the US Air Force (USAF) was established, and the Secretary of Defense, Louis E. Johnson, established a policy directing that the transportation of patients of the armed services would be accomplished by aircraft when air transportation was available, conditions were suitable for air evacuation, and there was no medical contradiction to air transport [2, 6]. In 1949, the USAF was given the official role of providing AE for the entire US military [5].

The Korean War

The unexpected start of the Korean War in 1950 caught the AE system as unprepared as the rest of the US military. There was no AE system set up in Korea, and there were few medical facilities located near airstrips anywhere in the Far East. Because of a lack of organizational infrastructure and available AE aircraft, the Army was required to develop a system of tactical AE in the Korean theater. Due to a critical shortage of combat-ready troops, the wounded were kept as far forward as possible so that they could be returned to combat as soon as they were physically able. In the early months of the conflict, most patients were evacuated by ship from Korea to Japan, even though empty cargo planes were available [1]. With the establishment of the Far East Air Force, the logistics of establishing an operational AE system was made a top priority [1]. Without adequate dedicated AE aircraft, the concept of retrograde aeromedical airlift again presented the best solution. After offloading personnel and cargo near the forward battle area in central Korea, Air Force rescue aircraft (C-54/C-46/C-47) were used to transport casualties further south in Korea or to Japan. In the first 6 months of the war, more than 30,000 casualties were evacuated by air. As the fighting became more intense, more than 10,450 combat casualties were airlifted between January 1 and 24, 1951 [1].

By fall 1952, the C-124 Globemaster became the primary air cargo aircraft, almost completely replacing the C-54. When configured for AE, the much larger C-124 accommodated 127 litters or 200 ambulatory patients. It also had the advantage of a shorter enplaning and deplaning time and required a smaller medical aircrew than the C-54. Unfortunately, because of its size, the C-124 could not land in Pusan, South Korea to evacuate patients from this area. Instead, the smaller C-46 aircraft, which carried a maximum load of 26 patients, was used for intratheater AE in Korea and Japan [1]. By the conclusion of the Korean War in 1955, the USAF AE system was again capable of safely moving a large number of casualties within the theater and back to the United States (Fig. 2.4). This system was also attributed to the decrease in the death rate of the wounded during the Korean War, which was 50% less than that seen during World War II [1, 6].

Pre-Vietnam War

In the years immediately after the Korean War, the peacetime AE system continued to serve the US Department of Defense by transporting military and civilian patients from the overseas theaters back to the United States [1]. A new aircraft, the Convair C-131A Samaritan, became the first airplane designed specifically for AE (Fig. 2.5). This first fully pressurized twin-engine transport was designed as a "flying hospital ward," complete with air conditioning and oxygen for patients, and had the capability to carry bulky medical equipment, such as the iron lung, chest respirator, and incubator [7]. The Samaritan accommodated 40 ambulatory or 27 litter patients or a combination of both [2].

Vietnam War

In 1964, the United States entered the Vietnam conflict. Again, the peacetime AE system had to be built up to meet the wartime needs of the US military. Initially, C-118 and C-130 cargo aircraft were used to evacuate patients within Vietnam and to offshore islands. When the C-141 Starlifter jet-powered cargo aircraft became available in 1965, it was given the AE mission in addition to its primary cargo mission. By 1967, the Pacific Air Forces aeromedical evacuation system had 17 operating locations throughout the Pacific. The C-118 became the workhorse for in-theater AE, allowing the C-130 to concentrate on the cargo mission [1].

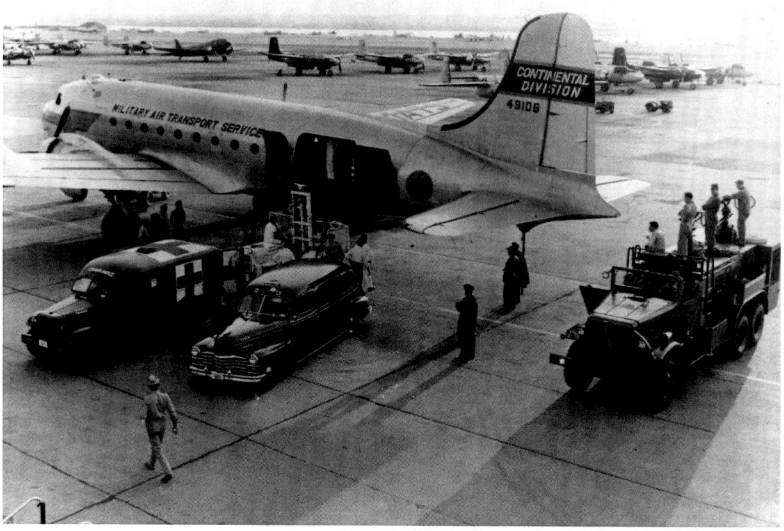

Fig. 2.4 The Douglas C-54 Skymaster was used for aeromedical evacuation during the Korean War. (US Air Force photo)

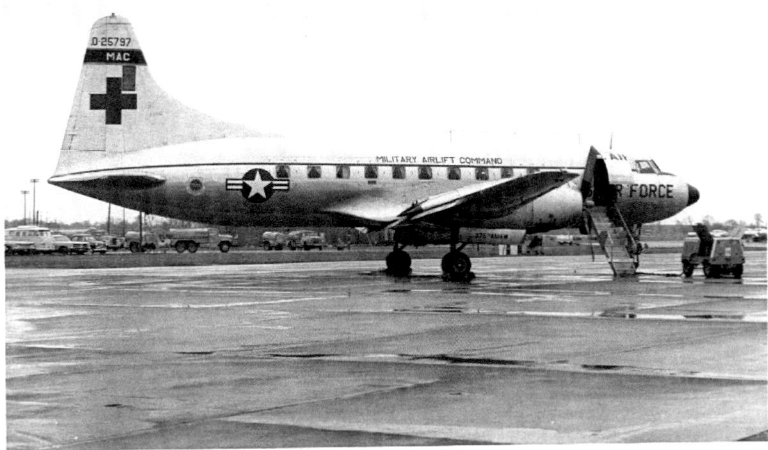

Fig. 2.5 The Convair C-131A Samaritan was used by the US Military Airlift Command aeromedical evacuation during the Vietnam War. (AFMS History Office)

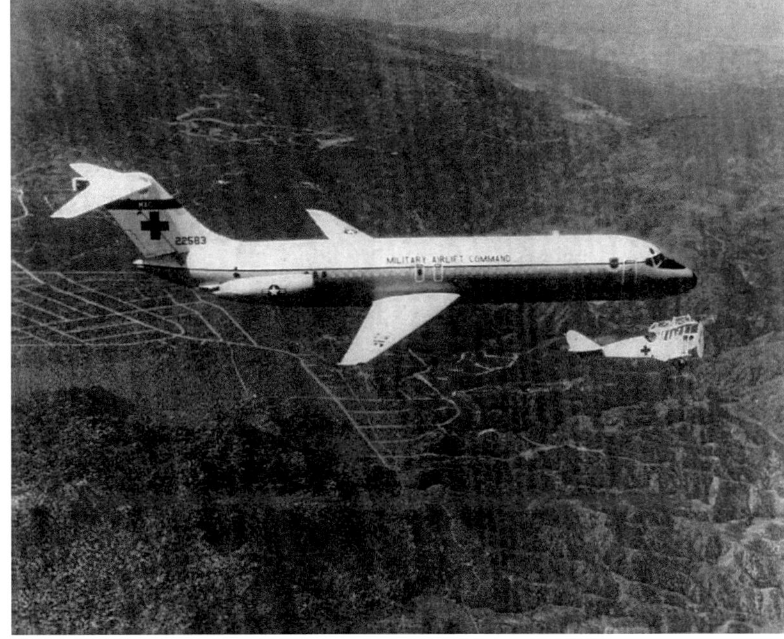

Fig. 2.6 Early biplane to sophisticated jet: C-9A Nightingale with Curtiss JN-4 Jenny. (USAF photo, 311th Human Systems Wing Archives, Brooks AFB, TX)

In 1968, the C-9A Nightingale made its debut as a state-of-the art medium-range, twin-jet aircraft used almost exclusively for the AE mission [1]. The Nightingale was a modified version of the McDonnell Douglas Aircraft Corporation's DC-9 and could carry 40 ambulatory patients, 40 litter patients, or a combination of both (Fig. 2.6).

However, the character of the combat in Vietnam made tactical AE especially important. Small transport aircraft, such as the C-123, would arrive at small airstrips carrying cargo. Within minutes, the aircraft would be unloaded and reconfigured to carry patients. The number of patients transported by the USAF AE system during the Vietnam War was astounding. During the 1968 Tet Offensive, 688 patients were processed within the Pacific aeromedical evacuation system on a single day. In May 1968, 12,138 casualties were evacuated from Vietnam on 154 AE missions. By 1969, the Military Airlift Command (MAC) AE system evacuated an average of 11,000 casualties per month. An all-time single-day high of 711 patients was moved out of Vietnam on March 7, 1969. In the closing months of 1969, patient movements began to decline to less than 7500 per month [1, 8].

During the Vietnam War, many advances were made in AE [1]. However, it was determined that wartime casualties did not do as well if prematurely placed on long flights. For this reason, patients were stabilized in combat hospitals and then transported to offshore islands nearby for definitive treatment. Patients were allowed to convalesce and then were either returned to duty or transported back to the United States for prolonged treatment. The average stay in-theater prior to long-distance AE was more than 1 week [8, 9]. Notably, however, the US Army created a "Burn Team," which provided clinical guidelines and personnel to move burned patients, with patients often arriving at a hospital for definitive treatment in the second postburn day [10].

In 1975, USAF AE participated in a humanitarian mission called Operation Babylift to transport orphans out of Saigon to be adopted by US families. During the first mission, the C-5A Galaxy, which was being used for transport, was forced to return to Saigon and crash-landed due to mechanical problems, killing three of the AE crew, five of the flight crew, nearly all of the children, and many of the attendants [11]. While the tragedy was used to inform the AE processes, Operation Babylift flights resumed on civilian aircraft, and over the next few weeks, nearly 3000 orphans were transported—all during the single month of April 1975 [11].

A Worldwide Aeromedical Evacuation Network

In the years following the Vietnam War, the Air Force MAC developed a worldwide peacetime AE network that relied on the use of the dedicated AE platform, the C-9 Nightingale, as well as military cargo planes such as the C-141 Starlifter and C-130 Hercules [12]. Four active duty AE squadrons and 28 Reserve and Guard units maintained the peacetime AE system and remained on standby for any worldwide contingency, and all AE missions were centrally coordinated and tracked through MAC headquarters at Scott Air Force Base (AFB) in Illinois [12]. This AE network transported 250 to 300 patients a day [13] and was primarily designed to transport patients following an accident or disaster, deliver critical medical equipment, and transport military beneficiaries to specialized medical appointments at larger military medical centers [12].

A specialized neonatal transport team was designed and based out of Wilford Hall USAF Medical Center in San Antonio, TX, to transport neonatal infants delivered at military hospitals worldwide that needed more intensive, neonatal intensive care unit (NICU) level care. This NICU team pushed the boundaries of the medical technology of the day, developing the first portable extracorporeal membrane oxygenation system, which successfully transported an infant with severe neonatal respiratory failure from Travis AFB in California back to Texas [14].

The USAF AE system also participated in other noteworthy military and humanitarian missions over the following years. In 1977, active and Reserve AE units assisted in the transport of those injured in a B-747 collision in the Canary Islands. In 1983, more than 400 wounded were evacuated from Grenada during Operation Urgent Fury, and hundreds of wounded were evacuated from Panama in Operation Just Cause in 1989. A mobile aeromedical staging facility (MASF) was first used in Panama, with over half of the casualties processed through the MASF during the first 24 hours [2].

In the final months of 1990, however, medical planners for Operation Desert Storm began to project the need to aeromedically transport up to 2,520 patients per day [15]. In response, the Air Force prepositioned 17 aeromedical staging facilities, 149 AE crews, and 23 AE liaison teams and control centers—although it was later noted that the actual number of personnel, equipment, and supplies would not have been adequate for that number of casualties [15]. Casualty numbers were significantly lower than anticipated, but nearly 15,000 patients were aeromedically evacuated from theater, less than 3% of which were due to combat injuries [12]. Although hailed as a "complete success" without any in-flight deaths [2], there were many lessons learned from the development of that robust AE infrastructure, given that between 43% [15] and 60% of the AE patients [12] initially arrived at the wrong location and required a significant amount of last-minute coordination to ensure they received the appropriate level of care. This was primarily attributed to technical issues with the patient regulation system, limited training for personnel, and a lack of coordination among the services [15].

An additional need to update the AE system was identified to be able to provide care to critically ill and injured patients during transport without requiring the use of the limited in-country medical resources. This was highlighted with the inability to quickly evacuate critically injured combat casualties from military operations in Somalia in 1993 [16]. In response, the development of a dedicated Critical Care Air Transport Team (CCATT) was finalized in 1993 to be able to augment the AE crew and provide this advanced capability. The first CCATTs were officially deployed in support of operations in Bosnia in 1995 [16].

Following the lessons learned from the First Gulf War (Operation Desert Shield/Storm), Panama (Operation Just Cause), Somalia, and the development of CCATTs, the Air Mobility Command (AMC; formerly MAC) undertook a major analysis, reengineering, and overhaul of the entire AE system [2, 17]. The comprehensive multicommand AE Tiger Team Report was signed in the fall of 2000 [18]. Two critical components of the report were "AE is a mission, not a platform" and "movement of stabilized patients," which became the new model for AE—a change from expecting the use of specific AE airframes or the requirement to move stable patients. It was also determined that AE should be considered as an operational (nonmedical) mission to ensure the appropriate resources and planning were integrated into the broader air campaign planning process. As a result, all AE personnel and functions were transitioned from within the medical infrastructure of the AMC Surgeon General (AMC/SG) to the AMC Director of Operations, although AMC/SG retained oversight and responsibility for clinical care [2].

The retirement of the C-9A Nightingale and the C-141B Starlifter also impacted the reengineering and analysis work of the AE system. As a result, aircraft were no longer dedicated only to the AE, but rather the AE system aligned with the mobility approach of common user, multiuse lift platforms. All the available airframes were analyzed, and the KC-135 was identified as a short-term fix to meet the intertheater requirements [2]. Modifications that would adapt the refueler aircraft into a more suitable patient transport platform came in the design and development of the patient support pallets. Additionally, there was a focus on requirements-based missions and mixing cargo and patients [2], thereby fully optimizing available resources and enhancing efficiency.

This decision led to significant changes at AMC headquarters and throughout the AE system, as duties, personnel, and resources were transitioned to new work areas. Changes to command and control included embedding AE control teams in the Air Mobility Division inside the Air Operations Centers and AE cells in the Air Mobility Operations Control Centers around the world [18]. AE squadrons were no longer specified by their aircraft qualifications (e.g., C-9, C-130, or C-141 units) but were now able to perform AE missions on all appropriate mobility airframes. AE squadrons became part of the Operations Group, directly under the Wing commander [2].

Clinical care standards were adopted using the National Flight Nurses Association principles [19], and medical equipment continued to be employed that enabled conversion of mobility aircraft into flying hospitals. Patient staging capabilities were also refreshed and reengineered as part of the AE Tiger Team analysis [2]. The MASFs were leaned and the larger contingency ASFs (CASFs) were bundled into smaller building blocks and repackaged.

All these changes impacted training for the entire AE system. The transition to universal qualification necessitated writing new AF instructions and recrafting the training pipelines of the Flight Nurse and AE Technician courses, which moved from Texas with the USAF School of Aerospace Medicine to Wright-Patterson AFB, Ohio.

CCATTs, which had proven successful in providing critical care capability during operational deployments, were integrated into AE operations upon deployment as part of the AE squadrons, which necessitated learning at all levels on how best to utilize and employ these vital assets [2]. The ability to expand AE capability by adding specialty teams, such as the NICU and burn teams, was also an important element of the system and paved the way for subsequent specialty teams, including an Acute Lung Rescue Team using extracorporeal membrane oxygenation [20].

The events of September 11, 2001, however, accelerated the transition to this new view of AE. AE leaders made the bold decision to implement the new recommendations with the anticipated deployment of troops to Afghanistan, and operational deployments of AE crews and personnel began in late 2001 with the new configurations and composition recommended in the AE Tiger Team report.

Operation Iraqi Freedom/Enduring Freedom

As contingency and war operations evolved in Afghanistan and then Iraq, the AE system continued to evolve and mature to meet the needs of the sick and injured. In Iraq, the terrain was relatively flat and smaller in geography, enabling manageable response rings that enabled transport of freshly wounded and injured from the point of injury directly to combat hospitals. By contrast, Afghanistan was larger, with more varied terrain, and proved challenging to the integrated medical evacuation plan that had developed in Iraq. Planners found it more challenging to place medical assets/response assets within "golden hour circles" to continue the swift transport of casualties to trauma care. Weighing the cost in airframes, the need for operational speed and agility, as well as limited personnel and resources, led to additional ingenuity and multitasking of crews and airframes to meet requirements [21, 22].

The medical evacuation system used to support the North Atlantic Treaty Organization (NATO) coalition in Afghanistan encompassed a variety of resources, including US Army Medical Evacuation (MEDEVAC) and USAF Guardian Angels/pararescue specialists, and focused on unregulated casualty movement either from the point of injury or from the initial stabilization locations to further definitive care (Fig. 2.7). Patient Evacuation Coordination Cells, a NATO construct [23], were used in the regional command centers and had the responsibility for the early unregulated phase of patient movement within theater, while the Joint Patient Movement Requirements Center guided patient movement for those regulated casualties on AF mobility aircraft, both intratheater (in country) (Fig. 2.8) and intertheater from Afghanistan to Germany and back to the United States [22].

Although ongoing military operations continued in Iraq and Afghanistan, the AE system during Operation Iraqi Freedom and Operation Enduring Freedom has been identified as a revolution in military medicine [24]. The integrated use of CCATT (Fig. 2.9) and Burn Flight Team, close coordination with the Joint Patient Movement Requirements Center and international partners, as well as the use of the C-17 Globemaster III aircraft (Fig. 2.10), has resulted

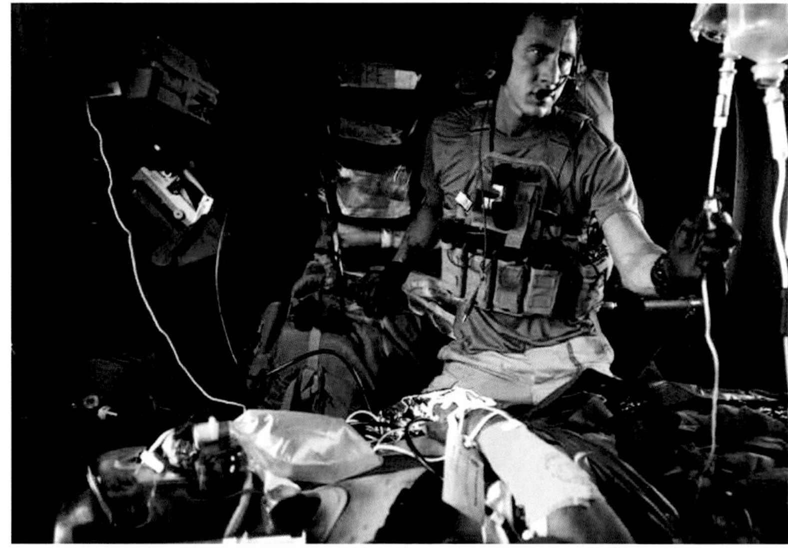

Fig. 2.7 USAF Pararescueman cares for a patient in an HH-60G Pave Hawk helicopter in Helmand Province, Afghanistan. (US Air Force photo/Staff Sgt. Shawn Weismiller)

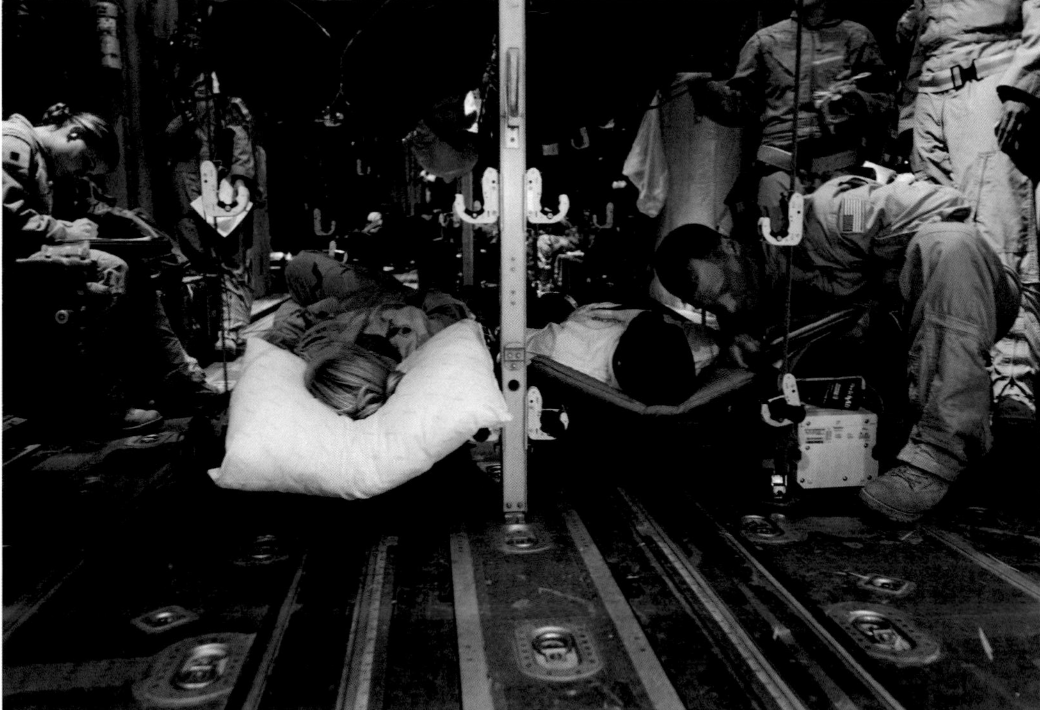

Fig. 2.8 USAF Flight Technician cares for patients on a C-130 during an intratheater AE mission to transport patients from Kandahar Airfield to Bagram Airfield in Afghanistan. (US Air Force photo/Staff Sgt. Shawn Weismiller)

in a majority of patients arriving at US-based hospitals for definitive care within 3–4 days of injury [24]. These rapid transport times for AE patients decreased the number of deployed medical assets required in-country to adequately treat combat casualties.

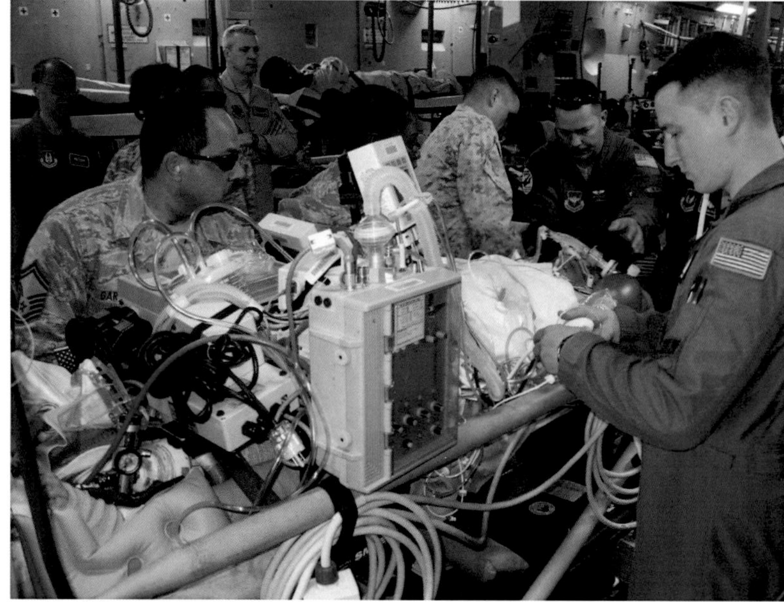

Fig. 2.9 A USAF Critical Care Air Transport Team prepares a severely wounded soldier for AE from Ramstein Air Base, Germany, to Walter Reed National Military Medical Center, Maryland. (Defense Department photo/Donna Miles)

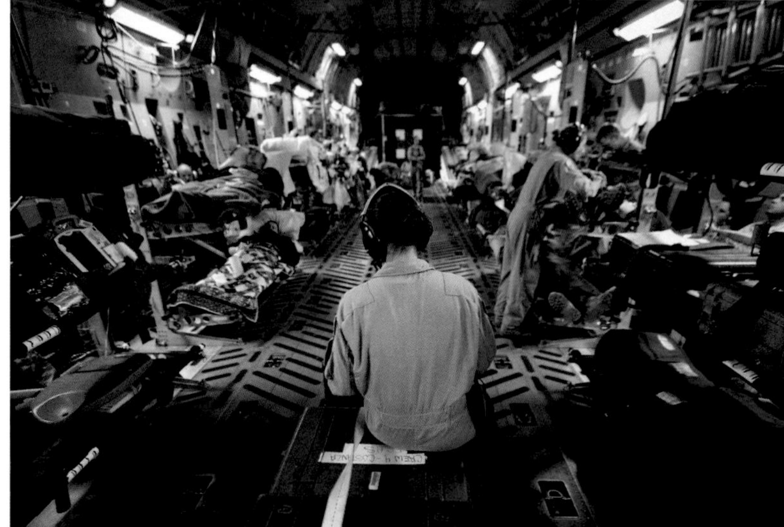

Fig. 2.10 A USAF Flight Crew cares for patients on a C-17 during an AE mission from Bagram Air Field, Afghanistan, to Ramstein Air Base, Germany. (US Air Force photo by Senior Airman Chris Willis)

Aeromedical Evacuation Today

Today, the Commander of the US Transportation Command (USTRANSCOM), located at Scott AFB in Illinois, is the single manager for patient movement [25]. To accomplish that mission, the Global Patient Movement Requirements Center exists to oversee patient movement around the world, including AE missions to Antarctica [26] and the Pacific (Fig. 2.11). AMC works closely to provide the military AE capability required by USTRANSCOM, to include ensuring that training and resources are available for AE missions and patient staging needs [27].

Training for AE nurses and technicians is accomplished at the US Air Force School of Aerospace Medicine at Wright-Patterson AFB, OH, and consists of a 20-day phase of classroom learning, 5-day survival training, and then a 27-day field training course that includes initial flight qualification [28]. This intensive schedule ensures the graduating AE crew members are

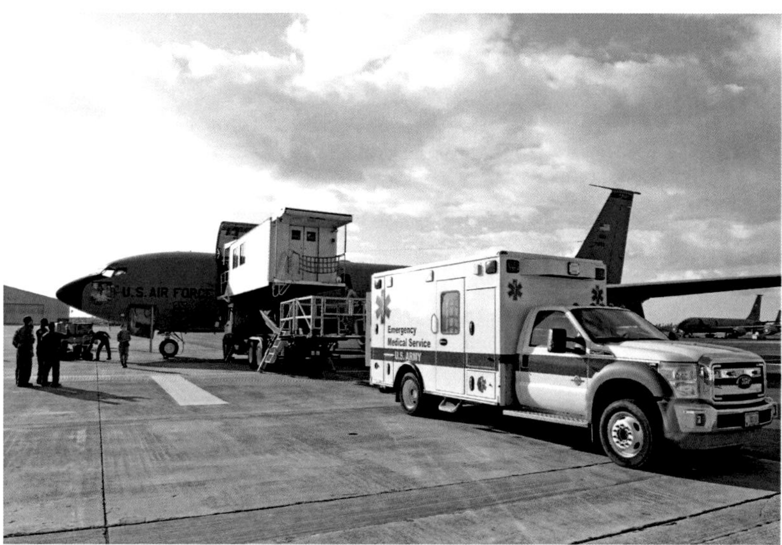

Fig. 2.11 AE Patients are offloaded from a KC-135R using a High Deck Patient Loading Platform (HDPLP) vehicle at Hickam Air Force Base, Hawaii. (US Air National Guard photo by Tech. Sgt. Annie Edwards)

fully qualified once assigned to their first duty station [29].

In response to emerging clinical needs, additional capabilities have also been added to AE, including a 3-member Tactical Critical Care Evacuation Team (TCCET) and TCCET Surgical Augmentation [28]. The development of the TCCET was based on the findings from a British model of a physician-led medical emergency response team in Afghanistan that was associated with improved outcomes for severely injured casualties [30]; this team also provides the ability to send advanced medical assets directly where they are needed. Another emerging clinical need was the potential movement of patients who had been exposed to Ebola, which resulted in the development of a clinical protocol that would safely allow the transport of multiple patients requiring contact precautions [31]. It is anticipated that other future gaps will continue to result in the modification of current AE protocols to meet both operational and patient needs.

The Future of Aeromedical Evacuation

Aeromedical evacuation has evolved based on the need to respond to changes in injury or illness patterns that occur in locations without a well-developed medical infrastructure. Providing AE capability in an immature theater may be challenging, but striving for a rapid response anywhere in the world is impossible. Increasing medical capability and using any available military aircraft have historically been the way to decrease the time needed to get to definitive care. In some cases, this has included augmenting the medical expertise of the AE crew with specialty teams, as well as developing new medical equipment that can provide a higher level of care than is available at the sending site. Another important capability that will need to be advanced in the future is the need to address the interoperability of equipment, aircraft platforms, and the clinical skills of international partners. With increased partnerships and collaborations supporting military operations around the world, having multiple teams waiting for a specific AE mission in a central location may not be the best option for the patient. A system that can incorporate military, civilian, and international aircraft and integrate healthcare devices and levels of care from different countries will need to be further developed to ensure timely, but safe, patient care.

The continued advancement of unmanned and remotely piloted vehicles is another key development that will impact the future of AE. Remotely piloted (unmanned) systems have been routinely used in recent conflicts in Southwest Asia, and

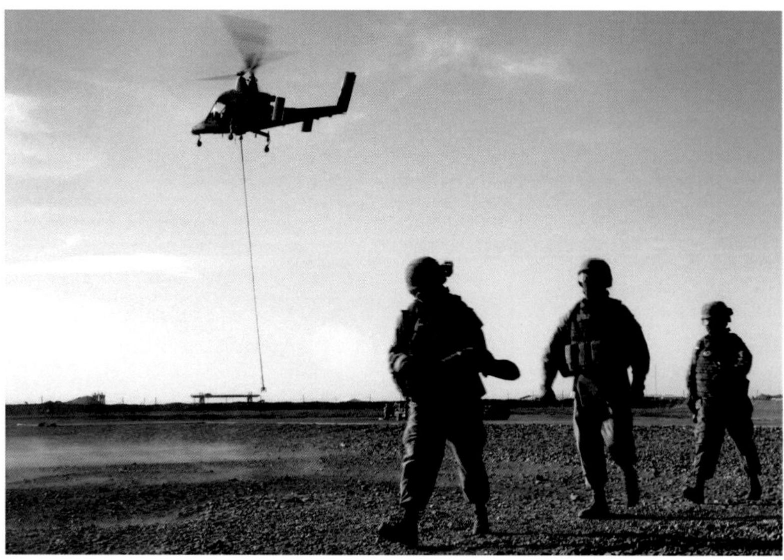

Fig. 2.12 Marines with Combat Logistics Battalion 5 return from familiarizing themselves with the downward thrust of a Kaman K1200, or K-MAX, unmanned helicopter during initial testing in Helmand Province, Afghanistan, May 22, 2012. (US Marine Corps photo by Cpl. Lisa Tourtelot)

the military currently maintains thousands of unmanned aircraft that accomplish a wide variety of missions [32]. Of note, the US Marine Corps successfully utilized a remotely piloted helicopter from 2011–2014 to transport cargo to and from outlying operating bases in Afghanistan (Fig. 2.12) [33]. While none of these platforms are currently designed to move patients, as the technology continues to develop it is anticipated that will be a key capability moving forward. In fact, NATO formed a working group to define safe ride standards for casualty evacuation using unmanned aerial vehicles as a way to anticipate what would be required to safely move patients [34]. Although there is concern about the safety of using unmanned aircraft to transport patients, it is interesting to note that the issues are much the same as when it was initially proposed to use aircraft during the initial development of AE. Given examples from the past, it is only a matter of time until AE includes unmanned aircraft as a potential platform that could be used to move an ill or injured patient in the future.

Conclusion

Today's contingency operations and battlefields continue to be challenging and require radical innovation as AE professionals continually seek new and creative ways to improve survival and quality of life for those entrusted to their care. Whether in an urban setting cut off from outside resources, or isolated locations in the mountains or jungles, remote islands far from the reaches of high quality care, or contested areas where civilian care or contract medical services cannot reach, the military health system must continue to evolve and innovate. Supporting many of these innovations have been the clinicians, researchers, and scientists who asked questions, gathered data, established programs of research to improve the knowledge and evidence for decisions, and advocated for solid and rigorous quality improvements.

As history has demonstrated, AE will continue to evolve as new challenges arise and technology advances. It is a testament to the passion and creativity of the AE system and flight crews that they continue to push the boundaries of what is possible to ensure patients receive the best possible medical care, regardless of where they are in the world. From the beginning development of aircraft through the use of the latest technology, providing the appropriate level of care throughout a patient's journey, is a hallmark of AE.

References

1. Department of the Air Force, Office of the Surgeon General. A concise history of the USAF aeromedical evacuation system. Washington, DC: U.S. Government Printing Office; 1976. p. 1–26.
2. Green B. Challenges of aeromedical evacuation in the post-Cold-War era. Aerosp Power J. 2001;15(4):14–26.
3. Link ML, Coleman HA. Air evacuation mission. Medical support of the Army Air Forces in World War II. Washington, DC: US Government Printing Office; 1955. p. 357–412.
4. Air Force Association. Air Force fifty: a look at the Air Force, Air Force Association and commemorative Las Vegas reunion. Nashville: Turner Publishing Company; 1998. p. 95–6.
5. Mebane R. Timeline events in the history of air evac. Mr Makovec's aeromedical evacuation history index. 1999. http://www.ior.com/~jmakovedmakovedae_tmlne.htm.
6. Military Airlift Command. Anything, anywhere, anytime: an illustrated history of the Military Airlift Command, 1941–1991. Scott AFB, IL: Military Airlift Command; 1991. Accessed 14 Aug 2017. Available from http://www.amc.af.mil/Portals/12/documents/AFD-131018-047.pdf.
7. Funsch HF, Nareff MJ, Watkins PB. Wings for wounded warriors. JAMA. 1967;200(5):391–8.
8. Howard WG. History of aeromedical evacuation in the Korean War and Vietnam War [Thesis]. Ft. Leavenworth (KS): U.S. Army Command and General Staff College; 2003. Report No. ATZL-SWD-GD. Accessed 7 Aug 2017. Available from http://www.dtic.mil/dtic/tr/fulltext/u2/a416927.pdf.
9. White MS, Chubb RM, Rossing RG, Murphy JE. Results of early aeromedical evacuation of Vietnam casualties. Aerosp Med. 1971;42(7):780–4.
10. Kirksey TD, Dowling JA, Pruitt BA Jr, Moncrief JA. Safe, expeditious transport of the seriously burned patient. Arch Surg. 1968;96(5):790–4.
11. James BM. Angels flying out of hell: the 7,000-mile journey of the Operation Babylift orphans. Denver: Blueline Publishing; 2015.
12. Gunby P. Winged medical care ranges worldwide. JAMA. 1980;244(5):420–6.
13. Skolnick A. Desert storm: medical airlift was ready. JAMA. 1991;265(12):1497.. 1501
14. Cornish JD, Gerstmann DR, Begnaud MJ, Null DM, Ackerman NB. Inflight use of extracorporeal membrane oxygenation for severe neonatal respiratory failure. Perfusion. 1986;1(4):281–7.
15. Gebicke ME. Operation desert storm: problems with Air Force medical readiness. Washington, DC: General Accounting Office; 1993. GAO/NSIAD Publication 94–58.
16. Beninati W, Meyer MT, Carter TE. The critical care air transport program. Crit Care Med. 2008;36(7 Suppl):S370–6.
17. Howell FJ, Brannon RH. Aeromedical evacuation: remembering the past, bridging to the future. Mil Med. 2000;165(6):429–33.
18. Air Mobility Command, Medical Readiness and Aeromedical Evacuation Division, Plans and Programs Studies and Analysis Flight. Annex A: a brief history of aeromedical evacuation. Scott AFB, IL: Air Mobility Command; 2000. Aeromedical Evacuation Tiger Team Final Report.
19. Air and Surface Patient Nurses Association (ASTNA) Patient Transport. In: Holleran S, editor. Principles and practice. 4th ed. Salt Lake: R. Mosby/Elsevier; 2011.
20. Dorlac GR, Fang R, Pruitt VM, Marco PA, Stewart HM, Barnes SL, et al. Air transport of patients with severe lung injury: development and utilization of the Acute Lung Rescue Team. J Trauma. 2009;66(4 Suppl):S164–71.
21. Clarke JE, Davis PR. Medical evacuation and triage of combat casualties in Helmand Province, Afghanistan: October 2010–April 2011. Mil Med. 2012;177(11):1261–6.
22. Lane I, Stockinger Z, Sauer S, Ervin M, Wirt M, Bree S, et al. The Afghan theater: a review of military medical doctrine from 2008 to 2014. Mil Med. 2017;182(S1):32–40.
23. North Atlantic Treaty Organization Standardization Agency. Allied joint doctrine for medical evacuation: AJMedP-02. Brussels, Belgium: NATO Standardization Agency; 2008. Medical Standardization Document STANAG 2546. Accessed 28 Aug 2017. Available from http://www.coemed.org/database/stanags.
24. Blackbourne LH, Baer DG, Eastridge BJ, Renz EM, Chung KK, Dubose J, et al. Military medical revolution: deployed hospital and en route care. J Trauma Acute Care Surg. 2012;73(6 Suppl 5):S378–87.
25. Under Secretary of Defense for Personnel and Readiness. Patient movement (PM). Washington, DC: Department of Defense; 2012. Department of Defense Instruction 6000.11. Accessed 17 Aug 2017. Available from http://www.esd.whs.mil/Portals/54/Documents/DD/issuances/dodi/600011p.pdf.
26. Kriss F. Team McChord deploys to Antarctica for medical evacuation. 2013 May 16. Accessed 17 Aug 2017. Available from http://www.afrc.af.mil/News/Article-Display/Article/156211/team-mcchord-deploys-to-antarctica-for-medical-evacuation/.
27. U.S. Air Force. En route care and aeromedical evacuation medical operations. Washington, DC: Department of the Air Force; 2017. Air Force Instruction 48–307, volume 1. Accessed 17 Aug 2017. Available from http://static.e-publishing.af.mil/production/1/af_sg/publication/afi48-307v1/afi48-307v1.pdf.
28. U.S. Air Force. En route critical care. Washington, DC: Department of the Air Force; 2017. Air Force Instruction 48–307, volume 2. Accessed 17 Aug 2017. Available from http://static.e-publishing.af.mil/production/1/af_sg/publication/afi48-307v2/afi48-307v2.pdf.

29. O'Connell KM, De Jong MJ, Dufour KM, Millwater TL, Dukes SF, Winik CL. An integrated review of simulation use in aeromedical evacuation training. Clin Simul Nurs. 2014;10(1):e11–8.
30. Apodaca A, Olson CM Jr, Bailey J, Butler F, Eastridge BJ, Kuncir E. Performance improvement evaluation of forward aeromedical evacuation platforms in Operation Enduring Freedom. J Trauma Acute Care Surg. 2013;75(2 Suppl 2):S157–63.
31. Thoms WE Jr, Wilson WT, Grimm K, Conger NG, Gonzales CG, DeDecker L, et al. Long-range transportation of Ebola-exposed patients: an evidence-based protocol. Am J Infect Dis Microbiol. 2015;2(6A):19–24.
32. Winnefeld JA, Kendall F. Unmanned systems integrated roadmap FY2013-2038. Washington, DC: Department of Defense; 2014. Accessed 7 Aug 2017. Available from https://www.defense.gov/Portals/1/Documents/pubs/DOD-USRM-2013.pdf.
33. Taylor DP. Air trucks: K-MAX success in Afghanistan reveals potential to expand UAS capabilities. Seapower. 2016;59(3):38–9. Accessed 7 Aug 2017. Available from http://www.seapower-digital.com/seapower/april_2016?pg=40#pg40.
34. North Atlantic Treaty Organization, Science and Technology Organization. Safe ride standards for casualty evacuation using unmanned aerial vehicles. Neuilly-Sur-Seine: NATO STO; 2012. STO Technical Report TR-HFM-184. Accessed 7 Aug 2017. Available from https://www.sto.nato.int/publications/STO%20Technical%20Reports/Forms/Technical%20Report%20Document%20Set/docsethomepage.aspx?ID=2344&FolderCTID=0x0120D5200078F9E87043356C409A0D30823AFA16F6010066D541ED10A62C40B2AB0FEBE9841A61&List=92d5819c-e6ec-4241-aa4e-57bf918681b-1&RootFolder=%2Fpublications%2FSTO%20Technical%20Reports%2FRTO%2DTR%2DHFM%2D184.

3 Military Casualty Evacuation: MEDEVAC

Cord W. Cunningham, Donald E. Keen, Steven G. Schauer, Chetan U. Kharod, and Robert A. De Lorenzo

Introduction

The term Medical Evacuation (MEDEVAC) has been broadly used in the past to describe all battlefield and tactical movement of casualties within theaters of operation [1–3]. When the term is used in this broad perspective, MEDEVAC encompasses all aspects of the movement of patients: from the point of injury to the nearest medical facility, between medical facilities at different roles of care, and finally to the site of embarkation out of the theater.

A key component of MEDEVAC is the provision of ongoing casualty care. To assure the success of what is one of the most important missions of military medicine, all military medical providers need to be familiar with the basic concepts and components of tactical MEDEVAC.

The rigors of MEDEVAC results in 3 major challenges for military medical providers. The first is preparing patients for tactical evacuation with adequate stabilizing prehospital care best accomplished with adherence to tactical combat casualty care guidelines. Preparation for condition decompensation en route is essential. The second challenge is en route care, which is often limited by the availability of equipment and trained providers as well as the austere environment. A third challenge is the urgent need for thorough reassessment immediately during transitions and handoff of care between evacuation platforms and, if needed, intervention to correct urgent problems.

C. W. Cunningham (✉)
LTC (P), MC, FS, DMO, USA, Critical Care Flight Paramedic Program, Center for Prehospital Medicine, Army Medical Department Center and School Health Readiness Center of Excellence, Joint Trauma System Committee on En Route Combat Casualty Care, DoD EMS & Disaster Medicine Fellowship SAUSHEC, Joint Base San Antonio-Fort Sam Houston, San Antonio, TX, USA
e-mail: cord.w.cunningham.mil@mail.mil

D. E. Keen
MAJ, MC, FS, USA, Army Critical Care Flight Paramedic Program, Center for Pre-Hospital Medicine, U.S Army Medical Department Center and School, Joint Base San Antonio-Fort Sam Houston, San Antonio, TX, USA

S. G. Schauer
MAJ, MC, USA, US Army Institute of Surgical Research, San Antonio Military Medical Center, Joint Base San Antonio-Fort Sam Houston, San Antonio, TX, USA

C. U. Kharod
Col, USAF, MC, SFS (ret.), SAUSHEC Military EMS & Disaster Medicine Fellowship, Emergency Medicine, Uniformed Services University, Bethesda, MD, USA

Department of Emergency Medicine, San Antonio Military Medical Center, Joint Base San Antonio-Fort Sam Houston, San Antonio, TX, USA

R. A. De Lorenzo
LTC, MC, FS, USA (ret.), Faculty Development, Department of Emergency Medicine, University of Texas Health Science Center at San Antonio, San Antonio, TX, USA

W. W. Hurd, W. Beninati (eds.), *Aeromedical Evacuation*, https://doi.org/10.1007/978-3-030-15903-0_3

History of MEDEVAC

MEDEVAC owes its inception to Napoleon's surgeon-in-chief, Dominique Larrey, who introduced the "Flying Ambulances," which were horse-drawn carriages that entered the battlefields to retrieve and care for the wounded soldiers [4]. Battlefield evacuation continued to evolve during the American Civil War, when the first dedicated horse-drawn carts were used to clear casualties off the battlefield. Later, when motorized transport became available, trucks were used to haul the wounded. World War II saw the first widespread use of dedicated motorized field ambulances to transport casualties from the battlefield to medical facilities and between medical facilities.

Helicopters were introduced for tactical medical evacuation during the Korean War and the transfusions of blood and plasma were under the ostensible control of the pilot, since the Bell H13 helicopter did not carry nor have room for medical attendants [5]. The addition of dedicated medical aircrew was introduced and operational employment of MEDEVAC helicopters was further improved during the Vietnam War [6]. The term "Dustoff" was coined for these UH-1 Huey helicopters and their dedicated medical crews [7]. The modern inventory now includes a large number of specialized ground and air ambulances.

Throughout the history of MEDEVAC, important advances have continued to be made in both the speed and versatility of the vehicles used. This has resulted in dramatic decreases in the time it takes wounded soldiers to receive treatment—a fact often credited with the improved casualty survival rates. MEDEVAC was viewed as mainly serving the purpose of clearing the battlefield. Historically both ground and air ambulances were staffed with combat medics that held the certification level of Emergency Medical Technician-Basic (EMT-Basic) and flight medics with additional training including Advanced Cardiac Life Support (ACLS) and basic crewmember training resulting in familiarity with rotary wing aircraft. More thorough and specific training for aircrew and flight medics was and still is provided at the unit level via standards established in the Aircrew Training Manual for the HH-60 utility helicopters and the Critical Care Flight Paramedic Training Support Package [8].

Recent Initiatives

In 2012, Mabry and coauthors published a study showing a 66% reduction in 48-hour mortality when Critical Care Flight Paramedic attendants rather than EMTs were available for combat casualty MEDEVAC via air ambulances in Afghanistan (Fig. 3.1) [9]. In response, the 2012

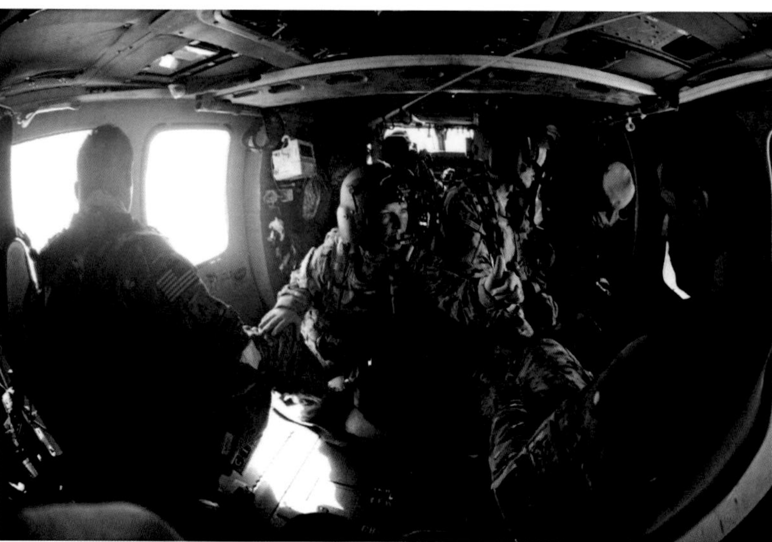

Fig. 3.1 A flight medic reassures patients in the back of an UH-60 M Black Hawk MEDEVAC helicopter in Logar province, Afghanistan. (US Army by Sgt. 1st Class Eric Pahon)

National Defense Authorization Act dramatically changed the level of training required for MEDEVAC using rotary- and fixed-wing aircraft to Critical Care Flight Paramedic [10, 11].

Air ambulance MEDEVAC of critically wounded combat casualties has benefitted greatly from increased training of prehospital providers and improvements in available medical equipment. This is in contrast to ground vehicle MEDEVAC, where limited medic training, sparse equipment, and austere conditions hamper the delivery of high-quality medical care [12].

Recently, the US Army began new training programs in an effort optimizing Prolonged Field Care (PFC), which is often necessary during lengthy ground evacuations when air MEDEVAC is not possible or when evacuation is delayed. These programs include the Expeditionary Combat Medic (ECM) program to enhance the skillset of combat medics, and the Enroute Critical Care Nurse (ECCN) program. These innovative solutions were intended to complement and enhance the capabilities of MEDEVAC in Afghanistan, especially for MEDEVAC of critical patients after damage control resuscitation by Forward Surgical Teams.

The increasing complexity of care and the trained providers available within the prehospital arena require more advanced medical oversight. The Army has guidance to perform both ground and air critical care evacuation, which is listed in the Army Uniform Task List. This capability requires similar evolution of the knowledge and skills of the command surgeon at the tactical level. Trauma surgeons have most recently filled the role of the Trauma Medical Director at the Role III theater hospital. This job title has been referred to as the "Trauma Czar" from around 2007 on but does not have an official doctrinal description or manning document slot.

The role of the Trauma Medical Director is to oversee all surgical care within the theater of operations and serve as the liaison to both the Combatant Command Surgeon's Office as well as to the Joint Trauma System focusing on clinical practice guideline (CPG) adherence. Through this oversight responsibility they also focus on the care of patients to the surgical Role II facility as well as from the Role II to the Role III, or occasionally from one Role III to another Role III, within the theater of operations. This responsibility frequently has them providing feedback and guidance to en route care providers.

Trauma surgery fellowships and general surgery residency do not have any prehospital rotations, education in Emergency Medical Services (EMS) direction, and potentially only have that exposure from prior military or civilian EMS experience. This leaves a capability gap that has been historically filled at the tactical level by physician assistants and general medical officers with very minimal formalized training in medical oversight, system quality analysis/improvement, protocol development, medic training/sustaining/skills verification, and system design. A recent *Military Medicine* article discussing the Army MEDEVAC blood transfusion program highlighted that physician oversight would ideally be performed by a full-time Prehospital Medical Director subspecialty trained in EMS [13]. This emphasis appears in the National Defense Authorization Act of 2017 as well. This Act lists EMS physicians as one of the five wartime medical specialties that requires a Secretary of Defense personnel management plan [14].

The US Department of Defense currently has only one graduate medical education training program dedicated to the creation of EMS specialists, or "prehospitalists," who are specifically trained in the skill areas identified above while also maintaining expertise in the delivery of critical care en route. The Military EMS & Disaster Medicine Fellowship, at Fort Sam Houston, Texas, is accredited by the Accreditation Council for Graduate Medical Education and trains US Army, US Air Force (USAF), and US Navy emergency physicians in the subspecialty of Emergency Medical Service medical direction. The graduates of this singular program, board-certified in EMS by the American Board of Emergency Medicine, are field-experienced physician thought-leaders helping shape the military landscape of battlefield medicine by incorporating civilian and military prehospital "best practices."

Contemporary Terminology

The meaning of the term Medical Evacuation (MEDEVAC) and Casualty Evacuation (CASEVAC) have evolved over the years. Originally, MEDEVAC was used to describe any patient movement on the battlefield. With the advent of patient transportation by rotary- and fixed-wing aircraft, many people began using the term to refer any patient movement, including long-distance transportation of patients by air, i.e., aeromedical evacuation (AE). *The term* Casualty Evacuation (CASEVAC) was originally used to describe the initial movement of patients in the tactical environment from the point of injury to initial medical care, in contrast to non-tactical (strategic) air transport of patients between medical facilities within the theater.

In modern usage, MEDEVAC is defined as all *regulated* patient movement by the US military (including Army, Navy, Marine Corps, Air Force, and Coast Guard) using predesignated tactical or logistic ground vehicles, aircraft (both fixed-wing and rotary), and watercraft medically equipped and staffed for en route care [2, 3]. MEDEVAC includes both movement of patients from the point of injury or illness to the nearest medical facility and movement of patients between medical facilities until the patient is ready for aeromedical evacuation to a fixed medical facility out of the theater. In most theaters, the final in-theater destination will be a fixed or contingency aeromedical staging facility (CASF). *In contrast, CASEVAC is defined as the unregulated movement of casualties by any land vehicles, aircraft, or watercraft* [2, 3]. The broad term *"Tactical Evacuation" refers to both MEDEVAC and CASEVAC* [3].

This chapter uses the traditional US Army definition of MEDEVAC as the regulated movement of casualties by ground or air from the battlefield to a medical facility and between medical facilities [1]. This chapter will focus on the most far-forward elements of MEDEVAC and examine the movement and en route care of patients from the point of injury or illness to a medical facility.

Tactical Combat Casualty Care (TCCC) refers to the standard of care in Prehospital Battlefield Medicine as described in the TCCC Guidelines published and updated by the Committee on Tactical Combat Casualty Care, a component of the US Department of Defense (DoD) Joint Trauma System. TCCC was originally conceptualized and published in 1996 by the Naval Special Warfare Command and the Casualty Care Research Center, Uniformed Services University of the Health Sciences [15]. The primary intent of TCCC is to provide the best possible care for casualties while taking into account tactical battlefield conditions. TCCC is currently taught as a DoD course to members of all branches of US armed forces.

MEDEVAC Principles

MEDEVAC is much more than the simple movement of casualties from the battlefield. In an effort to better understand the process, six basic principles of battlefield and tactical MEDEVAC have been identified (Table 3.1) [12]. The key principle is that MEDEVAC itself is a medical "intervention" or procedure subject to physician judgment. When and where a patient is evacuated, and by what means, should always be determined by a physician, either directly or through delegation by protocols and standing operating procedures. In contrast to civilian patient evacuation, military mission requirements and command approval are critical steps in the MEDEVAC decision-making process. Ultimately, of course, patient evacuation is a combatant command decision, but it should be made largely on medical recommendation [1].

"Speed and effectiveness" of transport is another important principle of MEDEVAC because it reflects the ultimate goal: the rapid transportation of casualties to a medical facility. The supporting principle of "proximity of resources" is a major challenge because the tactical environment is harsh and chaotic and limits

Table 3.1 Basic principles of battlefield and tactical MEDEVAC

Medical intervention
Speed and effectiveness
Proximity of resources
Medical care
Appropriateness
Precedence

the reach of evacuation assets. In most circumstances, the evacuation platform (e.g., vehicle or helicopter) will need to be relatively close to the anticipated concentration of casualties to ensure a rapid response.

The principle of "Medical Care" refers to the en route patient care provided (Fig. 3.2). This medical care is what separates merely moving casualties from MEDEVAC. The principle of "appropriateness" refers both to utilizing the best mode of

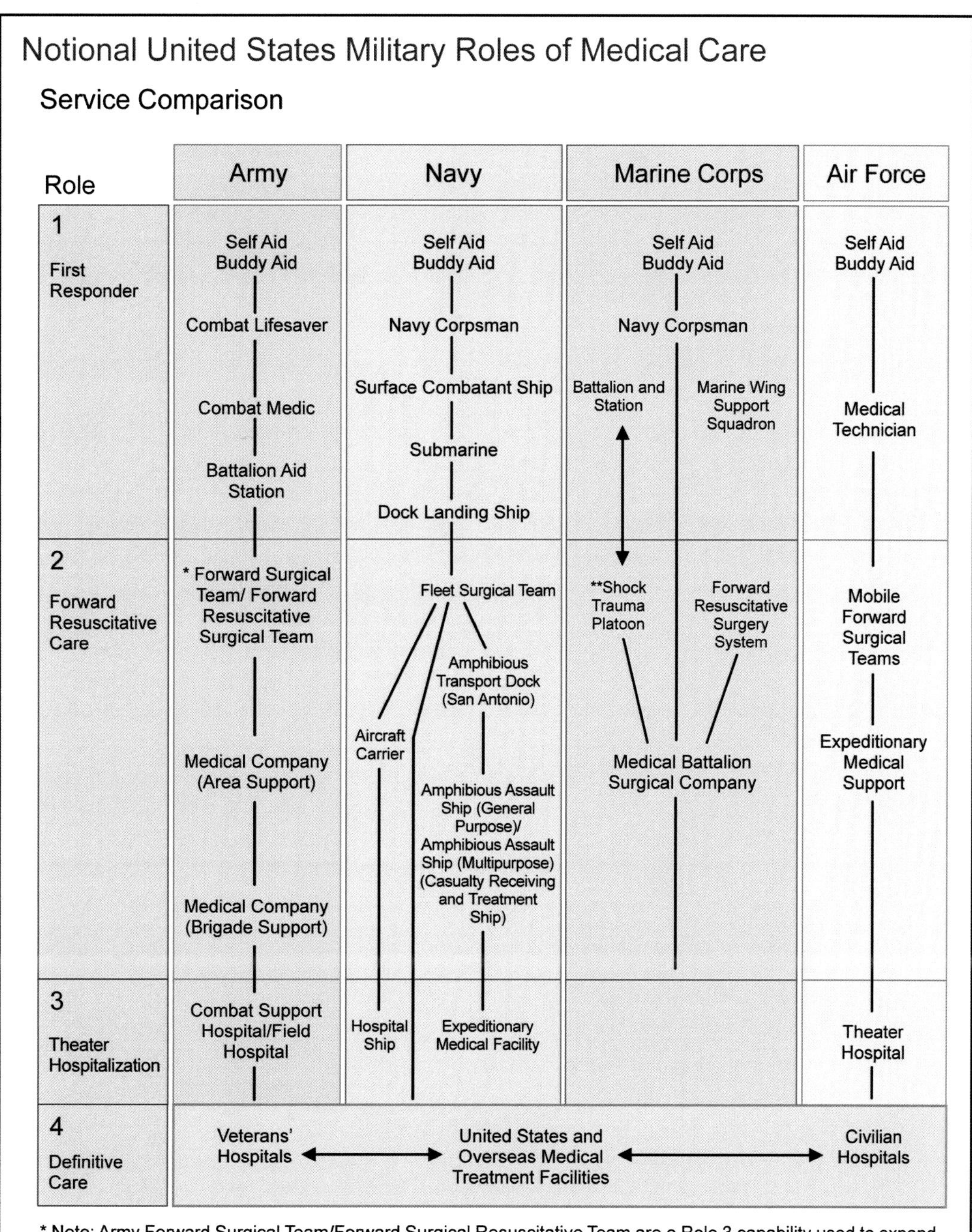

Fig. 3.2 US Military Roles of Medical Care. (Figure reprinted from Joint Health Services [2])

evacuation (e.g., ground or air) and bringing the casualties to the most appropriate medical facility, which is usually (but not always) the closest facility [16]. The principle of "precedence" refers to the categorization of patients by need for evacuation. Together, appropriateness and precedence support the triage concept, whereby casualties are sorted and resources conserved to maximize benefit. During a mass-casualty situation, medical providers frequently encounter a mismatch of patient needs and evacuation resources and therefore must make difficult triage decisions to assure the limited resources are utilized most effectively. Applying the principles of appropriateness and precedence will help deal with this mismatch.

Roles of Care

A basic understanding of the military roles of care system (Fig. 3.2) is needed to fully comprehend the concept of battlefield and tactical MEDEVAC [2]. This system describes a hierarchy of medical care and facilities designed to support the war fighting elements. Details of the US Army version are provided in Table 3.2 [16, 17]. Although these designations are current at the time of this writing, both military medical doctrine and nomenclature are continually changing.

Precedence

A key concept in the care provided to the casualty during evacuation is the MEDEVAC principle of precedence. Correctly choosing which casualty goes first and to which medical facility is central to providing good MEDEVAC. Individual precedence decisions made will impact the overall effectiveness of the evacuation effort. For this reason, medical commanders must ensure that precedence decisions are made by the most qualified medical provider, and in many cases this may not be the most senior or highest-ranking medical officer.

The US Army system uses 5 standard categories to determine MEDEVAC precedence (Table 3.3) [17]. "Urgent" patients need immediate evacuation and cannot tolerate a delay of more than 2 hours without significantly risking death or disability. The "urgent surgical" subcategory was created to emphasize the patient's need for acute surgical intervention, thus alerting the evacuation team to transport the patient to a surgery-capable facility. "Priority" patients are less likely to deteriorate and can tolerate an evacuation delay of 4 hours. "Routine" patients are unlikely to deteriorate and can tolerate an evacuation delay of 24 hours. "Convenience" patients are being evacuated by medical vehicle for medical convenience rather than necessity. NATO has removed convenience from its evacuation precedence categories but it is still deemed useful for the US Army operational environment [17]. These MEDEVAC precedence categories should not be confused with the standard NATO triage designations (i.e., immediate, delayed, minimal, and expectant), which identify treatment priorities rather than evacuation precedence.

These standard precedence categories are necessary to facilitate communication between the

Table 3.2 Roles of military medical care

Role	Military hierarchy	Personnel/facility	Type of care
1	Unit	Self/buddy aid	Tactical Combat Casualty Care (TCCC)
		Combat lifesaver	TCCC with some enhancements
		Combat medic	Emergency medical treatment
		Battalion aid station	Advanced trauma and medical management
2	Brigade/Division	Medical company, Forward Surgical Resuscitative Team (FRST) and Advanced Trauma Management Team	Damage Control Resuscitation and Surgery, Laboratory, Dental, preventive med and Combat Operational Stress Control (COSC)
3	Corps/Theater	Combat support hospital	Resuscitative surgery and medical care to stabilize and prepare for strategic Aeromedical Evacuation
4	Out-of-theater and Continental US	Fixed medical facilities	Restorative and rehabilitative care

Table 3.3 Standard US Army precedence categories for MEDEVAC

Priority level	Designation	Description
I	Urgent	Emergency cases that should be evacuated as soon as possible and within a maximum of 1 hour to save life, limb, or eyesight and to prevent complication of serious illness and to avoid permanent disability
IA	Urgent—surgery	Must receive far forward surgical intervention to save life and stabilize for further evacuation
II	Priority	Requiring evacuation within 4 hours or his medical condition could deteriorate to such a degree that he will become an urgent precedence or will suffer unnecessary pain or disability
III	Routine	Requiring evacuation within 24 hours, but whose condition is not expected to deteriorate significantly
IV	Convenience	Evacuation is a matter of medical convenience rather than necessity

Source: Adapted from USA data [16]

Table 3.4 US Army "nine-line" Medical Evacuation Request Form

1. Location of pickup site
2. Radio frequency and call sign
3. Number of patients by precedence (a) Urgent (b) Urgent surgical (c) Priority (d) Routine (e) Convenience
4. Special equipment required
5. Number of patients by type (litter and ambulatory)
6. Security of pickup site (wartime only)
7. Method of marking pickup site
8. Patient nationality and status
9. Nuclear, biologic, or chemical contamination (wartime only)
Terrain description (peacetime)

Source: Adapted from US Army data [16]

various elements in the evacuation chain. In the US Army MEDEVAC system, a nine-line Medical Evacuation Request Form is used (Table 3.4). The information is given to a supporting evacuation element, usually by radio, by reading the 9 lines of information in sequence [18].

Assessment and Ongoing Care

Assessment and care during tactical evacuation is a compromise between the provision of optimal care and the realities of a harsh, austere, often hostile battlefield environment. Assessment is limited by noise, movement, and light restrictions. Ongoing medical care is also hindered by equipment shortages, multiple casualties, and limited provider skills. Despite these limiting factors, effective assessment and care is possible in this environment.

MARCH: Care from Point of Injury through Initial Evacuation

The mnemonic "MARCH" is taught in the TCCC Course as an algorithm for care from the point of injury through initial evacuation. This care algorithm deviates somewhat from the "Airway, Breathing, Circulation, Disability, Exposure" (ABCDE) algorithm stressed by the American College of Surgeons Advanced Trauma Life Support training. Although the exact origin of the MARCH acronym is unknown, it likely came from the UK military about 2008 and was quickly incorporated into TCCC training. All military personnel providing prehospital care should become familiar with the MARCH algorithm:

- **M** represents massive hemorrhage, which must be immediately controlled. Immediate use of limb tourniquets in a "high and tight" hasty emplacement can prevent exsanguination from arterial limb bleeding while assessing for other life-threatening injuries. For severe bleeding not amenable to limb tourniquets in the axillary and groin regions, hemorrhage should be controlled by direct pressure, hemostatic dressings (e.g., chitosan or kaolin), and, when necessary, the use of junctional tourniquets.

- **A** represents airway management. For the unconscious casualty without orofacial injuries, initial airway management consists of positioning (e.g., head tilt, chin lift, and/or jaw thrust) or placement of a nasopharyngeal airway. For casualties with orofacial injuries with impending or current airway obstruction, conscious patients can be allowed to position themselves. Unconscious patients should be managed with a nasopharyngeal airway or surgical cricothyrotomy. Prior to evacuation of patients with unstable airways, a supraglottic airway or endotracheal tube should be placed.
- **R** represents respirations. Compromised ventilatory effort in the presence of an adequate airway should prompt evaluation for problems such as sucking chest wound or tension pneumothorax. A sucking chest wound should be addressed with a vented chest seal to prevent development of tension physiology and a tension pneumothorax needle should be decompressed with a needle or catheter at least a 14 gauge or larger in diameter. The effectiveness of tube or finger thoracostomy in the field remains under debate [19].
- **C** represents circulation. Radial pulses and mental status and radial pulses are used as indicators of adequate circulation. Unconscious patients should be evaluated for other less obvious sources of hemorrhage. The preferred resuscitative approach for patients with hemorrhagic shock is fresh whole blood; the simultaneous administration of fractionated blood products (packed red blood cells, platelets, and plasma) is discussed later under "Intravenous Fluid Resuscitation." Since 2010, 1–2 units of packed red blood cells have been placed on board evacuation platforms in active combat zones [11]. Also recommended is the immediate administration of tranexamic acid, an antifibrinolytic, in anticipation of multiple blood transfusions, which includes ongoing non-compressible bleeding, presentation in hemorrhagic shock, and major or multiple limb amputations.
- **H** represents hypothermia and head injury. Measures should be taken to avoid hypothermia, since it is one leg of the lethal shock triad, along with acidosis and coagulopathy. Care must be taken for patients with moderate (Glaucoma Coma Scale [GCS] 9–12) to severe (GCS 3–8) head injuries to prevent primary and secondary neurologic insults by maintaining systolic blood pressure (SBP) of $\geq$110 mm Hg, mean arterial pressure 80–110 mm Hg, end tidal CO_2 ($ETCO_2$) 35–40 mm Hg, and peripheral capillary O_2 saturation (SPO_2) >93% [14]. When serial examinations by MEDEVAC providers detect signs suggestive of intracranial hypertension (i.e., decreasing GCS, changes in pupillary size/reactivity, gross focal neurologic deficits) treatment with 3% saline prior to neurosurgical intervention has been recommended [16].

Other Mnemonics and Acronyms

In addition to MARCH, a number of additional mnemonics have been developed to aid in field medical care. The mnemonic PAWS focuses on Pain medication, Antibiotics, Wound care, and Splinting. The pre-transport checklist MITES has been developed by the Critical Care Flight Paramedic Standard Medical Operating Guidelines (Fig. 3.3) [11]. The SMEED (Special Medical Emergency Evacuation Device) is a tray-like device attached to the MEDEVAC litter to hold monitoring devices above the casualty's feet while still remaining visible and not adding to the width of the litter.

Ongoing Care

Patients should be continually reassessed while en route using the MARCH or expanded ABCDE algorithm (Table 3.5) with special focus on airway, breath, and circulation (ABC). Electronic physiological monitors (e.g., sphygmomanometer, pulse oximeter, and capnometer, etc.) should be employed when available (Fig. 3.4). When this type of equipment is unavailable, providers must rely on traditional inspection, palpation, and auscultation for assessment.

MITES CHECK

MEDICATIONS:

- ☐ Assure Appropriate Medications Given
- ☐ Necessary Medications Available For Transport?
- ☐ Note Meds Given (Name / Dosage / Time)

INVASIVE Procedures / IV Access:

- ☐ All Patients With At Least One Working Peripheral IV and/or IO Line
- ☐ Trauma / Emergent: At Least Two Working Peripheral IV / IO Line
- ☐ NG / OG On All Intubated Patients
- ☐ Chest Tube / Foley Catheter / etc., As Needed

TUBES & TOURNIQUETS:

- ☐ Note Size / Depth of ETT if Present
- ☐ Ensure Tubes Appropriately Secured (e.g., ETT, Chest, Foley, Wound)
- ☐ Evaluate Tubes for Displacement, Kinking, Clogging
- ☐ Ensure Heimlich Value or Working Suction To Chest Tube
- ☐ Note Location of Tourniquets and Time Placed
- ☐ Evaluate for Seepage From Tourniquet Areas and Augment PRN

EVERY VITAL SIGN:

- ☐ Document Full Set of Vitals (Including SPO_2 and $ETCO_2$, if applicable) and Monitor En Route
- ☐ Recheck As Appropriate

SECURE For Transport / Spinal Immobilization:

- ☐ Patient Status Adequate for Transfer?
- ☐ Hypothermia Precautions?
- ☐ At Least Two Litter Straps in place?
- ☐ Equipment Secured to SMEED and SMEED to Litter?
- ☐ Appropriate Spinal Precautions in Place?

Fig. 3.3 US Army Critical Care Flight Paramedic pre-transport checklist. (Reprinted from US Army MEDEVAC Critical Care Flight Paramedic Standard Medical Operating Guidelines [11])

Table 3.5 Principles of good prehospital care

Airway
Ensure patency and adequacy of airway
Breathing
Ensure adequacy of ventilation and oxygenation
Circulation
Ensure all bleeding is controlled
Provide appropriate fluid support
Disability and drugs
Monitor mental status and neurological response
Recheck splints and dressings
Administer appropriate medications
Extras
Keep casualty comfortable and warm
Provide reassurance and support
Ensure casualty is properly restrained against falls and crashes

Adapted from [3, 20]

The adequacy of both the airway and breathing can be roughly estimated by observing or palpating chest excursion. The traditional technique of breath sound auscultation is often impossible in the noisy tactical environment. Electronic monitoring is extremely useful in this environment, and pulse oximetry showing peripheral oxygen saturation >95% indicates satisfactory central oxygenation. In patients receiving supplemental oxygen, pulse oximetry allows accurate titration of flow rates to keep the saturation >95%, thus conserving scarce oxygen supplies [11]. In an intubated patient, electronic capnometry is another method to assure airway patency. Alternative manual methods include direct visualization of tube placement by laryngoscopy, an esophageal detector device, and observation of respirophasic condensation on the tube.

Although more advanced physiologic monitoring technologies are currently under development, pulse and blood pressure remain the primary indicators of circulatory status [20]. Electronic physiological monitors can reliably measure these parameters, even in the presence of

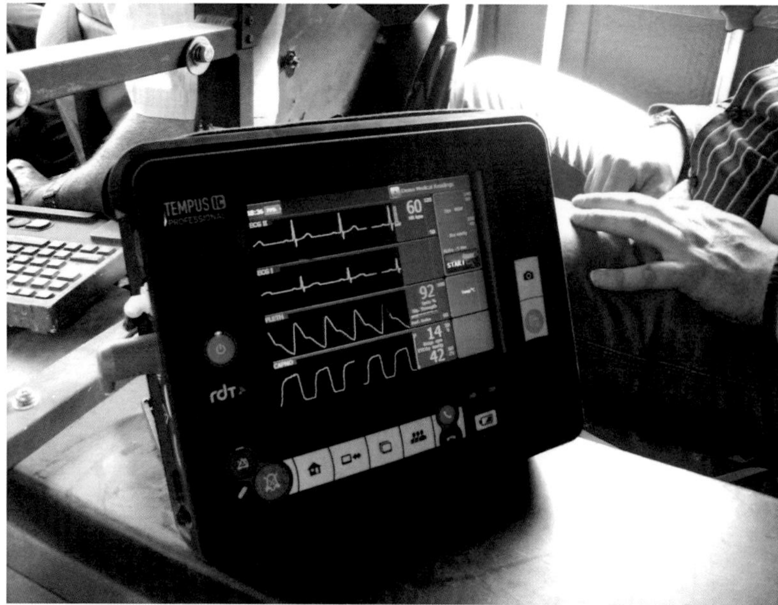

Fig. 3.4 Advanced patient monitors can transmit real-time patient telemetry data from moving tactical vehicles over tactical radios to forward medical treatment teams. (US Army Photo by Telemedicine and Advanced Technology Research Center)

significant noise and motion. Manually obtained pulse and blood pressure are more difficult to accurately obtain in the tactical environment. Capillary refill, indicative of peripheral vasoconstriction, is a reasonable alternative indicator of circulatory status that can be used in this environment. Refill time in excess of 3 seconds suggests circulatory compromise, and is best observed at a central location such as the forehead, neck, chest, or abdomen. Cold exposure can also prolong capillary refill, especially in the extremities [21].

Intravenous Fluid Resuscitation

The approach for administration of intravenous fluids to casualties in the field has recently undergone significant changes. Previously, the standard approach for patients suspected of having hemorrhagic shock was to administer massive amounts of crystalloid and colloid fluids in an effort to maintain a normal blood pressure. Recent trends in the care of penetrating injuries in the field have moved away from crystalloid fluid as the primary treatment approach for hemorrhagic shock since this approach can dilute clotting factors. Instead, administration of blood or blood products is recommended, using the following in descending order of recommendation: fresh whole blood (group O low titer preferred); blood component therapy (packed red blood cells, platelets, and plasma) in a ratio of 1:1:1; packed red blood cells plus plasma at 1:1, plasma; or packed red blood cells alone [22, 23].

The goal of ongoing damage control resuscitation during evacuation is systolic blood pressure ≥90–100 mm Hg with appropriate mentation (in the absence of head injury) plus urine output ≥0.5 ml/kg/hr. When prolonged field care is required, the current recommendation is to not allow sustained SBP <100 for ≥100 minutes. In some circumstances (e.g., burns, crush injuries) administration of crystalloid fluid is medically appropriate, especially when there is a delay of >2 hours before reaching definitive medical care and the primary condition being treated is not hemorrhagic shock.

Analgesia

Drug therapy in the field has come to play an increasingly important role in TCCC. Troops with mild to moderate pain are routinely trained with a "combat pill pack" containing acetaminophen and meloxicam (the only nonsteroidal anti-inflammatory that does not decrease platelet aggregation).

When injured patients have moderate to severe pain, the treatment goal is to relieve suffering rather than complete relief of pain, but without compromising hemodynamic or respiratory function. Patients not likely to develop shock or respiratory distress can be treated with buccal fentanyl. However, patients at risk for shock or respiratory depression should be treated with the dissociative anesthetic ketamine, given by the most expedient route (i.e., intramuscular, intranasal intravenous, or intraosseous) and re-dosed every 20–30 minutes as necessary [24]. Suboptimal dosing can result in partial dissociation with psychomimetic activation presenting as agitation, which can prove dangerous for both the patient and MEDEVAC crew. Undertreating pain for severely injured patients is inhumane.

Prophylactic Antibiotics

Prophylactic antibiotics are now routinely administered on the battlefield to casualties with penetrating injuries from bullets, fragments, blasts, and burns in an effort to decrease the risk of subsequent infection [25]. Early administration may be most effective and a number of different antibiotic regimens are recommended depending on the location and type of injury [25]. Tetanus prophylaxis with tetanus–diphtheria toxoid is also indicated for inadequately immunized casualties, most frequently civilians and foreign troops.

Chemical Agents Antidotes

Chemical or biologic attacks are extremely dangerous but thus far remain exceedingly unlikely in modern combat. Several known chemical warfare agents have antidotes or treatments that are effective if used promptly. For this reason, tactical medical providers must be familiar with atropine, pralidoxime, and diazepam for nerve agents; nitrites and thiosulfate for cyanide; and inhaled bronchodilators for pulmonary agents. Repeated dosing of these medications may be required throughout the evacuation chain. Biologic agents also remain a potential threat and the evacuation chain must be ready to begin drug treatment at the earliest possible time.

Transfer of Care

Eventually, the tactical MEDEVAC system must interface with the medical facility or the theater AE system. The effective transfer of care requires good communication between all elements, both verbal and written. Neither needs to be lengthy, but should highlight key aspects of the casualty's condition and treatment.

Completion of either one of two forms has become standard for written documentation of medical care before and during MEDEVAC: either the Department of Defense Form 1380 (DD1380) or the overprint of the Department of the Army Form 4700 (DA4700) entitled "Tactical Evacuation After Action Report & Patient Care Record." Both of these records are commonly referred to as "TC3 Cards" (for TCCC) or PCR/run sheet, and the TC3 card must be attached to the casualty in a prominent location prior to any MEDEVAC with the PCR completed at the conclusion of the MEDEVAC mission.

The DD1380 (Fig. 3.5) is an abbreviated document that includes basic demographic data, key physical findings, and treatment rendered using the "MIST" format: Mechanism, Injury, Signs/Symptoms, and Treatment. The DD1380 is more suited for shorter evacuations with less complicated injuries.

The DA4700 overprint (Fig. 3.6a, b) allows for much more detailed information. It allows documentation needed for more seriously injured casualties who have undergone damage control resuscitation and/or require MEDEVAC or AE between medical facilities.

Medical Regulating

Medical regulating refers to the coordination and control of patient movement to ensure their safe and efficient movement [2]. The medical regulation system identifies patients awaiting evacuation, locates appropriate and available receiving facilities, and coordinates patient transportation. The objectives of medical regulating are to (1) ensure an even distribution of patient load, (2) provide adequate beds and treatment capabilities for current and anticipated needs, and (3) ensure that patients requiring specialized care get to the appropriate facility.

Historically, medical regulation only became a concern prior to theater-level AE. However, as automated systems become more capable, medical regulation usually begins at the level of tactical MEDEVAC and sometimes at the point-of-injury. The Patient Evacuation Coordination Cell was initially established during Operation Enduring Freedom in Afghanistan at the Regional Command level to provide more unified casualty movement within and between medical treatment facilities. Establishment of a Patient Evacuation Coordination Cell within a brigade area of operations is the ultimate goal, which is at the operational level just above the tactical [16, 17].

The formalized system of medical regulating utilized by the US Transportation Command (TRANSCOM) as the lead command for patient movement is the TRANSCOM Regulating and Command & Control Evacuation System (TRAC2ES), which is generally not utilized until a casualty has reached a Role 3 medical treatment facility [2].

Transportation

The overall goal of MEDEVAC is the safe and effective movement of the casualties. MEDEVAC transportations modes can include manual carries, ground vehicles, aircraft, watercraft, or a combination of these depending on the circumstances.

EVAC CATEGORY: ______ BATTLE ROSTER #: ______

TACTICAL COMBAT CASUALTY CARE (TCCC) CARD

NAME (Last, First): ______ LAST 4: ______

DATE (DD-MMM-YY): ______ TIME: ______

UNIT: ______ ALLERGIES: ______

Mechanism of Injury: (X all that apply)

☐ Artillery ☐ Burn ☐ Fall ☐ Grenade ☐ GSW ☐ IED

☐ Landmine ☐ MVC ☐ RPG ☐ Other: ______

Injury: (Mark injuries with an X)

TQ: R Arm TYPE: ______ TIME: ______

TQ: L Arm TYPE: ______ TIME: ______

4.5 18 4.5 4.5 1 9 9 4.5 18 4.5 4.5 9 9

TQ: R Leg TYPE: ______ TIME: ______

TQ: L Leg TYPE: ______ TIME: ______

Signs & Symptoms: (Fill in the blank)

Time				
Pulse (Rate & Location)				
Blood Pressure				
Respiratory Rate				
Pulse Ox % O2 Sat				
AVPU				
Pain Scale (0-10)				

DD FORM (NUM), (DATE) Page 1 of 2

EVAC CATEGORY: ______ BATTLE ROSTER #: ______

Treatments: (X all that apply, and fill in the blank)

C: ☐ Extremity-TQ ☐ Junctional-TQ ☐ Pressure-Dressing

☐ Hemostatic-Dressing Type: ______

A: ☐ Intact ☐ NPA ☐ CRIC ☐ ET-Tube ☐ SGA Type: ______

B: ☐ O2 ☐ Needle-D ☐ Chest-Tube ☐ Chest-Seal Type: ______

C:

	Name	Volume	Route	Time
Fluid				
Blood Product				

MEDS:

	Name	Dose	Route	Time
Analgesic (e.g. Ketamine, Fentanyl, Morphine)				
Antibiotic (e.g. Moxifloxacin, Ertapenem)				
Other (e.g. TXA)				

OTHER: ☐ Combat-Pill-Pack ☐ Eye-Shield (☐ R ☐ L) ☐ Splint

☐ Hypothermia-Prevention Type: ______

NOTES: ______

FIRST RESPONDER NAME (Last, First): ______ LAST 4: ______

DD FORM (NUM), (DATE) Page 2 of 2

Fig. 3.5 Department of Defense Form 1380 (DD1380) Combat Casualty Care Card (TC3 Card), front and back

a

MEDICAL RECORD-SUPPLEMENTAL MEDICAL DATA

For use of this form, see AR 40-66; the proponent agency is the Office of the Surgeon General

REPORT TITLE
Tactical Evacuation After Action Report & Patient Care Record, *Page 1*

JTS APPROVED *(Date)*
(20141119) -V4.0

Event: Date ______ Time ____ | Time Zone ◯L ◯Z | MM (___) ______ | Pt # ____ of ____ | Tail to Tail ◯Y ◯N | Leg # ___ of ____

9-Line: Time ______ Platform ______ Dispatch Cat ______ Assessed Cat ______

Trauma MIST Report: *M=Mechanism of Injury, I=Injury, S=Signs & Symptoms, T=Treatments* / **Disease Diagnosis:** ______

M ______ I ______ S ______ T ______

Comments ______

Pickup: Time ____ Role ______ Other ______ Region ______ Other ______ Location ______

Dropoff: Time ____ Role ______ Other ______ Region ______ Other ______ Location ______

Capability ☐ EMT-B ☐ EMT-I ☐ EMT-P ☐ EMT-FPC ☐ RN ☐ CRNA ☐ PA ☐ MD/DO Other ______

Circulation-Hemorrhage Control

☐ Direct Pressure
☐ Hemostatic Dressing
☐ Kerlix Dressing
☐ Pressure Dressing
Other ______

Tourniquet
Prior TQ:
Reassess/tighten
◯Y
◯N
◯N/A

Time On ____ ☐ CAT ☐ SOFTT ☐ Other ______ ☐ RUE ☐ LUE ☐ RLE ☐ LLE # ___
Time On ____ ☐ CAT ☐ SOFTT ☐ Other ______ ☐ RUE ☐ LUE ☐ RLE ☐ LLE # ___
Time On ____ ☐ CAT ☐ SOFTT ☐ Other ______ ☐ RUE ☐ LUE ☐ RLE ☐ LLE # ___
Time On ____ ☐ CAT ☐ SOFTT ☐ Other ______ ☐ RUE ☐ LUE ☐ RLE ☐ LLE # ___
Time On ____ ☐ AAJT ☐ CRoC ☐ JETT ☐ SAM ☐ Other Junctional ______ # ___
TQ Comments ______

Airway

☐ Self ☐ NPA ☐ OPA ☐ Cric ☐ Trach ☐ ETT ☐ SGA Type ______

Tube Size ____ Pos ____ @ ____ Confirmed ☐BS ☐ Vis ☐ ETCO2

O2 Source ☐ NC ☐ NRB ☐ BVM ☐ Vent LPM ____

Intubated ☐ Prior to transport ☐ By transport crew **Suction** ☐ ETT ☐ Yaunker

Breathing

Needle Decompression
Time ____ ☐ R ☐ L ☐ Mid-ax ☐ Mid-clav
Time ____ ☐ R ☐ L ☐ Mid-ax ☐ Mid-clav
Time ____ ☐ R ☐ L ☐ Mid-ax ☐ Mid-clav
Time ____ ☐ R ☐ L ☐ Mid-ax ☐ Mid-clav

Chest Equal Rise and Fall
◯Y ◯N ◯N/A

Respiratory Effort
☐ Unlabored ☐ Labored
☐ Agonal ☐ Assisted

Chest Tube Time ____ ☐ R ☐ L

Vent Settings	Time	Mode	Rate	TV	FiO2	PEEP	PIP	ETCO2
Initial								
Change								
Change								
Change								

Annotate Injuries

(AMP)utation
(BL)eeding
(B)urn %TBSA ____
(C)repitus
(D)eformity
(DG)Degloving
(E)cchymosis
(FX)Fracture
(GSW)Gunshot Wound
(H)ematoma
(IMP)Impaled Object
(LAC)eration
(P)ain
(PP)Peppering
(PW)Puncture Wound
(SQA)Subcutaneous Air
(TBI)Suspect
Other ______

Circulation - Assessment

Rhythm / Ectopy
☐ NSR ☐ SVT
☐ ST ☐ VT
☐ SB ☐ VF
☐ PEA
☐ Paced
☐ Asystole
☐ A-FIB
☐ A-FLUT

Pulses
A, D, +1, +2, +3
RAD ____
BRAC ____
CAR ____
FEM ____
PED ____
TEMP ____

Circulation - Resuscitation

Transfusion Indication
☐ Amputation
☐ HR > 120
☐ SBP < 90

Blood Infusion Time	Component	ABO/RH	Unit Number	Exp. Date	Blood Age

IV Lines

Peripheral
Hand ☐ R ☐ L ga ___
Arm ☐ R ☐ L ga ___
EJ ☐ R ☐ L ga ___

IO Type / Site
☐ Fast-1 ☐ EZ IO Other ______
Humerus ☐ R ☐ L
Tibia ☐ R ☐ L
☐ Sternum

Central Line Location
☐ Triple lumen ______
☐ Cordis ______

Arterial Line
Wrist ☐ R ☐ L
Groin ☐ R ☐ L

PREPARED BY *(Name, Rank & Title)* | DEPARTMENT/SERVICE/CLINIC *(Treating Unit)* | DATE

PATIENT'S IDENTIFICATION *(Name: last, first, middle; grade; date; hospital or medical facility)*

Last Name ______ First Name ______ MI ___

BR# ____ Rank ____ Unit ______ Pt Cat ______

SSN ______ DOB ______ Gender ◯ M ◯ F Allergy ______ Other ______

☐ HISTORY/PHYSICAL ☒ TREATMENT
☐ DIAGNOSTIC STUDIES ☐ FLOW CHART
☐ OTHER EXAMINATION OR EVALUATION
☐ OTHER, Specify

DA FORM 4700, FEB 2003 EDITION OF MAY 78 IS OBSOLETE. **JTS TACEVAC AAR & PCR OP 05 (MCMR-SRJ) NOV 2014** APD PE v1.01ES

Fig. 3.6 (**a**) Front and (**b**) back of Department of the Army Form 4700 (DA4700) Tactical Evacuation After Action Report & Patient Care Record

b

MEDICAL RECORD-SUPPLEMENTAL MEDICAL DATA

For use of this form, see AR 40-66; the proponent agency is the Office of the Surgeon General

REPORT TITLE
Tactical Evacuation After Action Report & Patient Care Record, *Page 2*

JTS APPROVED *(Date)*
(20141119) -V4.0

Vital Signs

	Time	HR	BP	RR	SpO2	ETCO2	Temp	F	C	AVPU	GCS: Eyes 1-4	Verbal 1-5	Motor 1-6	Total	Pain 0-10
First			/					○	○						
			/					○	○						
			/					○	○						
Last			/					○	○						

PERRLA ☐ R Size (mm) ____ ☐ L Size (mm) ____

Field Ultrasound Results ____ Other Diagnostics ____

Additional Interventions

Foley Time ____ Comment ____ **Gastric Tube** Time ____ ☐ Oral ☐ Nasal Comment ____

Protection ____ ☐ Eye Shield ☐ Protective Eyewear ☐ Right ☐ Left Comment ____

Immobilization ____ ☐ C-Collar ☐ C-Spine ☐ Spine Board ☐ Pelvic Splint ☐ Pelvic Binder, Type ____
____ ☐ Splint, Type/Location ____

Warming ____ ☐ Hypothermia Prevention, Product ____
____ ☐ Hypothermia Prevention, Product ____

Other Interventions ____ ____
____ ____

Medications and Fluids *Route = IM, IN, IO, IV, PO, PR, SL, SQ*

Time	Drug / Fluid	Dose	Route

Medications and Fluids *Route = IM, IN, IO, IV, PO, PR, SL, SQ*

Time	Drug / Fluid	Dose	Route

Documents Received ☐ TCCC Card ☐ Patient Chart ☐ None Other ____

Narrative Summary of Care

Enroute Care Provider

Last Name	First Name	Rank	Capability	Signature

Email PCR to: usarmy.jbsa.medcom-aisr.list.jts-prehospital@mail.mil **MM (____)** ____

PREPARED BY *(Signature & Title)*

DEPARTMENT/SERVICE/CLINIC *(Treating Unit)*

DATE

PATIENT'S IDENTIFICATION *(Name: last, first, middle; grade; date; hospital or medical facility)*

Last Name ____ First Name ____ MI ____

BR# ____ Rank ____ Unit ____ Pt Cat ____

SSN ____ DOB ____ Gender ○ M ○ F Allergy ____ Other ____

☐ HISTORY/PHYSICAL ☒ TREATMENT
☐ DIAGNOSTIC STUDIES ☐ FLOW CHART
☐ OTHER EXAMINATION OR EVALUATION
☐ OTHER, Specify

DA FORM 4700, FEB 2003 EDITION OF MAY 78 IS OBSOLETE. **JTS TACEVAC AAR & PCR OP 05 (MCMR-SRJ) NOV 2014** APD PE v1.01ES

Fig. 3.6 (continued)

All members of the military medical team should have a general familiarity with the common transportation modes used for MEDEVAC.

Manual Carries

In combat and many military operations other than war, the manual carry is the primary means of moving casualties from the point of injury or illness to a point of safety where the medical evacuation can begin. Despite tremendous advances in many other areas of evacuation, manual carries remain almost unchanged over the centuries. While agility and finesse are essential to executing all manual carries, there remains no substitute for physical strength and endurance. Manual carries can be exhausting work and necessarily have a range limited to a few hundred or thousand meters.

Manual carries and drags may aggravate fractures and wounds because they offer little stable support for the casualty's body. Moving the casualty along the long axis of the body will minimize further injury to the casualty. Ongoing care is impossible during a manual carry. If possible, life-threatening bleeding should be controlled with a tourniquet prior to movement. Airway management, ventilation, and patient monitoring must be delayed until the casualty reaches a point of safety [1].

Litter Carries

Litter transportation offers modest improvements over manual carries. Some support and comfort is afforded the patient, and spinal immobilization, fracture splinting, oxygen therapy, and other static treatments can often be maintained during movement. Airway management, ventilation, and other dynamic care remains difficult to perform, however.

Litter carries have the additional advantage that the work of transporting a patient can be shared by two to four persons, markedly increasing the potential range of transportation. The obvious drawback, however, is that up to four persons are committed to moving one patient.

Litters are lightweight, portable, durable, and readily available on the battlefield. They are also widely used to move patients in and around medical facilities and on and off evacuation vehicles. Therefore, all military medical providers should be familiar with their use [1].

Ground Vehicles

Ground vehicles are the most common platform used to move casualties over relatively long distances on the battlefield. Current US military doctrine places dedicated ambulances in the warfighting maneuver units such as an armor or infantry battalion. In most scenarios, battlefield casualties will be carried or dragged several hundred meters to a point of relative safety (e.g., the casualty collection point) where a ground ambulance can pick them up. As a result, ground ambulances can be expected to get fairly close to the point of injury in many cases.

There are several ground ambulances in use today (Table 3.6). The M996 and M997 "Humvee" wheeled ambulances are built on the highly successful high-mobility multipurpose wheeled vehicle (HMMWV) chassis (Fig. 3.7). The HMMWV is organic to medical platoons of light-infantry battalions and most medical companies and can accommodate up to four litter patients.

The M113A2/A3 Armored Ambulance is a tracked armored personnel carrier (APC) modified to serve as an armored ambulance that can accommodate up to four litters (Fig. 3.8). It is a pre-Vietnam era design and suffers from thin armor, slow speed, and a jarring ride. It is organic primarily to medical platoons in armor and mechanized infantry battalions.

The US Army is hoping to completely replace the aging M113 with the M2A0 Armored Medical Evacuation Vehicle (AMEV), which is built on the M2/M3 Bradley fighting vehicle chassis (Fig. 3.9). The AMEV is also known as the Army Multi-Purpose Vehicle (AMPV) Ambulance Variant. The AMEV offers greater armor, speed, range, comfort, and room than the M113 and has provisions for onboard oxygen. In addition, it offers protection against chemical and biologic agents.

The Stryker, a wheeled armored vehicle for the Army's medium weight brigade, comes in a variety of configurations including an ambulance

Table 3.6 Ground vehicles and rotary wing aircraft used for MEDEVAC by the US Army

Platform	Description	Litter capacity
M996/M997	Wheeled ambulance, HMMWV chassis	2–4
M113	Tracked, armored ambulance	4
AMEV	Armored medical evacuation vehicle	4
Stryker	Wheeled armored medical evacuation vehicle (MEV)	4
RG-33 HAGA	Heavily Armored Ground Ambulance	3
UH/HH-60 Black Hawk	Twin-engine helicopter	6
UH-72 Lakota	Twin-engine light helicopter for noncombat MEDEVAC	1–2

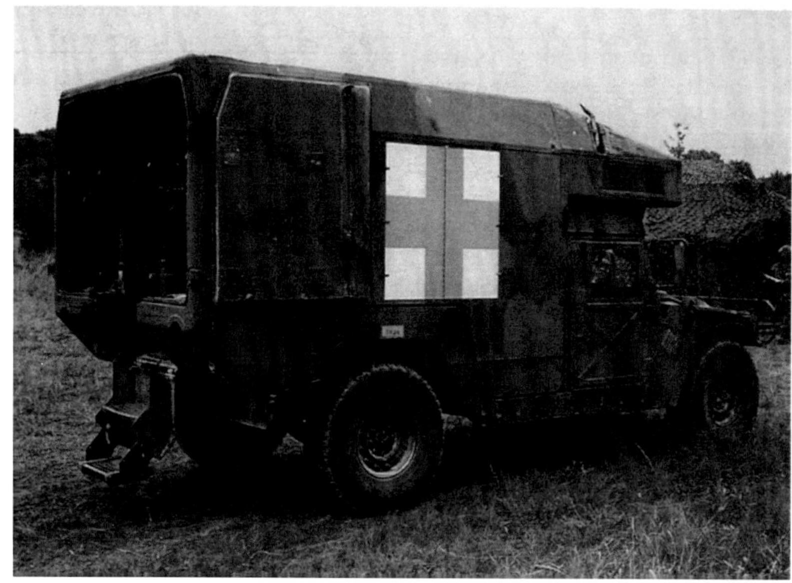

Fig. 3.7 The M997 wheeled "Humvee" ambulance is built on the high-mobility multipurpose wheeled vehicle (HMMWV). (Photo by LTC Robert De Lorenzo)

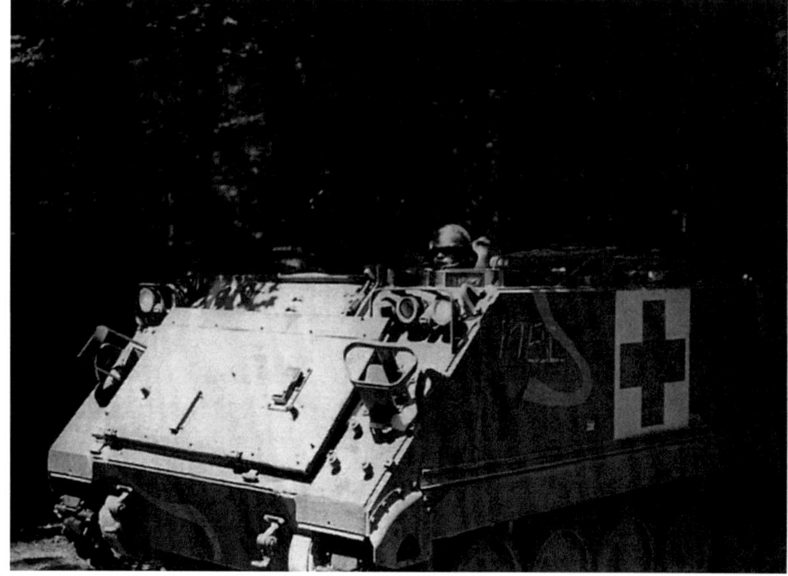

Fig. 3.8 The M113A2/A3 Armored Ambulance is a modified tracked armored personnel carrier (APC). (Photo by LTC Robert De Lorenzo)

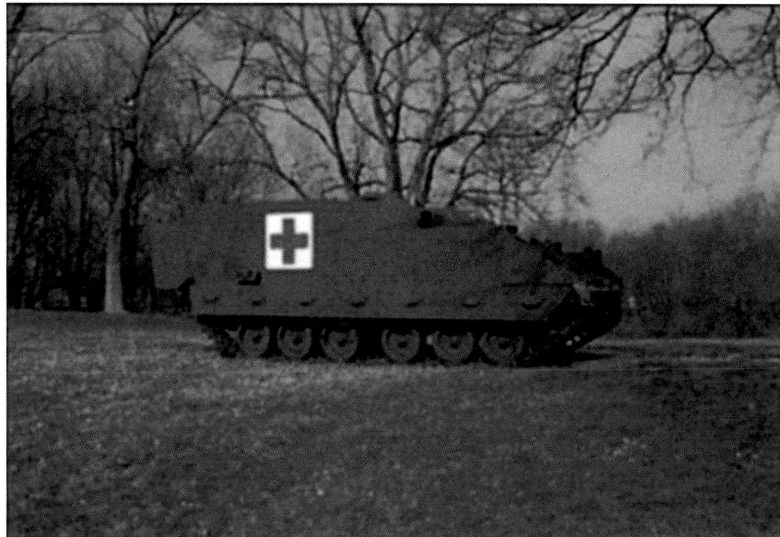

Fig. 3.9 The M2A0 Armored Medical Evacuation Vehicle (AMEV) is built on the M2/M3 Bradley fighting vehicle chassis. (Photo by LTC Robert De Lorenzo)

and offers a combination of protection, moderate weight, maneuverability, and speed that enhances versatility.

The RG33 Heavily Armored Ground Ambulance (HAGA) is a variant of the RG33L Mine Resistant Ambush Protected (MRAP) 6 wheel vehicles (Fig. 3.10). The primary mission of the RG33 HAGA vehicle is medical evacuation. The RG33 HAGA can transport three casualties on litters or be converted to provide seating for six (Fig. 3.11). It has rear steps that transform into a ramp for casualty loading. At time of publication there is an ambulance variant of the Joint Light Tactical Vehicle which is currently under development and field testing that will have a gross weight of about 9,000 lbs less than the MRAP with similar ballistic protection and is expected to be first fielded beginning in 2024 that will begin the phase out of both the HMMWV as well as the HAGA.

The challenge with all ground evacuation platforms is that their interior space is not designed for casualty care and complex medical interventions are nearly impossible to accomplish while moving at doctrinal evacuation speeds over uneven terrain.

Helicopters

Helicopter ambulances have been a high-visibility element of the MEDEVAC system since their introduction for this role during the Korean conflict. By the end of the Vietnam War, MEDEVAC by the UH-1 "Huey" helicopter DUSTOFF teams offered speed and versatility unmatched by ground platforms [7, 26]. Helicopters are largely unaffected by terrain and can reach remote areas inaccessible to ground vehicles. Disadvantages include the cost and their vulnerability to small-arms fire. This latter factor accounts for the doctrine of keeping helicopter pickup points a safe distance from direct hostile fire. For this reason, most casualties will still need to be carried to a point of safety by a combination of manual or litter carry and ground vehicle transportation prior to DUSTOFF. Currently, only the UH (or HH)-60 Black Hawk and to a lesser extent the UH-72 Lakota helicopters are used by the US Army for MEDEVAC (Table 3.6).

Blackhawk

For contemporary military air MEDEVAC, the UH/HH-60 Black Hawk helicopter has replaced the Huey (Fig. 3.12). This member of the Sikorsky S-70 helicopter family has a twin-engine and quad rotor blades, which result in improved range and speed compared to its predecessor. The Black Hawk has a capacity of six litter patients and is commonly fitted with a litter system called the Interim MEDEVAC Mission Support (IMMS) [7]. However, the IMMS is frequently removed during operations in Afghanistan to reduce overall

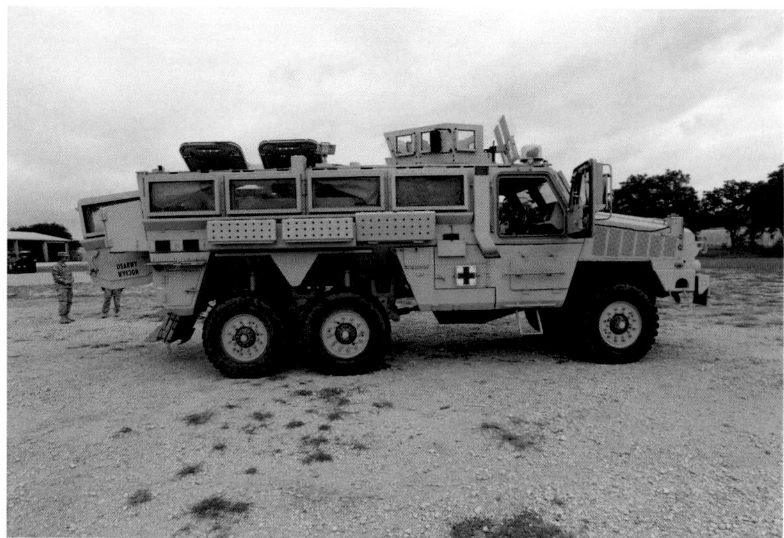

Fig. 3.10 The RG33 Heavily Armored Ground Ambulance (HAGA) is a variant of the six-wheeled Mine Resistant Ambush Protected (MRAP). (Photo by MAJ Donald Keen)

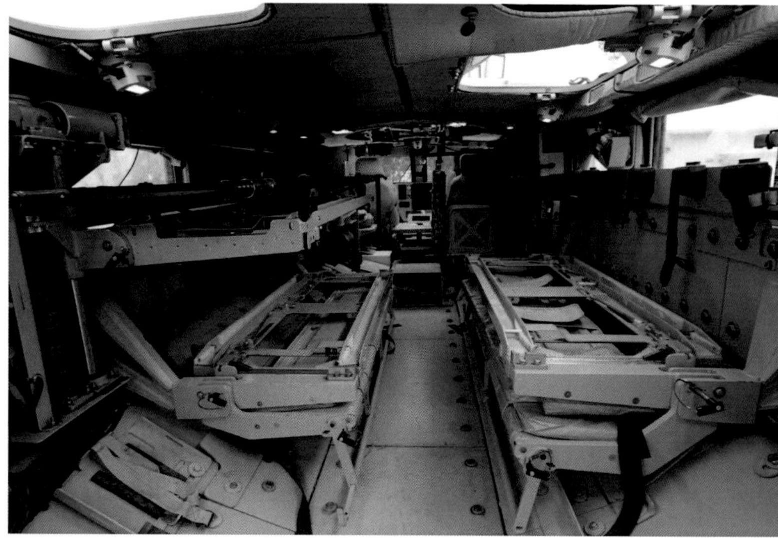

Fig. 3.11 The RG33 HAGA can transport three litter casualties or be converted to carry six ambulatory casualties. (Photo by MAJ Donald Keen)

weight in order to enable better lift parameters in the mountainous regions. The M model further improves the power and rotor system with wide-chord blades with 25% greater vertical rate of climb over the L model and a nearly fivefold increase from the A model.

The HH-60 M can be equipped with a medical evacuation mission equipment package (MEP) that has electronically controlled litter tray lifts and seats with the design requirement to be converted between litter and ambulatory seating within 2 minutes. These design innovations increased the possible number and complexity of in-flight medical procedures possible and preceded the Critical Care Flight Paramedic program.

Lakota

The UH-72 Lakota light utility helicopter is a military version of the Eurocopter EC145. The air ambulance version has the space to accommodate two litter patients (Fig. 3.13). However, because of limitation in its overall lift capabilities, carrying one litter patient with the provider and equipment is the more commonly used configuration. This airframe cannot be fitted with

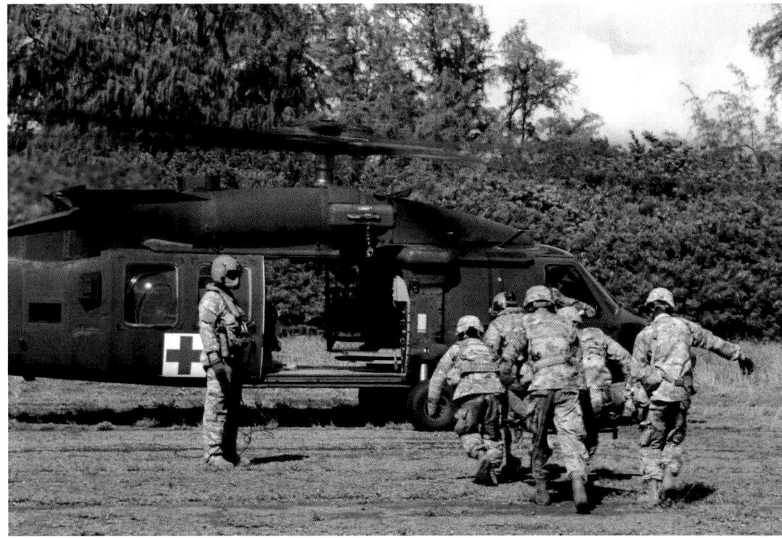

Fig. 3.12 Combat medics carry a simulated MEDAVAC patient toward a UH-60 Black Hawk helicopter during a training exercise. (US Army photo by Staff Sgt. Armando R. Limon)

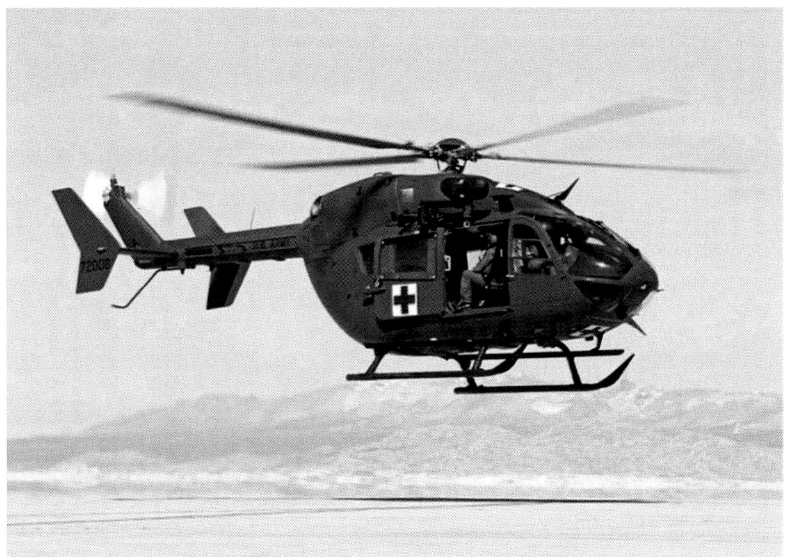

Fig. 3.13 UH-72 Lakota air ambulance. (US Army photo)

armor and subsequently has not been deployed in a combat setting.

Medevac Limitations

MEDEVAC, utilizing either ground or air vehicles, has a number of significant limitations. The first limitation is related to availability. Battlefields and disasters are fluid and dynamic situations, making it impossible to preposition MEDIVAC vehicles and crews where they will most be needed. Field medical providers must be prepared to acquire improvised transportation vehicles when dedicated ambulances are not available. Using nonmedical vehicles and personnel for CASEVAC—including trucks, buses, and nonmedical helicopters—is a well-recognized part of US Army medical contingency planning [1].

A second limitation of tactical MEDEVAC is the difficulty involved in providing en route and ongoing care. Both ground and air vehicles currently in use are cramped, noisy, poorly illuminated, and prone to vibration, jarring, and sway. Patient access, assessment, monitoring, and intervention are all more difficult in this environment.

A third, and perhaps the greatest, limitation is related to care providers. Most ground and air ambulances have one or two attendants assigned for up to six litter patients that in a combat situation could all be critical patients. If more than one patient requires intensive bedside care (e.g., active bag–valve–mask ventilation) the single attendant's capacity to provide care is exceeded. The level of training and experience of these medical technicians can vary dramatically, depending on location and mode of transportation.

References

1. Department of the Army. Casualty evacuation. Washington, DC: US Government Printing Office; 2013. Army Techniques Publication 4-25.13.
2. Joint Health Services. Joint Publication 4-02. Washington, DC: US Government Printing Office; 2017.
3. Department of the Army. Tactical combat causality care handbook. 2012. Available at: https://www.globalsecurity.org/military/library/report/call/call_12-10.pdf.
4. Ortiz JM. The revolutionary flying ambulance of Napoleon's surgeon. Army Med Dep J. 1998;4:17–25.
5. Driscoll RS. New York chapter history of military medicine award: US Army medical helicopters in the Korean War. Mil Med. 2001;166(4):290.
6. Mabry RL, De Lorenzo RA. Sharpening the edge: paramedic training for flight medics. US Army Med Dep J. 2011:92–100.
7. Dorland P, Nanney JDUSTOFF. Army aeromedical evacuation in Vietnam. Center of Military History United States Army. Washington, DC: U.S. Government Printing Office; 1982.
8. Department of the Army. Aircrew training manual, utility helicopter, H-60 series. Washington, DC: US Government Printing Office; 2013. Training Circular 3-04.33.
9. Mabry RL, Apodaca A, Penrod J, Orman JA, Gerhardt RT, Dorlac WC. Impact of critical care-trained flight paramedics on casualty survival during helicopter evacuation in the current war in Afghanistan. J Trauma Acute Care Surg. 2012;73(2 Suppl 1):S32–7.
10. Apodaca A, Olson CM Jr, Bailey J, Butler F, Eastridge BJ, Kuncir E. Performance improvement evaluation of forward aeromedical evacuation platforms in Operation Enduring Freedom. J Trauma Acute Care Surg. 2013;75(2 Suppl 2):S157–63.
11. U.S. Army MEDEVAC Critical Care Flight Paramedic Standard Medical Operating Guidelines. FY18 version. School of Army Aviation Medicine. Fort Rucker, Alabama. October 19, 2017.
12. De Lorenzo RA. Improving combat casualty care and field medicine: focus on the military medic. Mil Med. 1997;162:268–72.
13. Malsby RF 3rd, Quesada J, Powell-Dunford N, Kinoshita R, Kurtz J, Gehlen W, Adams C, Martin D, Shackelford S. Prehospital blood product transfusion by U.S. army MEDEVAC during combat operations in Afghanistan: a process improvement initiative. Mil Med. 2013;178(7):785–91.
14. US Congress. National defense authorization act for fiscal year 2017. Public Law 114–328—Dec. 23, 2016.
15. Butler FK Jr, Hagmann J, Butler EG. Tactical combat casualty care in special operations. Mil Med. 1996;161(Suppl):3–16.
16. Department of the Army. Army health services support to maneuver forces. Washington, DC: US Government Printing Office; 2014. Army Techniques Publication 4-02.3.
17. Department of the Army. Army health system support planning. Washington, DC: US Government Printing Office; 2015. Army Techniques Publication 4-02.55.
18. Department of the Army. Medical evacuation. Washington, DC: US Government Printing Office; 2014. Army Techniques Publication 4-02.2.
19. Butler FK Jr, Holcomb JB, Shackelford S, Montgomery HR, Anderson S, Cain JS, et al. Management of suspected tension pneumothorax in tactical combat casualty care: TCCC guidelines change 17-02. J Spec Oper Med. 2018;18(2):19–35. Department of the Army.
20. De Lorenzo RA, Porter RS. Tactical emergency care. Upper Saddle River: Brady (Prentice Hall); 1999.
21. Makreth B. Assessing pulse oximetry in the field. J Emerg Med Serv. 1990;15(6):12–20.
22. Vampire Program CCOP-01: Urgent resuscitation using blood products during tactical evacuation from POI. Joint Trauma System, San Antonio, Texas; 28 September 2016.
23. Butler FK, Holcomb JB, Schreiber MA, Kotwal RS, Jenkins DA, Champion HR, et al. Fluid resuscitation for hemorrhagic shock in tactical combat casualty care: TCCC guidelines change 14-01–2 June 2014. J Spec Oper Med. 2014;14(3):13–38.
24. Butler FK, Kotwal RS, Buckenmaier CC 3rd, Edgar EP, O'Connor KC, Montgomery HR, et al. A triple-option analgesia plan for tactical combat casualty care: TCCC guidelines change 13-04. J Spec Oper Med. 2014;14(1):13–25.
25. Infection Prevention in Combat-Related Injuries (CPG ID:24). Clinical practice guideline, Joint Trauma System, San Antonio, Texas; 8 August 2016.
26. Ayeni T, Roggenkamp N. The future of small navy ship sickbays and army aeromedical evacuation aircraft. Naval Postgraduate School Monterey, California; 2014 Dec.

Civilian Air Medical Transport

4

William Beninati, J. D. Polk, and William F. Fallon Jr.

Introduction

Civilian air medical transport represents a highly developed capability that has its roots in military air medical transport, including both medical evacuation (MEDEVAC) and long-distance aeromedical evacuation (AE). Advances in military clinical capabilities, crew training, transport equipment, aircraft, and control systems are translated into civilian advances, and vice versa. Like the military, civilian critical care transport services utilize ground, helicopter, and fixed-wing vehicles. In the military, transport requirements are driven by the organization of medical capability into increasingly sophisticated Roles of Care, formerly referred to as Echelons of Care (see Chap. 3). Similarly, civilian transport is driven by regionalization of medical care.

There are major differences between military AE and civilian air medical transport. Military operations require AE of casualties with both high and low medical acuity, whereas civilian air medical transport focuses almost exclusively on patients with critical illnesses or injuries. Cost is a dominant issue in civilian air medical transport and thus determining and documenting appropriateness of transport is an important aspect. This chapter will provide an overview of the current state of civilian air medical transport system and contrast it to the military MEDEVAC and AE systems from which it originated.

History

The development of civilian air medical transport in the United States resulted from a number of converging factors, but has its basis in the military. As discussed in Chap. 2 of this book, the history of military AE dates almost to the beginning of aviation, and the Army Air Corps provided large-scale fixed-wing AE in World War II. The large-scale use of helicopters for medical trans-

W. Beninati (✉)
Col, USAF, MC, CFS (ret.), Senior Medical Director, Intermountain Life Flight and Virtual Hospital, University of Utah School of Medicine, Salt Lake City, UT, USA

Clinical Associate Professor (Affiliated), Stanford University School of Medicine, Stanford, CA, USA
e-mail: bill.beninati@imail.org

J. D. Polk
LtCol, USAF, MC, CFS (ret.), National Aeronautics and Space Administration, Washington, DC, USA

Department of Policy, George Mason University, Fairfax County, VA, USA

Edward Via College of Osteopathic Medicine, Blacksburg, VA, USA

W. F. Fallon Jr.
LTC, MC, USA (ret.), Trauma Surgery & Surgical Critical Care, Summa Health System, Akron, OH, USA

Department of Surgery, Case West Reserve University School of Medicine, Cleveland, OH, USA

W. W. Hurd, W. Beninati (eds.), *Aeromedical Evacuation*,
https://doi.org/10.1007/978-3-030-15903-0_4

port began with MEDEVAC during the Korean War. The helicopter did provide rapid transport from a casualty collection point to a field hospital, but this "scoop-and-run" process provided no en route medical care since casualties were transported outside the helicopter cabin. By the Vietnam War, casualties were transported inside the helicopter, which ushered in the era of active management of the casualty during rotor-wing MEDEVAC. This forms the basis for modern civilian air medical transport.

As the military refined MEDEVAC, civilian developments were also occurring. In 1966, a report by the National Academy of Sciences acknowledged that injury was a neglected disease that causes substantial disability and loss of life [1]. At this same time, the Highway Safety Act of 1966 became law and established the basis for Emergency Medical Service (EMS) systems in the United States. Law enforcement agencies began utilizing helicopters for a variety of roles, which occasionally included air medical transport.

The development of the regionalized emergency medical care system during the 1970s was another major factor. This system was developed with the expectation that specialized regional centers would improve care for trauma victims [2]. For the system to be effective, air medical transport is required for trauma victims remote from these specialized centers to provide them with care within their time window of survivability.

The 1978 Airline Deregulation Act (ADA) had a profound effect on civilian air medical transport. One section of this law prohibited states from regulating air ambulance rates, routes, and services provided. Prior to ADA, the air ambulance industry was dominated by hospital-based systems, which were commonly not-for-profit and based at academic medical centers. Enactment of the ADA allowed substantial growth of private, for-profit, air ambulance systems. In the 10 years after this law went into effect, the annual number of patients transported by helicopter EMS increased by 35%, while the number of dedicated air ambulance helicopters increased by 88% [3].

This expansion of the US air medical transport system has created substantial controversy in the medical community. Proponents emphasize that it increases public access to lifesaving services. Critics contend that there is now an excess capacity in the industry that results in overuse of an expensive service. In addition, they maintain that the need to cover the substantial fixed costs of an air medical transport can lead to financial pressure to push operating limits, thus contributing to the observed increase in helicopter accidents [4]. The attention of the national media and the medical literature on both the high cost and frequent accidents have resulted in continued improvement of the industry.

An additional major factor driving evolution of air medical transport has been the continued advances in the level of clinical care available at major medical centers. In order to transport critically ill patients to major medical centers that provide lifesaving technology, equipment and expertise had to be developed to provide advanced en route ventilatory and circulatory support. Patients with respiratory failure are now routinely transported while receiving ventilator support, inhaled vasodilators, and extracorporeal membrane oxygenation (ECMO). Patients with cardiogenic shock are transported while receiving mechanical cardiac support with biventricular assist devices or full cardiopulmonary bypass. Critically ill newborns are now routinely transported while providing a high level of in-flight neonatal care.

Civilian air medical transport has become a major industry in the United States. The Association of Air Medical Services (AAMS) publishes the Atlas and Database of Air Medical Services, which provides comprehensive information about the distribution of civilian air medical transport in the United States. In 2017, the AAMS database included more than 300 air ambulance services that operated 1049 helicopters and 362 fixed-wing aircraft at 1065 bases [5].

Planning an Air Medical Transport

Patient transport to a higher level of care is appropriate whenever the attending physician caring for a patient identifies a care requirement that cannot be met at the current facility. When arranging to transport a critical patient, three principal steps must be completed:

Table 4.1 Comparison of medical transport modes

	Ground	Helicopter	Fixed-wing
Optimal range (in general)	0–50 miles	50–150 miles	Turboprop: >150 miles Jet: >300 miles
Cost	Low	High	High
Complexity	Low	High	High
Aeromedical Crew	Highly variable	Transport specialists	Transport specialists
Weather	Least weather dependent	Most weather dependent	Less weather dependent than helicopters
Transport safety	Significant concern	Significant concern	Higher degree of safety
Key advantages	Greatest availability Lowest cost	Flexibility with landing at scene and at hospital Speed of transport	High speed over long distances
Key limitations	Road conditions Traffic	Weather dependent	Requires an airport

1. Determine which hospital has the capability and the capacity to care for the patient, and secure acceptance by a physician there.
2. Arrange for transportation with the appropriate level of en route clinical care to optimize the chance for a favorable outcome.
3. Determine the mode of transportation that meets the urgency required by the situation.

The sending physician can consult with the receiving or medical control physician on these decisions, but no one can assume responsibility for the sending physician.

Once the sending physician has decided to transfer a patient, the first step is to determine the most appropriate receiving facility and secure an accepting physician [6]. The sending physician must then simultaneously determine the level of medical care required en route and the best mode of transportation: by ground, helicopter, or fixed-wing aircraft. For many patients, such as those with multiple trauma, or those requiring intervention for a stroke or myocardial infarction, the most important advantage that helicopters have over ground transportation is the decreased time required for transport to an advanced center. However, for other patients, continuing critical care, with no step-down in capability, is the most important aspect of the transportation. For example, if a patient in cardiogenic shock is on an intra-aortic balloon pump or ECMO device, the requirements for medical expertise and uninterrupted life support are more important than speed.

Several considerations must be taken into account in addition to medical care capability when considering air medical transport. Most important among these are transport distance, weather conditions, and ground traffic conditions. If fixed-wing aircraft are being considered, an additional factor is the time and expertise required for ground transport from the hospital to the airfield prior to the flight and vice versa at the end of the flight.

The relative strengths and weaknesses of the modes of transport are summarized in Table 4.1. The primary advantages of ground transport are availability, ability to operate in most weather conditions, relatively low cost, and simplicity. A limitation is speed of transport over large distances or through heavy automobile traffic. In addition, the medical capability of the crew can vary considerably depending on crew training and experience, e.g., Emergency Medical Technician-Basic (EMT-Basic) versus dedicated critical care transport teams, potentially including a physician. The safety of ground EMS is also a significant issue. Ambulance crashes have resulted in fatalities of patients and crew members, and ground ambulance crashes are the most common cause of death for EMS workers [7, 8].

A major advantage of helicopter transport is speed. When transportation greater than 45 miles is required, it is usually faster to dispatch a helicopter than to utilize ground EMS services already on the scene [9]. Another advantage of helicopter ambulances is the advanced medical capabilities usually possessed by aeromedical crew members. Disadvantages are the high cost, complexity, and weather limitations. Many specially equipped helicopter ambulances are able to operate in instrument meteorological conditions, and some even in icing conditions. As with ground EMS, helicopter accidents remain a major concern, with 22 incidents over a recent 2-year period. Fortunately, the number of such accidents has been on a downward trend for a number of years [10, 11].

Fixed-wing aircraft are generally most useful for transports greater than 150 miles, where the higher speed compared to ground and helicopter ambulances offsets the need for ground transport between the sending and receiving hospitals and the airport. Fixed-wing aircraft cabins are generally larger and support more advanced care compared to helicopters. In addition, fixed-wing aircraft are more likely to be instrument-flight capable, and are capable of flying over and/or around dangerous weather. Like helicopter ambulances, fixed-wing air ambulances are generally staffed by crews with advanced medical training and equipment. Fixed-wing aircraft also come with the highest price.

The safety of fixed-wing medical transport appears to be much better than both ground and helicopter ambulances. A study of the National Transportation Safety Board database found 54 fixed-wing air ambulance crashes over a 25-year period—a rate much lower than for helicopter ambulances despite the fact that fixed-wing air ambulances are much less commonly used than helicopters [12].

Patient Preparation for Air Transport

The first priority of the air medical transport crew is to evaluate the patient to be transported, whether this encounter is at an accident scene or in a hospital setting. The crew must quickly determine if the patient's condition is appropriate for immediate transport or if transport should be delayed so that the patient can be more thoroughly stabilized prior to transport.

Stabilization and immediate transport, sometimes referred to as "load and go," consists of rapid assessment, provision of immediate lifesaving care such as control of external hemorrhage or tension pneumothorax decompression, and expedient transport to a higher level of care. This strategy is most commonly utilized in the field or at smaller facilities, far from surgical and other advanced diagnostic and treatment options. Transport of stabilized patients does not eliminate the need for active monitoring, but decreases the chances of needing to perform additional interventions during transport. Common situations that call for this approach include exsanguinating truncal hemorrhage, intracranial hemorrhage with instability, and ST segment elevation myocardial infarction or stroke requiring emergent intervention.

The preferred approach in many situations is to stabilize a patient prior to air medical transport, sometimes referred to as "stay and play." This approach is possible when time is less critical for the patient's condition and transporting the patient without proper preparation increases the risk of complications during transport. Situations that should be effectively treated prior to transport include serious external hemorrhage, unstable airway, or normothermic cardiac arrest prior to return of spontaneous circulation. For patients with highly complex ongoing care that is susceptible to error (e.g., mechanical cardiac support), the aeromedical crew should use a deliberate, checklist-driven approach to prepare the patient for transport.

Helicopter Ambulances

Many community hospitals rely on the local helicopter air medical services for transporting patients because they can land on or adjacent to both accident sites and hospitals (Fig. 4.1). In general, twin-engine helicopters are preferred for their increased load capacity and added safety compared to single-engine models (Table 4.2). Helicopters with larger engines can carry heavier payloads and have a greater range, which can vary from 300 to more than 500 statute miles.

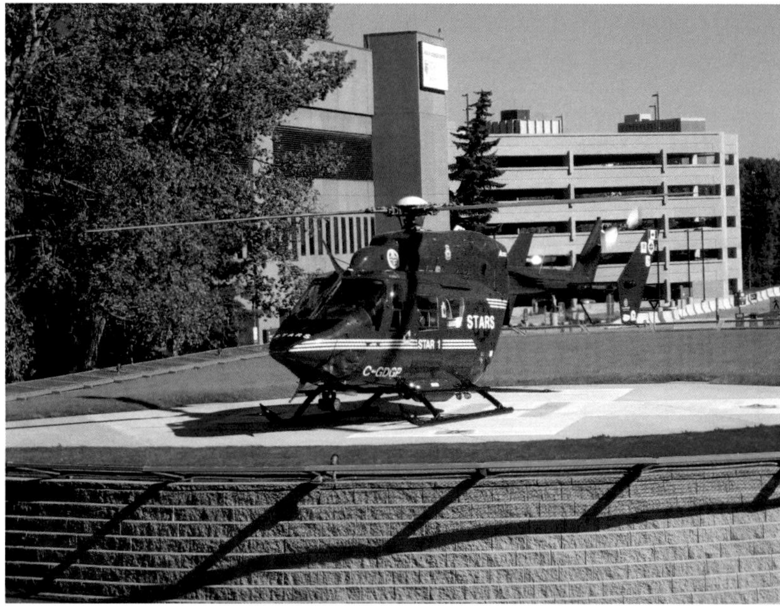

Fig. 4.1 The BK 117 helicopter is a twin-engine medium utility–transport helicopter developed and manufactured by Messerschmitt-Bölkow-Blohm (MBB) of Germany and Kawasaki of Japan. (Photo by Swmolnar, used with permission. https://commons.wikimedia.org/wiki/File:STARSFMC.jpg)

Table 4.2 Comparison of helicopters commonly used for civilian medical transport

	Bell 206	Bell 222	Eurocopter Dauphin	Eurocopter BO-105	Eurocopter BK-117	Sikorsky S-76B
Engine configuration	Single	Twin	Twin	Twin	Twin	Twin
Range (statute miles)	369	434	578	345	324	403
Maximum cruise speed	127	156	183	149	153	178
Maximum takeoff weight (lb)	4450	8250	9369	5511	7385	11,700
Useful load (lb)	2163	4874	4341	2643	3545	7623
Rotor diameter (ft)	37	42	39	32	43	44
Passenger compartment interior (ft^2)						
Length	6.7	9.2	8.0	14.1	9.4	7.9
Width	3.9	4.2	6.3	4.6	4.9	5.5
Height	3.8	4.8	4.5	4.1	4.2	4.5

Helicopters equipped to fly under instrument flight rules (IFR) in the clouds are preferred over those that can only fly by visual flight rules (VFR) with visual reference with the ground [13]. Modern IFR equipment includes global positioning satellite (GPS) apparatus that allows the pilot to accurately proceed directly to the exact location of a distant medical facility or accident site, regardless of darkness or inclement weather.

A copilot is another helpful asset, which unfortunately is not standard for many helicopters. A second set of hands and eyes, especially at an uncontrolled landing site or adverse weather conditions, can be invaluable. Emergency Medical Service (EMS) ground crews are trained to wait for the "thumbs-up" from the pilot to ensure safe approach to the running aircraft. In this respect, the second pilot adds another set of eyes for safety in and around the operating aircraft.

The type of aircraft utilized will depend on the mission profile of the air medical transport service. In a hot desert environment in Arizona where sunshine predominates, a single-pilot helicopter with only VFR capability is adequate for a service. In areas that are prone to low clouds and snow, such as Washington state or near the Great Lakes, larger aircraft with IFR capability and/or a second pilot are more often utilized.

Many hospital-based helicopter air medical services utilize smaller helicopters, such as the

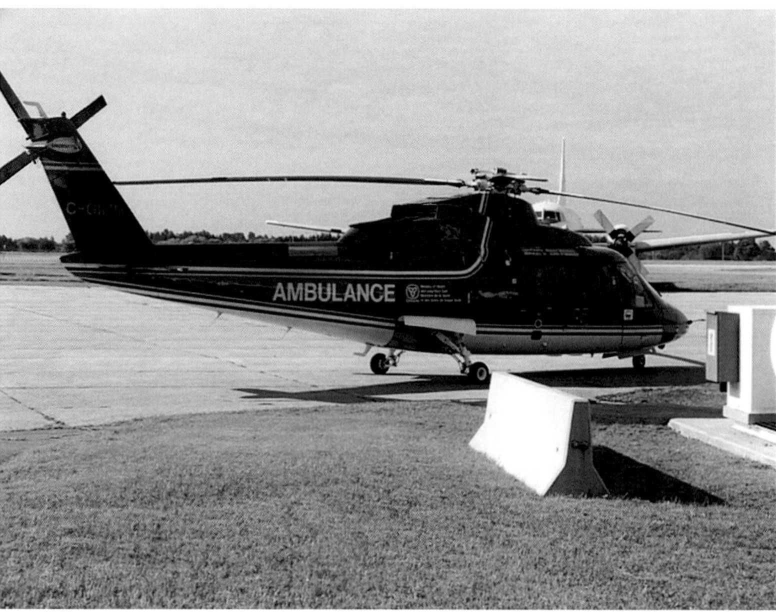

Fig. 4.2 The Sikorsky S-76A helicopter is a medium-sized twin-engine helicopter with four-bladed main and tail rotors and retractable landing gear manufactured by the Sikorsky Aircraft Corporation. (Photo by Ahunt, used with permission. https://commons.wikimedia.org/wiki/File:SikorskyS-76AC-GIMM.JPG)

BK 117 helicopter (Fig. 4.1). However, the dual-pilot, IFR-equipped Sikorsky S-76 helicopter has proven to be a versatile aircraft for transporting several trauma patients or for handling complex equipment needs such as dual isolettes, balloon pumps, and ECMO machines (Fig. 4.2).

Budgetary restraints also have an impact on which type of helicopter is used. Twin-engine helicopters with two pilots and advance avionics are obviously more costly to operate. The cost of parts, fuel, and refurbishment continues to rise as reimbursements for critical care transports have decreased. The result is that many hospitals have switched to less costly airframes or have gotten out of the business of air medical transport altogether.

The optimal use of helicopters for EMS remains controversial, and is the subject of much study and debate about both their efficacy and cost-effectiveness. A trauma database study included 61,909 patients transported by helicopter and 161,566 patients transported by ground and used propensity score-matching in a multivariable regression model [14]. This study found a small but statistically significant survival advantage for helicopter over ground transport, with absolute risk reductions of 1.5% for transport to a Level I trauma center and 1.4% to a Level II center. A subsequent meta-analysis of this topic included 34 studies comparing survival with ground versus helicopter EMS [15]. There were no randomized controlled trials, and the evidence was too weak overall to make any conclusion. A cost-effectiveness analysis was performed using a model built from multiple large data sets on trauma outcome and cost [16]. Helicopter transport of trauma patients would have to yield a 17% reduction in mortality to cost less than $100,000 per quality-adjusted life year (QALY) or a 33% reduction to cost less than $50,000. To achieve reductions of this magnitude, triage would have to be carefully applied to the decision to use a helicopter. Currently the US Centers for Disease Control (CDC) [17] and professional groups have published guidelines for prehospital use of helicopters for trauma patients [18, 19]. These guidelines, based on the available evidence, incorporate the CDC field triage criteria, are general in their guidance, and leave substantial latitude up to on-scene personnel.

Fixed-Wing Aircraft

While some helicopters have a range of around 300–500 miles, the range for fixed-wing turboprop or jet aircraft varies from hundreds to thousands of miles. Fixed-wing aircraft also travel at much greater speeds. A helicopter must rely on its main rotor for both generating lift and creating forward thrust for flight, thus reaching a practical limit of around 200 knots. In contrast, a modern Learjet routinely cruises at 400 knots, decreasing the time taken to travel long distances by more than half. Fixed-wing aircraft do, however, have several drawbacks compared to helicopters.

The greatest disadvantage of fixed-wing aircraft is that they require an airport. This means an additional ground ambulance trip to and from the airport on both the referring and receiving sides of the transport.

A second drawback is that loading and unloading of the patient into and out of a fixed-wing aircraft is more difficult compared to a helicopter, many of which have been extensively modified with patient transport in mind. Because high-speed flight limits engineering options, most civilian fixed-wing aircraft modified for air medical transport (e.g., Learjet) are still relatively difficult to load and unload with a litter patient. In these relatively small aircraft, the doors and cabin are so narrow that a litter must be rotated 30 degrees about its long axis to be loaded. Unfortunately, some patients or equipment may not be able to tolerate these movements. Fortunately, large military aircraft (e.g., C-130, C-17, KC-135) used for AE do not share these problems.

It should be noted that some companies use their fixed-wing aircraft only part time for air medical transport. For economic reasons many companies use their aircraft to move business people when not moving patients. A certain amount of time may be needed to convert their aircraft to a medical configuration and acquire the appropriate aeromedical crew. In these cases, the referring physician should ensure that the air medical transport service complies with Federal Aviation Regulation Part 135 for air taxi operation and is accredited by the Commission on Accreditation of Medical Transport Systems. Most large tertiary-care hospitals have fixed-wing air medical transport services they utilize on a frequent basis, and thus will be able to recommend a particular service to the referring physician.

The air medical transport of US Department of Defense (DoD) military medical beneficiaries during peacetime is arranged through the Global Patient Movement Requirements Center, which is a joint service agency operating under the US Transportation Command (USTRANSCOM). This center is responsible for coordinating military AE between theaters (e.g., from Europe to the United States) throughout the continental United States and from nearby offshore locations such as Puerto Rico.

It is extremely important to give the USTRANSCOM officer as much information about the patient and requirements as possible so that the appropriate decision can be made whether to utilize military or civilian aircraft. USTRANSCOM maintains a list of commercial providers that meet the appropriate professional standard, including the specific medical capabilities of each provider. The airlift demands on the military since 2001 have been so high that air medical transport of military medical beneficiaries has been largely relegated to civilian agencies contracted through USTRANSCOM.

Aeromedical Crew Configurations

The composition of an aeromedical flight crew is designed to safely carry out transport of the patient or patients and manage any adverse sequela that may result from either the disease process or the act of transporting the patient. The type of mission being flown determines the specific makeup of the crew. However, for both logistic and economic reasons, physicians are often not part of the crew of routine air medical transport flights. In any case, the diversity of skills found in mixed crews (physician–nurse, nurse–paramedic, and nurse–respiratory therapist) may be more advantageous than crews of like training (nurse–nurse, paramedic–paramedic).

Physician–Nurse Crews

Several air medical transport services that operate from a tertiary-care facility have an aeromedical crew consisting of a physician and critical care nurse. This crew mix is often necessary to care for the types of patients who are routinely transported to a level-one trauma and burn center and cardiac surgical referral centers. Advanced training and expertise are required to operate medical devices such as intra-aortic balloon pumps, ECMO devices, and biventricular assist devices, and to care for complex trauma casualties during flight.

The presence of an on-board physician adds certain procedural expertise and a broad knowledge base that can be particularly useful in the complicated patient [20]. It also eliminates the need to contact base physicians for decision-making authority or permission to give certain drugs. In a study of more than 5000 helicopter air medical transports in a service with a physician and a comparable service with paramedics, the physicians did not extend scene time [21]. However, they were more likely to pronounce death on scene and to evaluate and discharge the patient without transport. If the transport service does not have an on-board physician, the referring physician carries the bulk of responsibility and liability for the patient during transport until the patient is received by the accepting physician.

Nurse-Only Crews

Not all patients need an on-board physician. Many services use a crew consisting of two critical care flight nurses. This is particularly useful for helicopter services, which provide mostly interhospital, ICU to ICU transfers. Typically, air medical flight nurses have at least 3 years of prior critical care or emergency medicine experience, and many are certified emergency medical technicians or paramedics.

Nurse crews require medical control by a physician. This is ideally achieved using written protocols that allow the nurse to operate and perform medical duties under the license of the physician medical director. Another important aspect of medical control is the ability of the nurse to directly communicate with a physician when needed.

Nurse–Paramedic Crews

Many helicopter air medical transport services use a practical and cost-effective paramedic-nurse crew. The paramedic brings valuable and practical prehospital treatment experience to the team that complements the critical care background of the flight nurse. This crew mix is advantageous when the majority of flights are accident scene transports, but is less suited for interhospital transport of critically ill patients, where additional physiology and medical knowledge is advantageous. An attempt to remedy this situation has been made by the development of the "critical care paramedic." Unfortunately, a paramedic with this advanced training cannot be considered an equivalent replacement for a critical care nurse or a physician. Again, medical control is required as with any crew in which a physician is not present.

Diagnoses of Patients Requiring Transport

The predominant peacetime indications for air medical transport are remarkably similar for the military and civilian populations. These include trauma, heart attacks, strokes, respiratory failure, sepsis, and obstetric emergencies. Likewise, many hospitals in both the military and civilian communities have specific limitations to the care they can provide based on their diagnostic and therapeutic capabilities and/or the experience level of their staff. For this reason, both military and civilian physicians often find it necessary to transfer patients to a higher level of care.

Trauma Patients

The evacuation of the trauma patient in peacetime usually falls into one of two categories: acute and convalescent. The acute phase usually refers to the aeromedical team responding to the scene of an accident (Fig. 4.3) or a smaller community hospital to provide emergent care and evacuation for the acutely injured patient. The care provided

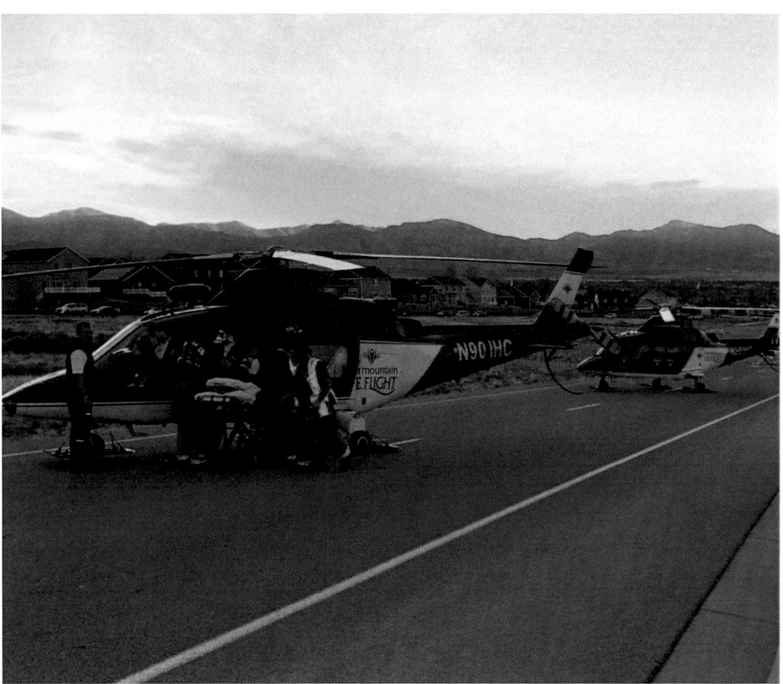

Fig. 4.3 Civilian air medical helicopters (Intermountain Life Flight) responding to a pedestrian accident. (Photo courtesy of Richard Dobson)

is consistent with the Advanced Trauma Life Support primary survey and treatment.

Scene stabilization is usually limited to airway interventions, control of gross hemorrhage, and spinal immobilization. Chest tubes, intravenous lines, blood infusion, and other modalities are usually initiated and continued in-flight to prevent delay in transport of the patient to a trauma center. The focused abdominal sonography for trauma (FAST) ultrasound exam has been developed as an essential inhospital tool for trauma evaluation [22]. Nearly 20 years ago, it was demonstrated that it was feasible to perform an in-flight FAST exam [23, 24], where there is the potential to rapidly identify patients with hemoperitoneum to expedite triage at the trauma center. This has not yet become an industry standard, but leaders in the trauma field continue to develop it as an air medical application, demonstrating a high specificity for hemoperitoneum and pneumothorax requiring intervention [25]. Thus, the aircraft and crew are an extension of the trauma team, bringing critical care skills to the patient in the field.

Hemorrhage control is perhaps the single most important aspect in the care of a trauma patient. If exsanguinating external hemorrhage is present and direct pressure is inadequate the aeromedical crew must quickly move to an appropriate adjunct. For extremity hemorrhage a tourniquet should be placed and tightened until the distal pulse is lost and bleeding stops. For hemorrhage from the scalp or anatomic junctions (groin or axilla) a hemostatic dressing can be applied. Pelvic fractures should be addressed with a pelvic binder applied appropriately over the femoral head. Civilian air medical transport programs are increasingly using prehospital blood products to initiate hemostatic resuscitation for massive hemorrhage during transport. A multicenter trial failed to draw conclusions about the efficacy of prehospital blood administration by air medical transport crews due to methodologic challenges with patient matching, but this trial did demonstrate the feasibility of the practicc [26]. Additional trials are ongoing.

Airway management is essential to the transport of severely traumatized patients. Aeromedical crews must be able to establish and maintain an airway in the most difficult patients, even in the vibrating, noisy, poorly lit environment of an aircraft in flight. Medications for rapid-sequence intubation are used frequently by the crews. If an airway cannot be established by the oral–tracheal route, the crew needs to be prepared to apply an extra-glottic airway. If this is inadequate, a surgical airway must be rapidly established. Other resuscitation measures utilized by aeromedical crews—such as chest tube placement, intravenous lines, thoracotomy equipment, ultrasound, and blood products—are all useless if the patient does not have a patent airway.

The second category of trauma patients requiring air medical transport is the convalescent category. These patients have already been stabilized and many times have already had surgery at the referring institution but require either specialized care or perhaps rehabilitation closer to home. Such patients rarely require acute interventions on the part of the flight crew but may need adjustments in their therapy or equipment to ensure safe travel and transport.

Cardiac Patients

Myocardial Infarction

Cardiac patients are among the most common critically ill patients transported by civilian air medical transport services. The most common cardiac patients requiring transfer are those with an acute myocardial infarction (MI) manifested by ST segment elevation, commonly referred to as "ST-elevation MI." These potentially unstable patients require transfer to centers that perform percutaneous coronary intervention (PCI), coronary artery bypass grafting, cardiac intensive care, and/or mechanical cardiac support.

Prior to flight, a standard MI treatment protocol should be followed, with therapies such as aspirin, nitroglycerin, beta-blockade, and anticoagulation. The decision to give pre-transport thrombolysis should be made in consultation with the accepting cardiologist and consider the anticipated time of transport and access to PCI.

The risk of in-flight cardiac decompensation for these patients is high. This can manifest by signs of decompensation such as hypotension, shock, pulmonary edema, hypoxia, florid heart failure, and/or dysrhythmias. For this reason, these patients should be transported with established intravenous access, and aeromedical crews must have readily available supplemental oxygen, intravenous fluids, advanced cardiac life-support drugs, defibrillator, and pacing capabilities. Advanced assessment of cardiac patients via in-flight echocardiography is now possible and may lend additional information as to contractility and wall-motion abnormalities in these patients. Although no prospective clinical trials have been published on this subject, a recent Danish observational study of >1500 patients with suspected ST-elevation MIs could not detect a significant beneficial effect of helicopter compared to ground transport on mortality or subsequent recovery [27].

Cardiogenic Shock

Patients in profound cardiogenic shock may require air medical transport while undergoing mechanical assistance in the form of an intra-aortic balloon pump, ECMO, or ventricular assist device (Fig. 4.4). The air medical transport crew must have special training in the use of these devices and have plans for contingencies, such as power failure in the aircraft. Centrifugal ventricular assist devices and some biventricular devices have mechanical mechanisms that can be used to maintain patient perfusion in the event of pump or power failure. Intra-aortic balloon pumps, however, will need manual inflation and deflation of the balloon to avoid thrombosis.

Dissecting Aortic Aneurysm

A symptomatic aortic aneurysm, usually related to atherosclerosis or hypertension, is another common indication for civilian air medical transport. Once a dissection has been identified, medical management must be immediately established to decrease the risk of extending the dissection. This is accomplished with effective beta-blockade to reduce shear stress on the vessel wall and blood pressure control using a rapidly titratable vasodilator such as nicardipine. The blood pressure target should be determined in consultation with the accepting surgeon. In-flight leaking or rupture manifests as increased pain and hypotension. The only effective method to sustain the patient long enough to get to the operating room is the targeted use of blood products and support with vasopressor agents.

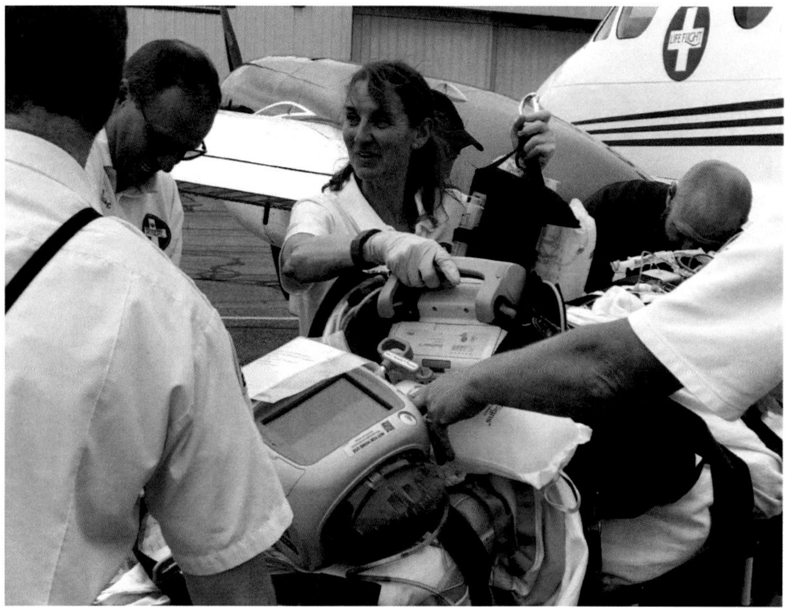

Fig. 4.4 Civilian aeromedical crew members loading a patient with a mechanical cardiac support device on a fixed-wing aircraft for emergency evacuation. (Photo courtesy of K. D. Simpson)

Post-cardiac Arrest

It is sometimes necessary to transport by air a patient who was recently resuscitated from cardiac arrest. The crew must have all necessary medications and equipment to carry out further resuscitation (e.g., defibrillators, airways, oxygen, suction, etc.) in the event the patient arrests in flight. If there is any question regarding need for cardioversion, it should be done prior to flight. If patients have not recovered neurologic function, controlled normothermia is indicated to increase the chance for an optimal neurologic outcome [28]. This equipment to control body temperature in a narrow range is not practical for use during air medical transport, and it is not clearly beneficial to attempt this [29]. However, the crew can monitor temperature and use patient coverings and the aircraft ventilation system to control the patient's temperature as closely as possible.

Stroke and Intracranial Hemorrhage

Patients with ischemic stroke are increasingly cared for in regionalized stroke systems as designated by The Joint Commission, often with telemedicine (i.e., "telestroke") support [30]. A major goal of these programs is to rapidly identify patients who will benefit from systemic thrombolysis, and to initiate this as soon as possible. Patients are then transported to higher-level stroke centers for ongoing care while the thrombolytic agent is being infused. The air medical transport crew must be thoroughly familiar with these agents to prevent dosing errors, and to identify and respond to complications. Other patients may be rapidly transported to a stroke center with thrombectomy capability for endovascular therapy. The aeromedical crew should be prepared to provide an emergency airway should the patient's condition deteriorate. Seizures should be anticipated and prepared for by having appropriate anticonvulsants available for use.

Patients with intracranial hemorrhage may need to be transferred by air medical transport so that they can receive either medical or surgical treatment. Patients with hemorrhagic stroke or intracranial hemorrhage secondary to trauma may be transferred so that they can receive emergency neurosurgical treatment. The aeromedical crew should ensure that the patient has a patent airway and an adequate gag reflex, and be prepared to provide emergent airway intervention if the patient deteriorates in-flight. A worsening neurological exam during flight is important information to the surgeon because it may indicate the need for expedient surgical intervention.

It is for this reason that routine chemical paralysis should be avoided unless warranted by the patient's condition. This will help the aeromedical crew identify a worsening neurological exam in a more expeditious manner.

Patients who have already had neurosurgery for head trauma, and who have residual intracranial air, are at risk of increased cerebral edema secondary to changes in atmospheric pressure during air medical transport using fixed-wing aircraft. Ventricular shunts and osmotic diuretics may decrease this risk. However, care must be taken to keep the cerebral perfusion pressure in a range of 60–70 mm Hg by keeping the mean arterial pressure high enough to avoid compromise of the cerebral perfusion pressure. For this reason, it is sometimes necessary to add a vasopressor to the patient's list of intravenous medications. This is discussed in detail in Chap. 12.

Pulmonary Patients

Patients with pulmonary disease can pose major challenges to the air medical transport crew. There are some important aeromedical considerations for patients with pulmonary disease, regardless of whether it is of medical or traumatic origin. The change in atmospheric pressure, especially during fixed-wing air medical transport, can be enough to cause significant worsening of oxygenation.

The first concern of the aeromedical crew should be maintenance of the patient's airway. Patients with a decreased mental status, heavy secretions, or labored breathing should be intubated prior to transport because their condition will almost certainly worsen at altitude. It has been demonstrated, in an analysis of US Air Force (USAF) transports, that using a lung-protective strategy for mechanically ventilated patients is associated with a reduction in complications, length of mechanical ventilation, and mortality [31]. Noninvasive positive pressure ventilation can be employed during transport, but this should be approached with great caution because the airway is not secured. It is difficult to adequately monitor the effectiveness of ventilation, or respond to further patient decompensation in the air medical transport environment. It is advisable to use a respiratory therapist as an additional crew member for these transports in order to more closely manage this therapy.

Pulmonary Trauma

The aeromedical crew should be vigilant in monitoring for signs of decreased oxygenation that may occur in the traumatized patient with chest injuries and be prepared to provide the necessary treatments. Placement of a definitive airway may be needed in patients with concomitant pulmonary injuries. Complications that arise from positive pressure ventilation must also be watched for and treated, especially in the traumatized patient. A significant air leak or a hemopneumothorax that develops in-flight will require placement of a thoracostomy tube if a qualified air medical transport crewmember is available.

Pneumothorax is an especially important issue for air medical transport patients because even a 20% pneumothorax at sea level will expand with altitude gain and may lead to total collapse of the lung. A traumatic pneumothorax of any size requires the placement of a chest tube with a Heimlich valve or pleural drainage system prior to air medical transport. Tension pneumothorax discovered in-flight should be treated and relieved by needle thoracostomy.

Obstetric Patients

Obstetric transport requires considerable skill and confidence on the part of the aeromedical crew (see Chap. 21). Urgent transfer of pregnant women in the second or third trimester of pregnancy is required whenever the referral facility is unable to provide the needed level of service to either the mother or imminent neonate. Indications for maternal transportation include preterm labor, premature rupture of membranes, eclampsia and preeclampsia, abruptio placenta, and placenta previa. Air medical transport crews who perform emergency obstetric transport must be ready to assist the mother and provide the initial neonatal resuscitation should a precipitous birth occur.

Certain careful considerations must be made before transporting the obstetric patient. A patient in active labor who is dilated beyond 6 cm should not be placed on the aircraft because the risk of precipitous delivery is higher and it is difficult to effectively assist the mother in the small environment of the aircraft. If the patient is in advanced labor, it is far safer to deliver the infant at the referral institution and then transport the mother and child post-delivery.

In all cases of emergency maternal air medical transport, the patient should be transported on a litter and receive oxygen supplementation. If there is any sign of maternal or fetal compromise, the patient should be in the left lateral Trendelenburg position. A large-bore intravenous catheter should be in place to allow the administration of fluid or blood in the event the patient requires aggressive resuscitation. In-flight portable ultrasound has been used to make fetal heart rate determinations, as it offers the advantage of being able to visualize the heart rate. Doppler techniques used in the past are limited due to the noise-filled aeromedical environment. External electronic fetal monitoring can be used. However, the medical utility of this has not been demonstrated because there is little that can be done in-flight in the event of an ominous tracing [32].

Pediatric Patients

Emergent transport of infants and children occurs for a number of reasons (see Chap. 22). Premature delivery is the most common indication for transportation of an infant. Common indications for urgent transport of older infants and children include trauma, sepsis, and airway compromise.

Neonatal Transportation

Safe transport of neonates requires specialized teams and equipment. The equipment and personnel necessary to accomplish this mission account for a large part of any flight program's budget, despite the fact that they may account for less than 25% of the volume of business. Dedicated air medical transport crew members trained solely for the transport and care of the neonate patient are ideal (Fig. 4.5). Neonatal

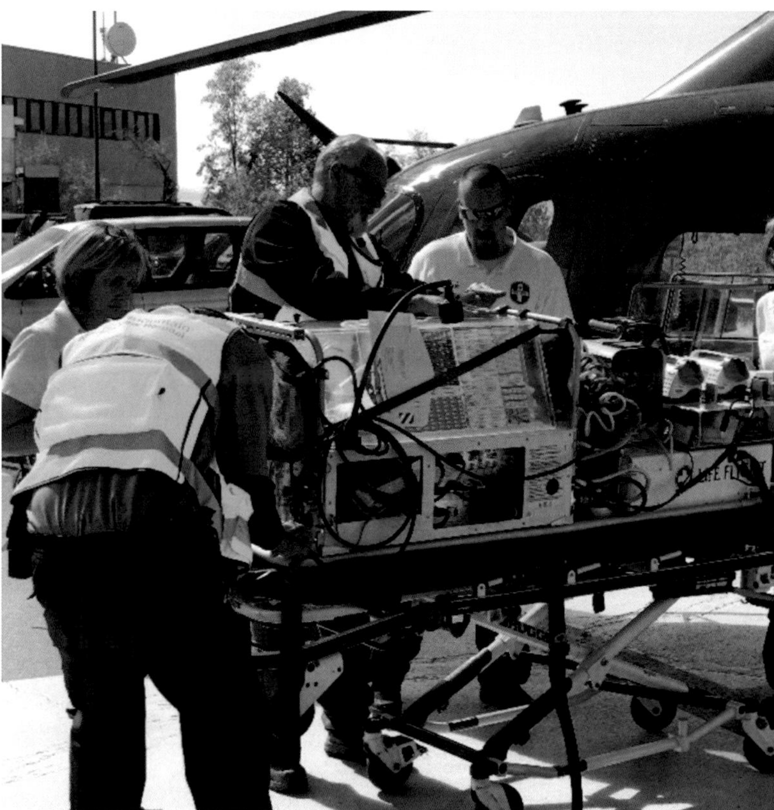

Fig. 4.5 A neonatal specialty team loading a patient in an isolette mounted to a standard transport litter. (Photo courtesy of K. D. Simpson)

nurses and physicians usually replace the routine adult or pediatric team members for these specialized transports.

The heavy and cumbersome equipment needed for neonatal transport (e.g., isolette, ventilator, and specialized supplies) adds significantly to the overall weight of the aircraft. Many small helicopters can carry only one incubator and thus require either multiple flights or multiple aircraft to transport twins or higher-order multiple births. Larger aircraft are capable of carrying twin isolettes and crews, but careful consideration of weight and balance on the part of the pilot(s) is needed. ECMO units or high-frequency jet ventilators require additional qualified personnel as well.

For neonatal transport, careful and thorough preflight preparation prior to air medical transport is important. Considerable time should be taken at the referral facility to achieve adequate stabilization and preparation for safe transport of the neonate. Optimization of ventilation, oxygenation, and temperature control is critical to successful air medical transport of the neonate. Environmental temperature, altitude, and travel distance are factors that are weighed in the clinical decision-making process by the neonatal flight crew and greatly impact the amount of time spent at the referral facility in preparation for transport.

Pediatric Trauma

After the first year of life, trauma is the leading cause of death in the pediatric population. Burns, smoke inhalation, drowning, blunt traumatic injury, spinal cord injury, child abuse and neglect, falls, and suicide collectively add to the epidemic number of pediatric deaths and disabilities that occur each year. It is not uncommon for children to engage in dangerous adult behaviors that put them at significant risk of death and serious injury. Of particular concern is the rise in penetrating trauma in the pediatric population related to gun and knife wounds associated with gang activities and drug-related violence.

There are specific differences in pediatric trauma that are of interest to the aeromedical crew. First, pediatric trauma patients are much more likely to sustain head injury than their adult counterparts. This is related to the fact that, in children, the head accounts for a large body surface area and relative weight in comparison to the remainder of the body. Secondary brain injury occurs as a result of hypoxia, hypercapnia, hypovolemia, seizures, and cerebral edema, all of which can lead to an increase in intracranial pressure (ICP). During air medical transport, cerebral perfusion can be optimized by intubation to ensure adequate oxygenation and maintain eucapnia.

The second important difference in children is that they do not show signs of hemodynamic decompensation until late in the course of the disease process. Hypotension is a late sign in the pediatric trauma patient, and thus tachycardia should be used in the child to gauge the need for fluid resuscitation. If needed, the aeromedical crew should begin fluid resuscitation with repeated boluses of blood products or isotonic crystalloid solution.

Pediatric Sepsis

The toxic-appearing child can have a rapidly progressive downhill course and thus warrants special consideration on the part of the flight crew. Emergency in-flight treatment consists of bolus intravenous fluid therapy, vasopressors, and broad-spectrum intravenous antibiotics. Sepsis care has been revolutionized by the application of bundles, with specific attention to timing of key resuscitation events [33]. The air medical transport crew can be full members of the sepsis resuscitation team by continuing, or even initiating, the sepsis bundle process during transport.

Pediatric Airway Compromise

The pediatric airway is short and small in comparison to the adult airway and thus is particularly susceptible to obstructions from conditions such as asthma, croup, epiglottitis, and foreign body. One millimeter of tissue edema decreases the pediatric airway lumen by a factor of 4. Unfortunately, the usual seatbelt harness by which we normally ensure safe transport in a seated position may prevent these patients from assuming a sniffing position when necessary.

Lethargy and bradycardia are ominous signs in this population and are precursors to impending respiratory arrest. Should a child with an airway problem begin to deteriorate, the flight crew must be prepared to obtain an emergency airway.

The crew must be capable of obtaining an emergent airway in a matter of minutes, most commonly by endotracheal or nasotracheal intubation. Transtracheal jet insufflation may be lifesaving in these patients if endotracheal intubation is impossible or impractical. Because carbon dioxide begins to accumulate immediately, this is a temporary solution, and retrograde intubation or completion of the surgical airway is necessary.

Other Applications of Civilian Air Medical Transport

Disaster Evacuation

The US homeland is subject to a range of natural and manmade disasters that include hurricanes, earthquakes, tornadoes, wildfires, terrorist attacks, industrial accidents, contagious disease outbreaks, and loss of critical infrastructure. Of these the most frequent and destructive are hurricanes. Among the characteristics of disasters are that they produce critically injured and ill casualties, and at the same time they have the potential to degrade and overwhelm patient care resources at the disaster site. For this reason, critical care evacuation capability is imperative in the disaster response. The American College of Chest Physicians has published guidelines for the evacuation of intensive care units, which acknowledge the value of air evacuation in distributing critical casualties [34].

For anticipated disasters such as hurricanes, it is possible to preemptively evacuate critically ill patients. This protects them from the risk of deterioration if there is loss of infrastructure from the disaster. This also makes critical care resources available for casualties generated by the disaster. Following the disaster, ongoing evacuation may be required as well. The use of military AE has the advantage of being able to simultaneously evacuate multiple casualties, and this has been employed effectively in multiple disasters, including hurricanes [35]. However, ongoing military operations limit the availability of DoD resources on short notice. In contrast, civilian air medical transport resources are distributed across the country, so the response time to a disaster in the US homeland can be short. The civilian aeromedical crews and aircraft bring a high level of capability that is in daily use moving critically ill and injured patients, which helps ensure the highest clinical standards are met. Typically, civilian air medical transport aircraft are not equipped for multi-casualty evacuation, but this limitation can be overcome by employing multiple agencies and aircraft.

Wilderness Search and Rescue

In the USA, wilderness search and rescue is performed by a patchwork of government and private organizations. This includes government agencies at the county, state, and federal level, EMS services, and volunteer groups. The civilian air medical transport services have characteristics that make them uniquely qualified to support these operations, with prior planning, coordination, and training [36]. Civilian air medical transport helicopters are able to cover large areas of terrain at a low altitude to facilitate the search for victims, and to rapidly reach victims that are away from roads. If a victim needs medical care, a civilian aeromedical crew brings advanced trauma and critical care resuscitation capability to their location. The helicopters are also able to shuttle additional rescuers to the victims' location and to evacuate victims, whether they require care or not. When a rescue is being conducted over terrain that blocks line-of-sight communication, civilian fixed-wing aircraft can serve as an airborne relay for critical communications. When there are multiple victims in a remote area, helicopters can be used to transport them to a nearby airfield so that fixed-wing aircraft can evacuate them for continued medical care.

In some circumstances, victims will be located in an area in which the helicopter cannot land nearby, in a position that makes them inaccessible

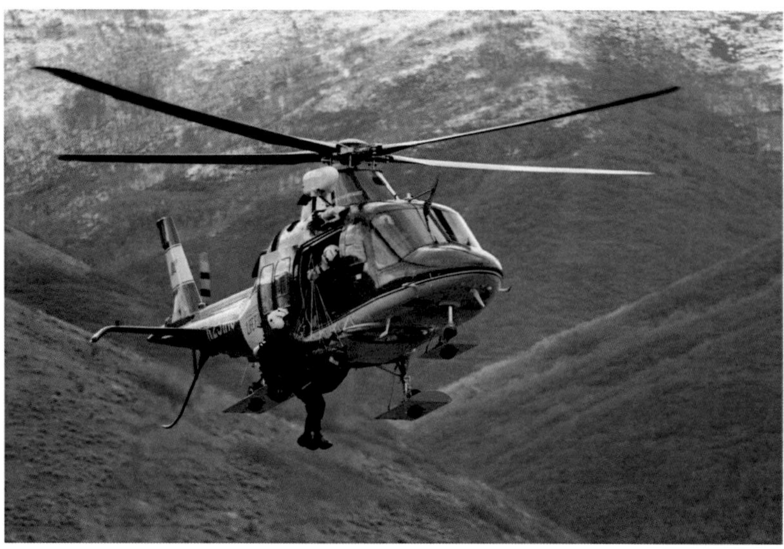

Fig. 4.6 An Intermountain Life Flight helicopter uses a lift hoist for a wilderness rescue. (Photo courtesy of K. D. Simpson)

to ground-based rescue teams. Helicopters provide several options for extracting victims from these situations, by hover load, long line, or hoist (Fig. 4.6). In the United States, such rescues are almost entirely a government function due to the cost and complexity of acquiring and maintaining the gear and the training requirement. In addition, such rescues are typically not covered by medical insurance, so reimbursement for the rescue is unlikely. This function can be provided by civilian air medical transport however. The Utah-based Intermountain Life Flight is the only US civilian program to have a Federal Aviation Administration (FAA) exemption for lift hoist rescue and it has maintained an active hoist program since 2001. In the first 10 years, Life Flight hoist-rescued 212 casualties, 68% of which required subsequent medical transport [37].

References

1. Committee on Trauma and Committee on Shock, Division of Medical Sciences. National Academy of Sciences, National Research Council. Accidental Death and Disability: The Neglected Disease of Modern Society. National Academies Press. 1966. https://www.ems.gov/pdf/1997-Reproduction-AccidentalDeathDissability.pdf. Accessed 30 Sept 2018.
2. Jurkovich GJ. Regionalized health care and the trauma system model. J Am Coll Surg. 2012;215(1):1–11.
3. Air ambulance: effects of industry changes on services are unclear. US Government Accounting Office. September 2010. https://www.gao.gov/products/GAO-10-907. Accessed 30 Sept 2018.
4. Habib FA, Shatz D, Habib AI, Bukur M, Puente I, Catino J, Farrington R. Probable cause in helicopter emergency medical services crashes: what role does ownership play? J Trauma Acute Care Surg. 2014;77(6):989–93.
5. Association of Air Medical Services. Atlas & Database of Air Ambulance Services (ADAMS). 2017. Alexandra, VA. http://www.adamsairmed.org/pubs/atlas_2017.pdf. Accessed 30 Sept 2018.
6. Shelton SL, Swor RA, Domeier RM, Lucas R. Medical direction of interfacility transports. Prehosp Emerg Care. 2000;4(4):361–4.
7. Centers for Disease Control, MMWR. Ambulance crash-related injuries among emergency medical services workers - United States, 1991-2002. 2003;52(8):154–6.
8. Maguire BJ, Hunting KL, Smith GS, Levick NR. Occupational fatalities in emergency medical services: a hidden crisis. Ann Emerg Med. 2002;40:625–32.
9. Diaz MA, Hendey GW, Bivins HG. When is the helicopter faster? A comparison of helicopter and ground ambulance transport times. J Trauma. 2005;58:148–53.
10. Nix S, Buckner S, Cercone R. A review of risk analysis and helicopter air ambulance accidents. Air Med J. 2011;33(5):218–21.
11. Hinkelbein J, Dambier M, Viergutz T, Genzwürker H. A 6-year analysis of German emergency medical services helicopter crashes. J Trauma. 2008;64(1):204–10.
12. Handel DA, Yackel TR. Fixed-wing medical transport crashes: characteristics associated with fatal outcomes. Air Med J. 2015;30(3):249–51.

13. Wuerz RC, O'Neal R. Role of pilot instrument proficiency in the safety of helicopter emergency medical services. Acad Emerg Med. 1997;4:972–5.
14. Galvagno SM Jr, Haut ER, Zafar SN, Millin MG, Efron DT, Koenig GJ Jr, Baker SP, Bowman SM, Pronovost PJ, Haider AH. Association between helicopter vs ground emergency medical services and survival for adults with major trauma. JAMA. 2012;307(15):1602–10.
15. Galvagno SM Jr, Sikorski R, Hirshon JM, Floccare D, Stephens C, Beecher D, Thomas S. Helicopter emergency medical services for adults with major trauma. Cochrane Database Syst Rev. 2015;12:CD009228.
16. Delgado MK, Staudenmayer KL, Wang NE, Spain DA, Weir S, Owens DK, Goldhaber-Fiebert JD. Cost-effectiveness of helicopter versus ground emergency medical services for trauma scene transport in the United States. Ann Emerg Med. 2013;62(4):351–364.e19. [Erratum in: Ann Emerg Med. 2014 Apr;63(4):411.].
17. Sasser SM, Hunt RC, Faul M, Sugerman D, Pearson WS, Dulski T, Wald MM, Jurkovich GJ, Newgard CD, Lerner EB, Centers for Disease Control and Prevention (CDC). Guidelines for field triage of injured patients: recommendations of the National Expert Panel on Field Triage, 2011. MMWR Recomm Rep. 2012;61(RR-1):1–20.
18. Doucet J, Bulger E, Sanddal N, Fallat M, Bromberg W, Gestring M, Emergency Medical System Subcommittee, Committee on Trauma, American College of Surgeons. Appropriate use of helicopter emergency medical services for transport of trauma patients: guidelines from the Emergency Medical System Subcommittee, Committee on Trauma, American College of Surgeons. J Trauma Acute Care Surg. 2013;75(4):734–41.
19. Thomas SH, Brown KM, Oliver ZJ, Spaite DW, Lawner BJ, Sahni R, Weik TS, Falck-Ytter Y, Wright JL, Lang ES. An evidence-based guideline for the air medical transportation of prehospital trauma patients. Prehosp Emerg Care. 2014;18(Suppl 1):35–44.
20. Garner A, Rashford S, Lee A, Bartolacci R. Addition of physicians to paramedic helicopter services decreases blunt trauma mortality (see comments). Aust N Z J Surg. 1999;69:697–701.
21. Roberts K, Blethyn K, Foreman M. Influence of air ambulance doctors on on-scene times, clinical interventions, decision-making and independent paramedic practice. Emerg Med J. 2009;26:128–34.
22. Scalea TM, Rodriguez A, Chiu WC, Brenneman FD, Fallon WF Jr, Kato K, McKenney MG, Nerlich ML, Ochsner MG, Yoshii H. Focused Assessment with Sonography for Trauma (FAST): results from an international consensus conference. J Trauma. 1999;46(3):466–72.
23. Polk JD, Fallon WF. The use of focused assessment with sonography for trauma (FAST) by a prehospital air medical team in the trauma arrest patient. Prehosp Emerg Care. 2000;4:82.
24. Polk JD, Fallon WF Jr, Kovach B, Mancuso C, Stephens M, Malangoni MA. The "Airmedical F.A.S.T." for trauma patients--the initial report of a novel application for sonography. Aviat Space Environ Med. 2001;72(5):432–6.
25. Press GM, Miller SK, Hassan IA, Alade KH, Camp E, del Junco D, Holcomb JB. Prospective evaluation of prehospital trauma ultrasound during aeromedical transport. J Emerg Med. 2014;47(6):638–45.
26. Holcomb JB, Swartz MD, DeSantis SM, Greene TJ, Fox EE, Stein DM, Bulger EM, Kerby JD, Goodman M, Schreiber MA, Zielinski MD, O'Keeffe T, Inaba K, Tomasek JS, Podbielski JM, Appana SN, Yi M, Wade CE, PROHS Study Group. Multicenter observational prehospital resuscitation on helicopter study. J Trauma Acute Care Surg. 2017;83(1 Suppl 1):S83–91.
27. Funder KS, Rasmussen LS, Siersma V, Lohse N, Hesselfeldt R, Pedersen F, Hendriksen OM, Steinmetz J. Helicopter vs. ground transportation of patients bound for primary percutaneous coronary intervention. Acta Anaesthesiol Scand. 2018;62(4):568–78.
28. Nielsen N, Wetterslev J, Cronberg T, Erlinge D, Gasche Y, Hassager C, Horn J, Hovdenes J, Kjaergaard J, Kuiper M, Pellis T, Stammet P, Wanscher M, Wise MP, Åneman A, Al-Subaie N, Boesgaard S, Bro-Jeppesen J, Brunetti I, Bugge JF, Hingston CD, Juffermans NP, Koopmans M, Køber L, Langørgen J, Lilja G, Møller JE, Rundgren M, Rylander C, Smid O, Werer C, Winkel P, Friberg H, Trial Investigators TTM. Targeted temperature management at 33 °C versus 36 °C after cardiac arrest. N Engl J Med. 2013;369(23):2197–206.
29. Arrich J, Holzer M, Havel C, Warenits AM, Herkner H. Pre-hospital versus in-hospital initiation of cooling for survival and neuroprotection after out-of-hospital cardiac arrest. Cochrane Database Syst Rev. 2016;3:CD010570.
30. Nguyen-Huynh MN, Klingman JG, Avins AL, Rao VA, Eaton A, Bhopale S, Kim AC, Morehouse JW, Flint AC. Novel telestroke program improves thrombolysis for acute stroke across 21 hospitals of an integrated healthcare system. Stroke. 2018;49:133–9.
31. Maddry JK, Mora AG, Savell S, Perez CA, Mason PE, Aden JK, Bebarta VS. Impact of Critical Care Air Transport Team (CCATT) ventilator management on combat mortality. J Trauma Acute Care Surg. 2018;84(1):157–64.
32. Haggerty L. Continuous electronic fetal monitoring: contradictions between practice and research [review]. J Obstet Gynecol Neonatal Nurs. 1999;28:409–16.
33. Seymour CW, Gesten F, Prescott HC, Friedrich ME, Iwashyna TJ, Phillips GS, Lemeshow S, Osborn T, Terry KM, Levy MM. Time to treatment and mortality during mandated emergency care for sepsis. N Engl J Med. 2017;376:2235–44.
34. King MA, Niven AS, Beninati W, Fang R, Einav S, Rubinson L, Kissoon N, Devereaux AV, Christian MD, Grissom CK. Evacuation of the ICU care of the

critically ill and injured during pandemics and disasters: CHEST consensus statement. Chest. 2014;146(4 Suppl):e44S–60S.
35. Lezama NG, Riddles LM, Pollan WA, Profenna LC. Disaster aeromedical evacuation. Mil Med. 2011;176(10):1128–32.
36. Grissom CK, Thomas F, James B. Medical helicopters in wilderness search and rescue operations. Air Med J. 2006;25(1):18–25.
37. Carpenter J, Thomas F. A 10-year analysis of 214 HEMS backcountry hoist rescues. Air Med J. 2013;32(2):98–101.

Part II

The Means

5 Aircraft Considerations for Aeromedical Evacuation

John G. Jernigan

Introduction

This chapter in the first edition of *Aeromedical Evacuation: Management of Acute and Stabilized Patients* began with the following sentence: "Any aircraft that can carry passengers can conceivably be used for aeromedical evacuation (AE), depending on the situation." That statement has been proven true over the past several years as the KC-135, the US Air Force's (USAF) primary refueling aircraft, has become one of the two strategic AE aircraft used by the USAF today. In contrast to the USAF approach, multiple civilian aircraft have been specifically configured for the special needs of AE.

It is impossible to discuss every aircraft used for AE throughout the world. Instead, this chapter will deal with the most important factors that must be considered in choosing the correct aircraft for the patient, including alternative methods of moving patients. To illustrate these important factors, this chapter includes a detailed discussion of the aircraft presently used by the USAF for AE, together with a detailed discussion of one civilian jet that is representative of the many aircraft used by the commercial air ambulance industry.

It is obvious why military medical personnel should be familiar with USAF aircraft used for AE. However, it is important for civilian medical personnel to be aware of both civilian and USAF aircraft used in AE, since in a disaster situation AE assistance is often provided by the Department of Defense (DoD) [1]. As the events of September 11, 2001 clearly showed, a requirement to move large numbers of casualties may arise suddenly, and the USAF AE system could prove crucial to meeting the patients' needs. The USAF AE system is a national treasure that has been called upon for more than 50 years to move casualties resulting from military operations (both armed conflicts and operations other than war) and civilian disasters beyond the local capability to respond. Although the DoD does not exist to compete with civilian air evacuation companies, the USAF AE system has moved more patients around the world than any other organization, including large numbers of civilians. In addition to aircraft specifics, this chapter will describe the capability of the USAF AE system.

Aircraft Selection for Aeromedical Evacuation

To select the best possible aircraft for any AE mission, both logistic and patient-related factors must be considered. Although patient-related factors are paramount, logistic factors may often

J. G. Jernigan (✉)
Brig Gen, USAF, CFS (ret.), Formerly Commander, Human Systems Center, Brooks Air Force Base, Texas, San Antonio, TX, USA

W. W. Hurd, W. Beninati (eds.), *Aeromedical Evacuation*,
https://doi.org/10.1007/978-3-030-15903-0_5

Table 5.1 Characteristics of aircraft used for aeromedical evacuation by the USAF

Characteristic	C-17	KC-135	C-130	C-21
Range (nautical miles without refueling)	6200	5000–11,000	2100	2300
In-flight refueling capability	Yes	Internal fuel transfer	Yes	No
Runway requirements				
Minimum (feet, approximate)	3500	7000	3500	4500
Minimally improved runways?	Yes	No	Yes	No
Maximum patient loads				
Ambulatory	54	8	80	6
Litter	36	15	74	2
Litter + ambulatory	36 + 54	24 + 30	50 + 30	1 + 2

Abbreviation: *USAF* United States Air Force

determine the type of aircraft needed (Table 5.1). These logistic factors include the number of patients (litter or ambulatory); the distance required for the particular AE mission; the runway length and runway surface condition at the AE sites of origin and destination; and competing requirements for the aircraft. Patient-related factors include the need for pressurization, the amount and type of special AE equipment needed, and the aspects of aircraft configuration that affect patient care. Depending on the situation, each of these factors can be critically important in making the ultimate decision on which aircraft or combination of aircraft best meets the particular requirements. The following is a detailed discussion of each factor.

Logistic Considerations

Number of Patients

The total number and complexity of patients is often the determining factor regarding which aircraft is used. If only one or two patients need movement, then virtually any aircraft is capable of meeting this need. The solution becomes more complex when large numbers of patients need to be moved from the same place, which is often the case during armed conflicts. Adding to the complexity of large patient movements is the fact that a tragedy is usually associated with such a requirement. In such instances, the airfield serving patients will also be involved with a dramatic increase in air traffic, which will limit the departure or arrival "slots" for AE missions. As a result, using multiple aircraft may not be a viable option, and a large aircraft (e.g., the C-17) may become the only solution to move large numbers of seriously wounded patients.

Distance

The distance required to move the patient from origin to destination will determine whether AE is the appropriate means and will also limit the choices of aircraft once that decision is made. In general, AE should not be considered unless the distance is too great to be accomplished by more readily available means of transport, e.g., ground ambulance or medical helicopter. Rarely is there a reason to consider AE for distances shorter than 300 miles.

Once it has been determined that AE is required, the type of aircraft capable of meeting the requirement becomes more limited. This is especially true for the USAF, which is often asked to accomplish missions that seem impossible at first glance. An example is the movement of critical burn patients thousands of miles without stops, e.g., moving a burn patient from Japan to San Antonio, TX. On the other hand, if the distance were short enough (e.g., less than 1000 miles), then virtually any of the aircraft used for AE, including all those discussed in this chapter, would suffice. Long-distance requirements can be met by the range of the aircraft or using en route stops.

Range is a crucial determinant because all aircraft have a finite distance they can fly with a full load and still arrive safely at the destination. The range for all USAF AE aircraft is more than a thousand miles (Table 5.1), but may be shorter for some civilian aircraft. In-flight aerial refueling can extend the range of certain USAF aircraft (e.g., the C-17) if the needs of the patients are critical. This is most frequently accomplished when moving severely injured patients from Japan or Korea to the United States. However, because of the difficulty, expense, and potential danger, in-flight refueling is rarely used for routine AE. That is one reason the use of the KC-135 in strategic missions is ideal. Its range, by internally transferring gas from its "flying gas station," is more than 10,000 miles!

Related to range is the cruise speed of the aircraft. Although the C-130 has a long range, its cruise speed is slow enough that the flight time differential between the C-130 and a jet aircraft over long distances makes the choice of a jet much more likely.

En Route Stops

En route stops is another way to increase the effective range for aircraft commonly used for AE. Assuming each leg is within their range, en route stops allow any aircraft to move patients over long distances. This method has been extremely important historically for the USAF in moving patients from the Western Pacific region to medical facilities in Hawaii. The use of en route stops is no longer a problem in the Pacific area due to the KC-135 becoming the primary AE aircraft in that theater.

If en route stops are used, the availability of medical care at the en route stop becomes extremely important. This consideration is crucial because aircraft frequently experience mechanical problems or weather constraints that prevent takeoff from the en route location. Therefore, a planned delay of 2 hours for refueling can easily turn into a delay of several days; so a plan for providing care to patients becomes critical.

Runway Length for Landing/Takeoff

Medical planners do not always have to consider runways and runway environments in their analyses, but runways can easily become the limiting factor in completing missions in austere environments. Runway environment is frequently a problem for the USAF, as it meets the needs of the DoD around the world, and often is the constraining factor that mandates the use of a specific aircraft (e.g., the C-130) when another aircraft would have been preferred. The C-17 can also operate on minimally improved runways. The C-9A could not, which is one of the primary reasons it was retired. This factor is rarely a problem for civilian moves from one large metropolitan area to another because the runways at the airports serving such cities are almost always long enough to meet the requirements of any of the aircraft described in this chapter.

Aircraft Availability

During armed conflicts, and sometimes during peacetime disasters, there are competing missions for a limited number of aircraft. That is certainly true of all the current USAF AE aircraft: the C-130, C-17, and KC-135 (transporting people and material, and refueling). The command center involved with the patient movement request will make the decision on which aircraft is used for each mission.

Patient-Related Considerations

The specific needs of the patients requiring transport must be added to the calculation of what aircraft to choose for each mission. These considerations include the need for altitude restriction, electrical support for equipment, supplemental oxygen, liter capability, cabin space, cabin noise, and cabin lighting. These patient-related considerations for transportation of stable and stabilized patients are compared for the USAF aircraft used for AE in Table 5.2.

Pressurization

One of the unique aspects of AE, when compared to ground and sea casualty transportation, is the issue of cabin pressure. Although most medical

Table 5.2 Patient-related considerations for US military aircraft currently used for aeromedical evacuation

Aircraft type	C-17	KC-135	C-130	C-21
Electrical outlets	115 volt	115 volt	Transformer	115 volt
Oxygen	Integral	Integral	PTLOX[a]	Oxygen canister
Litter loading capacity	Excellent	Requires special lift or ramp	Excellent	Difficult
Temperature control	Excellent	Moderate	Suboptimal	Excellent
Ambient noise level	70–80 dB	95–110 dB	95–110 dB	70–80 dB
Lighting	Excellent	Suboptimal	Suboptimal	Excellent

[a]Portable Therapeutic Liquid Oxygen System

conditions are unaffected by decreased pressure, there are several medical conditions (e.g., decompression sickness) that are adversely affected by cabin pressures lower than those found at sea level. It is extremely important that the flight crew (i.e., pilots) be made aware of any altitude restrictions that are required for medical indications during AE.

All modern aircraft used for AE are pressurized such that the cabin pressure is maintained between 6000 and 8000 ft (unless an unplanned decompression occurs). If a patient requires an altitude restriction, then an aircraft that is capable of pressurizing as close to sea level as possible is ideal. This is done primarily by limiting the en route cruising altitude.

Within the limitations of the patients' medical condition, it is important to keep cabin altitude restrictions to a minimum (i.e., allow a cruising altitude as high as possible). The reason for this is that the aircraft pays a huge price in terms of both speed and fuel to accomplish an altitude restriction. For example, the C-9A aircraft had a range of 2500 miles at a cruising altitude of 35,000 ft, but a range of only 2000 miles at 18,000 ft—the altitude required to maintain cabin altitudes near sea level. Further, ground speed is, in general, less at the lower altitude. The net result is that the mission takes longer and may require more en route stops, both of which can adversely affect the patients.

Electrical Aeromedical Evacuation Equipment

The range of capability provided by special equipment used to move patients has dramatically increased over the past several years. Types of equipment include electrical equipment, oxygen and ventilatory equipment, suction devices, and multiple other types of special equipment. These pieces of equipment are challenging to use in the AE environment for several reasons.

The use of electrical equipment is taken for granted on hospital wards but cannot be assumed on any AE mission, even those using well-designed AE aircraft. Although most equipment used in patient transport today is battery capable, the length of many AE missions exceeds even the longest battery capability. Most civilian aircraft used for AE, and the USAF's C-17 and KC-135, have existing electrical plug-in capability with the correct voltage/frequency used by medical equipment.

The other USAF transport aircraft that can be modified for AE (e.g., C-130) is not set up to use modern AE medical equipment on-board. The current solution is a bulky transformer that converts the aircraft-generated electricity to a usable voltage and frequency. The size and weight of this transformer become a constraint in itself.

Oxygen

The partial pressure of oxygen decreases exponentially as cabin altitude increases. Most aircraft used for AE maintain a cabin altitude between 6000 and 8000 ft during flight. For this reason, medical oxygen is often administered to AE patients. Individual patients can be given supplemental oxygen from existing capability on the aircraft or by using a portable oxygen canister.

In order to administer oxygen to a large number of patients, C-17 and KC-135 aircraft have been modified for AE so that patients can be connected directly to the existing aircrew oxygen system. This is not the case for the C-130.

When the C-130 is configured for AE, the work-around is the Portable Therapeutic Liquid Oxygen System (PTLOXS). This is a portable 10.0-liter liquid oxygen storage device that allows low pressure gaseous oxygen delivery and weighs approximately 80 lb when full. It is capable of supplying up to 8600 liters of gaseous oxygen at a maximum flow rate of 45 liters per minute at 50 psi.

Litter Loading Capacity

A crucial limiting factor in transporting litter patients by AE is the difficulty involved in loading litters into the aircraft. Civilian and military aircraft specifically designed for AE do not present a problem in this regard. The C-9A was designed with a retractable ramp that allows crew members to easily meet this requirement, but it has been retired. The size and slope of the rear entry ramp of the C-17 and C-130 are both more than adequate.

The KC-135 requires a K-loader (or similar equipment) to load litter patients, but this is not a problem since such equipment is always present in the theaters of operation where the KC-135 is used. The C-21 requires very careful loading of its litter patients because of the small entry door and the presence of a closet near the door.

Cabin Space

The cabin area must have adequate space for the medical crew to meet the needs of all patients. In general, this is not a problem with either the civilian or military aircraft used routinely for AE. However, the routine litter spacing for most military AE configurations is 21 inches, so meaningful procedures often require removing patients from their litter tiers and accomplishing the procedure on the floor. The small size of the C-21 cabin limits the amount of equipment that can accompany the patient and allow the medical attendant to use that equipment.

Temperature Control

Maintaining a comfortable temperature is important when transporting patients for long distances, as sick and injured patients may have difficulty regulating their core temperatures. Although commercial airliners sometimes have a difficult time trying to maintain the "ideal" temperature in all parts of the aircraft cabin, differences in various parts of these aircraft are negligible. Commercial AE aircraft accomplish uniform comfort reasonably well, but having a large supply of blankets is still a good idea for all missions.

However, the problem of temperature control is highly significant in the huge cabins of military transport aircraft. It is not unusual during AE in these aircraft for some patients to require several blankets, while others are shedding clothes to remain cool! Sensitivity of the medical flight crew to this problem can be vitally important. This is a major problem with the C-130 and the KC-135, although the short duration of most C-130 missions makes that less of a problem. The C-17 maintains temperature control almost as well as commercial airliners.

Cabin Noise Levels

The noise level during flight varies significantly for different aircraft. For the C-130 and KC-135, the noise level is approximately 95 to 100 dB during flight and thus ear plugs are required for all passengers and crew. For commercial AE aircraft, noise is considerably less (approximately 70–80 dB), but it is still a factor that needs consideration. Auscultation is extremely difficult during AE, even with stethoscopes specifically developed for this purpose. For this reason, alternative means of monitoring the patient have been developed, such as digital readout of blood pressure cuffs and pulse oximeters. Noise is much less a problem in the C-17 and C-21—around 75–85 dB.

Lighting

Lighting levels in aircraft cabins vary dramatically. The C-17 represents the benchmark for lighting, while the C-130 and KC-135 are poorly lit. AE crews must be aware of the lighting levels of the aircraft in which they will be flying so they can bring supplemental lighting on-board for those aircraft that require it.

United States Air Force Aircraft Utilized for Aeromedical Evacuation

This section will describe the general characteristics, strengths, and weaknesses of the USAF aircraft and a representative civilian aircraft commonly used for AE. In addition, ways to use other aircraft for AE in emergency situations are described.

C-130 Hercules

The C-130 has a truly unique role in the world of AE. Its versatility in takeoff and landing, together with its large capacity, makes it ideal for moving large numbers of patients from remote locations and poor runway conditions. Although there are some limitations that will be discussed in this section, it is safe to state that the USAF could not execute its worldwide mission, especially fighting the Global War on Terrorism, without the C-130.

Since its introduction to the USAF inventory in the 1950s, the C-130 has arguably become the most versatile aircraft ever developed (Fig. 5.1). Its roles are extremely diverse, extending far beyond the primary role of airlifting small loads of supplies and equipment to remote locations—a role it has executed in countless conflicts and civilian emergencies. It also flies into hurricanes to track motion and assess strength. It serves as a flying gunship, a role vital to Operation Just Cause in Panama and the war in Afghanistan. Finally, it has a role germane to this text: i.e., serving as the primary AE platform to reach patients in remote locations. The capability to land on virtually any cleared, semi-improved surface has made the C-130 a vital part of the USAF's ability to move any patient from any place at any time. An example of this was shown during the first Gulf War when the C-130 flew missions (fortunately few) into southern Iraq to move patients from the Army units attacking the enemy in that part of the desert. These missions required landing on a crude road, and could not

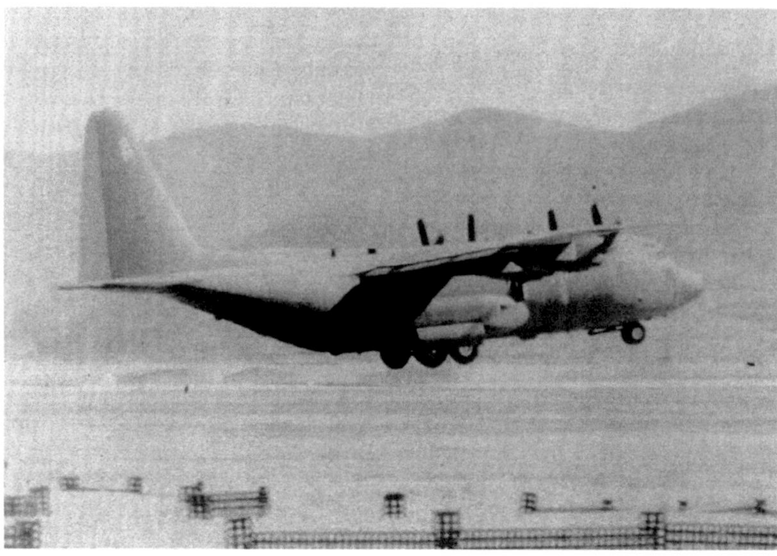

Fig. 5.1 C-130 Hercules. (USAF photo)

be accomplished with any other aircraft. It has continued that unique mission in many other locations during the Global War on Terrorism.

General Characteristics

The C-130J is a four-engine turboprop aircraft with a cruise speed of approximately 415 mph. It has a fuel capacity that allows it to cruise for approximately 10 hours, giving it a range potential of approximately 2100 miles. However, for the reasons described under weaknesses, the C-130 would only be used as a last resort to move patients over such a long distance. Its high wing configuration prevents debris from ruining the engines while operating in poorly improved airstrips. It has a short takeoff (3200 ft) and landing (2900 ft) capability unmatched by any other large aircraft.

Its maximum litter capacity is 74, and the litter stanchions (the supports into which the litters are placed) used in this role are kept on-board at all times. This factor adds incredible flexibility to the fleet of C-130 s as they operate in a variety of missions around the world.

Using web seats along the sides of the cabin, a maximum of 92 ambulatory patients could be moved. However, the discomfort and potential damage to patients would make such a configuration reasonable only for a short mission when no other alternative was available.

In military situations, such as an airfield under fire, the C-130 can also be floor loaded safely with 15 litters and approximately 30 ambulatory patients. The usual configurations for moving combinations of litter and ambulatory patients will be described at the end of this section.

Strengths

By far the greatest strength of the C-130 is its ability to land on short, minimally improved surfaces. Obviously, helicopters can also be used to pick up patients in similar situations, even with the total absence of any airstrip. However, the limitation of helicopters is the small number of patients that can be moved by each aircraft. So it is this one crucial strength that has kept the C-130 a vital member of the AE team for about 60 years and will likely remain in the role for many years to come. Medical planners simply would not have been able to develop a viable plan to move the projected casualties during the Gulf War without this capability. This same capability makes virtually any en route stop a viable option, so medical planners can use the C-130 for missions of extremely long distances. However, the weaknesses described later make such planning a last resort.

The patient movement capacity (i.e., potential for 74 litters or 92 ambulatory patients) makes the C-130 an ideal aircraft for medical planners as they attempt to minimize the number of far-forward AE missions required to support front-line troops in wartime. Although potential range (approximately 3500 miles) is a strength, the lack of comfort for the patient would make such a mission unlikely. The final strength of this aircraft is the ease of loading through the rear "clamshell" door. This wide open space allows crews to load large numbers of patients in approximately 20 minutes, including engine-running onloads (EROs). This procedure is only used at airfields under fire from the enemy or when ground time had to be minimized for another compelling reason.

Weaknesses

Noise is a major problem in the C-130 cabin, often making it necessary to shout within 18 inches of the listener to be heard. As a result, verbal communication between crew members is difficult and communication between medical crew and their patients is often impossible. Obviously, procedures requiring auscultation are impossible. Lighting is also extremely poor throughout the cabin, so medical crews must have a plan for providing lighting adequate enough for patient evaluation—especially with a full load of litter patients stacked 5 high. Electrical connections are available for attaching transformers (e.g., the transformer described earlier), but even with the transformer, electrical equipment support is extremely limited. The combination of limited space between litter stanchions and the effect of moderate turbulence, present on virtually every mission, makes care for patients extremely difficult. Simple care activities, such as feeding and taking vital signs, are easy, but more complex procedures are difficult. The only lavatory facilities available are a funnel that leads to the exterior of the aircraft, with a curtain for privacy, and a small chemical seat with a privacy curtain. There is no food service available, so boxed lunches are the only means of feeding patients. Climate control is poor, with cabin temperature rarely in the comfortable range. Neither patient oxygen nor suction is available, so both of these must be brought onto the aircraft for all missions requiring them. Finally, the C-130 cannot pressurize to sea level.

Configurations

The USAF uses four different configurations for the C-130 in its AE role [2]. The first provides 30 litter spaces with 46 web seats for ambulatory patients and AE crew (Fig. 5.2). This configuration provides the most space for the ambulatory patients, so it would be used when "stretching room" for ambulatory patients was important. The second configuration provides 70, 73, or 74 litter spaces with 6 seats for AE crews (Fig. 5.3a). This configuration is only used when a specific large load of litter patients is required. A third configuration provides 20 litter spaces with 44 sidewall seats, and this configuration would be used when space for medical equipment or cargo in the forward central portion of the cabin floor was required. The final configuration provides 50 litter spaces and 30 sidewall seats (Fig. 5.3b). This configuration is the one most commonly used in contingency or wartime operations because virtually any patient loads at the locations supported by the C-130 would include a combination of litter and ambulatory, with the majority being litter.

A unique feature of the C-130 is that all litter stanchion equipment needed to configure for AE is carried with each of the many (several hundred) C-130s deployed worldwide at any time. The total number of litter patients described in the aforementioned configurations depends on stacking five patients in each litter tier with approximately 21 inches of spacing between patients. Although the USAF practices this method of loading, the highest of the five patients is both difficult to load and virtually completely inaccessible for crew members to treat. Therefore, depending on circumstances, the medical crew director might well decide to load only four patients per upright station, thus giving more comfort to the litter patients and making nursing care more practical. Such a decision would only be made if all patients could be moved.

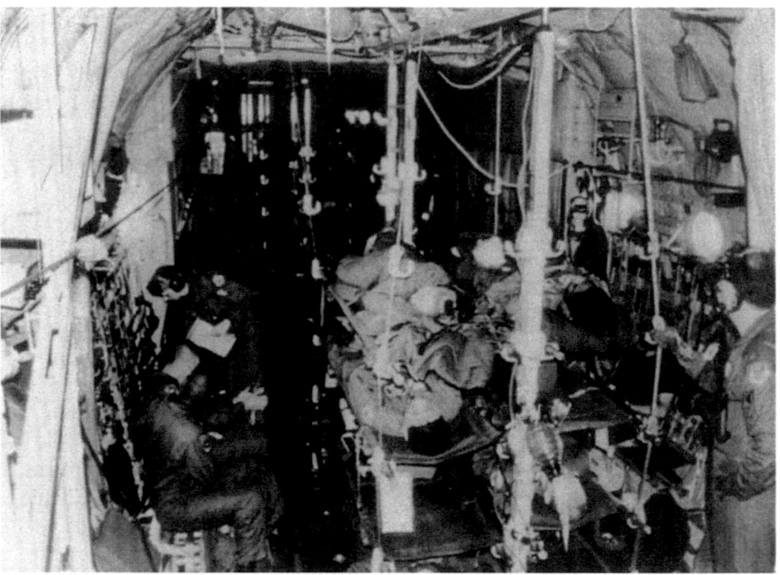

Fig. 5.2 Interior of C-130 Hercules configured for tactical AE

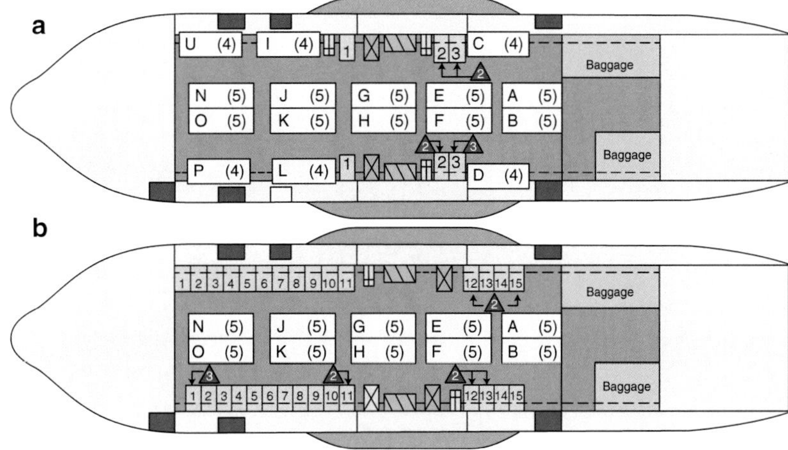

Fig. 5.3 Schematic of C-130 Hercules configured for (**a**) maximum litter patients and (**b**) tactical AE

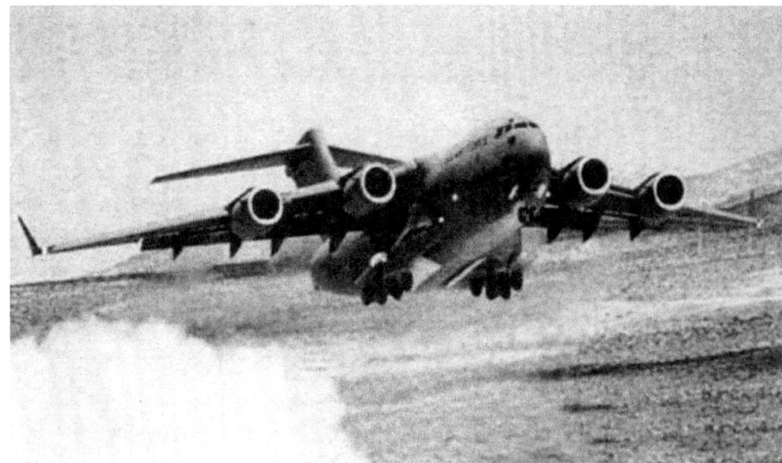

Fig. 5.4 C-17 Globemaster. (USAF photo by 1st Lieutenant Laurel Scherer)

Summary

From the strengths and weaknesses, it is obvious that the niche for the C-130 is moving patients out of "harm's way" from far-forward positions. Every effort will be made to minimize the length of these missions so the patients can be delivered to greater medical capability as soon as possible. Later transfer to another aircraft will be done if further movement is required. This aircraft will remain a vital part of the USAF inventory as long as this requirement exists and other aircraft cannot meet the need.

C-17 Globemaster

The C-17 is the newest transport jet in the USAF inventory and, among its other missions, it has the capability to perform the AE role. It has multiple strengths that make it ideal for this role. When the first edition of this book was published, it was unclear whether or not the C-17 would be used in the AE role because of competing needs for this aircraft. Fortunately it has proven highly capable in the strategic AE role, and it is currently one of the two strategic AE aircraft used in the AE role today.

General Characteristics

The C-17's incredible capabilities were first demonstrated during the initial deployment of troops to Bosnia in late 1995 (Fig. 5.4). Its primary mission is flying large loads—especially oversized loads—directly to minimally improved short runways. It is also designed to accomplish other missions, including AE and support of Army airborne units. Several problems have been identified over the past 15–20 years as the C-17 was used for AE, but these were easily fixed and the C-17 is firmly established as one of the two aircraft used for strategic AE.

Strengths

Virtually every previously described characteristic of an AE aircraft is a strength for the C-17. Perhaps its greatest strength is its unlimited range with aerial refueling. A close second is the ability to land on almost any semi-improved airfield. This combination makes it ideal for moving patients from almost any location directly back to the United States without en route stops. Its litter stanchions will accommodate 36 litter patients and a variable number of ambulatory patients depending upon the types of seats used (Fig. 5.5). Noise and lighting are almost as good as the C-9A and are certainly better than the C-130 or KC-135. The large clamshell doors make loading extremely easy. Cabin space is huge and the litter support structure gives excellent access to each patient. Comfort pallets are used to provide feeding and lavatory facilities. Climate control is better than either the C-130 or KC-135, but not as good as smaller cabins (e.g., the C-21). Pressurizing to sea level is possible with the usual mission constraints.

Weaknesses

Because the C-17 was not built primarily for AE, there is neither built-in oxygen nor suction. Like other large aircraft, climate control requires plenty of blankets to make sure all patients are warm enough. Undoubtedly the greatest weakness of the C-17 is the fact that there are relatively few airframes and its many potential uses frequently make it unavailable for the AE role.

Configurations

There are two configurations of the C-17 that are approved for AE. In one, there are only 3 litter tiers utilized, giving the capability to move 9 litter patients and 54 ambulatory seats on the periphery of the cabin. In the second configuration, there are 12 litter tiers, giving a total capacity of 36 litter and 54 ambulatory patients. In both configurations, up to 48 centerline seats can be added, but doing so makes the peripheral seats outboard of the litter stanchions unavailable. One obvious advantage of using the existing peripheral seats is that all C-17s can be configured this way without having seats available at the departure location.

Summary

In summary, the C-17 is a superlative aircraft for accomplishing the AE mission for all the reasons

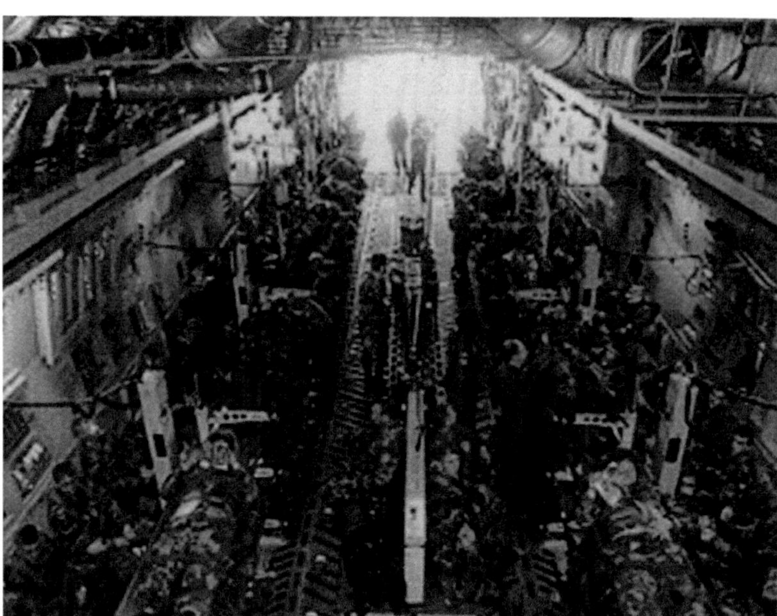

Fig. 5.5 Interior of C-17 Globemaster configured for tactical AE. (USAF photo)

listed under strengths, especially its speed, range, and short landing capabilities.

KC-135 Stratotanker

As mentioned in the opening of this chapter, any aircraft with a large enough cabin space can be used for aeromedical evacuation. The KC-135 certainly qualifies for that description, and it has been used in the AE role since December 2007 (Figs. 5.6 and 5.7).

It accomplishes this mission using a stacking litter system plus the seats it has always carried on its missions.

General Characteristics

The KC-135 has been the primary tanker for the Department of Defense for many years, but its AE role has existed only for the last 10 years. Since aerial refueling is a critical factor for many military operations, the KC-135 is present in virtually all areas of operation.

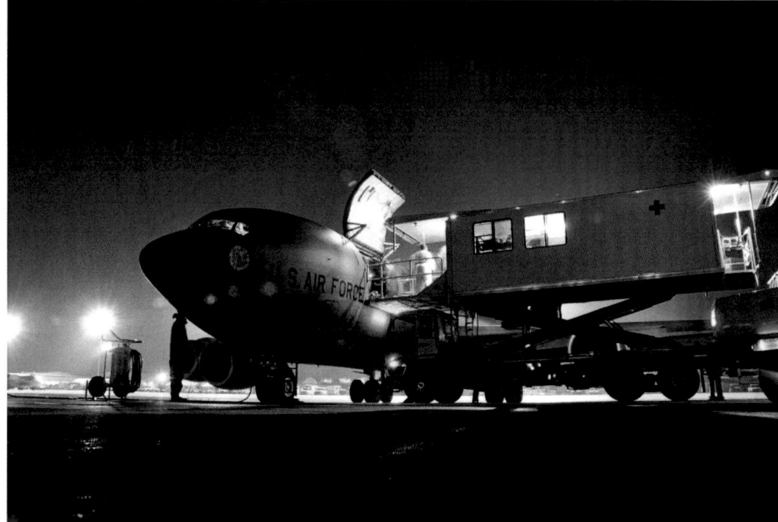

Fig. 5.6 A specialized transport vehicle is used to onload patients onto a KC-135 Stratotanker at Bagram Airfield, Afghanistan. (USAF photo by Lt. Col. Tyoshi Tung)

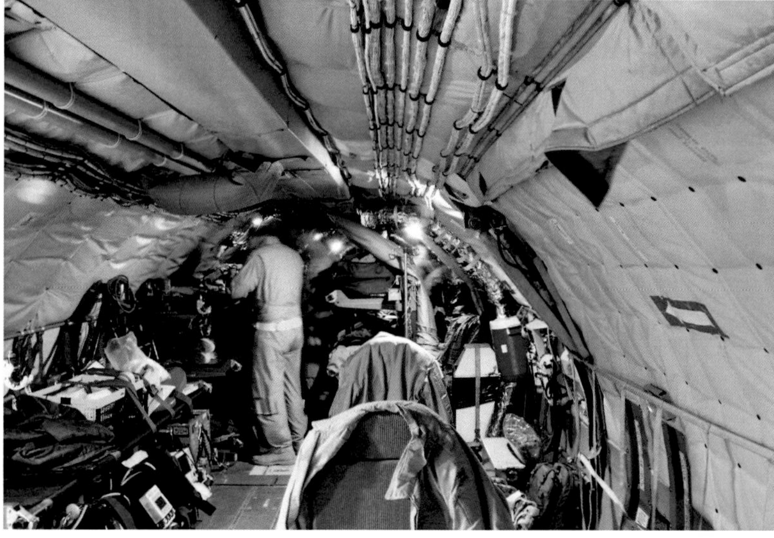

Fig. 5.7 KC-135 Stratotankers interior during an aeromedical evacuation mission. (USAF photo by Lt. Col. Tyoshi Tung)

Strengths

Its greatest strengths are the many active duty, Air National Guard, and AF Reserve Wings that fly the KC-135 and its range. Many USAF missions require tanker support, resulting in tankers deployed all over the world on a daily basis. This requirement can be shared with the many wings that fly this jet. Since the KC-135 is basically a flying gas station, it has a range of more than 10,000 miles when it internally transfers fuel.

Weaknesses

Since it was not designed for the AE role, it shares the same weaknesses of the C-130; i.e., loud noise levels, poor lighting, and poor temperature control. It has another unique weakness: It requires a K-loader or another lift device to lift patients up to the level of the loading area in the side of the jet. However, this is generally not a problem, since the KC-135 is almost always deployed at bases where K-loaders are plentiful.

Configuration

There are several different mixes of litter and ambulatory patients that are possible. However, the number of stacking litter systems that can be used on any mission is limited, so 8 litter patients plus 1 floor loaded litter is the current limit. The number of ambulatory patients depends on how many litter patients are being moved.

Summary

The KC-135 has proven itself as an AE aircraft. So much so that it is the primary strategic AE platform in the Pacific theater. It will continue in that role until it is retired sometime in the next few years as the KC-46A Pegasus replaces it. Even though the KC-46 is not yet operational, the USAF and Boeing have embraced AE as onc of its missions. They are designing patient oxygen and electric connections integral to the airplane and they have developed an AE configuration capable of moving up to 54 litter patients or a combination of 24 litter and 30 ambulatory patients.

C-21A Learjet

The C-21A (Fig. 5.8) is the military version of the Learjet 35A business jet. While the C-21A was not originally acquired for the AE role, it has proven itself highly effective in moving the right type of patient. The C-21A is located at multiple bases around the continental United States, which makes it readily available to move appropriate patients.

General Characteristics

The C-21A is a small twin-engine jet with a cabin large enough for 6 people or 1 litter plus 2 atten-

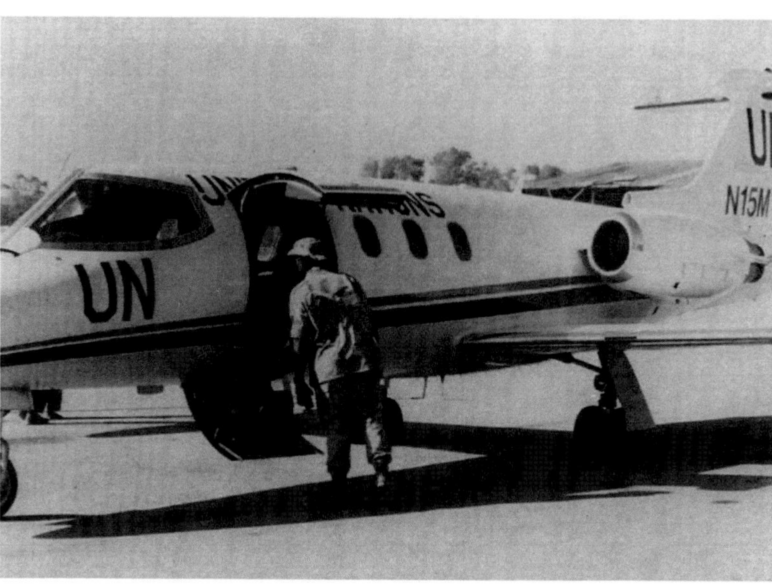

Fig. 5.8 C-21A Learjet (photo by Lieutenant Colonel John M. McNamara)

dants. The USAF procured it in the early 1980s with a primary role of moving high-ranking DoD personnel in peacetime and moving critical parts and people in war. In the late 1980s, AE was added to its missions. Several civilian air ambulance services use versions of the same Learjet, but all of these civilian jets have been specifically designed for the AE role.

Strengths

The C-21 requires little runway for takeoff or landing and can therefore move patients into or out of most locations. The range is about 2000 miles at a cruise speed of about 500 mph. This combination provides a capability to move patients throughout the United States. Noise is minimal and lighting is excellent. Because of the small size, climate control in the cabin is also excellent. A final strength is the ability to pressurize to sea level.

Weaknesses

Patient capacity is the greatest weakness, but that is usually not a problem because its mission is almost always picking up only one patient. It does not have equipment support, but batteries are adequate for its mission because flight times rarely exceed battery capability. Entry is a problem for adult litter patients because of a built-in closet near the door. Loading litter patients must be done carefully because of the small entry and the presence of a closet immediately in the way of the entry. Cabin space is extremely limited, and unlike all other USAF AE aircraft the crew cannot stand up in the cabin. The only lavatory is a chemical seat not readily available, and there are no feeding facilities. Finally, there is no oxygen or suction capability.

Configuration

If only ambulatory patients are being moved, the C-21 does not require any modification. It simply uses its existing four individual seats and two-person bench-type seat to move the patients and crew. If a litter or neonatal isolette is used, two seats on the same side are removed, and the litter or isolette is installed.

Summary

The C-21 is an excellent AE aircraft for specific patients. Its niche is newborns and ambulatory patients for whom quick transportation is most important, e.g., certain organ recipients. Its small entryway, relatively short range, and lack of room to fully utilize equipment for some patients will always limit its use.

Recently Retired Aeromedical Evacuation Aircraft: C-9, C-141, and the Civil Reserve Air Fleet

It is sad for me as an ex-Air Mobility Command Surgeon to write about the departure of these 2 aircraft and the Civil Reserve Air Fleet (CRAF) back-up program. But that is the reality of mission focus and with the impetus on using DoD funds in the best possible way.

The C-9A Nightingale was the face of aeromedical evacuation for more than 35 years, retiring in 2005. The C-9A, a modified version of the DC-9, was the only aircraft in USAF inventory specifically designed for the movement of litter and ambulatory AE patients. The C-9A had the capability to carry up to 40 litter patients or 40 ambulatory plus 4 litter patients. While its interior set the standard for meeting patient needs, there were a number of operational concerns that limited its effectiveness. For example, it had a relatively limited range, required improved runways for takeoff and landing, and the external noise of its low-bypass turbofan engines limited where and when it could land and take off. In the end the cost of replacing the engines of the entire fleet was too great to continue flying.

The C-141B Starlifter also was retired in 2006 after more than 40 years of service. Although this ubiquitous cargo aircraft was notorious for being relatively loud and cold at altitude, it was the workhorse of contingency AE related to it's range, speed, reliability, and availability. It could transport a relatively large amount of supplies into a warzone, and quickly reconfigure and transport up to 80 litter patients or a combination of 125 litter and ambulatory patients. The C-141B transported more than half a million patients during the Vietnam War. Again, the cost of maintaining this aircraft with its low-bypass turbofan engines was prohibitive, especially considering that the lift requirement could be met by the C-17 and KC-135.

The AE component of the Civil Reserve Air Fleet (CRAF) was canceled about 10 years ago. The cost of storing and maintaining the conversion kits that would have transformed CRAF Boeing 767s into AE platforms was surprisingly high. Furthermore, airlines signed up for AE CRAF were required to provide training for the crews who would serve on the 767s when called up. This became such a cost burden that airline companies stopped signing up for AE CRAF, resulting in AMC terminating the program.

Civilian Aircraft Utilized for Aeromedical Evacuation

The vast majority of civilian AE missions are moving only one patient [3]. They frequently make use of en route stops to move patients over long distances; e.g., moving patients from the Western Pacific to the United States. Almost all aircraft used by commercial AE companies have good temperature and noise control.

All reputable civilian air ambulance systems have access to the exact mix of doctors, nurses, and technicians needed to meet any patient's needs. A list of typical equipment that should be immediately available for aeromedical evacuation of stabilized litter patients is provided in Table 5.3. Three of the most commonly used aircraft are described as follows.

Table 5.3 Equipment commonly required for aeromedical evacuation of stabilized patients

Equipment
Electrical outlets with 115-V/60-cycle current
Oxygen
Oxygen monitor
IV pumps capable of supporting three lines per pump
Suction device
Defibrillator with pacing capability
End-tidal carbon dioxide monitor
Ventilator

Abbreviation: *IV* intravenous

Learjet 35 and 36

The Learjet 35 is among the most frequently used aircraft in civilian AE. This twin-engine jet carries 6 passengers at a cruising speed of 481 mph with a range of more than 3000 miles. The Learjet 36 is almost identical to the Learjet 35, except that it has a larger fuel tank, which extends its range by 500 miles but also reduces the passenger area length by 18 inches.

Most civilian companies who move patients by air use one of these twin-engine Learjet models to move one patient together with a medical attendant and one or two of their family members. The cabin is arranged so a medical attendant is seated beside the patient with access to all the medical equipment required to care for the patient. Since the vast majority of civilian requests to move a patient are for only one patient, this jet is ideal. In the continental United States, the company MedJet uses Learjet aircraft for around 90% of their moves.

The Learjet 35 is the civilian version of the USAF C-21A, so it has all of the strengths and weaknesses described in the discussion of the C-21A with one exception. Since the civilian version is not primarily designed to move distinguished visitors there is no need for a closet near the front of the cabin. Therefore, loading litter patients is easier, although still somewhat challenging.

Challenger 601-3R

The Challenger 601-3R is reflective of the wide variety of aircraft used to move patients in the civilian air ambulance industry (Fig. 5.9). It is highly capable as shown in the following discussion.

General Characteristics

This twin-engine jet is among the most capable jets serving the civilian AE mission, and is the only true wide-body aircraft used in the general aviation AE role today. With a cabin width of 8 ft 2 in, it is capable of seating ambulatory patients three or four abreast (Fig. 5.9). The cabin height of 6 ft 1 in allows for comfortable movement of patients and

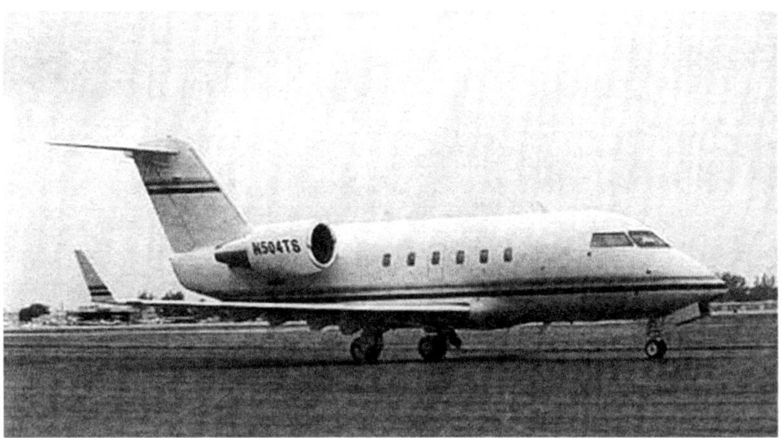

Fig. 5.9 Challenger 601-3R

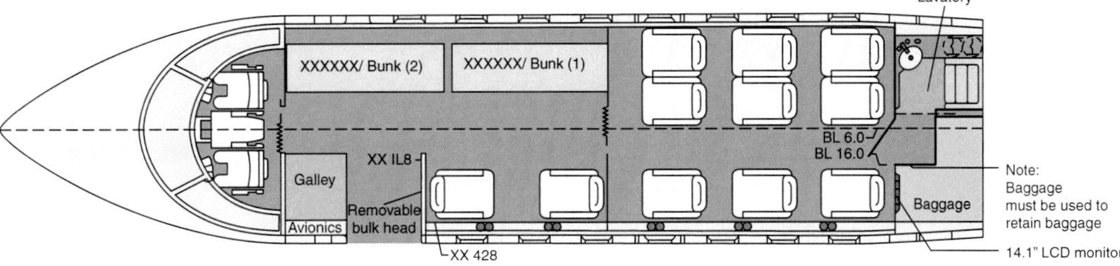

Fig. 5.10 Schematic of Challenger 601 configured for both litter and ambulatory patients

medical crew but is significantly shorter than any of the USAF aircraft previously described except the C-21. It has a cruise speed exceeding 500 mph and a range of 3400 nautical miles.

Strengths

The greatest strength of this airframe, as well as others used by the civilian air ambulance industry, is the robust list of equipment available for each mission and the outstanding crew-to-patient ratio. This ratio is possible because of the limited number of patients carried in most missions. Noise within the cabin is less than the C-9 and lighting is excellent. The cabin environment is easily temperature controlled, primarily due to its relatively small size.

Weaknesses

Although the Challenger 601 has a longer range than the C-9A, it is still not long enough for transoceanic missions without en route stops. Therefore, the same considerations described in using the C-9A for a transoceanic role apply to this aircraft. This airframe can move relatively few patients. The maximum capacity is 2 litters and up to 9 ambulatory patients, as long as none require extensive nursing care. Cabin space is adequate for crew movement but less than any of the USAF airframes described previously. Loading of litter patients is possible without undue tilting of the litter but is still more difficult than loading any of USAF aircraft.

Configuration

The configuration remains as shown in Fig. 5.10 for virtually all missions, although both litter positions in the intensive care part of the cabin are not used in all missions. The seats shown in the diagram can be used for either ambulatory patients or medical crew members, depending on the requirements of the patients.

Summary

The Challenger 601 is a highly capable AE airframe and is representative of the highest level of AE capability available in the general aviation environment. There are multiple other jet aircraft used in the commercial AE mission, including the Lockheed 731, the Hawker 3A, the Falcon 50, and the G-3, all of which have essentially the same strengths and weaknesses described above.

Commercial Airline Seats

For certain patients, the urgency to move may preclude waiting for a properly equipped and staffed AE airframe. In certain cases, commercial airline service can be used to meet the needs of a patient requiring medical transport who is not ill enough to require a flying intensive care unit.

Such patient transports are accomplished with the consent of the airline company by purchasing 2 side-by-side first-class seats. This allows the patient to rest appropriately on long flights and provides the medical attendant immediate access to the patient. This method has been used by commercial AE companies in the Western Pacific region, where multinational companies have small numbers of US citizens working in many nations separated by thousands of miles of ocean. Most of these countries lack Western-quality medical service but have airline service, thus making such moves practical with little delay.

Using this technique, one can safely move a patient for under $10,000, which compares favorably to a commercial AE service, which can cost as much as $50,000 to $100,000. Several airlines have stopped allowing litter patients on flights, so civilian companies (e.g., MedJet) use medium-range commercial jets to move patients via en route stops.

References

1. Guerdan BR. United States Air Force aeromedical evacuation—a critical disaster response resource. Am J Clin Med. 2011;8:153–6.
2. Department of the Air Force. C-130 Configuration and Mission Planning. Washington, DC: US Government Printing Office; 1997. MCI 11-258.
3. Tursch M, Kvam AM, Meyer M, Veldman A, Diefenbach M. Stratification of patients in long-distance, international, fixed-wing aircraft. Air Med J. 2013;32(3):164–9.

Preparation for Long-Distance Aeromedical Evacuation

6

Warren C. Dorlac, Phillip E. Mason, and Gina R. Dorlac

Introduction

The nature of combat and disaster casualty care, especially for trauma patients, can present extraordinary clinical and logistical challenges. Current US Department of Defense (DoD) doctrine emphasizes a tailored deployed medical footprint in theater, necessitating transfer of the casualty through staged, geographically disparate sites of care. Long-term care for casualties in theater is usually not possible because of limited clinical support facilities. Likewise, after natural or manmade disasters, it is unlikely that nearby medical facilities will be available to care for large numbers of recovering patients. As a result, patients must often be transported potentially long distances shortly after or even before they have received definitive care for their injuries.

W. C. Dorlac (✉)
Col, USAF, MC, FS (ret.), Trauma and Acute Care Surgery, Department of Surgery, Medical Center of the Rockies and the University of Colorado School of Medicine, University of Colorado Health, Trauma Services, Loveland, CO, USA
e-mail: Warren.Dorlac@uchealth.org

P. E. Mason
Lt Col, USAF, MC, Department of Surgery, San Antonio Military Medical Center, Fort Sam Houston, TX, USA

G. R. Dorlac
Col, USAF, MC (ret.), Critical Care Medicine and Pulmonary Disease, University of Colorado Health, Fort Collins, CO, USA

Transport of critical care patients can be fraught with complications and whenever possible is deferred until the patient is stable. Air transport multiplies those risks. For this reason, aeromedical evacuation (AE) of critically injured casualties should be approached as a procedure that exposes patients to additional risks brought on by the transport itself. When movement of critically ill patients is required, patient selection and pre-transport preparation become vital for minimizing transport-related complications [1].

Physiologic Stressors of Aeromedical Evacuation

The air transport environment is physiologically hostile to patients in a number of ways. Physiologic stressors common in the AE environment include hypoxemia, hypobarism, noise, vibration, temperature variations, decreased humidity, and acceleration/deceleration forces. Particularly during long-distance transports, the AE environment can make it difficult to recognize, diagnose, and/or treat a deteriorating patient. Each of these physiologic stressors can exacerbate illness and injuries, and should be appropriately addressed whenever possible. Johannigman et al. provide recommendations for addressing many of the physiologic stressors encountered during AE [2].

W. W. Hurd, W. Beninati (eds.), *Aeromedical Evacuation*,
https://doi.org/10.1007/978-3-030-15903-0_6

Hypoxia related to decreased altitude is the most profound physiologic insult to casualties during AE. Tissue hypoxia is a particular concern in the combat casualty with traumatic brain injury (TBI), extremity compartment syndrome, bowel anastomotic ischemia, burn wound, and soft tissue wounds that appear to be at increased risk of infection. Fortunately, oxygen supplementation is routinely administered to high-risk AE patients and oxygen saturation can be easily monitored.

The hypobaric environment at altitude is clinically significant because of the associated gas expansion. Upon ascent to cruising altitude, AE cabin pressure is typically maintained at an altitude equivalent of less than 8000 feet above sea level. This decrease in pressure results in an approximately 18% increase in the volume of any gas collection in the body. Unfortunately, even minimal expansion of trapped gas in some locations (intracranial, intraocular) can be dangerous or catastrophic. When absolutely necessary, flight altitude restriction can minimize hypobarism, but only a few military AE aircraft can maintain cabin altitude pressure near sea level using this technique (see Chap. 8).

The noise and vibration associated with AE can be significant stressors for both patients and medical attendants. Noise impedes both communication and situational awareness for staff as they monitor patients and life support equipment. Helicopters used for short-distance medical evacuation (MEDEVAC) and military cargo planes commonly used for long-distance military AE are well known for the excessive noise and vibration in their patient care environments. Noise levels should be mitigated for both AE patients and crew members through the use of hearing protection. The effects of vibration can be limited by padding litters and loading patients toward the center of the air frame away from the fuselage whenever possible.

Another stress of AE is variations in cabin temperature. At cruising altitude, outside ambient air temperature is well below freezing. In contrast to modern passenger jets, cargo aircraft temperature regulation can be suboptimal and temperatures have been known to fall below 55 °F. All patients should be closely observed for cold stress, and warming blankets should be available [2].

The relative humidity of cabin air at cruising attitude is low, particularly in cargo aircraft, and can increase the risk of patient dehydration. Throughout an AE flight, oral fluids should be provided, and intravenous fluid infusion rates should be liberal. Contact lens use should be discouraged and patients complaining of dry eyes should be offered eye lubrication. Ventilators used for AE should employ air humidifiers and heating devices.

Acceleration and deceleration forces during aircraft takeoff and landings increase gravitational forces by <1.0 G in an aft or fore direction respectively. These changes are insignificant for most AE patients. However, these forces can increase intracranial pressure (ICP) of patients with head injuries transported in a supine position. To minimize the effects of these forces, these patients should be loaded onto AE aircraft with their heads forward with the heads of their beds elevated 30° [2].

Preflight Assessment and Stabilization

The value of careful and thorough assessment and preparation of critically ill patients prior to long-distance AE cannot be overstated. AE crews and medical transport teams should make every effort to arrive at the patient's bedside with as much lead time as possible prior to departure (Fig. 6.1). When medical transport teams are co-located with the sending facility, sequential patient visits over a period of time will allow thorough preparation and assessment while avoiding excessive fatigue just prior to a long flight.

Unfortunately, logistical factors may limit preparation time, especially in a contingency environment. Thus, transport teams must be prepared to conduct a rapid assessment and preparation when required, and every effort should be undertaken to optimize preparation for all patients. The importance of adequate time for preflight preparation should also be recognized

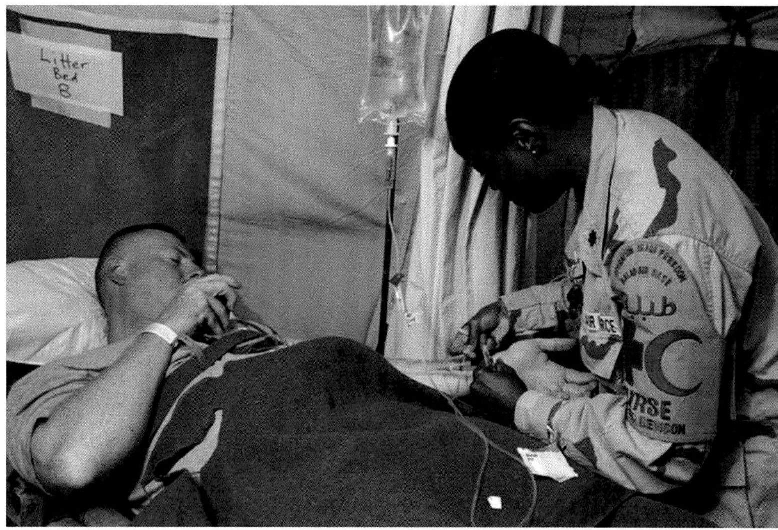

Fig. 6.1 A wounded US Army soldier being prepared for aeromedical evacuation (AE) at a Contingency Aeromedical Staging Facility at Balad Air Base, Iraq. (US National Archives photo)

by planners who assign missions to particular medical transport teams.

Prior to long-distance AE, all life-threatening concerns must be evaluated and stabilized. Each patient's history and clinical condition must be reviewed in a systematic fashion, with attention given to minimizing risks of AE transport. All invasive procedures that are likely to be needed should be accomplished prior to transport, since even minor or routine procedures will be more difficult or impossible to perform in the AE environment. For all patients, oxygenation and ventilation should be optimized, hemorrhage controlled, coagulopathy characterized and treatment initiated, contamination limited, and fractures stabilized prior to flight. Patients with borderline ventilator function should be intubated on the ground if there is more than a low likelihood intubation will be required en route. The approach to individual AE patients will vary depending on the level of care they have received prior to transport.

Equipment and Supplies

Medical equipment brought aboard an aircraft is required to have flight worthiness certification to ensure that the equipment does not interfere with aircraft avionics. In special cases, waivers can be obtained to use uncertified medical equipment during AE. In addition to flight safety, flight worthiness testing certifies that the equipment can perform at the decreased pressures associated with flight altitude. Some equipment, particularly ventilators, must be able to compensate for decreased ambient pressure to ensure appropriate tidal volumes.

The AE environment limits the ability to monitor patients because of noise and space limitations. Audible alarms are almost impossible to hear because of the noise of the AE environment. Monitors must be mounted so that their displays and alarm lights are clearly visible to medical providers. Newer equipment has been designed with improved visual interfaces to aid in earlier recognition of a patient's deteriorating condition. Some patients might have to be located out of the line of sight of AE crew members. The importance of carefully coordinating the exact plan for patient loading cannot be overemphasized.

Preflight Checklists

Pre-transport checklists have become an integral part of both military and civilian AE [3]. The dedicated and consistent use of checklists has been shown to decrease serious unexpected events during intrahospital patient transport by almost 50% [4]. AE checklists (Table 6.1) target potential complications.

Table 6.1 Long-range aeromedical transport checklist

Preflight
Begin AE documentation record
Review patient record
Examine patient, tubes; assess patency of lines
Review all medications (antibiotics, DVT chemoprophylaxis, seizure prophylaxis, pain meds, sedation meds, hypertonic saline, DDAVP, oral care)
Review I&Os
Review chest X-ray (for ETT, central line location, pneumothorax, pneumonia, chest tube placement)
Review monitoring plan ($ETCO_2$, EKG, pulse oximetry, ICP monitoring)
Oral-gastric tube placement (increased risk ileus/aspiration)
Review ventilator management plan:
FiO_2 and PEEP requirements
Lung protective strategy
$ETCO_2$
Measure/trend
Peak inspiratory pressure
Plateau pressure
Confirm blood analysis system function/calibration
Blood analysis system cartridges:
Type
Quantity
Calculate oxygen transport needs
Risk of abdominal compartment syndrome
Laboratory review:
HgB > 8.0
Lactate
Arterial blood gas
Intravenous access
Arterial line
Foley bladder catheter
Sedation plan
Pain management plan:
Consider peripheral pain catheter need
Antibiotic plan
Nutrition plan
Oral care plan
Need for contact precautions
Positioning concerns (enplaned head first, head of elevated, infection control)
Obtain all documentation and images
Communicate with transferring team
AT time of patient pickup
Medical records/images obtained
Reassess the patient for any changes:
Fit to fly determination? (Oxygenation, ICP monitoring, infection)
Ensure a secure airway:
ETT cuff location/cuff pressure
Place on transport ventilator:
HME
Obtain repeat arterial blood gases prior to movement
Altitude compensation required
Confirm sufficient oxygen for entire transport
SMEED setup
IV pumps:
Bleed air from bags/lines
Fluid type/rate
Suction devices:
Chest tubes
NG tube
Wound VAC
DVT prophylaxis: SCDs Low molecular weight heparin
Patient comfort:
Earplugs
Adequate litter padding
Eye protection need
Eye lubrication
Temperature regulation plan
Blood product needs assessment
Specific injuries
Traumatic brain injury:
Need for ICP monitoring:
ICP elevation treatment algorithm
EDV management plan
Head of bed elevation
Antiseizure meds
DDAVP for diabetes insipidus
Temperature control plan
Spinal cord injury:
Cervical spine collar padded (Miami J or Occian Back)
Need for vacuum spine board
Logroll plan
Positioning concerns (head of bed elevation)
Recent abdominal surgery:
NG to suction
Wound VAC to suction
Drains
Feeding tube
Burns:
JTS burn resuscitation document
Inhalation injury plan
Resuscitation plan
Resuscitation fluid type and sufficient volume

Table 6.1 (continued)

Check pulses
Need for escharotomy or fasciotomy
Extremity injuries:
Adequate pre-transport exam
Adequate pulses
Need for fasciotomy
Assess splint tightness
Avoid constricting circumferential dressings
Plan for exsanguinating bleeding (tourniquet availability)
Shock:
Vasopressors:
Type
Adequate supply
Fluid resuscitation plan
Pulse pressure variability:
Trend
Measurement

Abbreviations: *AE* aeromedical evacuation, *DDAVP* desmopressin, *DI* diabetes insipidus, *DVT* deep vein thrombosis, *EDV* electronic depressurizing valve, *EKG* electrocardiogram, $ETCO_2$ end-tidal carbon dioxide, *ETT* endotracheal tube, FiO_2 fraction of inspired oxygen, *HgB* hemoglobin, *HME* heat and moisture exchanger, *I&Os* patient intake and output, *ICP* intracranial pressure, *IV* intravenous, *JTS* Joint Trauma System, *NG* nasogastric, *PEEP* positive end-expiratory pressure, *SCD* sequential compression device, *SMEED* special medical emergency evacuation device; *wound VAC* vacuum-assisted wound closure device

General Preparation and Preventive Treatment

Tubes and Lines

The proper placement and function of all tubes, lines, and drains should be assessed prior to transport, since insertion of new lines and drains may be difficult or impossible in flight. The transport team should both aspirate and infuse fluid through all intravenous lines, inspect the arterial line waveforms and accuracy of blood pressure (BP), check that all drains are patent, and empty all collection systems prior to departure. Proper placement of endotracheal tubes (ETTs) should be verified by X-ray and all circuits examined for leaks. Urinary catheter collection systems should be placed prior to AE for all severely injured casualties in order to continuously and accurately measure urine output.

Gas-Filled Devices

Non-vented gas will expand at flight cabin altitude, as previously discussed. For this reason, ETT balloons and air splints must be monitored closely so that they maintain the recommended pressure of 20–30 mm Hg. ETT balloon expansion at altitude causes increases to as high as 80 mm Hg, and the resultant pressure on the endotracheal mucosa can result in ischemic injury. It is no longer recommended that ETT balloons be filled with water to avoid this problem, since nondistensible water has been shown to increase the risk of pressure necrosis of tracheal mucosal [5].

ETT balloons and air splints should be filled with air. The pressure of these devices should be recalibrated with a manometer before and after both aircraft ascent and descent. Newer methods of automatic ETT cuff pressure adjustment during changes in altitude have been tested successfully in altitude chambers [6]. Air within intravenous fluid bags should also be monitored closely during AE flights since its expansion can cause line disconnection or increased air pockets within the tubing.

Venous Thromboembolism (VTE) Prophylaxis

Venous thromboembolism (VTE) prophylaxis is recommended for trauma patients, unless it is contraindicated by their medical condition. Low molecular weight heparin is most commonly used for this purpose in trauma patients, including those with serious head injuries without progression of intracranial pathology on computed tomography (CT) or other anticoagulation contraindications such as coagulopathy or active bleeding [7]. Sequential compression devices (SCDs) are not commonly utilized during AE. If the patient arrives with SCDs in place, they should be discontinued if it cannot be verified that the pump device has been certified for air worthiness.

Pain Control

Pain and discomfort should be controlled throughout all phases of flight. Intubated patients are typically managed with sedative and narcotic infusions that allow titration during the mission. Patients with traumatic brain injury (TBI) may need augmentation of analgesics and sedatives to avoid the increases in intracranial pressure (ICP) caused by pain and external stimuli. In the event of increased ICP, a sedation bolus can be administered to verify that sedation is adequate.

Pain, particularly when related to bone fractures, is exacerbated by the motion and vibration associated with transport. Peripheral pain catheters or nerve blocks should be considered in all isolated extremity injuries as they provide improved pain relief [8].

Neuromuscular Blockade

Indications for neuromuscular blockade are generally the same is in the hospital. During high-risk periods where patient access and line of sight monitoring may be impaired, a bolus dose of a non-depolarizing agent may add some degree of protection from unexpected patient movement, self-extubation, or other harmful events.

Nutrition

Appropriate nutrition is an integral part of long-distance AE, which can be >10 hours in duration. Providing food and drink to conscious patients is a major task in a large AE mission.

Nutritional support for unconscious and semi-conscious trauma patients provided via enteral tube feeding (ETF) has been shown to be important. If ETF has been started prior to AE, it should be continued when feasible. In an effort to prevent aspiration, an oral gastric tube should be placed for continuous gastric decompression and an ETF advanced distal to the ligament of Treitz. These patients should be monitored closely during AE for abdominal distension due to either postoperative ileus or intestinal gaseous expansion that occurs at altitude [9].

AE patients receiving ETF should be placed in a semi-recumbent position with head elevated using a NATO litter backrest. These patients should also receive stress ulcer prophylaxis usually in the form of histamine-2 receptor antagonists or proton pump inhibitors [10].

Prevention of Hyperthermia and Hypothermia

The ambient cabin temperatures during AE can be difficult to monitor and control, as discussed earlier. While this is primarily a comfort issue in healthy passengers, hypo- and hyperthermia are physiologic stressors that should be avoided in all patients. For trauma patients, regular temperature monitoring and maintenance of normothermia is important to prevent secondary injury related to increased ischemia, inflammation, or edema. Mitigating the effects of low or high cabin temperatures during AE can be accomplished with blankets or external cooling techniques as necessary.

Temperature control appears to be particularly important in patients with traumatic brain injury (TBI). While induced hypothermia in severe TBI was once considered to be beneficial, the standard has become to maintain normothermia [11–14]. For TBI patients, in addition to hypotension and hypoxemia, hyperthermia has been shown to be an important predictor of mortality and is associated with increased ICP [4, 15, 16].

Preventing Compartment Syndrome

Soft tissue, particularly when injured, appears to be subject to edema related to the decreased cabin pressure associated with AE. For this reason, circumferential dressings should be avoided or closely monitored in flight to ensure that they do not become constricting, impairing venous return and eventually arterial flow. Tight-fitting casts should be bivalved prior to AE.

Compartment syndrome risk is high in combat patients exposed to blast or thermal injury, especially in those who are intubated and have received large crystalloid resuscitations. For patients discovered to have significantly increased compartment pressures, fasciotomy should be performed before transport [17].

Wound Care

Negative pressure wound therapy (wound VAC, vacuum-assisted wound closure device) has become the standard of care for the management of soft tissue wounds and is commonly used for trauma patients in the AE environment. The ability to troubleshoot these devices and repair leaks within the system is crucial to their success.

When maintenance of suction is not possible, the occlusive dressings should be removed and replaced with moist dressings, but this is far from ideal [18]. Open abdomen type of dressings will require continuous suctioning and thus the appropriate suction tubing and equipment will be required.

Respiratory Considerations

Critically ill patients should be routinely provided with therapeutic oxygen during AE. Some aircraft routinely used for AE (e.g., C-17, KC-135) are equipped to provide patient oxygen via the onboard aircraft system. However, other aircraft (e.g., C-130) do not have this ability, and oxygen for AE patients must be carried onboard in liquid or compressed gaseous form. Transport teams need to calculate the amount of oxygen required for the flight and coordinate as required to make certain it is available. One common approach is to use the most pessimistic assumptions when calculating AE oxygen requirements and then add 50–100% as a safety margin.

Patients with hypoxia at ground level are of special concern since oxygen partial pressure decreases in parallel to decreasing cabin pressure. Patients with borderline or worsening hypoxia should be intubated and placed on a ventilator prior to AE because deteriorating pulmonary status can be difficult to treat in flight. Similarly, extubation should be avoided immediately (12–24 hours) prior to transport as intubation during transport is challenging and tube placement is more difficult to confirm. Chest radiograph should be available on the day of transport to confirm proper endotracheal tube placement.

Monitoring of O_2 saturation and end-tidal carbon dioxide ($ETCO_2$) is required during AE in order to avoid hypoxia and fluctuations in partial pressure of carbon dioxide ($PaCO_2$) [19]. Continuous waveform capnography is also valuable as a visual monitor that instantaneously alerts the provider to certain maladies including endotracheal tube (ETT) dislodgment, airway obstruction, ventilator malfunction, and ventilator circuit disconnection. Ventilator-associated pneumonia prophylaxis should include oral care and elevation of the head of the litter. Subglottic suction device ETTs can be used, with intermittent syringe evacuation of the subglottic fluid collection.

Ventilator-Dependent Patients

For ventilated patients, two effective means of addressing hypoxia are increasing either fraction of inspired oxygen (FiO_2) or the positive end-expiratory pressure (PEEP). Although it was previously believed that higher levels of PEEP decrease cerebral perfusion pressure (CPP) by increasing thoracic venous pressure and thus increasing ICP, more recent studies have demonstrated that increasing PEEP decreases ICP and thus increases CPP [20]. Because PEEP is an effective means of treating pulmonary injury after trauma, appropriate use of PEEP is recommended during AE transport of critically ill patients [21]. Strict adherence to guideline tidal volume, peak inspiratory pressure, and PEEP during AE has been shown to result in a lower incidence of acute respiratory distress, acute respiratory failure, and ventilator-associated pneumonia [22].

Pneumothorax and Hemothorax

Pneumothorax and hemothorax are common after trauma and the majority of critical casualties with these conditions will be transported with chest tubes. Stable small pneumothoraces are often left untreated since they are unlikely to create a problem. However, AE will result in some degree of trapped gas expansion, which could adversely affect a trauma patient [23]. For this reason, standard US Air Force (USAF) practice is to decompress all pneumothoraces prior to movement in a fixed-wing aircraft. Once placed, chest tubes should not be removed within 24 hours of flight to minimize risks of symptomatic pneumothorax during the flight [24, 25].

Pre-transport evaluation of the patient with a chest tube should include review of that day's chest radiograph, chest tube output, and examination for air leaks. Chest tube drainage systems should be carefully secured during transport. Modern dry drainage systems use a dial to set suction pressure rather than a fluid column as was used in the previous wet systems.

Hemodynamic Considerations

Measuring blood pressure by auscultation in the AE environment is extremely difficult because of increased noise levels. Thus, automatic noninvasive blood pressure cuffs are routinely used. However, automated non-invasive blood pressure cuffs can be less accurate in the high-vibration environments of AE aircraft. For this reason, arterial lines are often employed in critically injured and ill patients for continuous blood pressure monitoring.

Hypovolemic casualties should be volume resuscitated prior to AE. If further transfusion is anticipated, blood products should be transported with the patient. While vasopressors can be used to support blood pressure, aggressive and balanced approach to blood product resuscitation is preferable [26]. As a result, AE flight crews increasingly carry blood products to obtain this survival advantage by adhering to the recommended 1:1:1 ratio of PRBC-plasma-platelets for transfusions [27].

In-flight point of care (POC) testing can over- or underestimate hemoglobin, so decisions to transfuse during AE should be based on a complete clinical assessment and not just a change in hemoglobin from POC testing compared to sending hospital laboratory results [28]. A baseline hemoglobin obtained on the POC device prior to transport for trending may prevent unnecessary transfusion.

Gastrointestinal Considerations

Patients who have recently undergone laparotomy will be more susceptible to gas expansion during ascent to altitude. The routine use of nasogastric tubes for non-intubated patients or orogastric tubes for intubated patients is recommended for these patients during AE.

Metabolic Considerations

Electrolytes

Electrolyte levels from the day of transport should be available for critical patients. Extreme electrolyte abnormalities should be corrected before transport. For less severe abnormalities, electrolyte replacement started before transport should be continued. If renal failure is of a concern and pre-transport dialysis is not available, alternative methods of electrolyte management may be necessary in flight.

Glycemic Control

Hyperglycemia and hypoglycemia are associated with increased mortality of critically ill patients. Hyperglycemia is common in critically ill patients and has been shown to exacerbate secondary brain injury and is an independent predictor of outcome [29]. Alternatively, hypoglycemia can also adversely affect outcome and is more common with tight glucose control (80–110 mg/dL) versus moderate control (120–150 mg/dL) [30]. For these reasons, moderate control of blood sugar (120–150 mg/dL) is recommended, and frequent checks during transport should be performed. Although the accuracy of older POC glucometers used for AE were affected by variable altitudes, humidity, and temperature, the newer blood analysis systems do not appear to have this problem [31].

Infectious Disease Considerations

During AE, extra precautions must be taken when transporting patients with serious infections to avoid cross-contamination of other patients and crew members. Most patients with infectious diseases can be safely transported by AE using basic infection control standard precautions, including hand hygiene and standard personal protective equipment. However, this is not the case with highly contagious, quarantinable diseases including cholera, diphtheria, infectious tuberculosis, plague, smallpox, yellow fever, viral hemorrhagic fevers, and severe acute respiratory syndromes. Patients with these diseases undergoing AE require additional transmission-based precautions (i.e., contact precautions, droplet precautions, airborne precautions) to protect the other patients, medical personnel, and aircrew and to fulfill international public health regulations (Fig. 6.2). More details can be found in Chap. 11.

Patients with known bacterial infections should be transported with a supply of appropriate antibiotics adequate to treat them until they reach the receiving medical facility. However, occasionally untreated patients might develop a clinical picture of sepsis syndrome during an AE flight. AE crews routinely carry a supply of broad-spectrum antibiotics, which can be started empirically based on the recommendations of the originating physician. However, AE crews do not routinely carry supplies necessary to collect cultures prior to initiating antibiotics during transport.

For trauma patients with open wounds, avoiding secondary infection becomes an important goal. Supplemental oxygen during AE is recommended for these patients, since it has been shown to significantly reduced bacterial growth in wounds [32]. Bathing of trauma patients with cloths impregnated with 2% chlorhexidine gluconate, a common military approach during the early years of recent Middle East conflicts, decreases bacterial colonization in surgical intensive care units (ICUs), but does not appear to decrease mortality [33, 34].

Avoidance of cross-contamination is an important goal in the AE setting, where multiple patients must remain in a confined space for a matter of hours. To adequately adhere to standard infection control guidelines, gowns and gloves (usually in marked excess of what is anticipated) are required. Typical body fluid precautions must be followed and sharps disposal containers used. Patients known to have highly contagious diseases are transported in isolation chambers.

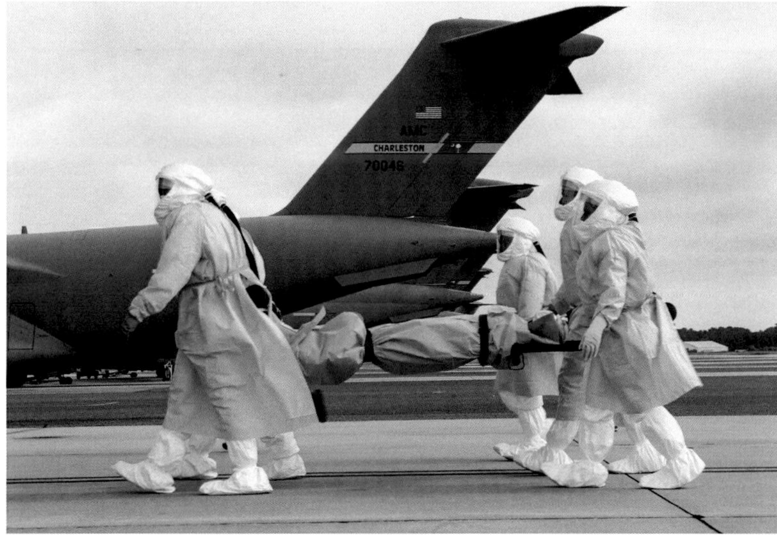

Fig. 6.2 Airmen transport a simulated infectious patient during an aeromedical evacuation (AE) training exercise at Joint Base Charleston, South Carolina. (US Air Force photo by A1C Joshua R. Maund)

Neurologic Injuries

Head Injuries

Traumatic brain injury (TBI) can result in significant cerebral edema, which is a major cause of morbidity and mortality in these patients. Cerebral edema in TBI has been attributed to blood-brain barrier leak (i.e., vasogenic edema), ischemia and inflammatory-ionic dysfunction (i.e., cellular edema), and loss of autoregulation leading to vascular engorgement [35]. Cerebral edema is exacerbated by hypoxia and hypotension and begins immediately post-TBI and reaches a peak by day 3–5 [36].

The hypobaric environment of AE appears to exacerbate cerebral hypoxia and perhaps worsen neuroinflammation [37]. Necessitating early movement may also factor into the transport timing decision. However, based on lack of contingency hospital capacity, the common co-existence of other injuries and other logistical considerations, military patients and disaster casualties with severe TBI are usually transported to a higher echelon of care as soon as possible.

A key principle of TBI care is to avoid hypoxia. Prehospital hypoxia, which is common in TBI patients, significantly increases mortality [38]. During AE transport TBI patients should be given supplemental oxygen and their oxygen saturation closely monitored using pulse oximetry. TBI patients determined to have borderline oxygenation should be intubated and placed on a ventilator prior to AE. However, it must be kept in mind that intubation can result in complications in patients with TBI, such as transient hypoxia, bradycardia, hypotension, and increased ICP [4].

Another key principle of TBI care is to avoid hypotension. Early hypotensive episodes following brain injury doubles the mortality and is likely to have a significant impact on long-term outcome. Hypotensive episode (mean arterial pressure [MAP] < 70) in TBI patients (Glasgow Coma Scale [GCS] ≤ 8) increases both morbidity and mortality [13]. For this reason frequent noninvasive blood pressure monitoring or continuous invasive blood pressure monitoring is highly recommended during AE transport of patients with severe TBI.

Seizures are a common complication of TBI. As a result, TBI patients are routinely given empiric prophylaxis with antiepileptics, which has been shown to significantly decrease the risk of seizure during the first week after injury [39]. This has led to the current recommendation of a loading dose of antiepileptics followed by 7 days of prophylaxis for TBI patients. Although phenytoin was most commonly used in the past, levetiracetam is now more commonly used due to its ease of administration.

Central diabetes insipidus (DI) is another common complication for patients with moderate/severe TBI [40]. The most common symptoms of DI include polydipsia, polyuria, and nocturia due to the defect in concentrating urine. Unrecognized, this can result in hypovolemia and hypernatremia. For this reason, monitoring of urine output for these patients during AE is critical. If electrolyte assessment is not available, treatment should be started based on clinical suspicion alone.

Treatment of DI consists of fluid replacement until urine output is decreased. When transporting patients with moderate/severe TPI, preflight AE preparation should include extra crystalloid fluids and a supply of desmopressin (synthetic vasopressin).

Intracranial Pressure Monitoring

Intracranial pressuring monitoring (ICP) is recommended for patients with severe TBI (GCS ≤ 8) who meet the following criteria [41, 42]:

- CT scan evidence of intracranial pathology
- No CT evidence of intracranial pathology but at least two of the following:
  - >40 years of age
  - Hypotensive episode with systolic blood pressure (SBP) < 90 mm Hg
  - Abnormal motor posturing (unilateral or bilateral)

The best estimate of cerebral blood flow is cerebral perfusion pressure (CPP), defined as the difference between the mean arterial pressure (MAP) and ICP:

Table 6.2 Increased intracranial pressure (ICP) treatment algorithm. (Goal: maintain ICP < 20–25 mm Hg)

1. Elevate head of bed >30°
2. Position head in midline
3. Decrease cervical collar tightness
4. Titrate $PaCO_2$ to 35–40 mm Hg
5. Treat hypoxia; maintain saturation ≥95%
6. Treat hypotension; maintain CPP > 60
7. Maintain sodium >145 mEq/L
8. Provide analgesic to treat occult pain
9. Sedate; limit external stimuli
10. Evacuate CSF if ventriculostomy present
11. Consider hyperosmolar therapy
12. Obtain head CT imaging once available
13. Consider treating subclinical seizure activity

Abbreviations: *CPP* cerebral perfusion pressure, *CT* computerized tomography, *$PaCO_2$*, partial pressure of carbon dioxide

$$CPP = MAP - ICP$$

The goal is to maintain CPP > 60 mm Hg (>90–100 mm Hg for severe TBI) by administering isotonic or hypertonic fluid and vasoactive agents when necessary [27, 41, 42]. A treatment algorithm for the management of elevated ICP is provided in Table 6.2.

Historically, mild hyperventilation was used in an effort to lower ICP by causing cerebral vasoconstriction. This practice is no longer recommended since hypocapnia is associated with a worse prognosis [13]. In an effort to avoid hyperventilation (PCO_2 < 25) in patients with severe TBI during AE, continuous end-tidal CO_2 monitoring by capnography is recommended [43]. More details about ICP monitoring can be found in Chap. 14. However, AE crews must be trained to competently use and troubleshoot ICP monitoring devices.

Spinal Cord Injuries

Cervical spine injuries should always be a concern in patients with multisystem trauma, particularly with TBI. Until cervical spine injury can be excluded by clinical examination and imaging, cervical spine protection is recommended [44]. In many cases, this will necessitate the prolonged use of a cervical collar. To reduce the risk of pressure ulcers in these situations, the DoD has approved use of padded Miami J or Occian Back cervical collars [45].

Unstable thoracic and lumbar spine injuries should be transported with the vacuum spine board rather than a rigid spine board due to concerns of decubitus ulcers [46]. During level cruise flight in the absence of turbulence, the vacuum may be released to provide additional protection against pressure injuries while allowing no more movement of the spine than would strict spine precautions in an ICU. However, any turbulence or other potential movement would necessitate reinstitution of vacuum for continuous immobilization.

Spinal blood flow should be maximized by maintaining adequate perfusion pressure. Toward this end, the recommended goal for MAP is 85–90 mm Hg for the first 5–7 days after injury. Norepinephrine is the vasopressor of choice once intravascular volume status has been restored [47].

Patients with unstable spinal injuries should be transported using vacuum spine boards. When a vacuum spine board is not available, an alternative approach is to use a standard, padded NATO litter with additional litter straps to support the mid-section and minimize the flexion and extension of the spine. For this approach, the litter is supported in the mid-section by strapping it to a second litter located above the patient.

Skeletal traction can be applied during AE using spring-loaded devices that measure tension and do not require weights, since free weights would not be stable in flight. However, prolonged skeletal traction is generally not practical during AE and external or internal fixation is preferred.

Administrative Considerations

Extensive regulations need to be followed for all USAF AE. Knowledge of these regulations is critical to avoid delays and allow for the safest possible movement. The streamed regulations for civilian AE differ according to the company providing the service, and are not included here.

Responsibility of Patient Outcome

The responsibilities for in-flight care and outcome are shared by the originating physicians, the AE medical crew, and specialty medical transport teams. The originating physicians should ensure that the patient's condition and ongoing care have been optimized for AE. The AE crew should also ensure this optimization to minimize the chances of the patient's condition deteriorating during flight. The AE crew and medical transport team carry out the clinical goals of the originating physicians and provide a thorough handoff to the receiving medical team.

Adherence to US Central Command Joint Theater Trauma System or Joint Theater System Clinical Practice Guidelines has been instrumental to care, and their knowledge and compliance by all medical care teams, including AE crews, are crucial to improved outcomes [48].

This specialized medical transport team approach for AE was pioneered by the US Army Burn Flight Team program, which has successfully transported burn patients by air for more than 60 years (see Chap. 21). More recently, the US Air Force (USAF) has developed Pediatric/ECMO transport teams. In one study, using specialized pediatric transport teams for interhospital transport has been shown to dramatically increase survival rates from 9% to 23% [49].

This led to the development of USAF Critical Care Air Transport Teams (CCATT) (see Chap. 9). CCAT teams are composed of critical care trained physicians, critical care nurses with current bedside experience, and actively practicing respiratory therapists who undergo specific training in the aeromedical transport of critically ill and traumatized patients. Expertise for CCATT team members in both in critical care and in AE are essential (Fig. 6.3).

Aeromedical Evacuation Crew and Medical Transport Team

A basic AE crew consists of flight nurses and flight medics trained in the aeromedical transport of stable patients. When a doctrinal decision was made to transport stabilized (i.e., potentially unstable) patients, specialized medical transport teams are used to augment the AE crews.

Aircraft Selection

Upon the retirement of the C-9A in 2005, the USAF no longer utilized dedicated AE aircraft (see Chap. 8). However, several aircraft are routinely reconfigured in the field for AE. Aircraft most commonly used for AE today include the KC-135, C-17, and C-130. These, and other less commonly used aircraft, vary substantially in

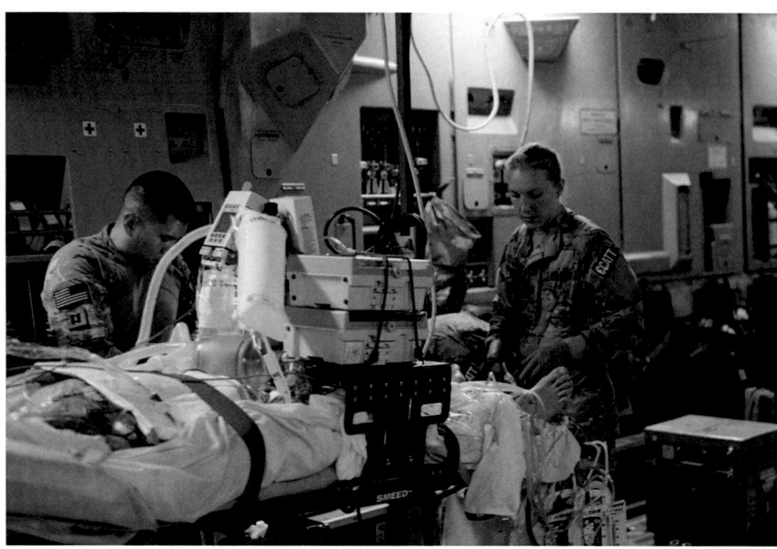

Fig. 6.3 Critical Care Air Transport Team (CCATT) members ensure that a patient is properly secured aboard a C-17 prior to aeromedical evacuation (AE) from Bagram Airfield, Afghanistan, to Ramstein Air Base, Germany. (US Air Force photo by Maj. Tony Wickman)

terms of electrical systems, patient oxygen supply, and temperature control.

The aircraft to be used for each AE mission is determined primarily by a number of non-clinical reasons to include aircraft availability, weather, terrain to be traversed, altitude, and distance to be flown. For extended ranges, other issues come into play such as midair refueling capability versus multiple en route stops for fuel. For select AE missions, clinical factors can also play a roll. Knowledge of the specific aircraft cabin altitude pressurization and oxygen supply are critical.

Selection of Receiving Facility

Careful selection of the receiving facility is extremely important. In some instances, closer facilities will have to be bypassed to reach a location with optimal capabilities—particularly subspecialty care. These capabilities may include imaging resources, a 24-hour operating room, hemodialysis, a burn center, or other subspecialty surgical care [42]. Mortality for severe TBI patients has been shown to decrease by 50% when they were taken directly to trauma centers with appropriate resources [50]. However, the adverse effects of longer transport times should also be considered.

Documentation

Prior to AE, hard copies of all documentation and imaging (reports as well as images) should be obtained and transported with the patient. A detailed discharge summary that includes all medications and their timing of administration is ideal. This is important because patients can be delayed or diverted to unintended locations en route and electronic medical record systems are not always available. Documentation of en route vital signs, medications, lab values, input/output, neurological examinations, and other care provided is often overlooked or done haphazardly. A detailed record of en route care can be vital to ongoing care and should be completed with a level of detail commensurate with the patient's condition.

Transportation to and from the Airfield

In the USAF AE system, specific aeromedical staging facilities and personnel are tasked with the somewhat complex mission of transporting patients to and from the airfield (see Chap. 7). Arrangements must be made for ground transport with sufficient space for the patient, transport team members, and equipment, as well as a sufficient oxygen supply and electrical power. This phase of transport presents unique challenges and can be at least as risky as the much longer in-flight portion of the patient movement. The process of moving patients into and out of vehicles is an opportunity for lines and other devices to become dislodged, kinked, or disconnected. Distractions, impaired patient access, and difficulties with line of sight monitoring are additional risks that should be planned for and mitigated.

Contingency Plans

Prior to each flight, the AE crew director in conjunction with the pilot in command should identify the available stop-off points en route to the final destination in case of aircraft diversion. This will necessitate determination of additional supplies and medications should contingency plans be activated.

References

1. Blakeman TC, Branson RD. Inter- and intra-hospital transport of the critically ill. Respir Care. 2013;58(6):1008–23.
2. Johannigman JA, Zonies D, Dubose J, Blakeman TC, Hanseman D, Branson RD. Reducing secondary insults in traumatic brain injury. Mil Med. 2015;180(3 Suppl):50–5.
3. Davis DP, Peay J, Sise MJ, Vilke GM, Kennedy F, Eastman AB, et al. The impact of prehospital endotracheal intubation on outcome in moderate to severe traumatic brain injury. J Trauma. 2005;58:933–9.
4. Davis DP, Koprowicz KM, Newgard CD, Daya M, Bulger EM, Stiell I, et al. The relationship between out-of-hospital airway management and outcome among trauma patients with Glasgow Coma Scale Scores of 8 or less. Prehosp Emerg Care. 2011;15(2):184–92.

5. Britton T, Blakeman TC, Eggert J, Rodriquez D, Ortiz H, Branson RD. Managing endotracheal tube cuff pressure at altitude: a comparison of four methods. J Trauma Acute Care Surg. 2014;77(3 Suppl 2):S240–4.
6. Blakeman T, Rodriquez D Jr, Woods J, Cox D, Elterman J, Branson R. Automated control of endotracheal tube cuff pressure during simulated flight. J Trauma Acute Care Surg. 2016;81(5 Suppl 2 Proceedings of the 2015 Military Health System Research Symposium):S116–20.
7. Fang R, Dorlac GR, Allan PF, Dorlac WC. Intercontinental aeromedical evacuation of patients with traumatic brain injuries during Operations Iraqi Freedom and Enduring Freedom. Neurosurg Focus. 2010;28(5):El1:1–7.
8. Buckenmaier CC 3rd, Rupprecht C, McKnight G, McMillan B, White RL, Gallagher RM, Polomano R. Pain following battlefield injury and evacuation: a survey of 110 casualties from the wars in Iraq and Afghanistan. Pain Med. 2009;10(8):1487–96.
9. Air Force Instruction 48–307, Volume 1, 8.17.6, from 9 January 2017.
10. Marik PE, Vasu T, Hirani A, Pachinburavan M. Stress ulcer prophylaxis in the new millennium: a systematic review and meta-analysis. Crit Care Med. 2010;38(11):2222–8.
11. Clifton GL, Allen S, Barrodale P, Plenger P, Berry J, Koch S, et al. A phase II study of moderate hypothermia in severe brain injury. J Neurotrauma. 1993;10:263–73.
12. Marion DW, Penrod LE, Kelsey SF, Obrist WD, Kochanek PM, Palmer AM, et al. Treatment of traumatic brain injury with moderate hypothermia. N Engl J Med. 1997;336:540–6.
13. Jeremitsky E, Omert L, Dunham CM, Protetch J, Rodriguez A. Harbingers of poor outcome the day after severe brain injury: hypothermia, hypoxia, and hypoperfusion. J Trauma. 2003;54(2):312–9.
14. Hifumi T, Kuroda Y, Kawakita K, Yamashita S, Oda Y, Dohi K, et al. Fever control management is preferable to mild therapeutic hypothermia in traumatic brain injury patients with Abbreviated Injury Scale 3-4: a multi-center, randomized controlled trial. J Neurotrauma. 2016;33(11):1047–53.
15. Jones PA, Andrews PJ, Midgley S, Anderson SI, Piper IR, Tocher JL, et al. Measuring the burden of secondary insults in head-injured patients during intensive care. J Neurosurg Anesthesiol. 1994;6(1):4–14.
16. Cooper PR, Golfinos JG, editors. Head injury. 4th ed. New York: McGraw-Hill; 2000. p. 239–40.
17. Ritenour AE, Dorlac WC, Fang R, Woods T, Jenkins DH, Flaherty SF, Wade CE, Holcomb JB. Complications after fasciotomy revision and delayed compartment release in combat patients. J Trauma. 2008;64(2 Suppl):S153–61; discussion S161-2.
18. Tuma M, El-Menyar A, Abdelrahman H, Al-Thani H, Zarour A, Parchani A, et al. Prehospital intubation in patients with isolated severe traumatic brain injury: a 4-year observational study. Crit Care Res Pract. 2014;2014:1–6.
19. Fang R, Dorlac WC, Flaherty SF, Tuman C, Cain SM, Popey TL, et al. Feasibility of negative pressure wound therapy during intercontinental aeromedical evacuation of combat casualties. J Trauma. 2010;69(Suppl 1):S140–5.
20. Huynh T, Messer M, Sing RF, Miles W, Jacobs DG, Thomason MH. Positive end-expiratory pressure alters intracranial and cerebral perfusion pressure in severe traumatic brain injury. J Trauma. 2002;53(3):488–92; discussion 492-493
21. Barnes SL, Branson R, Gallo LA, Beck G, Johannigman JA. En-route care in the air: snapshot of mechanical ventilation at 37,000 feet. J Trauma. 2008;64(2 Suppl):S129–134; discussion S134-135.
22. Maddry JK, Mora AG, Savell SC, Perez CA, Mason PE, Aden JK, Bebarta VS. Impact of Critical Care Air Transport Team (CCATT) ventilator management on combat mortality. J Trauma Acute Care Surg. 2018;84(1):157–64.
23. Braude D, Tutera D, Tawil I, Pirkl G. Air transport of patients with pneumothorax: is tube thoracostomy required before flight? Air Med J. 2014;33(4):152–6.
24. Majercik S, White TW, Van Boerum DH, Granger S, Bledsoe J, Conner K, Wilson E, Weaver LK. Cleared for takeoff: the effects of hypobaric conditions on traumatic pneumothoraces. J Trauma Acute Care Surg. 2014;77(5):729–33.
25. Sacco F, Calero KR. Safety of early air travel after treatment of traumatic pneumothorax. Int J Circumpolar Health. 2014;73:1–3.
26. Stephens CT, Gumbert S, Holcomb JB. Trauma-associated bleeding: management of massive transfusion. Curr Opin Anaesthesiol. 2016;29(2):250–5.
27. Murphy CH, Hess JR. Massive transfusion: red blood cell to plasma and platelet unit ratios for resuscitation of massive hemorrhage. Curr Opin Hematol. 2015;22(6):533–9.
28. Tsuei BJ, Hanseman DJ, Blakeman MJ, Blakeman TC, Yang SH, Branson RD, Gerlach TW. Accuracy of noninvasive hemoglobin monitoring in patients at risk for hemorrhage. J Trauma Acute Care Surg. 2014;77(3 Suppl 2):S134–9.
29. Prisco L, Iscra F, Ganau M, Berlot G. Early predictive factors on mortality in head injured patients: a retrospective analysis of 112 traumatic brain injured patients. J Neurosurg Sci. 2012;56(2):131–6.
30. Vespa P, McAnhur DL, Stein N, Huang SC, Shao W, Filippou M, et al. Tight glycemic control increases metabolic distress in traumatic brain injury: a randomized controlled within-subjects trial. Crit Care Med. 2012;40(6):1923–9.
31. Londeree W, Davis K, Helman D, Abadie J. Bodily fluid analysis of non-serum samples using point-of-care testing with iSTAT and Piccolo analyzers versus a fixed hospital chemistry analytical platform. Hawaii J Med Public Health. 2014;73(9 Suppl 1):3–8.
32. Earnest RE, Sonnier DI, Makley AT, Campion EM, Wenke JC, Bailey SR, Dorlac WC, Lentsch AB, Pritts

TA. Supplemental oxygen attenuates the increase in wound bacterial growth during simulated aeromedical evacuation in goats. J Trauma Acute Care Surg. 2012;73(1):80–6.
33. Evans HL, Dellit TH, Chan J, Nathens AB, Maier RV, Cuschieri J. Effect of chlorhexidine whole-body bathing on hospital-acquired infections among trauma patients. Arch Surg. 2010;145(3):240–6.
34. Mohr NM, Pelaez Gil CA, Harland KK, Faine B, Stoltze A, Pearson K, Ahmed A. Prehospital oral chlorhexidine does not reduce the rate of ventilator-associated pneumonia among critically ill trauma patients: a prospective concurrent-control study. J Crit Care. 2015;30(4):787–92.
35. Unterberg AW, Stover J, Kress B, Kiening KL. Edema and brain trauma. Neuroscience. 2004;129(4):1021–9.
36. Bareyre F, Wahl F, McIntosh TK, Stutzmann JM. Time course of cerebral edema after traumatic brain injury in rats: effects of riluzole and mannitol. J Neurotrauma. 1997;14(11):839–49.
37. Goodman MD, Makley AT, Huber NL, Clarke CN, Friend LA, Schuster RM, Bailey SR, Barnes SL, Dorlac WC, Johannigman JA, Lentsch AB, Pritts TA. Hypobaric hypoxia exacerbates the neuroinflammatory response to traumatic brain injury. J Surg Res. 2011;165(1):30–7.
38. Chi JH, Knudson MM, Vassar MJ, McCarthy MC, Shapiro MB, Mallet S, et al. Prehospital hypoxia affects outcome in patients with traumatic brain injury: a prospective multicenter study. J Trauma. 2006;61(5):1134–41.
39. Temkin NR, Dikmen SS, Wilensky AJ, Keihm J, Chabal S, Winn HR. A randomized, double-blind study of phenytoin for the prevention of post-traumatic seizures. N Engl J Med. 1990;323(8):497–502.
40. Silva PP, Bhatnagar S, Herman SD, Zafonte R, Klibanski A, Miller KK, et al. Predictors of hypopituitarism in patients with traumatic brain injury. J Neurotrauma. 2015;32(22):1789–95.
41. Brain Trauma Foundation. Guidelines for the management of severe traumatic brain injury 3rd edition. J Neurotrauma. 2007;24(Supp 1):S1–106.
42. ACS TQIP best practices in the Management of Traumatic Brain Injury. American College of Surgeons Trauma Quality Improvement Program. January 2015.
43. Walsh BK, Crotwell DN, Restrepo RD. American Association for Respiratory Care Clinical Practice Guidelines: capnography/capnometry during mechanical ventilation. Respir Care. 2011;56(4):503–9.
44. Hills MW, Deane SA. Head injury and facial injury: is there an increased risk of cervical spine injury? J Trauma. 1993;34(4):549–53; discussion 553-554
45. Tescher AN, Rindflesch AB, Youdas JW, Jacobson TM, Downer LL, Miers AG, et al. Range-of-motion restriction and craniofacial tissue-interface pressure from four cervical collars. J Trauma. 2007;63(5):1120–6.
46. Rahmatalla S, DeShaw J, Stilley J, Denning G, Jennissen C. Comparing the efficacy of methods for immobilizing the thoracic-lumbar spine. Air Med J. 2018;37(3):178–85.
47. Streijger F, So K, Manouchehri N, Gheorghe A, Okon EB, Chan RM, Ng B, Shortt K, Sekhon MS, Griesdale DE, Kwon BK. A direct comparison between norepinephrine and phenylephrine for augmenting spinal cord perfusion in a porcine model of spinal cord injury. J Neurotrauma. 2018;35:1345.
48. Eastridge BJ, Costanzo G, Jenkins D, Spott MA, Wade C, Greydanus D, Flaherty S, Rappold J, Dunne J, Holcomb JB, Blackbourne LH. Impact of joint theater trauma system initiatives on battlefield injury outcomes. Am J Surg. 2009;198(6):852–7.
49. Orr RA, Felmet KA, Han Y, McCloskey KA, Dragotta MA, Bills DM, et al. Pediatric specialized transport teams are associated with improved outcomes. Pediatrics. 2009;124(1):40–8.
50. Härtl R, Gerber LM, Iacono L, Ni Q, Lyons K, Ghajar J. Direct transport within an organized state trauma system reduces mortality in patients with severe traumatic brain injury. J Trauma. 2006;60(6):1250–6; discussion 1256

Aeromedical Patient Staging

7

Lisa Diane DeDecker and William W. Hurd

Introduction

Aeromedical patient staging refers to the immediate pre- and post-flight medical care, preparation, and ground transportation for patients undergoing aeromedical evacuation (AE) [1]. Staging personnel assist AE flight crews as they enplane and deplane these patients with all required medical supplies and equipment. In many cases, these patients are transported with their personal baggage and/or medical/nonmedical attendants. Patient staging also includes the administrative processing required for any patient movement within the worldwide AE system.

Aeromedical patient staging is carried out on a daily basis at US military aeromedical staging facilities in the continental United States (CONUS) and throughout the world. In addition, the military AE system is prepared to set up and effectively operate staging facilities in combat operation theaters and on very short notice at the site of natural or manmade disasters.

This chapter will describe the various types of staging facilities, their organization, and the numerous services they provide. In addition, typical AE launch and recovery missions will be described.

L. D. DeDecker (✉)
Lt Col, USAF, NC, CFN (ret.), En Route Critical Care Program, Division of En Route Medical Care, Headquarters Air Mobility Command, Command Surgeon's Office, Scott Air Force Base, IL, USA
e-mail: lisa.dedecker.1@us.af.mil

W. W. Hurd
Col, USAF, MC, SFS (ret.), Chief Medical Officer, American Society for Reproductive Medicine, Professor Emeritus Department of Obstetrics and Gynecology, Duke University Medical Center, Durham, NC, USA

Formerly, CCATT physician and Commander, 445th ASTS, Wright-Patterson Air Force Base, Dayton, OH, USA

Aeromedical Staging Facility

An aeromedical staging facility and its personnel include all the elements required for aeromedical staging. A patient-staging facility temporarily maintains and supports patients as they transit the AE system [1]. When required, staging personnel provide short-term complex medical-surgical nursing care to these patients and are prepared to provide limited emergent interventions. A staging facility also must provide all the tasks routinely performed by an air passenger terminal.

The length of stay in a staging facility ranges from 2 to 72 hours. Holding times differ depending on the size of the facility. A large facility will often lodge en route ambulatory patients for up to 3 days, while inpatients are cared for in the host medical treatment facility (MTF) until time for transport to the flight line [1]. In an operational setting, a staging facility must be prepared to

W. W. Hurd, W. Beninati (eds.), *Aeromedical Evacuation*,
https://doi.org/10.1007/978-3-030-15903-0_7

provide around-the-clock nursing care to seriously injured patients immediately prior to an AE flight [2]. On the other end of the spectrum, a ten-bed mobile staging facility must restrict patient holding times to a matter of hours due to the limited amount of space and supplies in the equipment package [3].

Staging personnel must be prepared to provide complex medical/surgical nursing care for patients in the AE system with a wide range of medical conditions, including traumatic injury, cardiac, respiratory, gastrointestinal, genitourinary, neurological, and multi-system illnesses. Skill and experience are often required in managing multiple intravenous and central lines, administering numerous intravenous medications and blood products, performing wound irrigations and dressing changes, and assisting with placement and management of chest tubes. Additionally, knowledge of flight considerations for trauma and medical patients and the stresses of flight is crucial in a staging facility.

A staging facility is not designed to provide care to critically ill patients. These patients will remain at an MTF until immediately before AE. These patients are transported under the care of a Critical Care Air Transport Team (CCATT) and transported from the MTF to the AE aircraft with the assistance of staging vehicles and personnel (see Chap. 9). When the staging facility is located at a significant distance from its host MTF, a flight surgeon or family practice physician is often assigned to the staging facility to assist in stabilizing patients.

Types of Patient-Staging Capability

Four relatively distinct types of staging facilities have been described: (1) in-garrison, which is attached to an MTF and is there permanently; (2) ten-bed mobile; (3) the larger staging facilities that are assembled based on anticipated patient flow, usually 50–100 beds; and (4) disaster staging facilities [1, 4]. Although many of their basic roles are identical, their administrative structure and the details of their strengths and capacities differ considerably.

In-Garrison or Fixed Staging Facility

A fixed staging facility is a designated, numbered unit, attached to a host MTF for administrative and logistical support [1]. They are located in dedicated buildings and staffed by active duty personnel augmented by Air Reserve Component personnel. Like all staging facilities, its primary purpose is to provide continuing nursing care and administrative processing for patients traveling in the AE system on a 24-hour basis. These patients can be inpatients or outpatients who are (1) entering the AE system from a collocated or nearby MTF, (2) arriving from a distant MTF for care proximate to the staging facility, or (3) stopping temporarily at the staging facility en route in the AE system from one MTF to another [1].

Currently, fixed staging facilities are located at Andrews Air Force Base, Maryland; Travis Air Force Base, California; and Lackland Air Force Base, Texas. Although each is co-located with an MTF, the facility at Andrews serves as the primary East Coast hub for aeromedical evacuation and sends a majority of inbound AE patients to Walter Reed National Military Medical Center [5], and Travis serves as the primary West Coast receiving hospital.

Contingency Staging Facilities

Contingency staging facilities fulfill the same roles in the AE system as in-garrison or fixed staging facilities. However, in a contingency, the staging facility differs in that it is not part of a medical wing's permanent mission and only remains in operation as long as patient flow mandates its need during a contingency operation [1]. These facilities can be created in the continental United States or deployed overseas [6, 7].

They are attached to a host MTF for administrative and logistical support, but may be geographically separated from the MTF if necessary to support AE mission requirements. Usually they are set up in either a building of opportunity or tents, often located at or near an airfield that can accommodate AE aircraft. They are designed to be able to support non-critical patients traveling in the AE system, as previously described, for up to 72 hours. However, the usual length of stay for a patient in a contingency scenario is <12 hours. Contingency staging facilities are commonly staffed by Air Reserve Component personnel from an Aeromedical Staging Squadron (ASTS).

Ten-Bed Mobile Staging Facility

A ten-bed staging facility is an air and ground transportable holding facility that is deployed and staffed by medical group personnel, including nurses, medical technicians, and administrative personnel trained in aerospace physiology and the stresses of flight [8]. The purpose is to "receive patients, sustain life, and administratively process patients who are to be moved in the Tactical Aeromedical Evacuation System" [9]. AE missions are almost exclusively generated in support of patients that need to move due to battle injuries.

A Tactical Aeromedical Evacuation System is designed to evacuate patients using US Air Force (USAF) assets from locations within a military area of operation (or a disaster area) to an MTF outside the area [9]. It includes an AE control team, a ten-bed mobile patient-staging capability, an AE liaison team (AELT), and the AE crew members. The AELT provides an interface between the patient stage and the initiating forward MTF, and a physician from a collocated or nearby MTF clears patients for AE.

A ten-bed patient-staging facility, staffed by medical personnel trained on the AE system, provides ongoing medical care to patients and prepares them for AE, both medically and administratively. It is set up in a tent facility or a structure of opportunity (such as a hangar) usually adjacent to the flight line. Ten-bed staging facilities were set up in the Louis Armstrong New Orleans International Airport after Hurricane Katrina in 2005 (Fig. 7.1) [10], and in Haiti after the 2010 earthquake [3]. At George Bush Intercontinental Airport in Houston after Hurricane Harvey in 2017 [11], the US Department of Defense (DoD) set up a disaster aeromedical staging facility. Numerous patient-staging capabilities have been set up and taken down depending on patient flow in a number of combat zones.

Deployment planning and preparation is essential to support operations during contingencies. Planners must account for messing, billeting, fuel, an operation site, and other support requirements for deployed medical elements. When notified of an event, equipment and supplies must be ready and prepared for transport. Medical squadrons have checklists and/or flowcharts to document procedures for deployment of personnel and cargo. These squadrons maintain fully trained staging personnel that are ready to deploy.

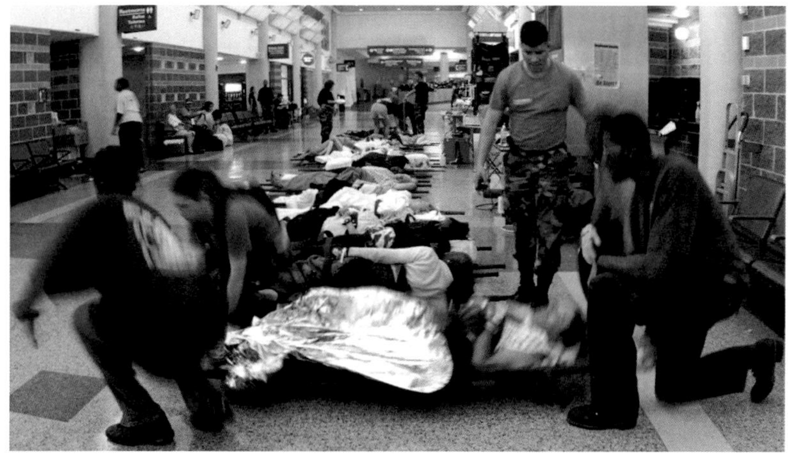

Fig. 7.1 A mobile staging facility set up in a passenger terminal at the Louis Armstrong New Orleans International Airport shortly after Hurricane Katrina in 2005. (US Air Force photo by Master Sgt Jack Braden)

Patient-staging packages are assembled based on the size needed for the patient flow expected. The smallest is designed to hold ten patients. Larger patient-staging assemblages are designed to hold 50 patients for an average of 3–5 hours and have the ability to process and transport >100 patients per day to AE aircraft [9]. The smaller facilities will occasionally have to process patients that have not been regulated prior to reaching their facility. They often temporarily hold both ambulatory and stable litter patients. With the addition of a CCATT, they will sometimes host critical care patients as well.

Disaster Staging Facilities

A disaster staging facility is similar in structure to a contingency staging asset but is set up as part of a disaster response by DoD after the state or territory has requested assistance [4, 12]. Disaster staging facilities are set up by AF personnel in collaboration with the Federal Emergency Management Agency (FEMA), the lead coordinating agency for federal emergency assistance within the Department of Homeland Security (DHS). For CONUS disasters, DoD and the Department of Health and Human Services (DHHS) team up to provide patient staging and critical care patient holding at the Aerial Port of Embarkation (APOE).

The primary purpose of a disaster staging facility is to accept patients from civilian hospitals, to stage them and prepare them for flight, and to transport the patient to the military AE aircraft [12]. Similar to a ten-bed staging capability, patients transported to a disaster staging facility may not be regulated until they arrive at the staging facility, depending on the nature of the disaster.

A disaster staging facility, like the mobile ten-bed facility, can be set up in a tent facility or a structure of opportunity (such as a hangar) and is usually located at the airport nearest to the site of a natural or manmade disaster that has generated more casualties than the nearby MTFs can manage [11]. In the FEMA organization, an Aeromedical Transport Officer is in charge of all patient care and clinical aspects of the air medical transport service and supports the disaster staging facility when deployed [4]. DoD uses a Director of Patient Stage Operations to ensure the smooth running of the disaster staging facility.

Patient-Staging Personnel and Duties

The personnel assigned to a patient-staging facility vary greatly depending on the type and location [1]. However, every patient stage has a number of standard duties necessary to assure successful AE. Ideally, all patients should be appropriately entered into the AE administrative system, i.e., "regulated." They must be provided with supportive medical care and nutrition before and after AE. Each patient must be medically cleared for AE by a flight surgeon prior to each flight and their condition reassessed after each flight. Each patient's medical conditions and the care they receive must be clearly documented on the patients' record so that care can continue uninterrupted during flight and upon reaching the receiving MTF. AE patients must undergo a security inspection and be briefed about what to expect prior to each flight. Finally, patients must be safely transported to and from the flight line along with their required medical equipment, baggage, and medical/nonmedical attendants.

Administration

The Chief of Medical Staff of the host MTF provides medical oversight for all things medical in any patient-staging capability larger than the ten beds. For larger capabilities, the MTF administrators provide necessary logistic support, including supplies and security.

The senior person directing patient-staging capability is designated as the Flight Chief or Squadron Commander, depending on the organization [1]. This person can be a physician, nurse, or administrator. In addition to overseeing all communication and clinical aspects of the patient stage, the flight chief/commander supervises and directs the utilization of all resources allocated to the stage. This includes coordinating appropriate medical care for all en route patients with the MTF commander or the appropriate medicine squadron. The Staging Flight Chief/Commander provides daily situational reports to the MTF commander or AE system command and control.

Patient-Staging Training

The Staging Flight Chief/Commander is also responsible for arranging ongoing training to all assigned personnel. The AE staging mission is a unique role, and a thorough understanding of its intricacies by personnel is important to assure successful AE. Patient-staging training exercises are routinely conducted with simulated patients using staging and AE equipment and supplies and actual ground vehicles and aircraft. Patient-staging personnel are required to perform strenuous work, often in an austere environment, so maintaining physical fitness is a necessity.

Communications

Patient-staging command and control center must maintain close communication with operations managers. This is usually performed by a staging facility or AE clerk. All patient movement activity must be coordinated through either the Global Patient Movement Requirements Center (GPMRC) or a Theater Patient Movement Requirements Center (TPMRC)/Aeromedical Evacuation Control Team (AECT), depending on the type and location of the staging facility [1].

Patient Regulation

Patient regulation refers to the coordination of each patient's medical requirements with available AE personnel, airlift assets, and MTF capability and capacity at both the originating and receiving ends of the AE continuum. Regulation also includes monitoring of patient movement within the AE system. Interacting with the patient regulation system is an important staging facility responsibility, and staging facility or AE clerks must enter all patient information into the US Transportation Command (USTRANSCOM) Automated Information System. However, all patient-staging facilities must be flexible enough to be able to transport unregulated patients when required.

Flight Surgeons

A flight surgeon is a military medical officer practicing in the clinical field of aerospace medicine. Those involved in any aspect of AE must have a thorough understanding of the effects of flight on human illness and the special requirements and limitations of medical care provided during AE [13].

Flight surgeons play an integral part in patient staging and AE patient care. All patients preparing for AE must be medically cleared, and a flight surgeon is available on a 24-hour basis to evaluate patients in the facility. Prior to an AE flight, ambulatory patients are routinely evaluated in the facility, whereas litter patients can be evaluated either in a co-located MTF or after arriving at the staging facility. The flight surgeon reviews the patient's record, prescribes treatment and diet, and addresses any current medical complaints, and verifies that everything is documented on the patient's record. Each patient is "cleared for AE" if the flight surgeon determines the patient can begin or continue travel in the AE system or returned to an MTF for further treatment. Litter patients arriving on an AE flight are evaluated by a flight surgeon once they arrive at the staging facility or MTF.

When patients remain in a staging facility, a flight surgeon evaluates and documents each patient's condition every 24 hours and consults with medical specialists as needed. If the flight surgeon determines that a patient is no longer stable enough to proceed with AE, the patient will be returned to an MTF for further evaluation and treatment.

Critical patients are handled differently in the AE system. These patients are managed by a CCATT or similar specialty team (see Chap. 9). They remain in an MTF prior to AE whenever possible and are transferred from the MTF directly to the flight line. CCATT patients arriving on an AE flight are transported directly from the aircraft to an MTF. However, in austere environments, critically ill patients and their CCATT teams sometimes remain in a staging facility before or in between AE flights.

Flight surgeons are assigned administratively to either the responsible MTF or the staging facility. Fixed and contingency staging facilities with large patient volumes will often have flight surgeons assigned to the unit and might have other physicians assigned as well to help evaluate and stabilize patients while in the staging facility. Mobile staging facilities do not usually have flight surgeons directly assigned. For these highly mobile units, patients are cleared for AE by a flight surgeon assigned to the originating MTF or by a remote flight surgeon after reviewing clinical details provided electronically by an onsite nurse.

Nursing Services

A patient-staging facility senior nurse supervises all attached nurses and medics assigned to nursing services [1]. The chief nurse is also responsible for nursing training and patient flow within the staging facility. They also assign a staging facility team chief for each AE launch and recover mission and are responsible for the success of each mission.

Nursing services personnel take care of the medical and personal needs of AE patients while they are in the staging facility. They document all patient care in the patient's record upon admission, at least once a shift, and upon discharge from the staging facility. These nurses are also responsible for daily accountability of patient narcotics. Outpatients deemed compliant and competent to self-medicate may carry and self-medicate with controlled and non-controlled medications.

Pharmacy

Pharmacy personnel are employed at staging facilities that are 50 beds or larger in size. They must obtain and dispense authorized pharmaceuticals included in the staging facility stock list from the host MTF pharmacy [1]. They must ensure that the AE patients have enough prescription drugs to reach their destination. Patients should have a 3-day supply of medications intratheater movement and a 5-day supply for intertheater movement. In rare cases, staging personal will be required to obtain total parenteral nutrition or other special pharmaceuticals for en route AE patients staying overnight in a staging facility.

Nutrition and Hydration

Staging facilities must coordinate nutrition services for patients. This service can be provided by the host MTF or can be intrinsic to the facility. Staging facility requirements can vary considerably depending on the acuity of the patients served and the length of time they remain in the facility.

When patients arrive at a staging facility, food allergies are noted and diet orders are ascertained before administering meals, snacks, or beverages. Each patient's nutritional status is assessed and documented, including intake patterns, appetite, ability to chew/swallow/digest, time of last meal, and fluid intake. Litter patients are assisted with preparation, positioning, and eating as necessary. This will usually include elevating their heads or assisting them in attaining a sitting position.

Patient hydration is a very important consideration before and during an AE flight since the low relative humidity during flight increases fluid loss. All AE passengers should be offered fluids at least every 2 hours throughout the transport period unless their diet orders include food or fluid restrictions.

Security

Anti-hijacking Procedures

All staging facilities must carry out anti-hijacking precautions for all AE patients and passengers according to US Air Force

Instructions and Federal Aviation Administration directives [1]. Patients and passengers must first be informed about baggage restrictions and prohibitions, including the prohibition on bringing weapons, explosives, and large volumes of liquids onboard the aircraft. All patients, attendants, and baggage placed aboard aircraft must be carefully checked by staging personnel to ensure inappropriate items (e.g., guns, knives, and ammunition) are not carried onto AE flights. In the rare circumstance that a passenger is authorized to carry a weapon onboard, the aircrew must be notified.

All patients and attendants, their hand-carried items, and their hold baggage must be screened with a handheld or walkthrough metal detector, X-ray machine, or by a physical check (Fig. 7.2). Air Force Instructions also require all psychiatric patients to be carefully checked to ensure they do not have any weapons or any other forbidden items that can be used as a weapon or incendiary device [1]. Before each AE mission launch, the staging security team must provide the AE medical crew director (MCD) with a signed Certificate of Security Check.

Facility Security

Security within the immediate area for patients and personnel resources at each medical site is a medical responsibility. The flight chief/commander is responsible for ensuring force protection measures are taken to protect his/her unit and can request assistance from co-located security forces, depending upon threat level and requirements. During disasters, local law enforcement will assist with perimeter security.

If a patient arrives at the staging facility with weapons, they should be properly cleared and transferred immediately to the patient's unit or a family member. When not possible, the staging facility may temporarily store cleared weapons until the patient's unit or family can accept responsibility. Each staging facility must have processes in place to handle weapons.

Manpower

Physically moving litter patients along with their medical equipment and baggage is a core requirement of a staging facility. This responsibility, along with assisting ambulatory patients, is shared by the majority of personnel when not performing other duties, including medics, security and administrative personnel, nurses, and physicians. Ambulatory patients require only direction and supervision when enplaning and deplaning. Litter patients, in contrast, require a great deal of physical effort to safely load and unload from AE aircraft. The team chief, under the direction of the AE medical crewmembers and aircraft loadmasters, organizes and supervises

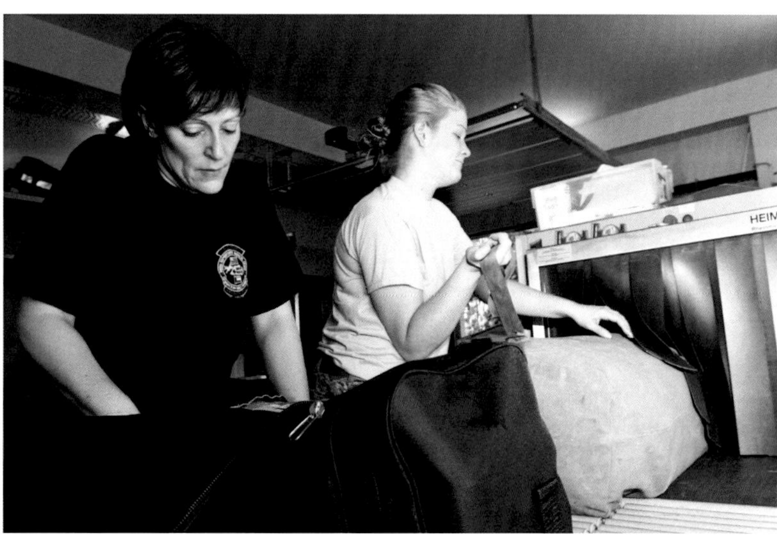

Fig. 7.2 Patient's baggage being screened prior to an aeromedical evacuation (AE) flight at a contingency staging facility at Ramstein Air Base, Germany. (US Air Force photo by Senior Airman Nathan Lipscomb)

these processes. Safety and efficiency are both important priorities.

Baggage

Patients can always bring a small hand-carried bag for personal items for use during travel and overnight stops. If a patient is authorized to self-medicate, staging facility personnel will ensure the patient's medications are in his/her hand-carried baggage. Checked baggage is often allowed, depending on the type and location of the staging facility.

Ground Transportation

A relatively unique role of patient-staging personnel is to transport all AE patients, medical and nonmedical attendants, medical equipment, and baggage from the facility to the flight line, sometimes under challenging conditions. For an AE launch, this involves transporting ambulatory and litter patients from the facility to the flight line via ground transportation (van, ambulance bus, or ambulance) and loading them onto the aircraft during an AE launch. For AE recovery, these elements must all be done in reverse order.

In order to accomplish this, an MTF vehicle control officer serving as the liaison with the vehicle operations flight associated with the host MTF must first obtain all required vehicles [1]. Routine driver maintenance must be performed on all assigned vehicles. In addition, personnel must be appropriately trained to operate vehicles and obtain certification for flight line vehicle operation.

The primary goal during each AE launch and recovery is to minimize patient discomfort and avoid further injury. However, assuring completion in time to allow on-time aircraft departures and avoiding aircraft damage are also extremely important.

The manner in which patients are transported—ambulatory or litter—is determined prior to transportation by an experienced flight nurse (i.e., patient movement clinical coordinator) at the Global Patient Movement Requirements Center (GPMRC) based on the recommendations of the sending physician (Table 7.1).

Table 7.1 Aeromedical evacuation categories used by the US military

Inpatient
Category 1: Psychiatric
Litter
1A Severe: requiring restraints, sedation, and close observation
1B Intermediate severity: potentially dangerous, but not presently disturbed, who requires sedation; restraints should be available
Ambulatory
1C Moderately severe: cooperative and reliable under observation
Categories 2 and 3: Medical/surgical
Litter
2A Immobile litter patient: unable to move unassisted
2B Mobile litter patient: able to move unassisted under emergency circumstances
Ambulatory
3A Patients going for treatment or evaluation: all medical and surgical conditions excluding drug or alcohol abuse
3B Recovered patients returning to station
3C Patients with drug or alcohol abuse going for treatment
Category 4: Infants and children <3 years old
Ambulatory
4A Infant or child going for treatment traveling in an aircraft seat
4B Infant or child returning from treatment traveling in an aircraft seat
Litter
4C Infant requiring an incubator
4D Infant or child going for treatment traveling by litter
Ambulatory outpatients
4E Infant or child, ambulatory outpatient
Outpatient
Category 5: Outpatient adults and children >3 years old
Ambulatory
5A Patient going for treatment or evaluation: all medical and surgical conditions excluding drug or alcohol abuse
5B Patient with drug or alcohol abuse going for treatment
5C Psychiatric patient going for treatment
Litter
5D Patient going on litter for comfort for treatment or evaluation: all medical and surgical conditions excluding drug or alcohol abuse
5E Patient returning from treatment going on litter for comfort
Ambulatory
5C Patient returning from treatment
Nonpatient
Category 6: Attendant
6A Medical attendant
6B Nonmedical attendant

Source: Adapted from Department of the Air Force

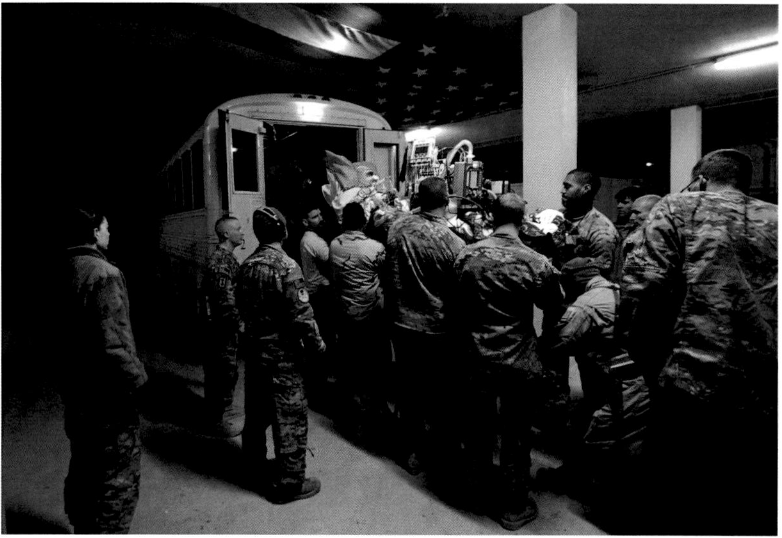

Fig. 7.3 Patients being loaded onto a bus for transportation to the flight line at a contingency staging facility at Bagram Airfield, Afghanistan. (US Air Force photo by Senior Airman Chris Willis)

Litter patients must be carefully moved from the staging facility onto the bus or ambulance (Fig. 7.3), transported to the flight line, and finally onto the AE aircraft for every launch and unloaded for every recovery. Both the litter carriers and patients are at risk of injury during transportation, as is obvious to anyone who has ever carried a litter. The patient-staging personnel are at risk of musculoskeletal injury when moving patients to the awkward places often found in both ground vehicles and aircraft.

The task is complicated by the variation in AE aircraft configuration, as discussed in Chap. 5. In addition, the hardware that secures patient litters can cause injury to the litter carrier's fingers and hands. To minimize these risks, staging facility personnel must be well trained in patient movement techniques so that they are familiar with proper movement techniques and the various ground vehicles and aircraft configurations, and be prepared with appropriate personal protective equipment.

Logistics

For the larger staging facilities, the host MTF provides logistical support services [1]. The ten-bed facilities often receive logistical support from the host air base or host nation. However, when deployed to austere environments, they should maintain approximately 7 days' worth of supplies and equipment. In high-volume situations, supplies and equipment should be re-inventoried every day or every shift.

Final Preparation for Aeromedical Evacuation

Patient Preparation

All personnel, nurses, medics, and assigned flight surgeons are responsible for patient preparation, which is critical to ensure continuity of care and safe AE. Proper preparation for AE includes verifying that the patients have the proper amount of prescribed medications, medical equipment, supplies, briefings, and security measures. A thorough review of each patient's condition and requirements is crucial. A hand-off is used to assist in communication and serves as a checklist to assure correct documentation paperwork, supplies, equipment, meals, and X-rays accompany the patient (Table 7.2).

Patient Identification

All travelers in the AE system are required to carry government identification (e.g., passport, driver license) and an AE identification wristband

Table 7.2 Typical incoming aeromedical evacuation mission report information

Number of patients added or canceled and reason for cancelation
Number of critical care cases
Blood was transfused en route
Ambulance requirements on arrival
Patients with conditions requiring special room accommodations or care
Family member traveling with a patient
Amputee needs for wound wash or operating room visit for dressing change
Mental health patients' concerns

supplied by either the MTF or the staging facility. This includes patients and their medical attendants, whether they are active duty members, dependents, retirees, or civilians. The AE identification wristband should include last name, first name, original MTF, destination MTF, date of birth, patient status, blood type, and allergies. All patients with allergies should have a separate wristband listing specific allergies,,that is, medications, foods, and latex.

Valuables

Patients and their nonmedical attendants should be encouraged not to carry valuables (e.g., large amounts of cash, checks, and jewelry) while in the AE system. Whenever possible, patient valuables should be secured with the next of kin, or sent by registered mail to their emergency contact or destination MTF.

Cane and Crutches

Crutches and canes must accompany patients who require such items. AE patients who are unable to walk without crutches and those whose condition prevents them from using available aircraft seats will be classified and transported as litter patients.

Medical Records

All AE patients must have a DD Form 602, Patient Evacuation Tag, or AF Form 3899, Aeromedical Evacuation Patient Record, in which medical personnel document the care provided. In addition, a copy of all available medical records (clinical records, outpatient treatment records, X-rays, and any other pertinent patient information) should be transported with the patient in an envelope. The outside of each patient envelope should be labeled with the patient's name, patient classification, self-administering medications (or not self-administering status), allergies, last four numbers of Social Security number, nationality if not a US citizen, organization, date of departure, and destination.

Medical and Nonmedical Attendants

In some cases, AE patients will be accompanied by medical or nonmedical attendants. Medical attendants are responsible for providing care to their patient throughout the transport period. Nonmedical attendants provide emotional support and help with the activities of daily living. All attendants must remain within line of sight of the patient they accompany at all times unless relieved by staff. With prior approval, attendants can return in the AE system to their point of origin without the patient. Attendants are prohibited from carrying weapons, unless the attendant is assigned to guard a prisoner patient.

Equipment

Litter Preparation

Military litters are designed for short-term transportation of non-ambulatory patients. For long-distance AE, litters need to be prepared with a mattress, two blankets, two sheets, one pillow and pillowcase, two litter straps, and any additional items required for patient needs or weather (Fig. 7.4). This is particularly important in cold environment and for patients wearing hospital pajamas, since the cabin temperature can be quite low and the patients will be exposed to weather during transfer between aircraft, ground vehicles, and staging facility or MTF.

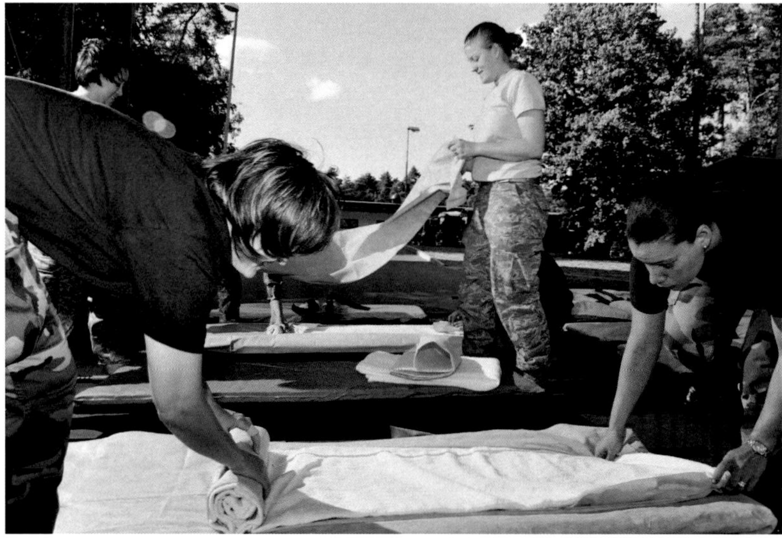

Fig. 7.4 Litters being prepared prior to aeromedical evacuation at a contingency staging facility at Ramstein Air Base, Germany. (US Air Force photo by Senior Airman Nathan Lipscomb)

Patient Movement Items

Patient movement items (PMIs) refer to specific medical equipment (e.g., ventilators, patient monitors, and pulse oximeters) and durable supplies pre-positioned at MTFs and staging facilities that can be exchanged with equipment brought in with the patient. The purpose of PMI is to allow the same equipment to stay with patients in the AE system without degrading the capacities of the CCATT team, the MTF, or the staging facility [14]. It also allows for the replacement of malfunctioning equipment and seamless supply of additional needed supplies en route.

Typical Aeromedical Evacuation Missions

Staging facilities command and control entities are given daily updates on the scheduled AE flight departures and arrivals from the AE control team. This list can be updated up to several times daily.

The flight chief/commander will hold a morning conference to discuss the daily missions planned for that day with the team chiefs and NCOs who will assign the appropriate number of personnel to each launch and recovery mission. The transportation NCO will coordinate with the MTF vehicle control officer to arrange for appropriate number of vehicles and drivers.

Aeromedical Evacuation Mission Launch

Three hours before the AE mission launch, the team chief will review the number of ambulatory and litter patients and their reported conditions and brief all staff members involved in each aspect of the mission. The staging facility team chief will report how many patients will be transported from the staging facility to the flight line and how many additional patients will be transported directly from the MTF to the flight line. A plan will be made as to when to begin the process to allow the schedule AE flights to depart at the scheduled time.

Two hours before the AE mission's scheduled departure time, all staging facility personnel assigned to the AE launch will report to duty. For a mission that requires deplaning a fully loaded C-17 with both ambulatory and litter patients, the crew will include a team chief with at least ten staging personnel and liaison officers. The team chief, flight surgeon, and AE medical crew director determine what order and position the patients will be loaded. A mission brief will then be performed with all launch personnel.

As the buses and ambulances arrive on the flight line, they are carefully parked in the appropriate positions for the aircraft type (Fig. 7.5). Patients are then enplaned as expediently as possible. This is particularly important when the

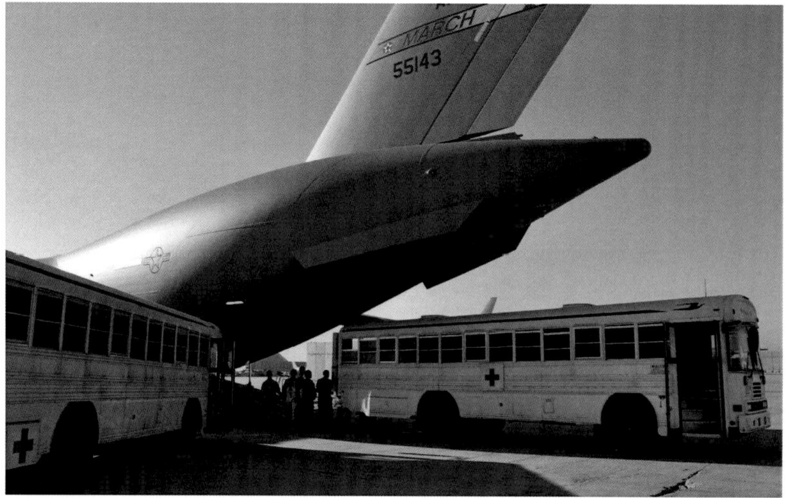

Fig. 7.5 Contingency staging facility personnel positioning patient buses in preparation to enplane patients on a C-17 Globemaster III at Bagram Airfield, Afghanistan. (US Air Force photo by TSgt Shawn David McCowan)

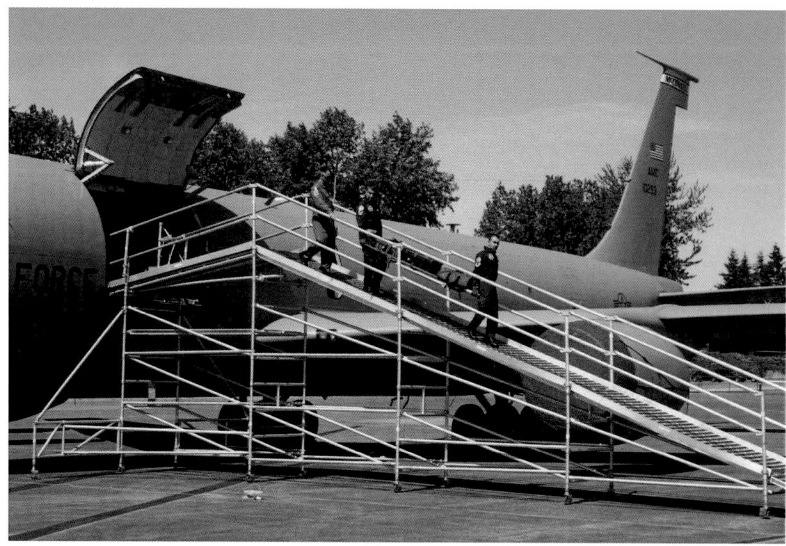

Fig. 7.6 Turkish contingency staging facility personnel members carrying aeromedical evacuation equipment on a litter down the KC-135 Patient Loading System ramp at McChord Air Force Base, Washington. (US Air Force Photo by Tech. Sgt. Scott T. Sturkol)

ambient temperature on the ramp is especially high or low, since the inside temperature of the aircraft will quickly equilibrate with the temperature when the doors are opened for loading.

The type of aircraft will dictate the method of enplaning ambulatory and litter patients. The KC-135 requires a relatively steep ramp or a special mechanical loader to deplane patients from the elevated side cargo door (Fig. 7.6). For both the C-17 and C-130, both ambulatory and litter patients are deplaned down a ramp via the aft cargo door. All patients are then transported to the staging facility or directly to the prearranged MTF.

Aeromedical Evacuation Mission Recovery

Three hours before the AE mission arrival, the Charge Nurse reviews the latest report of the patients' conditions since the AE mission departed. To be properly prepared for the arrival of a mission, all staff members involved in each aspect of the mission must review the latest available information regarding vital clinical and administrative information before AE mission arrives. The team chief in conjunction with a flight surgeon will determine which patients will be transported directly from the flight line to a

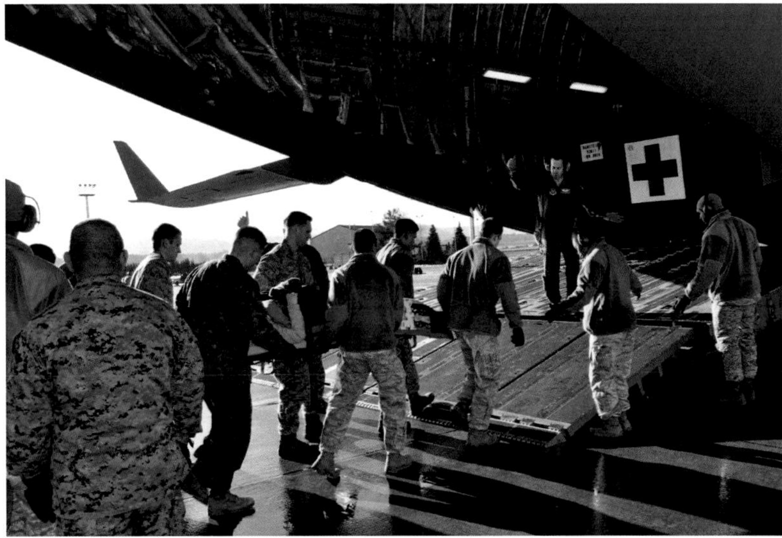

Fig. 7.7 Contingency staging facility personnel at Ramstein Air Base loading a patient onto a 445th Airlift Wing C-17 Globemaster III bound for Joint Base Andrews, Maryland. (US Air Force photo by Capt. Elizabeth Caraway)

receiving MTF and which en route AE patients will be transported to the staging facility where they will remain until their next AE flight departs.

Two hours before the plane's arrival, all personnel assigned to meet the mission at the flight line will report to duty. For the average mission, this might include a flight surgeon, ten staging personnel including a team chief, additional personnel from the MTF, liaison officers, and volunteers. The team chief will assure the availability of an appropriate number of vehicles, drivers, spotters, and other necessary personnel. A mission brief of the entire group will be performed with latest clinical picture and the flight surgeon will clarify any clinical questions that arise.

Prior to the plane's landing, the transportation NCO will arrange for the appropriate type and number of transport vehicles (e.g., buses, ambulances) from the staging facility and all receiving MTFs to be positioned. However, the final determination will be made for each patient after the aircraft has landed, since patient destinations can change while in flight due to changes in patient condition, medical capability changes, and other administrative reasons.

Once the aircraft has landed and parked on the ramp, several things must happen simultaneously. The flight surgeon or senior nurse discusses every patient onboard to determine if their condition has changed in flight such that they need to be transported to an emergency room for stabilization rather than to the prearranged MTF or staging facility. The staging facility team chief speaks with the AE medical crew chief and loadmasters aboard the aircraft to determine the best way to arrange the vehicles to expedite the patient offload. Priority is usually given to critical care patients.

The patients are then deplaned in an expedient manner (Fig. 7.7). Similar to patient loading, the staging facility team must remember that the inside temperature of the aircraft quickly equilibrates with the temperature when the loading doors are opened and the last patients to deplane can be significantly stressed when the ambient temperature on the ramp is uncomfortably high or low. Again, the type of aircraft will dictate the method required for deplaning ambulatory and litter patients.

References

1. Department of the Air Force. Air Force Instruction 48–307. En route care and aeromedical evacuation medical operations. Washington, DC: US Government Printing Office; 2017.
2. Dick A. Aeromedical staging facility staff to reach major milestone in warrior care. Air Force News. 2009. Available at https://www.af.mil/News/Article-Display/Article/118782/aeromedical-staging-facility-staff-to-reach-major-milestone-in-warrior-care/.

3. Stuart JJ, Johnson DC. Air Force disaster response: Haiti experience. J Surg Orthop Adv. 2011 Spring;20(1):62–6.
4. Federal Emergency Management Agency. Position qualifications for public health, healthcare, and emergency medical services; Aeromedical transport officer. FEMA 509 v20130717. September 2016.
5. Markfelder G. Helping wounded warriors return home US Army Public Affairs, 2011. Available at: https://www.army.mil/article/69125/helping_wounded_warriors_return_home.
6. Lostumbo MJ, McNerney MJ, Peltz E, Eaton D, Frelinger DR, Greenfield VA, et al. Overseas basing of U.S. military forces: an assessment of relative costs and strategic benefits. Arlington: National Defense Research Institute. Rand Corporation; 2013.
7. McCowan SD. CASF: staff, volunteers send heroes home. US Air Force News, 2012. Available at: https://www.af.mil/News/Article-Display/Article/110734/casf-staff-volunteers-send-heroes-home/.
8. Berry ML. USAF improving interface between aeromedical evacuation and enroute systems. Air Command and Staff College. Air University, Maxwell Air Force Base, Alabama; 2002. Available at: http://www.dtic.mil/dtic/tr/fulltext/u2/a420660.pdf.
9. US Army Medical Course MD0752-101. US Army Medical Department Center and School. Department of Healthcare Operations. Fort Sam Houston, Texas. Available at: https://www.scribd.com/document/7867950/US-Army-Medical-Course-MD0752-101-Patient-Accountability-Branch.
10. Lopez T. Air Force MASF last stop for some hurricane victims. US Air Force News, 2005. Available at: https://www.af.mil/News/Article-Display/Article/133485/air-force-masf-last-stop-for-some-hurricane-victims/.
11. Martinez J. Aeromedical team at Scott AFB joins response to hurricane Harvey. US Air Force News, 2017. Available at: https://www.af.mil/News/Article-Display/Article/1298809/aeromedical-team-at-scott-afb-joins-response-to-hurricane-harvey/.
12. Crane SS. State, federal teams prepare for hurricane season. Scott Air Force Base News, 2012. Available at: https://www.scott.af.mil/News/Features/Display/Article/162481/state-federal-teams-prepare-for-hurricane-season/.
13. Hurd WW, Montminy RJ, De Lorenzo RA, Burd LT, Goldman BS, Loftus TJ. Physician roles in aeromedical evacuation: current practices in USAF operations. Aviat Space Environ Med. 2006;77(6):631–8.
14. Joint Chiefs of Staff. Joint Publication 4-02. US Government Printing Office, Washington DC; 2017.

Military Aeromedical Evacuation Nursing

8

Elizabeth Bridges and Melissa A. Buzbee-Stiles

Introduction

The backbone of military aeromedical evacuation (AE) is provided by a highly trained group of qualified flight nurses (FNs) and aeromedical evacuation technicians (AETs) serving in US Air Force Active Duty, Reserve, and National Guard units. To transport critically ill and injured patients, they are augmented by specialized teams, including Critical Care Air Transport Team (CCATT) and Acute Lung and Burn teams. A central tenet of AE is that level of clinical care required will be maintained throughout the duration of patient movement. In collaboration with en route patient staging personnel and other ground-based providers, FNs and AETs are responsible for the en route care of more than 90% of evacuated patients. This chapter presents some of the unique aspects of nursing care for AE patients in addition to some of the growing body of research related to en route nursing care [1–4].

E. Bridges (✉)
Col, USAF, NC (ret.), Biobehavioral Nursing and Health Informatics, University of Washington School of Nursing, University of Washington Medical Center, Seattle, WA, USA
e-mail: ebridges@uw.edu

M. A. Buzbee-Stiles
Maj, USAF, NC, En Route Medical Care Division, Office of the Command Surgeon, Headquarters Air Mobility Command, Scott Air Force Base, IL, USA
e-mail: melissa.a.buzbeestiles.mil@mail.mil

Military Aeromedical Evacuation

Education, Training, and Sustainment

Flight nurses and AETs undergo initial and ongoing education and training to achieve and maintain "universal qualification" for any AE platform approved for patient movement (e.g., C-130, C-17, KC-135) [5]. Initial ground training includes flight physiology, exposure to an altitude chamber to learn the effects of hypoxia and barometric pressure changes, and aspects of patient care organized around the stresses of flight. Ground-based simulators are used for training for each aircraft. These simulators (aircraft fuselage) are designed to mimic the AE environment (space, noise, lighting). Additional simulators are used for training on ground transport (e.g., AMBUS). Examples of required content and competencies for AE crew members (AECMs) are outlined in Table 8.1 [6, 7] and include not only the medical aspects of care but also aircraft-specific training and crew responsibilities and safety.

Recent US Military Experience

Between 2001 and 2014, there were 210,863 military AE patient movement requests (PMRs), reflecting the transport of 137,433 individual patients (Fig. 8.1) [8]. These patients were

W. W. Hurd, W. Beninati (eds.), *Aeromedical Evacuation*,
https://doi.org/10.1007/978-3-030-15903-0_8

transported on 81,869 flights. Most of these patients receive en route care from a standard AE crew consisting of two FNs and three AETs, with approximately 2% transported by a specialty team, including CCATT, Burn, Lung Transport, and Neonatal teams [9]. The number of patients transported per flight varies by route but ranges from a median of 13 (IQR 13) to 32 (IQR 15), with approximately 50% of the patients on litters. In AE, these patients onload and offload simultaneously, which have implications for handoff and safety.

Table 8.1 Example of curriculum for aeromedical crew members

Initial qualification [6]	Semiannual continuation flying requirements [7]
Flight physical	Mission management
Physiological training	Oxygen, electrical, communication, and lighting systems
Anti-hijacking	Aircraft/floor load litter configuration
Initial crew resource management	Rapid decompression
Aircraft training (C-130, C-17, KC-135)	Fuselage fire/smoke and fumes elimination
Cardiopulmonary resuscitation	Emergency landing/ditching
Medical equipment review	Door warning light illuminated in-flight
Aircrew flight equipment	Cardiac/respiratory emergences
Emergency egress training	Neurological/medical emergencies
Local survival/combat survival training	Maxillofacial, neck, and eye trauma
Water survival training	Abdominal and genitourinary emergencies
Medical survival, evasion, resistance, and escape training	Orthopedic and vascular emergencies
	Pediatric management
	Acceptance/transfer of medical care
	Contingency engines running onload or offload

Unlike a hospital where patients are cared for on nursing units focusing on a unique population, there is a wide variation in the diagnoses of AE patients. From 2001 to 2012, the major diagnostic categories for AE patients were musculoskeletal injuries (primarily back and knees), non-battle injuries (sprains and fractures), mental health disorders (e.g., adjustment reactions, mood disorders, anxiety disorders, and post-traumatic stress disorders), and general "signs and symptoms" (primarily respiratory) [10, 11]. The diversity of diagnoses is further exemplified using data from 2009 (Table 8.2), which was a period of high operational tempo. During this period there were a high number of patients requiring care for orthopedic injuries, mental health, general surgery, neurosurgery, and neurology as well as more unique care requirements including obstetric and pediatric patients. The variety of patients, and the unique en route aspects of their care, has implications for the ongoing education and training of FNs and AETs [12]. The AE crew members must be knowledgeable in the general care of these patients, the interface between the patient's diagnosis, and the en route care environment (e.g., stresses of flight) and the risk for en route adverse events.

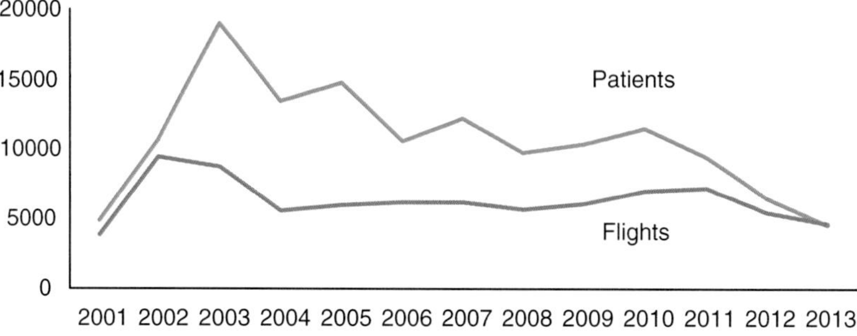

Fig. 8.1 Number of regulated aeromedical evacuation (AE) patients and flights during operation Enduring Freedom from September 2001 through December 2014

Table 8.2 Distribution of the primary medical specialty care required by the USAF Aeromedical Evacuation patients in 2009

Specialty	Number of patients[a]	Specialty	Number of patients[a]
Orthopedic surgery	2207	Nephrology	142
Psychiatry	1573	Otorhinolaryngology	141
General surgery	1219	Medical oncology	139
Neurosurgery	864	Hand surgery	131
Neurology	723	Colorectal surgery	113
Internal medicine	602	Spinal surgery	83
Cardiology	327	Oral surgery	76
Ophthalmology	297	Burns	74
Pulmonary disease	244	Obstetrics	66
Urology	244	Dermatology	59
Gastroenterology	217	Pediatrics	56
Gynecology	169		

[a]Patients often required multiple care by multiple specialties.

To further illuminate the breadth of knowledge required by FNs and AETs, Table 8.3 provides an example of 13 patients transported from the combat zone to Germany on a single mission. Two of the patients were cared for by CCATT, and the remaining 11 were cared for by the AE crew. The diagnoses range from cardiac arrhythmias (implications for en route hypoxia and gravitational forces), infectious disease with fatigue, a dental disorder (risk for barodontalgia due to gas expansion at altitude), mild traumatic brain injury (risk for hypoxia), and several severely injured patients being transported within days of injury and surgery (en route pain management exacerbated by vibration, risk for hypoxia, risk for exacerbation of a pneumothorax due to gas expansion, risk for compartment syndrome).

Aeromedical Evacuation Mission Preparation

Flight nurses and AETs are responsible for all aspects of mission planning. Each patient has been medically validated for flight by a flight surgeon. Mission preparation is more extensive than focusing solely on the medical/transport aspects of a single patient. The number of patients who can be transported varies depending on the aircraft. For example, the C-130, which is a turboprop aircraft, can transport a maximum of 138 passengers, with the capacity for up to 97 litters, and the C-17 can transport up to 102 passengers, with up to 36 litters on stanchions. This capability was demonstrated during disaster response evacuations ahead of Hurricane Rita, when 1169 patients were transported on 16 missions in a single day, with passenger loads ranging from 40 to 120 patients and nonmedical attendants.

Mission preparation requirements [13] include readiness not only for patient care but also consideration of aircraft unique requirements (location of oxygen outlets or need for portable oxygen, electrical outlets, airflow in the cabin); medical emergency response plans, ensuring special equipment and supplies are onboard the aircraft; and logistical aspects of en route care (e.g., how much electricity is required for all the equipment, calculation of oxygen requirements, and estimated weight of patients, crew, and equipment). A load plan is created by a FN based on multiple factors including patient care requirements (e.g., litter versus ambulatory), special equipment (oxygen, suction, external fixator), specialty care teams (e.g., CCATT, Burn), and infection prevention considerations. In addition to the load plan, mission planning documents for each flight include spreadsheets for calculation of required oxygen, electricity, and a separate spreadsheet with exact times for each phase of

Table 8.3 Summary of 13 patients transported on a single mission

1.	Spontaneously resolving palpitations
2.	Continuous headache
3.	Day 3. MVA—back "popped"—lumbar disc injury
4.	Day 1. Landmine blast. Traumatic BKA. s/p washout. RUE laceration, R gluteal laceration, soft tissue injury to LLE. PAN CT no traumatic abnormality identified within the head, face, neck, chest, abdomen, pelvis, cervical, thoracic, or spinal fracture. Pain 8/10 w/out meds, 4/10 with meds
5.	Day 1. Sustained shrapnel injury to neck. DX: Right zone II Injury, s/p removal of retained frag, neck exploration. No airway or esophageal injury identified fragment removed. Initial GCS 15, current GCS 15
6. CCATT	Day 2. IED blast. Injuries included open lower extremity fracture, right tibial plateau fracture, right distal tibia/fibula fracture, right midfoot fracture, right metatarsal fracture × 4, left distal fibula fracture, left calcaneal fracture, fractures to both distal upper extremities, including left ulnar fracture. L5 burst fracture (unstable) per CT scan. Pt has external fixators to bilateral lower extremities. GCS on arrival 15. No MACE. Respiratory status: Intubated. Sedated with propofol and fentanyl. Appears comfortable
7.	Day 2. Gunshot wound to the right forearm, fractured radius: soft tissue derangement, no other trauma. Radial nerve damage
8.	Day 11. MVA vs IED blast. Blast came through gunner hatch. No LOC. Originally presented with low back pain only and then developed persistent headache with decreasing MACE 20/30 and persistent tinnitus in the left ear
9.	Day 0. Right hemothorax. Pt suffered injury from suicide bomber (vest) with shrapnel wound to the right chest with right hemothorax. Injury occurred at 0555 (Day 0), GCS 15. Lacerations to posterior thighs. Pain 5/10 premed, 2–3/10 post meds
10.	Male with fatigue during past few months. Pt sent to medical officer for positive HIV screen on blood drive in the country. Autoimmune infectious disease suspected
11. CCATT	Day 0. Evacuated to Role 3 IED blast at 0730Z. Pt arrived here at Role 3 at 1230Z. Pt presents with penetrating injury to the left neck, right thigh, and chest and piece of metal in the right ventricle presently okay. Piece of metal entered the heart through venous system. Patient needs immediate flight to Germany for possible cardiac intervention
12.	Day 0. Transferred to Role 3 with RUE distal humerus fracture and multiple shrapnel wounds to the right upper extremity and bilateral lower extremities s/p suicide bomber explosion. Arrived in stable condition. RUE 9/10 pain with movement, 6/10 after meds. Went to OR for external fixator of right humerus. Radial nerve intact, ulnar nerve possible dysfunction. Good sensation and movement. Compartment syndrome considered. GCS 15/15. Current VS: 137/78, 87, 16, 98% on RA. Pain 7/10 before meds, now 3/10 after meds. CT not functioning. C-spine cleared clinically
13.	History of maxillofacial dental symptoms prior to deployment. Dentist recommends evacuation to home base secondary to pain, bone loss, periodontal disease, and erosion. Pain 7/10 w/out meds, 4/10 w/meds

Abbreviations: *BKA* below the knee amputation, *C-spine* cervical spine, *CCATT* Critical Care Air Transport Team, *CT* computed tomography, *DX* diagnosis, *GCS* Glasgow Coma Scale, *HIV* human immunodeficiency virus, *IED* improvised explosive device, *LLE* left lower extremity, *LOC* loss of consciousness, *MACE* Military Acute Concussion Evaluation, *MVA* motor vehicle accident, *OR* operating room, *PAN CT* wide field-of-view computed tomography protocol covering the body from the head to the pubic symphysis, *R* right, *RA* room air, *RUE* right upper extremity, *VS* vital signs

mission planning, including preflight mission planning, time to alert the medical crew, crew briefs, time to start loading patients on the aircraft, and time for aircraft takeoff (wheels up).

A separate launch crew is generally responsible for preparing the aircraft, which includes transitioning the cargo compartment from transporting equipment and supplies to the preparation to receive patients (Fig. 8.2). Of note, unlike civilian air medical transport, there are no US military aircrafts dedicated solely to patient transport.

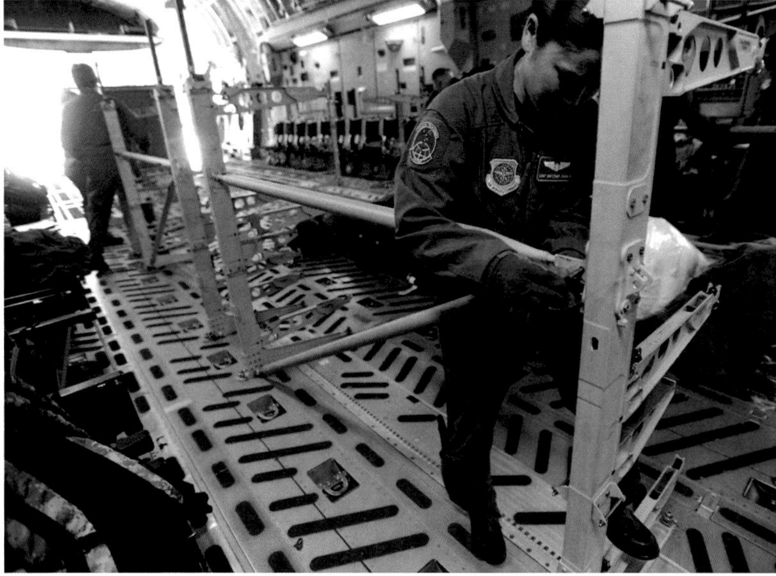

Fig. 8.2 Configuring the aircraft with litter stanchions. (US Air Force photo by Master Sgt. Rick Sforza)

Patient Preparation

Once the patient is medically validated for flight by a flight surgeon, preflight preparation is performed by nurses either in the hospital or staging facility. The focus of this activity is to ensure the patient is prepared for transport and has all required medications and supplies. The AE crew or launch team are responsible for verifying that the patient is ready for transport along with additional administrative requirements, such as anti-hijacking, securing patient belongings and patient identification documents, and ensuring the patient is appropriately clothed for the flight. For each patient, a 57-item Patient Transfer Checklist is completed for this purpose at the medical facility sending the patient and verified by staging facility prior to departure.

Handoff

During the transport of a patient from the warzone to the United States, the patient may experience as many as 14 handoffs. The challenge of a handoff is magnified in the AE environment when large numbers of patients may be transported simultaneously. On arrival at a destination, the AE crew may provide handoffs to multiple teams (e.g., patients transported to multiple locations or by multiple methods). To ensure the transfer of critical information, standard documentation (Fig. 8.3a, b) has been created to facilitate the handoff, drawing on the SBAR mnemonic: Situation, Background, Assessment, Recommendation, or Request [14].

Patient and Crew Safety

Patient safety during en route care is the highest priority for AE crew members [15, 16]. Similar to hospital-based programs, the AE system has a robust patient safety tracking system, with the collection of reports on close calls, near misses, and safety incidents integrated as a standard in post-flight debriefs. Examples of these incidents unique to en route care include medication issues (medication discontinued before flight but given to nurse during handoff), equipment malfunctions or is missing, patient not correctly prepared for flight or not secured on the litter, and human factors (team not strong enough to lift a litter).

The prevention of injuries in AE crew members is of great importance. The role is physically challenging. AE crew members must be able to load and unload litter patients and configure the aircraft (Fig. 8.4), including setting up stanchions or pull-

AEROMEDICAL EVACUTION (AE) PATIENT HANDOFF CHECKLIST

I (Identify)	**DATE/TIME:**	**CITE #:**	**PATIENT NAME:**	**AGE:**	**RANK:**
	ORIGINATING FACILITY:		**DESTINATION FACILITY:**	**PATIENT CLASSIFICATION:**	

	HANDOFF TO AE CREW BY FACILITY / **REPORT BY:**	**HANDOFF BY THE AE CREW**
S (Situation)	**Diagnosis:** ___ **Date of injury/admission:** ___ **Date of surgery:** ___ **Current status:** ☐Alert/Oriented ☐Confused/Disoriented ☐Responds to verbal ☐Responds to pain ☐Unconscious **Patient onload method:** ☐Unassisted ☐Crutches/cane ☐Litter **Code status:** ☐DNR **Attendant:** ☐Medical ☐Non-medical	☐**No change in status/situation** **Status change:** ☐A/O ☐Confused ☐Verbal ☐Pain ☐Unconscious **Pt offload method:** ☐Unassisted ☐Crutches/cane ☐Litter **Other information:**
B (Background)	**Allergies:** ☐NKDA ☐List: ___ **Medications:** ☐None ☐Self-Administered ☐Given to Flight Nurse ☐See 3899 for list **Recent:** Pain Meds/Route/Time Given (zulu) ___ Antiemetic/Route/Time Given (zulu) ___ Antibiotics/Route/Time Given (zulu) ___ Other Meds/Route/Time Given (zulu) ___ **Other pertinent information/history:**	☐**No change in medication** **Inflight:** Last Pain Meds/Route/Time Given (zulu) ___ Last Antiemetic/Route/Time Given (zulu) ___ Last Antibiotics/Route/Time Given (zulu) ___ Other Meds/Time Given (zulu) ___ **Other information:**
A (Assessment)	**Vitals:** BP ___ P ___ R ___ SpO2 ___ T ___ **Time:** ___ **Pain level:** ___/10 **Location:** ___ **Airway:** ☐No devices ☐Trach ☐ Other: ___ **Breathing:** ☐Spontaneous ☐Labored ☐Assisted **Oxygenation:** ☐Room Air ☐NC ☐NRB **Rate:** ___LPM **Circulation:** ☐Adequate ☐Altered (location): ___ **IV:** ☐0.9% NS ☐LR ☐D5W ☐Other: ___ **Rate:** ___mL/hour ☐Packed RBCs ☐Saline Lock **Location:** ___ ☐Fluids brought onboard w/ patient ☐Tubing/fluids/medications labeled **Devices:** ☐ Suction ☐ Orthopedic device ☐ NG tube ☐ ProPaq ☐ Zoll ☐ Restraints ☐ Foley ☐ Chest tube ☐ IV pump ☐ Cast ☐ KCI wound vac x ___ ☐ SCDs ☐ Feeding tube ☐ Drain ☐ Epidural ☐ PCA pump ☐ Peripheral Nerve Block ☐ Other: ___ **Pain equipment safety check:** ☐Site: ___ ☐ Line patent ☐ Pump functional ☐ Right Medication ☐ Right infusion rate ☐ Tubing unclamped **Wound vac safety check:** ☐Site(s): ___ ☐ Tube unclamped ☐ Pump functional **Abnormal labs:** ☐H/H ☐Cardiac enzymes **Other pertinent information:**	**Last Vitals:** BP ___ P ___ R ___ SpO2 ___ T ___ **Pain level:** ___/10 **Location:** ___ **Airway:** ☐No change ☐Changed to: ___ **Breathing:** ☐No change ☐Changed to: ___ **Oxygenation:** ☐No change ☐Changed to: ___ at ___LPM **Circulation:** ☐No change ☐Changed to: ___ **IV:** ☐No change ☐Changed to: ___ at ___mL/hour **Devices:** ☐ No change ☐ Changed to/issues during flight: **Device safety checks completed:** ☐ Yes ☐ No* ** If "No" is checked, please explain why below.* **Other information:**
R (Recommendation/Request)	**Specific inflight orders/instructions for AE Crew (*AF 3899, Section III: Other Orders*):**	☐**Inflight orders/instructions accomplished** **Other information:**
Standard Patient Preparation Items Completed? ☐ Yes ☐ No ***** See back of checklist*****		

* This form is not a part of the patient's permanent medical record. PERSONAL DATA, Privacy Act 1974 (5 U.S. C. 557a), 01 August 2000 AFVA 205-15

AEROMEDICAL EVACUTION (AE) PATIENT HANDOFF CHECKLIST (BACKSIDE)

STANDARD PATIENT PREPARATION ITEMS
(TO BE COMPLETED BY THE ORIGINATING FACILITY/CASF/ASF PRIOR TO ARRIVING AT THE AIRCRAFT)

TASK	DESCRIPTION	SUPPORTING REGULATION
Medication ☐ **N/A**		
☐ Adequate supply of medications given to the patient or flight nurse	Role 2 to Role 3 (i.e. Bastion to Bagram) movements in combat operations theater: ***1-day minimum***; Role 3 to Role 4 (i.e. Bagram to LRMC) movements: ***2-day minimum***; inpatients from OCONUS MTF to port of entry MTF CONUS (i.e. LRMC to Bethesda): ***2-day minimum***; inpatients from OCONUS MTF to other locations in CONUS with RON: ***3-day minimum***; all outpatient movements OCONUS to CONUS: 5-day minimum; CONUS to CONUS movements: ***1-day minimum***.	AFI 44-165, *Administering Aeromedical Staging Facilities*, para 2.5.3., 2.10.3.1., 2.10. 2.10.4, 2.10.7., 2.12.5.; AFI 41-301, *Worldwide Aeromedical Evacuation System*, para 4.4.; USTRANSCOM Memorandum, *Medication Administration, Self-Medicating Patients and Controlled Substance Accountability within the Patient Movement System*, dated 17 May 2010.
☐ Patient is pre-medicated prior to flight	• Pain medication within 1 hours of departure (if applicable) • Antiemetic (if applicable) • Medication that would be scheduled to be given during patient loading and through 1 hour after takeoff (if applicable)	
☐ Patient medication verified	• Medication delivered to the aircraft is for the right medication for the right patient with the right time/frequency of administration annotated on it and in the right form for route of administration • All medications are verified with order on AF Form 3899/DD Form 602 • All medications have been documented and timed on MAR/PMR	
Equipment ☐ **N/A**		
☐ Working condition confirmed	Equipment must work properly and battery must be fully charged prior to leaving facility.	AFI 41-301, *Worldwide Aeromedical Evacuation System*, para 8.2.
☐ Approved for flight ☐ Equipment waiver obtained	Originating MTF must use only flight-certified medical equipment for use on AE missions. All "approved equipment" questions must be directed to GPMRC or appropriate theater AECC/TPMRC.	
☐ All auxiliary parts present	Power cords/adapters, canisters, litter brackets/securing device, tubing	
Supplies ☐ **N/A**		
☐ Adequate amount of supplies given to the patient or flight nurse	Role 2 to Role 3 (i.e. Bastion to Bagram) movements in combat operations theater: ***1-day minimum***; Role 3 to Role 4 (i.e. Bagram to LRMC) movements: ***2-day minimum***; inpatients from OCONUS MTF to port of entry MTF CONUS (i.e. LRMC to Bethesda): ***2-day minimum***; inpatients from OCONUS MTF to other locations in CONUS with RON: ***3-day minimum***; all outpatient movements OCONUS to CONUS: 5-day minimum; CONUS to CONUS movements: ***1-day minimum***.	AFI 44-165, *Administering Aeromedical Staging Facilities*, para 2.6.3., 2.10.7.; AFI 41-301, *Worldwide Aeromedical Evacuation System*, para 4.4.; USTRANSCOM Memorandum, *Medication Administration, Self-Medicating Patients and Controlled Substance Accountability within the Patient Movement System*, dated 17 May 2010.
Documentation		
☐ Documentation verified	• Physician has signed the AF 3899/DD Form 602 • Flight surgeon has cleared the patient; documented on form • AF Form 3899/DD Form 602, medical record, x-rays placed in an envelope affixed with completed DD Form 2267 or with the following information: patient's name, rank/status, SSN, nationality (if not a US citizen), organization, date of departure, and destination) • Military ID card with the patient or in envelope listed above • ID bracelet on patient with last name, first name, middle initial, cite #, and date of birth (printed/typed)	AFI 44-165, *Administering Aeromedical Staging Facilities*, para 2.2.8.1.5, , 2.5.3., 2.9., 2.10.7., 2.12.5; AFI 41-301, *Worldwide Aeromedical Evacuation System*, para 4.3., 4.8; USTRANSCOM Policy Letter, dated 9 October 2009.
Anti-hijacking/Baggage		
☐ Completion confirmed	• Patients, attendants, and their baggage are inspected with a hand-held or walk-through metal detector, x-ray machine, or physical check for weapons or explosives. • All baggage is tagged appropriately and baggage manifest is provided to the AE crew.	AFI 44-165, *Administering Aeromedical Staging Facilities*, para 2.8.2.1, 2.8.1.5., 2.12.4.2., 2.13.; AFI 41-301, *Worldwide Aeromedical Evacuation System*, para 2.11.1., 4.2., 4.6.3.

Fig. 8.3 SBAR Handoff tool for AE. (**a**) Front side. (**b**) Back side. The checklist includes the critical information and provides other preflight tasks with a description and supporting regulations

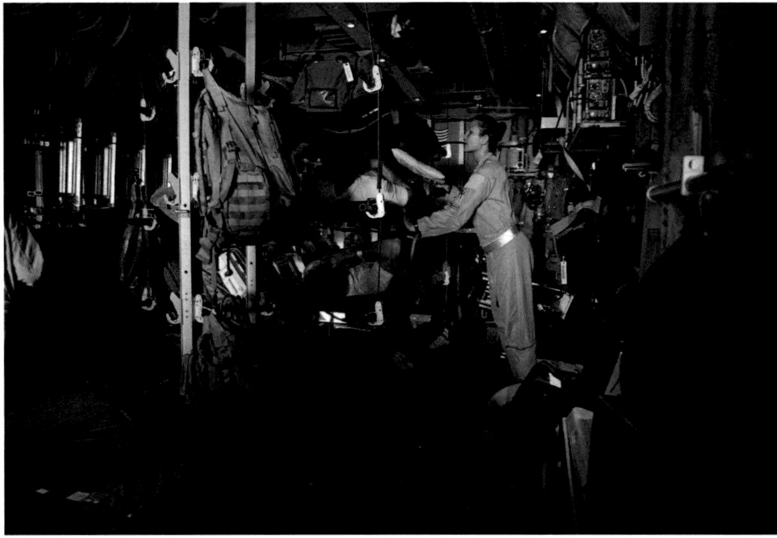

Fig. 8.4 The behind-the-scenes physical challenges of AE. An AET prepares to escort patients off a C-130 Hercules after reaching their final destination. (US Air Force photo/ Staff Sgt. Marleah Miller; 130,720-F-SI788–120.JPG)

ing straps from the top of the aircraft, running lines, and securing equipment [17]. As a part of ongoing training, there is an emphasis on crew safety, including correct lifting and movement techniques, which is essential in this physically challenging environment. The potential effect of this training was demonstrated by the findings that AE crew members had a lower incidence of musculoskeletal injuries compared to non-AE counterparts [18, 19].

Crew fatigue is also a safety concern. A study [20] of Critical Care Air Transport Team members found that a majority used strategies to mitigate fatigue (e.g., caffeine, exercise, energy drinks) and that they experienced a decrease in perceived alertness. However, the altered alertness was not manifested as a decrease in vigilance. Of note, none of these individuals received fatigue management training. This study, which integrated subjective and objective data [21], needs to be replicated in the larger population of FNs and AETs and emphasizes the need for education specific to fatigue management.

Psychological Risks to Crew Members

The provision of en route care may have psychological sequelae. A survey of 188 AE and CCATT personnel found that CCATT members were 3.22 times more likely than AE personnel to endorse symptoms consistent with post-traumatic stress disorder (PTSD) [22]. Among these individuals, 14% of CCATT providers (7/50) and 4.4% (6/138) of AE personnel met symptom criteria for PTSD. Despite the physical, emotional, and professional challenges of en route care, en route patient staging personnel, FNs, and AETs consistently voice devotion, a high level of commitment and mission focus, and a passion for safely bringing home our warriors [23, 24]. Key factors that may underpin the paradox between the challenges and devotion to the role include the unique demands of the role, personal autonomy and control, the availability of resources including fellow crew and leadership, and intrinsic motivation. Further exploration of these factors is needed to mitigate the challenging aspects of this unique role.

Stresses of Flight and Aeromedical Evacuation Patients

The cornerstone of in-flight nursing care is the identification of AE patients at increased risk related to the stresses of flight and implementing strategies to mitigate these risks (Table 8.4).

Barometric Pressure Changes

Military aircraft used for AE routinely maintain a cabin air pressure equivalent to 8000 feet above sea level. At this altitude, the volume of air increases by approximately one-third. This

Table 8.4 Nursing interventions to mitigate the stresses of flight

Stressor	High-risk patient populations	Nursing interventions
Decreased oxygen at cruise altitude	Cardiopulmonary disease, traumatic brain injury (TBI), anemia	Supplemental oxygen, pulse oximetry monitoring, request cabin altitude restriction
Decreased barometric pressure	Patients at high risk for entrapped air (i.e., ear, sinus, gastrointestinal tract, pulmonary), trauma, postsurgical, decompression exposure	General care considerations include venting colostomy bags, controlling intravenous fluid flow, naso- or orogastric tube for gastric decompression, high-flow oxygen (decompression sickness), request cabin altitude restriction, preflight decongestants
Thermal Stress	Burn, postsurgical, infants/small children, elderly, diabetic, traumatic brain injury, patients with orthopedic devices	Maintain comfortable temperature level (coordinate with flight crew), thermal (space) blankets, ice packs, warmed/cooled fluids, fan/air movement devices
Decreased humidity	Infants/children, elderly, trauma, burn, gastrointestinal, urologic, postsurgical, pregnancy, dental/maxillofacial	Dehydration and immobility may be risk factors for venous thromboembolism. Frequent offering of water and physical activity/range or motion or ambulation. Nasal spray, eye drops, topical rehydration agents, intravenous fluids, oral hygiene
Increased noise	Auditory illness/injury, infants/children, elderly, mental health, TBI/neuro, pregnancy	Hearing protection, positioning away from wheel well/engines, alternate communication options, amplified assessment devices
Vibration	Orthopedic, postsurgical, trauma, infants/children, elderly, TBI/neuro, gastrointestinal, maxillofacial, auditory/visual, burn	Extra padding, position changes, frequent ambulation, pain control, antiemetics, elevate the head of bed, maintain head alignment
Gravitational Forces	Neuro/TBI, pregnancy, trauma, orthopedic, infants/children, elderly, postsurgical	Elevate the head of bed, load head first, extra padding, antiemetics, maintain head alignment, intracranial pressure monitoring, range of motion extremity exercises to prevent venous stasis
Fatigue	All stresses of flight induce fatigue to some degree Neuro/TBI, cardiac, pulmonary, postsurgical, pregnancy, infants/children, elderly, mental health	Attempt to maintain treatment schedule consistent with destination, sleep medications, litter for comfort, attempt to control other stresses of flight to prevent exacerbation of fatigue, dimming cabin lights

increases the risk for in-flight complications related to the expansion of entrapped air. Everyone who flies is at risk of complications from expanding air in the inner ear.

AE patients at increased risk for the expansion of entrapped air include those with a pneumothorax, pneumocephalus, postabdominal surgery, entrapped ocular air, as well as individuals at risk for decompression injuries. For some patients, a flight surgeon may order that the aircraft fly with a lower cabin altitude (i.e., cabin altitude restriction) to mitigate these effects [25, 26]. Although ocular air is identified as a potential indicator for cabin altitude restriction, research addresses only civilian transport 14 days after the injury or surgery. There is no research on the effects of altitude on patients with acute ocular injury. Other specific conditions affected by the hypobaric environment of AE are considered later in this chapter.

Hypobaric Hypoxia

The partial pressure of oxygen (PaO_2) decreases as pressure decreases, as defined by Dalton's Law of partial pressures. This results in decreased partial pressure of O_2 (PaO_2) in arterial blood, which is routinely estimated by pulse oximetry, which measures peripheral capillary oxygen saturation (SpO_2). During ascent from sea level to 5000–8000 feet, SpO_2 decreases by 2–4% in healthy individuals [27, 28]. In individuals with cardiopulmonary disease, the SpO_2 can decrease 33% or more [29]. A study of ambulatory combat casualties found that 85% had occult hypoxemia (SpO_2 < 90%) without dyspnea or tachycardia and 34% had at least 1 desaturation to <85% [30]. In another study, all nine seriously injured casualties evacuated after the bombing of the *USS Cole* had an SpO_2 > 92% at sea level but were found to have SpO_2 < 85% with ascent to altitude without reports of dyspnea [31]. One of these patients with a pulmonary blast injury had an SpO_2 of 50%. All patients were treated with supplemental oxygen and achieved an SpO_2 > 92%. As a result of these and other studies, supplemental oxygen should be considered for all trauma patients transported via military AE.

Anemia (Hgb < 8 g/dL) increases the risk of hypobaric hypoxia for patients with impaired perfusion [30, 32, 33]. According to military standards, all patients with acute anemia (<9 g/dL) receive supplemental O_2 during flight [6]. There are nomograms and standard equations available to estimate the en route oxygen requirements [6]:

$$\text{Required FiO}_2 = \text{FiO}_2\left(\text{PB}_1 - 47\right)/\left(\text{PB}_2 - 47\right)$$

For example, if a patient was receiving 30% oxygen at sea level (PB_1 = 760 mm Hg), with ascent to 8000 feet (PB_2 = 564 mm Hg), they would require 40% oxygen to maintain the same PaO_2:

$$\text{Required FiO}_2 = 0.3\left(713\right)/\left(517\right) = 0.4$$

Noise

Ambient noise onboard the aircraft inhibits the ability to communicate and perform assessment skills, such as auscultation [34]. The ambient noise levels on military aircraft routinely used for AE are approximately 80–100 dB for the turboprop C-130 and 86 dB for multi-jet engine C-17. At these noise levels >85 dB, shouting is required to be heard from more than 3 feet away, and above 90 dB speech is not possible. For this reason, all AE patients are provided hearing protection (noise reduction rating 29 dB), and the AE crew wear noise-reducing communication headsets.

Aircraft noise has a negative effect on the provision of patient care resulting in both increased errors and omissions—a medical aircrew education is designed to mitigate these effects. In a study of en route pain, it was noted that AE patients were reticent to talk to the AE crew who were wearing headsets [35]. Active noise reduction headphones with interconnection cables enhance communication between providers and simulated patients under AE conditions [36]. However, such headsets are not routinely available during military AE.

Noise interferes with the ability to perform a physical assessment. The heartbeat cannot be auscultated with a traditional stethoscope when the ambient noise level is >85 dB [37, 38]. Since noise levels on most military aircraft used for AE exceed this level, stethoscopes are rarely used in the air during AE missions. Alternate methods of assessment are used in critically ill patients such as pulse oximetry, capnography, and ultrasound. A potential solution under development is a noise-immune stethoscope [39, 40].

Ambient aircraft noise is an even greater problem for patients transported with electronic devices, such as ventilators and intravenous pumps, since audible alarms cannot be heard. As a result, AE crews must focus their attention on visual alarms and other condition indicators. A study evaluated the care provided by CCATT providers during a cardiac arrest scenario under conditions consistent with flight on a C-17 with simulated aircraft noise (86 dBA) and hypobaric hypoxia (8000 feet) [34]. These investigators demonstrated that care for critically ill patients was significantly affected by both noise and altitude-induced hypoxemia, regardless of the experience of the providers.

Thermal Stress

There is limited research on thermal stress during en route care or solutions to minimize the risk of hyperthermia or hypothermia. Two studies [41, 42] described the thermal environment and human response to the thermal environment onboard cargo aircraft configured for AE (C-130,

C-141, C-17). No description of the thermal environment on the KC-135 or any other aircraft used for AE has been reported. In the C-130 during winter months, temperature throughout the aircraft was 22–24 °C, with airflow greatest in the back top and bottom litter tiers. Thermal comfort was lowest in the back/bottom litter tier, which was correlated with both ambient temperature and air flow.

In the C-17, the temperature in the back of the aircraft decreased from an average of 20 °C ± 0.6 °C (68 °F) to a nadir of 12.6 °C ± 0.6 °C (54.7 °F) at 45 minutes into the flight compared to the front of the aircraft where the temperature decreased from preflight 20.6 °C ± 0.6 °C to a 14.7 °C ± 0.5 (58.5 °F) at 30 minutes of flight and 15.2 °C ± 0.4 °C (59.4 °F) at 45 minutes of flight.

The temperature change varies based on ground temperature. If ground temperature was greater than 25 °C, there was a significant decrease in cabin temperature over the first hour of flight. In contrast if ground temperature was less than 15 °C, there was minimal change in cabin temperature.

Results from a study in the C-141 aircraft, which is no longer in the US Air Force (USAF) inventory, are relevant to current aircraft [42]. In healthy subjects, there was a relationship between ambient temperature and exposed skin temperature and thermoregulatory vasoconstriction, which was slightly higher with lower ambient temperature. These results demonstrate the potential iatrogenic effects of a colder environment on patients who have impaired thermoregulation (i.e., elderly, neonates, burns). There was also an association between the ambient temperature and thermal sensation/aversiveness, reflecting increased discomfort with lower temperatures. These findings emphasize that consideration should be given to placement of patients at increased risk for thermal stress, the need to frequently reassess the patients comfort and to provide thermal comfort measures. However, there are no reports of adverse events associated with this thermally stressful environment, including the effects of high ambient temperature on patient outcomes.

Currently hypothermia prevention involves the use of the Hypothermia Prevention Kit (HPMK) [43–45], which includes a radiant blanket, warming pad, and head cover. This strategy has been shown to maintain core body temperature in a hemorrhagic shock model under a temperature of 2 °C with a 3.6 m/sec airflow. Of note, the use of a wool blanket alone did not prevent hypothermia in severe hemorrhagic shock at 10 °C (50 °F), demonstrating the need for active versus passive warming [46]. An aspect of hypothermia prevention unique to AE or high-altitude care is that the Ready-Heat blanket relies on oxygen as a part of the thermal reaction, with decreased heat production above 7000 feet [47].

Gravitational Forces

Gravitational forces (Gs) in military aircraft used for AE are greatest during takeoff, landing, and banking. In healthy seated patients facing forward (i.e., standard airline configuration), changes in horizontal G forces are small, with takeoff (acceleration) resulting in +0.4 G and landing (deceleration) in −0.1 G. Banking <40° increases vertical forces by only +0.15 Gs. In supine patients, changes in horizontal G forces depend on the direction of the patient's head, and military AE patients are routinely loaded with their heads toward the front of the aircraft. These small changes in G forces can be of concern in high-risk patients, particularly those with severe traumatic brain injury and cardiac disease.

A unique case report in a patient with a biventricular assist device (BiVAD) demonstrates the effects of gravitational forces [48]. The patient was transported on a civilian fixed wing aircraft in a supine position with head forward and the BiVAD pump at knee level. During takeoff (30 seconds of climb), BiVAD flow was decreased 33%, with a return to baseline when the patient flexed their calf muscles. During landing, deceleration increased flow, which resolved within 30 seconds after completion of braking. The hemodynamic changes were thought to reflect gravitational effects in a patient with probable hypovolemia.

Gravitational forces may also increase aspiration risk in seriously ill patients [49–51]. Current standard of practice [52] is to administer enteral nutrition through a post-pyloric tube, with correct tube position (past the ligament of Treitz) confirmed by radiography. Follow-up includes monitoring and documentation of the tube length, and quantity and pH of the aspirate should also be examined to determine proper placement. Auscultation over the abdomen for an air bolus is no longer recommended as a method to verify proper tube placement. To decrease aspiration risk in high-risk patients, the flight surgeon can order backrests for litter patients.

Decreased Humidity

In commercial aircraft the humidity is estimated to decrease to approximately 10–40% [53]. In the C-17 cargo aircraft, the humidity decreased to 5% within 30 minutes of ascent to altitude [42]. There are no studies on the effect of decreased humidity on patients, although dehydration may be a risk factor for venous thromboembolism, airway compromise, and the maintenance of moist dressings. A primary intervention is the supplementation of water intake for all patients and crew.

Vibration

There is limited research on the effects of vibration on patients, except for ground-based studies on the effects of vibration during transport in a military helicopter and ambulances in models of spinal cord injury. These studies found no differences in functional outcomes. An important secondary finding was that inflammatory mediators were highest in the first 2.5–6 hours post-injury, which may have implications for the timing of transport. An observational study by Hatzfeld [35] did not find increased pain associated with vibration during takeoff. However, further research is needed to evaluate the effect of vibration during transport on an AMBUS or K-loader on patients with vertebral or orthopedic injuries, as the latter group reported the highest pain scores upon arrival to the aircraft [54]. It is also not known if vibration increases the risk for compartment syndrome.

General Patient Transport Considerations

As a general rule, all medical conditions have potential for deterioration. In addition, AE intensifies many of the risk factors associated with this deterioration. Anticipation of potential complications is imperative to ensuring the safe transport of AE patients. As there are few absolute contraindications for AE, medical flight crew members must be keenly aware of the general risks associated with air evacuation across a wide spectrum of medical conditions.

Preflight Assessment

A preflight assessment is critical in identifying any potential complications early and determining the patient's suitability for flight. Each patient should be screened for risk factors for issues commonly experienced during AE, such as nausea, motion sickness/vertigo, psychological stress and anxiety, tissue expansion (especially in orthopedic and traumatic cases), venous stasis, respiratory disturbances/hypoxia, and increased pain. When appropriate, premedicating patients for flight for pain, nausea, or anxiety should be considered to maintain adequate comfort.

Pain Management

The delivery of optimal pain management as the patient moves across the continuum of care is a challenge, particularly during the handoff periods. For example, in a study of patients transported from the hospital to the aircraft, there was limited documentation of pain status preflight or upon arrival to the aircraft [54]. Patients with orthopedic injuries with external fixators had the highest pain scores (with external fixator

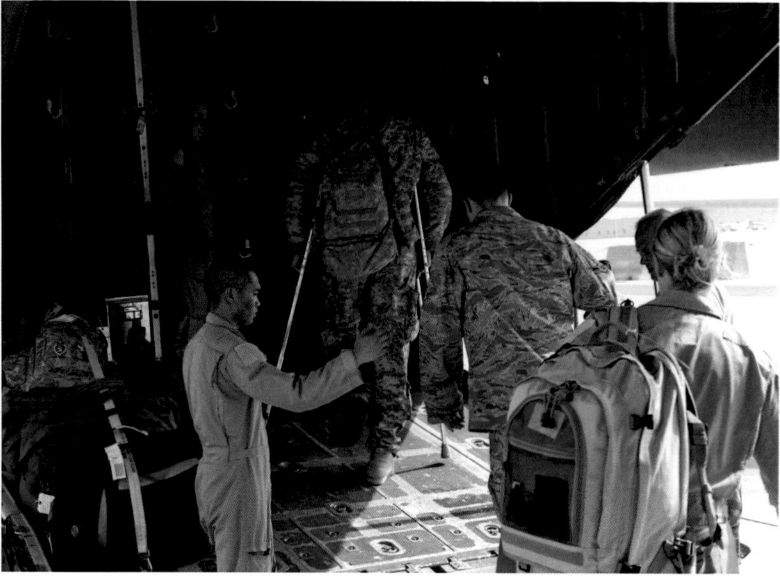

Fig. 8.5 Patient boarding aircraft on crutches demonstrates the challenge of balancing effective pain management and safety. (US Air Force photo/ Staff Sgt. Robert Barney http://www.af.mil/News/Photos.aspx?igphoto=2000487356)

8.7 ± 1.1/without 2.8 ± 2.8, $p = 0.012$). These results were similar to another study of patients with extremity trauma [55].

Adequate preflight preparation is important, particularly in light of the fact that >50% of patients self-administer pain medications [56, 57]. Preflight preparation for in-flight pain management should strive to adequately address the effects of known stressors as discussed above and timing issues related to flight; i.e., during ascent when FNs are not able to administer analgesia [58].

A human factors/systems engineering analysis of en route pain management [59] recommended the creation of a standardized education brochure and the creation of a pain management plan document for each patient. The timing of medication administration relative to the phases of transport is also a challenge [6]. In Gentry's study [54], the time from hospital departure to aircraft lift off ("wheels up") was 110 ± 42 minutes (range 56–240 minutes). In this small study, the four patients with severe pain all received a narcotic (Dilaudid, morphine, or Percocet) approximately 1 hour before hospital departure. The timing of the preflight medication suggests there may have been inadequate analgesia during the extended period when the patients were being transported from the hospital to the aircraft and during take-off and ascent to altitude. Given that many patients are ambulatory, the timing of analgesic administration must also be considered in the context of patient safety (Fig. 8.5).

During flight, higher pain scores were reported by trauma patients compared to patients with medical or psychiatric diagnoses [56, 57, 60, 61]. A challenge is to accurately assess pain as military combat casualties are stoic and reluctant to take pain medications. In an observational study, pain levels >3 were nearly always due to the patient's reluctance to ask for pain medications, which are further complicated as approximately 50% of these patients self-administered their medication [35, 62]. A unique nursing challenge onboard the aircraft is access to narcotics, as the single narcotics box is carried by an FN. A task timing study found that 7% of the FN's time was used to access the narcotics box. Given that analgesics are the most commonly administered medication during flight, the addition of another narcotics box, or a single box in a fixed location, may decrease the nurses travel time and fatigue [59].

Epidural Analgesia/Peripheral Nerve Block

The Joint Trauma System Clinical Practice Guideline: Pain, Anxiety, and Delirium recommend a multimodal strategy for pain management [63]. One aspect of a multimodal approach is the use of epidural analgesia or a peripheral nerve block (PNB) catheter during transport [64]. Analysis of 84 combat casualties who suffered a limb amputation found decreased opioid consumption and a lower rate of intubation in the casualties who received regional anesthesia during the en route phase of care [65]. To mitigate risk associated with regional anesthesia, patients must wait at least 24 hours before being manifested for transport if they have experienced a complication related to the epidural or PNB catheter. Additionally, they must have the epidural or PNB in place and running without complication for at least 4 hours before transport to minimize the chance of side effects, such as local anesthetic toxicity. Intravenous or oral analgesics may be used for breakthrough pain. Patients with an epidural or PNB to the lower extremity may ambulate, but they should be considered a fall risk due to potential motor weakness.

Conditions with Important Aeromedical Evacuation Implications

Ear Block

Ear block is one of the most common complications of human flight. Patients at increased risk for ear block include those with upper respiratory infections, or post ear-nose-throat surgery may experience pain caused by air trapped behind the tympanic membrane. In addition to standard therapies (yawning, chewing gum), procedures for manually clearing ear blocks have been established utilizing high-pressure bursts of air via the bag-valve-mask.

Pneumothorax

AE for patients with pneumothorax is an important issue for AE patients because even a small pneumothorax at sea level will expand during flight and can cause significant pulmonary complications. For this reason, an untreated pneumothorax is considered a contraindication to flight. A patient with a traumatic pneumothorax of any size requires the placement of a chest tube with a Heimlich valve prior to AE.

Management of a patient with a chest tube is an important aspect of AE nursing care. In the confined space on an aircraft, it is difficult to avoid the creation of a dependent loop in the tubing. The effect of different tubing position was studied in an animal model [66]. When the tubing had a dependent loop, there was significantly less fluid drained compared to coiled on litter, straight on litter, or lifted and drained every 15 minutes. Internal tube pressure was significantly higher in the dependent loop with/without lifting and draining. The optimal position for the tubing is coiled or straight on the litter, but when this is not possible, lifting and draining the tube every 15 minutes improves function. Because of the risk of a rapid decompression, the chest tube system must have an integrated one-way valve or a Heimlich valve.

Orthopedic Injuries

Orthopedic and soft tissue injuries are common in the AE system. Adequate monitoring of neurovascular status, peripheral pulses, capillary refill, and motor functions—both preflight and at altitude—are paramount. Closed injuries are at increased risk for tissue damage or compartment syndrome due to barometric pressure changes. Frequent reassessment throughout the flight is required. Flexible splints are the recommended method of stabilization as they allow tissue expansion. If casts are used, the AECM should ensure the cast is bivalved. Open fractures are frequently stabilized using external fixators. Assessment of the pin sites and external dressings is conducted in addition to neurovascular checks. If swelling occurs, it may be necessary to loosen the outer dressing to prevent disruption in circulation. Every effort should be made to protect the device from points of vibration or where it may be inadvertently jarred.

Postabdominal Surgery

There is minimal research on en route care and adverse events associated with expansion of abdominal gas. Older studies in humans and animals did not find any sequelae associated with gas expansion with ascent to altitude, although standards [6] recommend consideration of gastrointestinal decompression in at-risk patients. CCATT clinical practice guidelines [67] identify an open abdomen as a possible indication for negative pressure wound therapy; however, there are no studies or guidelines specific to its use in AE.

Typical preflight/in-flight considerations include assessing the patient's previous or current disease processes, including abdominal surgical history, intestinal complications, ulcerative colitis, kidney or cardiopulmonary disease, as well as pregnancy or stroke. Consideration must be given to the effects of altitude when determining the plan of care during transport. Key interventions include the use of nasogastric tubes to reduce distension, pain management, and intravenous (IV) fluids as required to maintain hemodynamics. Other considerations include supplemental oxygen, special diet or nil per os (NPO) status, intake/output monitoring, antiemetics, and comfort measures (i.e., litter for comfort, backrest, etc.).

Psychiatric Conditions

Mental health diagnoses are among the most common diagnoses in evacuated patients [10, 68]. The stresses of flight should be considered in caring for these patients, since their condition can be exacerbated by fatigue, noise, and hypobaric hypoxia.

Examples of en route care include using of strategies to enhance communication with the patient as needed (i.e., having the patient wear a communication headset), ensuring adequate rest, and ruling out hypoxia as a cause of mental status changes. High-risk patients should be transported with an experienced mental health provider. En route safety considerations may include placing the patient on the lowest litter tier away from emergency exits and equipment and the flight deck. The potential need for sedation and restraints should be addressed preflight.

Positional Pressure Injuries

The en route care phase is a period of increased risk for pressure injuries due to restrictions on turning and repositioning the patient. In a study of CCATT patients transported between 2008 and 2012, 164 patients had documentation of a pressure injury within 3 days of transport. A particularly high-risk group are patients with an unstable thoracolumbar fracture, who may be transported by CCATT in a vacuum spine board or a standard litter with/without the foam mattress [69, 70]. Among these patients, the incidence of pressure injuries ranged from 9.3% [71] to 13% [72], which is higher than the 5% incidence observed in all CCATT patients [73, 74]. A limitation is that there are no data available on the incidence of pressure injuries in AE patients.

A challenge in AE for pressure injury prevention is the size of the litter (24 × 72 inches), which limits repositioning. The standard AE mattress has good pressure redistribution characteristics in the supine position (occiput: 38 ± 11, sacrum 32 ± 4 mm Hg, heels 49 ± 12 mm Hg) [75]. The use of a blanket as padding causes an increase in interface pressure and is not recommended [76]. Recently, two strategies were evaluated that may be useful in AE: Mepilex (Mölnlycke Healthcare AB, Götenborg, Sweden), a multi-layer dressing on the sacrum and heels, and LiquiCell (LiquiCell Technologies, Inc.), a pad containing a series of bursa-like pouches containing a thin layer of low-viscosity fluid positioned between the sacrum and head [77]. Neither strategy decreased skin interface pressure or was associated with differences in skin blood flow or tissue oxygenation on the sacrum or heels compared to the standard AE mattress alone, suggesting that their mechanism of injury may be a reduction of friction and shear. Given that Mepilex has been associated with a decreased risk of pressure injuries in high-risk patients [78–80], its prophylactic use during AE should be considered. Steps to mitigate friction, shear, and increased skin temperature and moisture during transport need to be evaluated.

Venous Thromboembolism

Several of the known stresses of flight increased the risk of venous thromboembolism (VTE).

Three major en route risk factors for VTE are dehydration, hypobaric hypoxia, and prolonged immobilization in a seated, but not supine position [81–87]. A limitation of all the studies that identified these risks was that they were conducted with healthy patients undergoing commercial transport rather than acutely ill or injured patients. Trauma patients are known to be at increased risk for VTE during the first 48 hours post-injury. Although this time period often coincides with time of AE transport, increased VTE for these patients risk attributable to AE remains uncertain [88]. In addition to thromboprophylaxis for patients at increased VTE risk [89], general en route nursing care that might help minimize VTE risk includes offering patients water frequently and encouraging mobilization or the performance of range-of-motion exercises.

Acute Coronary Syndrome

ACS represents one of the most common medical reasons for evacuation. A unique aspect of military AE is the need for transport of ASC patients during the acute phase. General civilian recommendations are to avoid travel for 2–4 weeks after a major cardiovascular event [90–95]. In contrast, patients undergoing military AE may be transported within hours of resolution of chest pain.

The two most common en route adverse events for patients with ACS are the unanticipated need for supplemental oxygen and recurrence of chest pain. These adverse effects are related to hypobaric hypoxia, but the effect of gravitational forces, cold, and fatigue also increases risk for these patients [93]. Hypobaric hypoxia may also increase pulmonary artery pressure, which may exacerbate pre-existing pulmonary hypertension and right-sided heart failure [96–98].

Prior to AE, a flight surgeon will risk stratify patients with ACS and identify the required level of en route care [99]. For example, a patient at low risk for coronary artery disease (i.e., less than three risk factors, negative cardiac enzymes, and no ECG changes) can be transported by routine AE. A patient at intermediate risk (i.e., negative cardiac enzymes, ECG changes) will require en route cardiac monitoring and supplemental oxygen; consideration should be given to a medical attendant or CCATT transport. A high-risk patient (e.g., one with hemodynamic instability, pulmonary edema, and sustained ventricular tachycardia) will require CCATT transport.

In-Flight Cardiac Arrest

When a cardiac arrest occurs onboard the aircraft, the patient is cared for in accordance with the American Heart Association Advanced Cardiac Life Support guidelines [6, 100]. However, the austere and cramped AE environment requires a number of adaptions and increased precautions.

When cardiac arrest is diagnosed in a litter patient, cardiopulmonary resuscitation should be initiated on the litter and defibrillation attempted before movement to the aircraft deck. Although transferring the patient to the aircraft deck improves patient access, the time it takes delays performance of compressions and the return of spontaneous circulation. The effectiveness of cardiac compression in a litter patient can be quickly improved by placing a backboard between the patient and the mesh litter [101].

During cardiac defibrillation, environmental awareness is critical to avoid inadvertent injury to air crew or nearby patients in the cramped AE environment. Defibrillating a patient on a litter with aluminum handles is ideal. If the patient is on a liter with ferric metal handles or on the metal aircraft deck, a blanket should be placed between the patient and the deck [13].

In-Flight Death

Deaths en route must be handled according to international law. If there is a physician onboard the flight, he/she may pronounce the patient dead. The time of death should be recorded in Zulu time and information relayed to the aircraft commander who will notify the appropriate ground command before arrival. If no physician is onboard, the AE medical crew director should notify the aircraft commander of the suspected death who will in turn notify the appropriate ground command before arrival. A physician will routinely meet the aircraft to pronounce the patient dead.

Disclaimer The views expressed in this chapter are those of the authors and do not necessarily represent the official position or policy of the US Air Force, the US Department of Defense, or the US government.

References

1. Schmelz JO, Bridges EJ, Duong DN, Ley C. Care of the critically ill patient in a military unique environment: a program of research. Crit Care Nurs Clin North Am. 2003;15(2):171–81.
2. Bridges E. Facilitation of evidence-based nursing practice during military operations. Nurs Res. 2010;59(1 Suppl):S75–9.
3. Bridges E, Biever K. Advancing critical care: Joint Combat Casualty Research Team and Joint Theater Trauma System. AACN Adv Crit Care. 2010;21(3):260–76.
4. Hatzfeld JJ, Dukes S, Bridges E. Chapter 3: innovations in the en route care of combat casualties. Annu Rev Nurs Res. 2014;32(1):41–62.
5. US Air Force. AFI11-202 V2 Aircrew standardization/evaluation program; 2010.
6. US Air Force. Air Force Instruction 48–307, Volume 1. Health services: en route care and aeromedical evacuation medical operations. Secretary of the Air Force; 2017.
7. US Air Force. Air Force Instruction 11-2AE, Volume 1: Aeromedical Evacuation Aircrew Training. Washington, DC: Secretary of the Air Force; 2013.
8. Bridges E, Mortimer D, Dukes S. Aeromedical evacuation registry. Aviat Space Environ Med. 2016;87(3):309.
9. Rasmussen TE. The military's evolved en route care paradigm: continuous, transcontinental intensive care. JAMA Surg. 2014;149(8):814.
10. Armed Forces Health Surveillance Center. Surveillance snapshot: medical evacuations from Operation Enduring Freedom (OEF), active and reserve components, U.S. Armed Forces, October 2001–December 2011. MSMR. 2012;19(2):22.
11. Patel AA, Hauret KG, Taylor BJ, Jones BH. Non-battle injuries among U.S. Army soldiers deployed to Afghanistan and Iraq, 2001-2013. J Saf Res. 2017;60:29–34.
12. De Jong MJ, Dukes SF, Dufour KM, Mortimer DL. Clinical experience and learning style of Flight Nurse and Aeromedical Evacuation Technician students. Aerosp Med Hum Perform. 2017;88(1):23–9.
13. US Air Force. Air Force Instruction 11-2AE, Volume 3: Aeromedical Evacuation (AE) operations procedures. Washington DC: Secretary of the Air Force; 2014.
14. Dufour KM, Dukes S. Enhancing patient safety through improved patient handoffs. Aviat Space Environ Med. 2014;85(3):297–8.
15. McNeill MM, Pierce P, Dukes S, Bridges EJ. En route care patient safety: thoughts from the field. Mil Med. 2014;179(8 Suppl):11–8.
16. Connor S, Dukes S, McNeill M, Bridges E, Pierce P. En route patient safety: a mixed-methods study. School of Aerospace Medicine Wright Patterson Afb Oh;2014. ADA600951.
17. Fouts B, Serres J, Dukes S, Maupin G, Wade M, Cowgill M. Quantification of ergonomic risks associated with aeromedical evacuation tasks. MHSRS; 2014.
18. Serres JL, Fouts BL, Dukes SF, Maupin GM, Wade ME. Records review of musculoskeletal injuries in aeromedical evacuation personnel. Am J Prev Med. 2015;48(4):365–71.
19. Fouts BL, Serres JL, Dukes SF, Maupin GM, Wade ME, Pohlman DM. Investigation of self-reported musculoskeletal injuries on post-deployment health assessment forms for aeromedical evacuation personnel. Mil Med. 2015;180(12):1256–61.
20. Serres J, Dukes S, Wright B, Dodson W, Parham-Bruce W, Powell E, et al. Assessment of fatigue in deployed critical care air transport team crews. Wright Patterson AFB, OH: Air Force Research Laboratory, 711th Human Performance Wing; July 2015.
21. Cicek I, Serres JL. Safe-to-fly test and evaluation of fatigue research study test devices. Aviat Space Environ Med. 2014;85(4):473–9.
22. Swearingen JM, Goodman TM, Chappelle WL, Thompson WT. Post-traumatic stress symptoms in United States Air Force aeromedical evacuation nurses and technicians. Mil Med. 2017;182(S1):258–65.
23. Pierce P. Focus group patient safety concerns and solutions: unexpected findings. Aviat Space Environ Med. 2014;85(3):297.
24. Pierce P, McNeill M, Dukes S. An occupational paradox: why do we love really tough jobs. Crit Care Nurs. 2018;38(2):52–8.
25. Maupin G, Butler W, Smith D. Descriptive analysis of patient transports with a cabin altitude restriction: 2001-2014. Aviat Space Environ Med. 2016;87(3):321.
26. Butler WP, Steinkraus LW, Burlingame EE, Fouts BL, Serres JL. Complication rates in altitude restricted patients following aeromedical evacuation. Aerosp Med Hum Perform. 2016;87(4):352–9.
27. Cottrell JJ, Lebovitz BL, Fennell RG, Kohn GM. Inflight arterial saturation: continuous monitoring by pulse oximetry. Aviat Space Environ Med. 1995;66(2):126–30.
28. Geertsema C, Williams AB, Dzendrowskyj P, Hanna C. Effect of commercial airline travel on

oxygen saturation in athletes. Br J Sports Med. 2008;42(11):877–81.
29. Muhm JM, Rock PB, McMullin DL, Jones SP, Lu IL, Eilers KD, et al. Effect of aircraft-cabin altitude on passenger discomfort. N Engl J Med. 2007;357(1):18–27.
30. Johannigman J, Gerlach T, Cox D, Juhasz J, Britton T, Elterman J, et al. Hypoxemia during aeromedical evacuation of the walking wounded. J Trauma Acute Care Surg. 2015;79(4 Suppl 2):S216–20.
31. Alkins S. Long-distance air evacuation of blast-injured sailors from the U.S.S. Cole. Aviat Space Environ Med. 2002;73(7):678–80.
32. Mora AG, Ervin AT, Ganem VJ, Bebarta VS. Aeromedical evacuation of combat patients by military critical care air transport teams with a lower hemoglobin threshold approach is safe. J Trauma Acute Care Surg. 2014;77(5):724–8.
33. Johannigman J, Gerlach T, Cox D, Britton T, Elterman J, Rodriquez D Jr, et al. Relationship of hemoglobin to arterial oxygen desaturation during aeromedical evacuation. Air Force Research Laboratory 711th Human Performance Wing U.S. Air Force School of Aerospace Medicine Aeromedical Research Department; 2015. AFRL-SA-WP-SR-2015-0007.
34. McNeill M. Critical care performance in a simulated military aircraft cabin environment: University of Maryland; 2007.
35. Hatzfeld J, Dukes S, Serres J. Factors that impact pain management in Aeromedical Evacuation: an ethnographic approach. Aviat Space Environ Med. 2014;85(3):270.
36. Iyer N, Romigh G. Real-time patient-provider communication system for en route patient care. Aerosp Med. 2016;87(3):198.
37. Houtsma AJ, Curry IP, Sewell JM, Bernhard WN. A dual-mode noise-immune stethoscope for use in noisy vehicles (ADA481444). Fort Rucker Al: Army Aeromedical Research Lab; 2006.
38. Houtsma AJ, Curry IP, Sewell JM, Bernhard WN. Dual-mode auscultation in high-noise level environments. Aviat Space Environ Med. 2006;77:294–5.
39. Cho T, Kelley A, Simmons J, Gaydos S, Estrada A. Assessment of the noise immune stethoscope in a clinical environment: United States Army Aeromedical Research Laboratory, Warfighter Health Division; 2014.
40. Fouts B, Wilson M, Eaton K, Serres J. Investigating the usefulness of noise immune stethoscope technology in the en route care environment. ASMA; 2016.
41. Walsh M. Thermal environment of litter positions and human responses onboard Hercules C-130 aircraft, The University of Texas Graduate School of Biomedical Sciences; 1998.
42. Bridges E. Thermal stress and the human response to thermal stress with litter position on the C-141 Starlifter and C-17 Globemaster II. Bethesda, MD: TriService Nursing Research Program; 1 August 2005.
43. Joint Theater System. Joint Theater Trauma System Clinical Practice Guideline: Hypothermia Prevention, Monitoring, and Management. 2012; http://www.usaisr.amedd.army.mil/cpgs/Hypothermia_Prevention_20_Sep_12.pdf. Accessed 5 May 2017.
44. Schmelz J, Bridges E, Sanders S, Wallac MB, Shaw T, Kester N, et al. Preventing hypothermia in critically ill patients during aeromedical evacuation – Chillbuster® and reflective blanket. Paper presented at: 110th Annual Association of Military Surgeons of the United States meeting, Karen Rieder Poster Session, November 15, 2004, Denver, CO.
45. Bridges E, Schmelz J, Evers K. Efficacy of the Blizzard Blanket or Blizzard Blanket plus Thermal Angel in Preventing Hypothermia in a Hemorrhagic Shock Victim (*Sus scrofa*) under operational conditions. Mil Med. 2007;172(1):17–23.
46. Nesbitt M, Allen P, Beekley A, Butler F, Eastridge B, Blackbourne L. Current practice of thermoregulation during the transport of combat wounded. J Trauma. 2010;69(Suppl 1):S162–7.
47. McKeague AL. Evaluation of Patient Active Warming Systems (PAWS). MHSRS; 2012.
48. McLean N, Copeland R, Casey N, Samoukovic G, Quigley R. Successful trans-Atlantic air ambulance transfer of a patient supported by a bi-ventricular assist device. Aviat Space Environ Med. 2011;82(8):825–8.
49. Jansen JO, Turner S, Johnston AM. Nutritional management of critically ill trauma patients in the deployed military setting. J R Army Med Corps. 2011;157(3 Suppl 1):S344–9.
50. Turner S, Ruth MJ, Bruce DL. "In flight catering": feeding critical care patients during aeromedical evacuation. J R Army Med Corps. 2008;154(4):282–3.
51. Stankorb SM, Ramsey C, Clark H, Osgood T. Provision of nutrition support therapies in the recent Iraq and Afghanistan conflicts. Nutr Clin Pract. 2014;29(5):605–11.
52. AACN. Practice alert: initial and ongoing verification of feeding tube placement in adults. Crit Care Nurse. 2016;36(2):e8–e13.
53. Grün G, Trimmel M, Holm A. Low humidity in the aircraft cabin environment and its impact on well-being – results from a laboratory study. Build Environ. 2012;47:23–31.
54. Gentry C, Frazier L, Ketz A, Abel L, Castro M, Steele N, et al. Preflight/enroute pain management of trauma patients transported by USAF AE from Operation Enduring Freedom. Paper presented at: the 116th Annual Meeting of AMSUS, the Society of Federal Health Professionals, San Antonio, TX. 2010.
55. Buckenmaier CC 3rd, Rupprecht C, McKnight G, McMillan B, White RL, Gallagher RM, et al. Pain following battlefield injury and evacuation: a survey of 110 casualties from the wars in Iraq and Afghanistan. Pain Med. 2009;10(8):1487–96.

56. Bridges E, Dukes S, Maupin G. Assessment of pain: a safety consideration within aeromedical evacuation. Military Health Sciences Research Symposium; 2014.
57. Bridges E, Dukes S, Serres J. Assessment of pain in less severely ill and injured aeromedical evacuation patients: a prospective field study. Mil Med. 2015;180(3 Suppl):44–9.
58. Hatzfeld J, Serres J, Dukes S. Factors that impact pain management in aeromedical evacuation: an ethnographic approach. Crit Care Nurs. 2017; in press
59. Gallimore J. Systems and human factors evaluation to improve pain management during the air evacuation process. Wright State University; 2016. AFRL-SA-WP-TR-2016-0004.
60. Pfennig P, Bridges E. Pain management in operational aeromedical evacuation. Paper presented at: 79th annual scientific meeting of the Aerospace Medical Association 2008; Boston, MA.
61. Dukes S, Bridges E, Maupin G. Retrospective review of the pain management of aeromedical evacuation patients. Aviat Space Environ Med. 2014;85(3):269.
62. Hatzfeld J, Dukes S, Serres J. Understanding pain management in the aeromedical evacuation system. Aviat Space Environ Med. 2014;83(3):269–70.
63. Buckenmaier CC, McKnight GM, Winkley JV, Bleckner LL, Shannon C, Klein SM, et al. Continuous peripheral nerve block for battlefield anesthesia and evacuation. Reg Anesth Pain Med. 2005;30(2):202–5.
64. Carness JM, Wilson MA, Lenart MJ, Smith DE, Dukes SF. Experiences with regional anesthesia for analgesia during prolonged aeromedical evacuation. Aerosp Med Hum Perform. 2017;88(8):768–72.
65. Schmelz JO, Johnson D, Norton JM, Andrews M, Gordon PA. Effects of position of chest drainage tube on volume drained and pressure. Am J Crit Care. 1999;8(5):319–23.
66. Joint Trauma System. CCAT Negative pressure wound therapy clinical practice guideline. 2013; http://usaisr.amedd.army.mil/cpgs/CCATCPGNegativePressureWoundTherapyDec2013.pdf.
67. Wilmoth MC, Linton A, Gromadzki R, Larson MJ, Williams TV, Woodson J. Factors associated with psychiatric evacuation among service members deployed to Operation Enduring Freedom and Operation Iraqi Freedom, January 2004 to September 2010. Mil Med. 2015;180(1):53–60.
68. Joint trauma system clinical practice guideline: cervical and thoracolumbar spine injury evaluation, transport and surgery in the deployed setting (CPG ID:15). 2016. Accessed 20 June 2017.
69. Bridges E. Vacuum spine board testing report: skin interface pressure on vacuum spine board compared to standard spinal immobilization methods. Brooks AFB, TX; 2009.
70. Bebarta V. Critical Care Air Transport Team (CCATT) short term outcomes with spinal fractures moved with the vacuum spine board between 2009 and 2010. Paper presented at: MHSRS 2011.
71. Mok JM, Jackson KL, Fang R, Freedman BA. Effect of vacuum spine board immobilization on incidence of pressure ulcers during evacuation of military casualties from theater. Spine J. 2013;13(12):1801–8.
72. Dukes S. Risk factors for pressure ulcer development in CCATT patients. Military Health System Research Symposium; 2014; Fort Lauderdale, FL.
73. Dukes S, Maupin G, Thomas M, Mortimer D. Pressure injury development in patients treated by Critical Care Air Transport Teams: a case-control study. Crit Care Nurse. 2018;38(2):30–6.
74. Bridges E. Comparison of peak skin interface pressure on prototype aeromedical evacuation mattress: USAF; 16 Aug 2005.
75. Bridges EJ, Schmelz JO, Mazer S. Skin interface pressure on the NATO litter. Mil Med. 2003;168(4):280–6.
76. Bridges E, Whitney J, Burr R, Tolentino E. Reducing the risk for pressure injury during combat evacuation. Crit Care Nurse. 2018;38(2):38–45.
77. Call E, Pedersen J, Bill B, Black J, Alves P, Brindle CT, et al. Enhancing pressure ulcer prevention using wound dressings: what are the modes of action? Int Wound J. 2015;12(4):408–13.
78. Santamaria N, Gerdtz M, Sage S, McCann J, Freeman A, Vassiliou T, et al. A randomised controlled trial of the effectiveness of soft silicone multi-layered foam dressings in the prevention of sacral and heel pressure ulcers in trauma and critically ill patients: the border trial. Int Wound J. 2015;12(3):302–8.
79. Brindle CT, Wegelin JA. Prophylactic dressing application to reduce pressure ulcer formation in cardiac surgery patients. J Wound Ostomy Continence Nurs. 2012;39(2):133–42.
80. Bendz B, Rostrup M, Sevre K, Andersen TO, Sandset PM. Association between acute hypobaric hypoxia and activation of coagulation in human beings. Lancet. 2000;356(9242):1657–8.
81. Bendz B, Sandset PM. Acute hypoxia and activation of coagulation. Lancet. 2003;362(9388):997–8.
82. Crosby A, Talbot NP, Harrison P, Keeling D, Robbins PA. Relation between acute hypoxia and activation of coagulation in human beings. Lancet. 2003;361(9376):2207–8.
83. Hodkinson PD, Hunt BJ, Parmar K, Ernsting J. Is mild normobaric hypoxia a risk factor for venous thromboembolism? J Thromb Haemost. 2003;1(10):2131–3.
84. Bradford A. The role of hypoxia and platelets in air travel-related venous thromboembolism. Curr Pharm Des. 2007;13(26):2668–72.
85. Schobersberger W, Schobersberger B, Partsch H. Travel-related thromboembolism: mechanisms and avoidance. Expert Rev Cardiovasc Ther. 2009;7(12):1559–67.
86. Venemans-Jellema A, Schreijer AJ, Le Cessie S, Emmerich J, Rosendaal FR, Cannegieter SC. No effect of isolated long-term supine immobilization

or profound prolonged hypoxia on blood coagulation. J Thromb Haemost. 2014;12(6):902–9.
87. Hutchison TN, Krueger CA, Berry JS, Aden JK, Cohn SM, White CE. Venous thromboembolism during combat operations: a 10-y review. J Surg Res. 2014;187(2):625–30.
88. Joint trauma system clinical practice guideline: the prevention of deep vein thrombosis. 2012; http://www.usaisr.amedd.army.mil/cpgs/Prevention_of_Deep_Venous_Thrombosis_24_Apr_12.pdf.
89. Essebag V, Halabi AR, Churchill-Smith M, Lutchmedial S. Air medical transport of cardiac patients. Chest. 2003;124(5):1937–45.
90. Wang W, Brady WJ, O'Connor RE, Sutherland S, Durand-Brochec MF, Duchateau FX, et al. Non-urgent commercial air travel after acute myocardial infarction: a review of the literature and commentary on the recommendations. Air Med J. 2012;31(5):231–7.
91. Thibeault C, Evans AD, Dowdall NP. AsMA medical guidelines for air travel: fitness to fly and medical clearances. Aerosp Med Hum Perform. 2015;86(7):656.
92. Smith D, Toff W, Joy M, Dowdall N, Johnston R, Clark L, et al. Fitness to fly for passengers with cardiovascular disease. Heart. 2010;96(Suppl 2):ii1–16.
93. Ross D, Essebag V, Sestier F, Soder C, Thibeault C, Tyrrell M, et al. Canadian Cardiovascular Society consensus conference. Assessment of the cardiac patient for fitness to fly: flying subgroup executive summary. Can J Cardiol. 2004;20(13):1321–3.
94. Aerospace Medical Association Medical Guidelines Task Force. Medical guidelines for air travel, 2nd ed. Aviat Space Environ Med. 2003;74(5 Suppl):A1–19.
95. Turner BE, Hodkinson PD, Timperley AC, Smith TG. Pulmonary artery pressure response to simulated air travel in a hypobaric chamber. Aerosp Med Hum Perform. 2015;86(6):529–34.
96. Smith TG, Talbot NP, Chang RW, Wilkinson E, Nickol AH, Newman DG, et al. Pulmonary artery pressure increases during commercial air travel in healthy passengers. Aviat Space Environ Med. 2012;83(7):673–6.
97. Smith TG, Chang RW, Robbins PA, Dorrington KL. Commercial air travel and in-flight pulmonary hypertension. Aviat Space Environ Med. 2013;84(1):65–7.
98. Steinkraus LW. The patient with acute coronary syndrome. 2008.
99. Link MS, Berkow LC, Kudenchuk PJ, Halperin HR, Hess EP, Moitra VK, et al. Part 7: adult advanced cardiovascular life support: 2015 American Heart Association Guidelines update for cardiopulmonary resuscitation and emergency cardiovascular care. Circulation. 2015;132(18 Suppl 2):S444–64.
100. Bridges E, Schmelz J, Woods S, Harrington I. Efficacy of CPR on the NATO and decontamination litter with and without a backboard. Am J Crit Care. 2004;13(3):257.

9 Critical Care Air Transport: Patient Flight Physiology and Organizational Considerations

William Beninati and Thomas E. Grissom

Introduction

Critically ill or injured patients need to be cared for in a critical care environment as soon as possible to optimize survival and recovery. Once established, this environment should continue uninterrupted, including during transport, until the critical illness resolves. However, there are special challenges to maintaining a critical care environment during aeromedical evacuation (AE), particularly over long distances far from medical backup. To meet this challenge, the Critical Care Air Transport Team (CCATT) program was developed.

This chapter will review the physiologic effects of flight as they apply to critical care and describe the CCATT medical members and the equipment they utilize during AE. In addition, this chapter will outline some of the most important information gained from extensive CCATT experience since the inception of the program.

W. Beninati (✉)
Col, USAF, MC, CFS (ret.), Senior Medical Director, Intermountain Life Flight and Virtual Hospital, University of Utah School of Medicine, Salt Lake City, UT, USA

Clinical Associate Professor (Affiliated), Stanford University School of Medicine, Stanford, CA, USA
e-mail: bill.beninati@imail.org

T. E. Grissom
Col, USAF, MC (ret.), Department of Anesthesiology, R Adams Cowley Shock Trauma Center, University of Maryland School of Medicine, Catonsville, MD, USA

Patient Flight Physiology and Stressors of Flight

Aerospace medicine has long been concerned with the effects of altitude and flight stresses on the performance of the aircrew. Only in the last two decades has it focused deeply on the effects of these factors on the care and outcome of critically ill and injured patients transported within the long-distance AE system. These stresses impact not only the patient but those managing their care as well.

Beyond a simple assessment of the environmental factors, other aspects of AE often magnify the potential problems of aeromedical transportation. As discussed in Chap. 5, fixed-wing military aircraft used for most AE missions do not protect patients and medical crew members from the stresses of flight to the same degree that commercial airliners protect passengers. The duration of exposure also plays a negative role in the impact of these stressors on both patients and crew members.

This section will review the classic flight stressors—including decreased barometric pressure, temperature, noise, vibration, decreased humidity, acceleration, and fatigue—and their potential impact on patient physiology and care delivery. An understanding of altitude physiology and related disease- or injury-specific considerations is important for preparing patients for AE and for anticipating and responding to problems

W. W. Hurd, W. Beninati (eds.), *Aeromedical Evacuation*,
https://doi.org/10.1007/978-3-030-15903-0_9

that arise in-flight. Subsequent chapters explore in more depth the effects of these stressors on specific conditions.

Barometric Pressure Changes

The most prominent environmental consideration in AE operations is the impact of changes in barometric pressure on oxygen delivery and gas expansion. The acceptable altitude range in which physiological functions are minimally impaired is limited to a fraction of the Earth's atmosphere. Modern aircraft are pressurized to maintain a cabin pressure at cruising altitudes equivalent to <8000 feet above sea level, an environment wherein most normal individuals can function without impairment [1]. However, medically impaired patients are at risk for progressive decompensation at these pressure altitudes without appropriate medical support. Movement of patients through the AE environment requires an understanding of the classic *gas laws* and an application of their principles as they apply to normal and abnormal physiology:

- *Boyle's Law* – The volume of gas is inversely proportional to the pressure surrounding it, as long as the temperature remains constant as in the human body. This law explains why a balloon expands as it ascends and also why a volume of trapped air expands in a body cavity when the pressure around it is reduced. A given volume can expect to increase by almost 20% at the cabin pressure altitude of 8000 feet commonly maintained by military cargo aircraft.
- *Dalton's Law* – The total pressure of a mixture of gases is equal to the sum of the partial pressures of each gas in the mixture. Although oxygen makes up 21% of the atmosphere at all attitudes, at sea level the partial pressure of oxygen (PO_2) is 160 mm Hg but decreases to 120 mm Hg at a cabin altitude of 8000 feet. This law explains why decreased cabin pressure at aircraft cruising altitudes reduces the available oxygen and increases the risk of hypoxia in compromised patients.
- *Charles' Law* – The pressure of a gas decreases proportionally as temperature decreases, as long as the volume remains constant. Consequently, the decreased cabin air temperature that often occurs in military cargo aircraft at altitude can lead to a decrease in the pressure within oxygen cylinders.
- *Henry's Law* – The amount of a gas in a solution decreases as the partial pressure of that gas over the solution decreases. This law explains why nitrogen bubbles can come out of solution in body tissues during ascent and lead to altitude-induced decompression sickness in susceptible patients, for example, those who have been scuba diving recently.

Hypoxia

Hypoxia can be defined as deficiency in the amount of oxygen reaching the tissues sufficient to cause impairment of function [2]. In the AE environment, hypoxia can have delirious effects on both patients and medical personnel. Many patients requiring AE frequently have one or more factors that predispose them to developing hypoxia. A decrease in barometric pressure with a reduction in the inspired partial pressure of oxygen may be enough to push the "stabilized" patient over the edge. In a classic study looking at casualties being transferred from Vietnam to other locations, 95 of 201 postoperative surgical patients developed a PaO_2 of <60 mm Hg when flying at cabin altitudes between 3000 and 7500 feet [3].

Hypoxia Categories

Hypoxic hypoxia occurs as a result of a decrease in the partial pressure of oxygen in the lungs or of other conditions that reduce the diffusion of oxygen across the alveolar-pulmonary capillary membrane. This is the most common type reported in flying personnel exposed to a lowered partial pressure of oxygen at high altitude. Additional causes include ventilation perfusion defects, airway obstruction, and apnea. Partial compensation through an increase in tidal volume and respiratory rate can be seen starting at

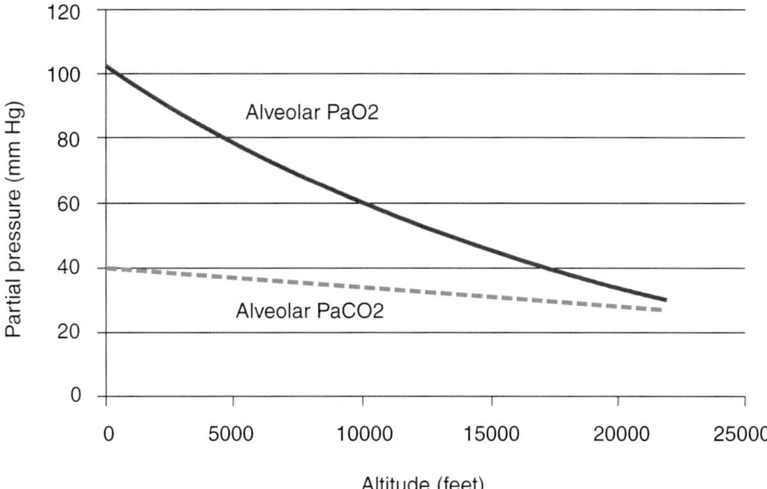

Fig. 9.1 Partial pressure of alveolar PaO_2 and $PaCO_2$ during exposure to altitude. (Adapted from [2])

5000 feet (1500 m) with a resulting drop in $PaCO_2$ (Fig. 9.1). Additional compensation occurs through increases in heart rate and cardiac output resulting in a decrease in the arteriovenous oxygen difference with an elevation in mean capillary oxygen tension [2].

Modern pressurized aircraft, including commercial airliners, rarely exceed a cabin pressure altitude of 8000 feet [4]. Because alveolar partial pressure of oxygen (PaO_2) at that altitude is approximately 70 mm Hg (O_2 saturation >90%), the majority of patients and normal passengers would be minimally affected at that cabin pressure. A small study looking at 29 patients with known or suspected ischemic heart disease requiring AE demonstrated that 5 (17%) of these patients dropped their oxygen saturation (SaO_2) to <90% [5]. The average cabin altitude during the flights was 6900 feet (2108 m) in a C-9A aircraft. In all cases, the addition of 4 L/min of oxygen corrected their oxygen desaturation.

Hypemic hypoxia occurs when there is a reduction in the capacity of blood to carry a sufficient amount of oxygen. This includes blood loss (anemic hypoxia), dyshemoglobinemias, excessive smoking, and carbon monoxide poisoning. For medical personnel and patients who smoke tobacco products, the formation of carboxyhemoglobin through the inhalation of carbon monoxide will make the individual more susceptible to this type of hypoxia. Typically, military aircrew members who donate blood are grounded for 72 hours following blood donation due to the reduced hemoglobin level. The impact of the reduced partial pressure of oxygen on the oxygen-carrying capacity of blood with reduced barometric pressure is illustrated in Fig. 9.1.

At a sea-level equivalent cabin pressure of 760 mm Hg, with a PaO_2 of 102 mm Hg, hemoglobin (Hb) of 15 g/dL, and SaO_2 of 98%, each 100 mL of blood carries approximately 20 mL of oxygen. This is reduced to 19 mL per 100 mL of blood due to venous admixture with unsaturated blood. The content drops by one half when the hemoglobin drops from 15 to 7 g/dL; however, the extraction remains constant at 5–6 mL of oxygen per 100 mL of blood. Thus, the venous saturation drops from 75% to <50%, leaving no reserve for additional oxygen demands when there is an associated drop in inspired oxygen.

Stagnant hypoxia occurs when there is a reduction in total cardiac output, pooling of the blood, or restriction of blood flow reducing oxygen delivery. This includes problems commonly found in critically ill or injured patients such as congestive heart failure, shock, and patients receiving positive pressure ventilation that impairs venous return. This concept can be extended to specific organ systems such as the development of cerebral vasoconstriction and reduced blood flow that occurs with hyperventilation. The use of supplemental oxygen is necessary in patients with stagnant hypoxia, especially in the presence of other hypoxia risk factors such as altitude or reduced carrying capacity.

Histotoxic hypoxia occurs when the utilization of oxygen by the body tissues is hindered. This includes carbon monoxide poisoning, cyanide poisoning, and excess alcohol ingestion. For the AE patient, this is not in general a contributing factor except in specific cases of known exposure, such as burn victims (carbon monoxide) and cyanide (sodium nitroprusside) toxicity.

Gas Expansion

Changes in barometric pressure produce effects beyond hypoxia. According to Boyle's Law, a volume of gas is inversely proportional to the pressure surrounding it (Fig. 9.2). This resulting gas expansion can adversely affect not only patients but also the medical crew and equipment as well. The end product of gas expansion in patients and crew can be pain that will affect mission performance or actual tissue damage.

The terms used to describe the effects of barometric pressure changes include dysbarism, barotrauma, and decompression sickness. *Dysbarism* refers to the general topic of pressure-related injuries. *Barotrauma* refers to the direct injuries that are a result of the mechanical effects from an applied pressure differential. Finally, *decompression sickness* relates to the complications associated with the evolution of dissolved gas from tissues and fluids of the body.

The most common sites of trapped gas disorders in the typical patient or medical crew member involve the ears, sinuses, gastrointestinal tract, and, rarely, teeth. When considering the potential for problems with the air transport of patients, you may need to consider other areas, including medical equipment and air introduced into other anatomic sites as a result of injury or operation.

Barotitis media or "ear block" is an acute or chronic trauma of the middle ear caused by the difference of pressure between the air in the tympanic cavity and mastoid air cells and that of the surrounding atmosphere. During ascent, expanding gas within the tympanic cavity is vented. The eustachian tube usually functions as a one-way valve to allow this gas to escape from the middle ear. On descent, however, the volume within the middle ear contracts, causing the tympanic membrane to retract. Active opening of the eustachian tube using positive pressure from the nasopharynx or using the jaw muscles usually suffices to equalize the pressure differential: yawning, swallowing, or the Valsalva maneuver.

This process of expansion and contraction can cause significant complications if the normal corrective procedures are ineffective or impaired. Severe pain, nausea, vertigo, tinnitus, perforation of the eardrum, and bleeding can occur with an associated temporary impairment of hearing.

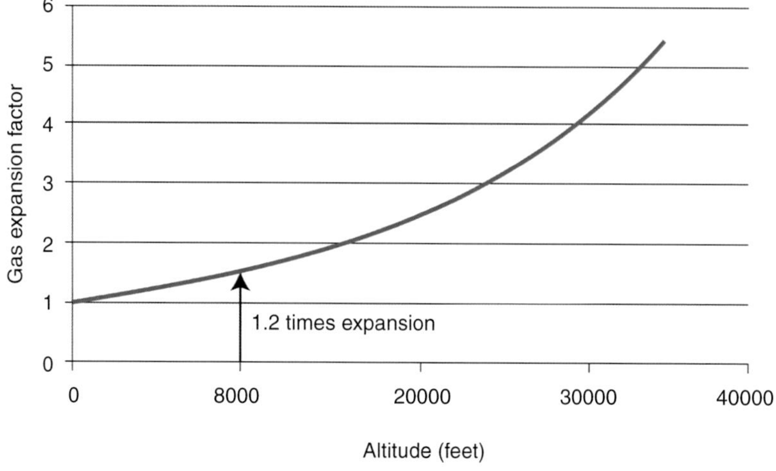

Fig. 9.2 Impact of altitude on gas expansion. At the highest cabin altitude expected during flight in a pressurized aircraft (8000 feet), gas expands to 1.2 times the original volume

Medical crew members should be aware of the early symptoms of barotitis media. In patients or crew with congestive symptoms, topical vasoconstrictors such as 0.25% phenylephrine spray may be beneficial when used 15 minutes before descent or takeoff. Severe symptoms should be reported to the director of the aeromedical crew because the aircraft may have to increase altitude again to allow equalization of pressure in the middle ear before reattempting descent. Finally, politzerization may be required to equalize pressures. This involves the delivery of pressurized air using a handheld compression device (Politzer bag) or compressed air through the nose to open the eustachian tube. Instrumentation of the nasal passages should be undertaken cautiously in patients with coagulopathy or platelet disorders due to the risk of hemorrhage.

The implications of gas expansion and barotitis media are less clear for the comatose, psychotic, or disoriented patient. Do not forget to evaluate those patients who have been nasotracheally intubated or who have nasogastric tubes in place because they are prone to develop edema and eustachian tube dysfunction. You should observe patients for evidence of increased irritability or agitation during descent, which may accompany the discomfort associated with increased middle-ear pressures. Direct examination of the tympanic membrane for significant retractions may rule out this problem.

Barosinusitis occurs when there is obstruction of airflow that normally passes in and out of the sinus cavities without difficulty. The presence of an upper respiratory infection may produce swelling of sinus mucosal membranes that will obstruct normal venting. On ascent, this will produce pain or pressure below (maxillary), above (frontal), or behind the eyes. More commonly, problems occur during descent. The use of the Valsalva maneuver will frequently provide at least temporary relief. Vasoconstrictors and return to a higher altitude may also be necessary. When considering the AE patient, barosinusitis may occur in patients with abnormal nasal pathology or inflammation such as facial trauma or nasal instrumentation (intubation, nasogastric tubes).

Barodontalgia occurs when trapped air in abscesses, dental fillings, or caries expands, resulting in severe pain during ascent. This is an uncommon problem and can be confused with barosinusitis involving the maxillary sinuses. In the case of barodontalgia, only one tooth is usually involved, whereas several of the upper teeth on the affected side are symptomatic with maxillary barosinusitis. Therapy is limited to descent and pain control with appropriate follow-up.

Barogastralgia or gas expansion in the gastrointestinal tract is rare in healthy passengers and crew at cabin altitudes <8000 feet where gas expansion is typically 1.2 times the volume at sea level (Fig. 9.2). Passengers or crew who eat hasty, large meals with foods known to produce gas, or carbonated beverages, may on occasion experience problems related to gas expansion.

Patients immediately post-abdominal surgery or with gastrointestinal problems such as bowel obstructions, ileus, or motility problems are at increased risk for symptoms related to expansion of bowel gas during AE. Symptoms can include abdominal pain, belching, flatulence, nausea, vomiting, shortness of breath, or vasovagal reaction symptoms. Preflight placement of a nasogastric tube should be accomplished in these patients and be left unclamped for passive drainage or intermittent suction as appropriate during flight.

Intrathoracic air presents a special consideration because it is contained within a space with limited distensibility (see Chap. 16). The management of the patient with a pneumothorax requires the medical crew to consider several issues. Even patients with an asymptomatic pneumothorax can develop significant decompensation with gas expansion inside the thorax.

An untreated pneumothorax is considered a contraindication to movement by aircraft except in situations with both the absence of respiratory compromise and the ability to maintain cabin altitude equal to that at the point of origin. Even under these circumstances, the medical team should have the capability to provide definitive treatment should the patient's condition change, because the process that caused the pneumothorax may have the potential to continue and progress to tension physiology independent of cabin pressure.

The safest approach for all patients with pneumothorax is preflight placement of a chest tube attached to an appropriate collection system. All chest tubes should be connected to a rigid, nonglass collection system with a Heimlich or other one-way valve. Water levels should not be changed during ascent or descent, although the suction level, if used, should be checked frequently.

When patients will be requiring AE, chest tubes should be left in place before flight even if they could otherwise be removed. If a chest tube has been recently removed in a patient requiring AE, an occlusive dressing should be applied to the chest tube site, and a chest X-ray obtained to exclude recurrence of the pneumothorax. Air Force Instructions specify a minimum of 24 hours should elapse between removal of a chest tube and air transport [6].

Current guidelines for commercial air travel suggest a 2-week delay after radiographic resolution of a traumatic pneumothorax before flying. To assess this guideline, Majercik et al. examined radiographic and physiologic changes in 20 patients with traumatic pneumothorax treated by chest tube (70%) or supplemental oxygen (30%) under hypobaric conditions with exposure to pressures equivalent to altitudes of 8400 or 12,650 feet [7]. Patients were evaluated for a mean of 19 hours following chest tube removal with chest radiographs at a baseline altitude of 4500 feet, at target altitude, and after return to baseline barometric pressure. There was a slight increase in pneumothorax size at altitude, but no cardiopulmonary changes or tension physiology was noted at altitude. When seen, pneumothorax sizes returned to baseline on recompression. Until these findings are confirmed in larger studies, placement of a chest tube is still recommended for all patients with a pneumothorax prior to AE.

Intracranial air is one of the rare areas of gas expansion that can be potentially devastating (see Chap. 12). Whether it is from a penetrating injury, surgery, or diagnostic study, the presence of intracranial air requires close monitoring of the air transport patient. If the patient needs to be moved, the medical crew should consider maintaining cabin pressure equivalent to the point of origin. In addition, the presence of a cerebrospinal fluid leak from the ears or nose raises theoretical concern for drawing in air or bacteria during descent.

Medical equipment that contains air can also be adversely affected by gas expansion. Items such as military anti-shock trousers (MAST) and pneumatic splints may become excessively distended on ascent or may not function as intended with volume loss during descent.

Endotracheal tube cuff management presents a particular problem. Cuff expansion at decreased barometric pressures can result in excessive pressure on the tracheal mucosa, and rapid decompression could theoretically lead to tracheal injury or rupture. Stoner and Cooke demonstrated this in 1974 using an animal model and suggested that endotracheal tubes with pressure-regulating valves on the pilot balloon or foam cuffs be used to avoid the problems related with cuff expansion (Fig. 9.3) [8].

In the past, it was recommended that saline be used to expand the cuff during AE since pressure-related expansion would be minimal. Figure 9.4 shows the cuff pressure response from 0- to 15,000-feet altitude with air, saline/air, and saline. Saline expansion is no longer recommended because there is a steep volume-pressure response curve in commonly used endotracheal tubes (Fig. 9.5)—an excess pressure can damage the tracheal mucosa.

We currently recommend that the endotracheal and tracheostomy tube cuffs be inflated with air to the minimal pressure required to prevent a leak during ventilation and then monitor and adjust cuff pressure during transport [6]. This will minimize the risk of tissue damage, air leak, or aspiration around the cuff due to gas expansion and compression during all phases of AE flight.

Other equipment considerations include distention of balloon bladder catheters, intravenous (IV) solution bags, aortic balloon pumps, and mechanical ventilators. When using mechanical transport ventilators during AE, special attention

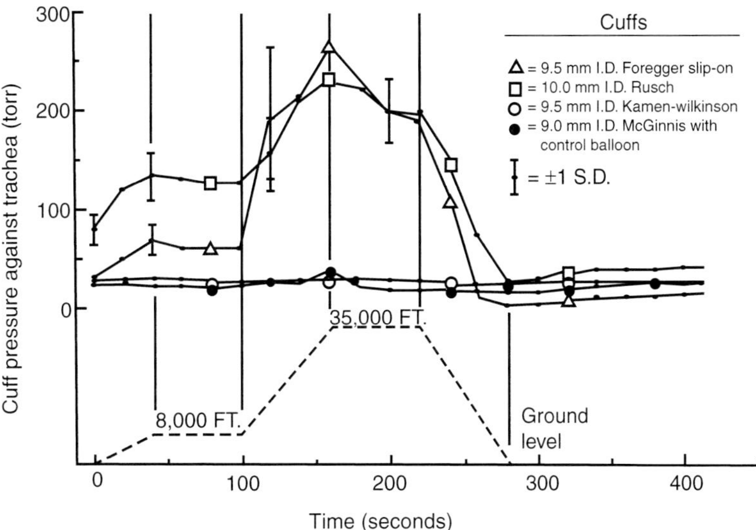

Fig. 9.3 Changes in tracheal wall pressure associated with changes in altitude for air-inflated cuff (Foregger and Rusch), foam cuff (Kamen-Wilkinson), and pressure-regulated cuff (McGinnis) endotracheal tubes in an animal model. (Reprinted with permission Stoner and Cooke [8])

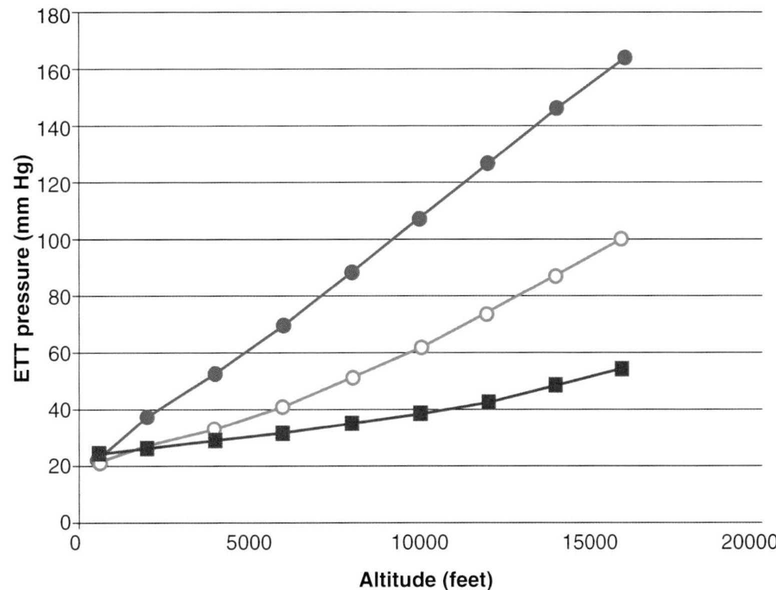

Fig. 9.4 Changes in mean cuff pressure associated with changes in altitude for a standard 8.0-mm ID endotracheal tube (ETT, Portex) with air (solid blue circles), saline plus 2 cc air (open green circles), and saline (solid red squares)-filled cuff using a laryngeal model

should be paid to the delivered tidal volume since volume increases as the cabin pressure decreases. While some ventilators have automatic compensation, others do not (Fig. 9.6) [9, 10].

Cabin Pressurization at Cruising Altitude

To reduce the problems associated with hypoxia and gas expansion, fixed-wing aircraft used for AE maintain cabin pressurization using engine bleed air. In some aircraft, the pilot can regulate cabin pressure and ventilation by varying the amount of air forced into the cabin and adjusting the overflow while correcting for the known leak rate. Malfunction of this system, or aircraft structural damage, may result in a loss of cabin pressure or decompression. The cabin volume, size of the defect, altitude, and pressure differential will then impact on problems related to the decompression.

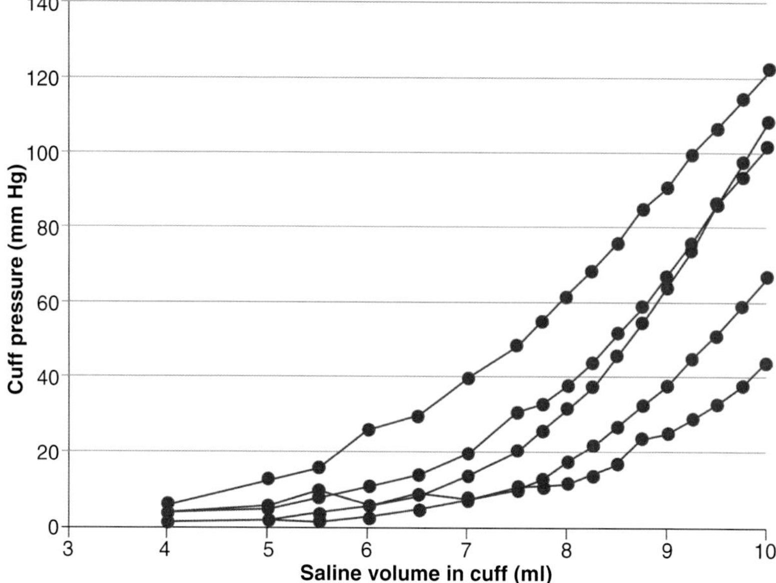

Fig. 9.5 Pressure responses for saline-inflated endotracheal tube cuffs in a laryngeal model. (Unpublished data courtesy of the author)

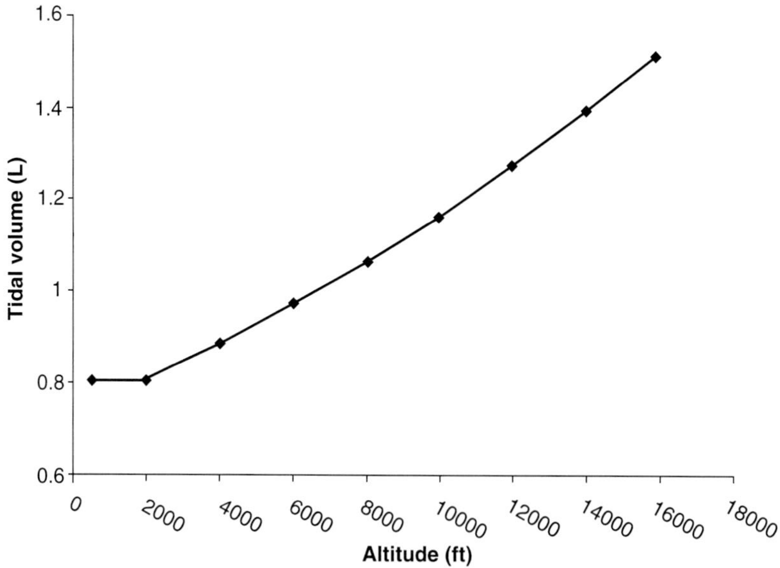

Fig. 9.6 Effect of changing altitude on the tidal volume delivered by the Impact 750 transport ventilator when not recalibrated following changes in ambient pressure

Aircraft use different cabin pressurization schemes as is illustrated with two *former* USAF AE platforms. The C-9A, a dedicated AE aircraft, which has been retired by the USAF, could maintain a constant cabin pressure (isobaric system) as aircraft altitude increased. With this type of system, the pressure differential between cabin pressure and ambient pressure increases with altitude. The C-9A maintained a pressure slightly greater than ambient pressure while ascending to 8000 feet and then maintained 8000 feet through its certified ceiling. The C-141, on the other hand, used an 8.6-psi isobaric-differential pressurization system. The cabin altitude remained at sea-level or ground-level pressure until the aircraft reached 21,000 feet. Above this level, the system maintained a pressure differential of 8.6 psi to the service ceiling of the aircraft. For example, at 40,000 feet the ambient pressure is 2.72 psi with a cabin pressure of 11.3 (8.6 + 2.72) psi. This corresponds to an altitude of 8000 feet.

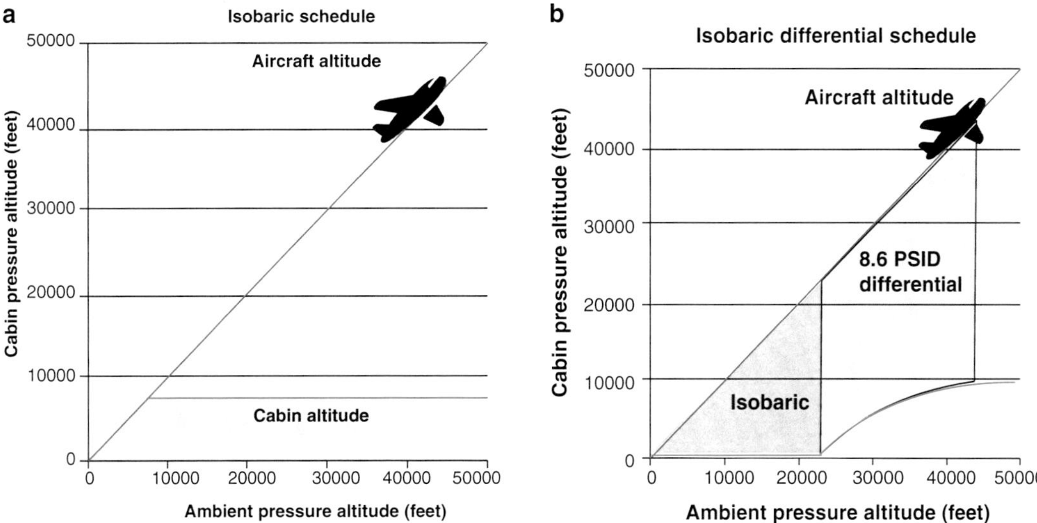

Fig. 9.7 Comparison of (**a**) isobaric and (**b**) isobaric-differential aircraft pressurization schedules. (Adapted from [2])

Figure 9.7a, b graphically demonstrates these two pressurization schemes.

Altitude Restrictions

Military and civilian aircraft can uniformly maintain standard cabin pressure altitude equivalent to <8000 feet above sea level at cruise altitudes. However, patients with a PaO_2 ≤60 mm Hg (90% saturation) at sea level usually exhibit symptoms of hypoxia above 2000–4000 feet cabin altitude. The standard treatment for all patients with oxygenation problems is oxygen supplementation.

Patients with decreased pulmonary perfusion and those with cardiac conditions should be routinely administered supplemental oxygen and closely monitored during AE flights. In addition, patients with chronic obstructive pulmonary disease (COPD) should be administered low-flow oxygen therapy (1–2 L/min) via nasal cannula or 24–31% Venturi mask to regulate the delivered oxygen concentration [11]. In the most serious cases, patients should be intubated and mechanical ventilation initiated prior to AE.

Flight altitude restriction is a treatment approach reserved for critical patients for whom adequate oxygenation cannot be maintained by medical means alone. The decision to grant a request for altitude restriction is a decision made by operational controllers based on several non-medical considerations. To maintain sea-level cabin pressurization, fixed-wing military aircraft used for AE must fly at altitudes much lower than their normal cruise altitudes. Flying at lower altitudes increases their fuel consumption, decreases their range, and increases the probability of turbulence. Thus, cabin altitude restrictions necessitate the use of alternate routes that lengthen air miles flown, delay delivery of critical casualties to a higher level of care, and increase time and cost of flight.

Temperature

Aircraft cabin temperature fluctuates considerably depending on the outside air temperature, which decreases by 6 °F for every 1000 feet increase in altitude or about 1 °C per 100 m. Unfortunately, most military refueling and cargo aircraft used for AE have suboptimal cabin temperature control systems with delayed response of aircraft temperature controls. As a result, inside aircraft temperature can often vary from 15 °C to 25 °C during winter flights and from 20 °C to >35 °C during summer flights. This problem is compounded by the necessity of opening large aircraft loading doors at en route stops.

These wide temperature variations require the medical crews to be aware of cabin temperature changes in relation to patient care/comfort and medical crew performance. The effects on patients of increased or decreased cabin temperatures can be magnified by other flight stresses, including vibration and dehydration. In addition, there can be degradation of equipment performance at the extremes of temperature.

Noise

Noise represents one of the more troublesome stresses encountered during AE operations. Cabin noise levels in commercial aircraft vary as a function of the distance from the engines. They can reach 105 decibels during takeoff and landing and are usually around 85 decibels at cruise altitude. In military aircraft used for AE that were not originally designed for passenger travel (i.e., KC-135, C-130), the noise levels are usually much higher.

Prolonged noise exposure during AE flights can have a number of undesirable effects on patients and crew members including (1) degraded communications and patient evaluation, (2) temporary auditory threshold shifts (auditory fatigue), (3) permanent threshold shifts (sensorineural hearing loss), and (4) fatigue.

AE crew members must rely on other means to communicate with each other and monitor and assess the patient's condition. Interference with effective communications between providers and between the medical crew and the conscious patient makes it difficult to detect small changes in patient symptoms or condition. During flight, it is impossible to auscultate for breath sounds and audible equipment alarms cannot be heard. Close observation of the patient and the use of visual alarms must be used in place of the usual forms of patient interaction and assessment.

Auditory fatigue induced by noise is frequently accompanied by a feeling of fullness, high-pitched ringing, buzzing, or a roaring sound (tinnitus) in the ears. These symptoms usually resolve within a few minutes of noise cessation but may take hours in some circumstances. Most of the significant symptoms of noise exposure, such as nausea, disorientation, and fatigue, in general occur with exposure to noise levels in excess of those seen during AE missions.

It is recommended that all patients and AE crew members use hearing protection during patient transport operations. Patients are supplied with ear plugs, while crew members use communication headsets. While these headsets allow communication between crew members, they make it even more difficult for the medical crew to communicate with patients.

Vibration

Vibration, like noise, is inherent in all transport vehicles and may interfere with patient assessment and some routine physiological functions. The most common sources of vibration during AE are the engines and wind. When in direct contact with a source of vibration, mechanical energy is transferred, some of which is degraded into heat within those tissues that have dampening properties. The whole-body response to sustained vibration is a slight increase in metabolic rate that is similar to mild exercise. Low-frequency vibration may also promote the onset of fatigue, irritability, and motion sickness [12]. In conjunction with the other stresses of flight, the overall effect is magnified.

Because there is little that the pilot or crew can do to eliminate or decrease the amount of vibration, care should be taken in minimizing its effects. Patients should be properly secured, encouraged, and assisted with position changes and provided with adequate padding and skin care. Special care should be taken in the movement of neonates because they may be more susceptible to direct injury from both noise and vibration [13]. In addition, vibration may cause dysfunction of activity-sensing pacemakers, although other types of pacemakers should not be affected [14].

The potential deleterious effects of vibration extend to the equipment used during transport. Although evaluation of several pulse oximetry units demonstrated their capability to function in the flight environment, they are sensitive to motion and may display artefactual readings on occasion [15, 16]. Similarly, noninvasive blood pressure (BP) monitors will work well under most in-flight circumstances; however, they are still subject to the same accuracy limitations seen in the hospital [17].

Decreased Humidity

One of the more subtle stresses of flight is a decrease in cabin humidity. As altitude increases and air cools, moisture in the air decreases significantly. Thus, the fresh air supply drawn into the aircraft cabin comes from a very dry atmosphere. This dry air also replaces the moisture-laden cabin air such that the relative humidity is <10–20% on most commercial flights [4].

Medical crew will develop chapped lips, scratchy or slightly sore throat, hoarseness, and general moisture loss. The patient with respiratory complaints or who is already dehydrated may have more significant problems. Patients requiring oxygen should receive humidified gas, and fluid intake of both the crew and patients should be monitored to minimize problems with dehydration.

Acceleration

The patient effects of acceleration, expressed as multiples of gravitational force (Gs), are negligible under most circumstances during AE. Changes in G-forces in the longitudinal axis (fore and aft) are potential issues only during takeoff and landing. The implications for patient care are mostly theoretical. However, flight-induced G-forces can be important in regard to routine operations, accident prevention, and accident survival.

Federal regulations stipulate that each item of mass inside the cabin that could injure an occupant be restrained when subjected to load factors seen during flight. This includes all medical equipment and monitoring devices. Care should be taken to secure all equipment bags opened during flight to prevent injury in the event of turbulence or during landing-related deceleration.

The primary AE concern about G-forces involves positioning for patients with either traumatic brain injury (see Chap. 12) or poor myocardial function (see Chap. 19). These changes are only slightly >1.0 G in the direction away from acceleration or toward deceleration, and any clinical significance of these G-force changes has yet to be demonstrated. As a result, the current recommendation is to load these patients into AE aircraft in the orientation determined best for en route care. The effects of longitudinal G-forces also can be mitigated by elevating the head of the bed so that the patient's head is above the heart.

Fatigue

Patient and AE crew member fatigue is the end product of all the physiological and psychological stresses of flight discussed previously. Performance degradation with loss of attention and decrease in reaction time can be a significant contributor to decreased operational capability. This problem is often made worse by self-imposed stress such as the use of over-the-counter drugs, prescription medications, caffeine, exhaustion, alcohol, tobacco, and poor dietary habits. Although the hours worked by AE crew members on flying status are limited by military regulations (e.g., mandatory crew rest), CCAT team members are classified as operational support fliers and can on occasion be required to work long hours.

Critical Care Air Transport Teams

History

In the period following the Vietnam War, and the end of the Cold War, it became necessary for the US Air Force to plan for the large-scale transport of unstable casualties. The casualty management system of prior eras was focused on stabilizing casualties at high-capacity field hospitals positioned near the anticipated locations of conflict. Casualties were treated and returned to duty or managed to convalescence and evacuated when they were no longer critically ill or injured [18]. This period of convalescence typically lasted multiple weeks for casualties treated during the Vietnam War [19].

A major shift occurred in the medical support of deployed military forces following the Vietnam War and the end of the Cold War. The rapidly shifting, asymmetrical way contemporary military forces deploy makes it highly unlikely that high-capability, high-capacity medical facilities will be nearby. As a result, casualties are treated in lightweight mobile medical and surgical facilities designed to provide rapid stabilization and treatment and moved within a matter of hours or days via AE—often long distance in nature. Many of these stabilized casualties have a considerable risk of becoming unstable during transport.

When it became necessary to evacuate unstable casualties, the AE system added critical care resources from the sending facility on an ad hoc basis. This included physicians and other personnel, along with supplies and equipment. The inclusion of physicians as medical attendants meant that during AE, casualties could receive new diagnoses, treatments could be adjusted, and new treatments started.

The nidus for change came when several incidents from the 1980s through the early 1990s called upon the AE system to move stabilized but relatively unstable casualties on short notice: This included the 1983 Marine barracks bombing in Beirut, the 1989 Panama invasion, and the 1993 Battle of Mogadishu including the publicized Black Hawk Down incident [20, 21].

The lack of integral critical care transport capability in the USAF AE system was immediately identified as a challenge when providing medical support for these operations. The medical teams that deployed with these rapidly developing military operations could be highly capable, but they had to be small and mobile to permit rapid deployment. Therefore, it was difficult or impossible for these small teams to either sustain critical casualties in place or send limited medical personnel to accompany casualties during AE. In Panama it was necessary for emergency physicians to accompany unstable casualties during long-range AE back to Texas [20]. In Mogadishu, Somalia, the deployed rangers were supported by an Army Combat Support Hospital with three general surgeons [21]. One of the four surgeons assigned to this hospital was absent at the time of the Battle of Mogadishu because he had been required to accompany a shark attack casualty during AE back to Germany. This degraded the ability to provide care to the 34 combat casualties who required 56 procedures over a 48-hour period. The experience in Operation Desert Storm demonstrated that even in a mature operation, with high-capacity/high-capability deployed medical forces, there was a need for physicians to actively manage potentially unstable patients during AE.

The solution adopted by the AE system was to develop the integral capability for critical care transport in the form of the Critical Care Air Transport Team (CCATT) program [22]. CCAT teams differed from AE crew members in that they have current critical care experience and specific training, supplies, and equipment to execute the critical care transport mission during AE. These CCATTs were not designed to function independently but rather to supplement the AE crew by accompanying critically ill or injured casualties during AE.

As experience with the AE of potentially unstable casualties grew, it was apparent that we needed to develop a better understanding of effects of air transport on critically ill patients and the equipment required to care for such patients. Thus, an essential requirement for CCATT members is a thorough understanding of patient flight physiology and the effects of flight on critically ill patients.

Critical Care Air Transport Team Members

In 1994 the USAF developed the CCATT program to provide the intrinsic capability to rapidly

Table 9.1 Goals of the Critical Care Air Transport Team (CCATT) program

Establish the need for transport and the optimal destination
Pre-transport clinical optimization of the casualty
Prevention of delays during transports—except as required to optimize casualty care
Provision of a safe transport environment for patient and staff
Provide a level of care during transport at or above that available at the sending facility
Safe delivery to the appropriate level of care

evacuate casualties that had been stabilized but who remain unstable [22]. Each CCAT team consists of a physician, nurse, and cardiopulmonary technician. Each team is designed, supplied, and equipped to manage three high-acuity patients or six lower acuity patients [23]. The goals of the CCATT program are listed in Table 9.1.

The USAF has developed a robust process to ensure team members are qualified to perform the critical care transport mission [22, 23]. CCATT physicians are fully trained in critical care and/or a related specialty such as anesthesiology or emergency medicine. The nurses have both training and experience in critical care or emergency nursing. The cardiopulmonary technicians have extensive training and experience in the technical aspects of cardiology, pulmonology, and respiratory therapy. Each team member undergoes additional training and equipment familiarization during the USAF CCATT Initial and Advanced courses. When not deployed as part of a CCATT, team members are expected to be active clinically in a hospital critical care environment.

The USAF was required to develop programs to teach and sustain this knowledge for CCATT members. The CCATT Initial Course teaches team members how to operate in the aeromedical environment. The CCATT Advanced Course includes a higher level of clinical training in casualty management, and it integrates lessons from recent operations in the context of integrative training exercises. Essential elements of CCATT sustainment training include periodic training flights, operational exercises, and medical readiness training.

Critical Care Air Transport Team Equipment

The care and monitoring of critically ill and injured casualties in the aeromedical environment requires the use of electronic biomedical equipment. The goal is to create an environment of critical care to the highest level possible and at least to the level of the sending facility. The major pieces of equipment required to accomplish this are physiologic monitors, mechanical ventilators, infusion pumps, and point-of-care lab testing devices. There is an increasing use of ultrasound across the air transport industry as well, although this is of uncertain benefit at this time.

The medical logistics system provides the CCATT program with a standardized set of supplies and equipment with which to carry out their mission [23]. The supplies, medications, and select equipment items are listed on the CCATT allowance standard, which can be updated as required by changes in care standards.

Patient Movement Items

The CCATT crews use patient movement items (PMI), which are medical equipment and supplies required to support patients during AE. PMI include standardized pieces of electronic equipment that are shared between field hospitals and evacuation teams.

A key strength of the PMI system is the ability to swap similar equipment items at the time of patient handoff between care teams. This has the potential to reduce errors from reprogramming ventilators and infusion pumps during these busy handoffs, allowing the CCATT members and receiving medical personal to focus more attention on the patient and less on the equipment. The deployed pools of PMI also provide an inventory of devices that can readily replace damaged or malfunctioning equipment. This allows CCATTs to remain fully equipped after every mission.

Airworthiness Testing

It is essential that all medical equipment used undergo airworthiness testing, and the equipment should not be used until a device is certified as safe and effective. Devices that function in an intensive care unit (ICU) on the ground may not function when exposed to stresses of flight. These stresses include altitude, temperature changes, and vibration. The aeromedical environment also increases the risk of physical damage, while devices are moved. Electromagnetic radiation from radiofrequency (RF) transmitting equipment found on the airframe can interfere with the proper function of these electronic devices. In addition, the medical devices may produce emissions that interfere with the communication and navigation systems found on the aircraft. In 1989, 70% of neonatal transport equipment failed military-specific testing for potentially excessive electromagnetic interference (EMI) [24].

The airworthiness testing requirement applies to all military and civilian air medical transport, and multiple laboratories provide the testing. The testing procedures evaluate the impact of vibrations, acceleration/deceleration, rapid barometric pressure changes, and wide temperature shifts on a variety of medical devices. Testing requirements are less stringent in the civilian community, although recommendations exist for equipment used in air ambulances [25].

Equipment Power Requirements

One of the more noteworthy considerations in the AE environment is the need to obtain appropriate power sources in AE aircraft for biomedical equipment. Unlike commercial power, which provides 110 VAC at 60 Hz, many fixed-wing aircraft operate on 110 VAC at 400 Hz or 12-V DC, while rotary-blade aircraft in general operate on 28-V DC systems. For AE flights, aircraft power must be converted to conventional 110 VAC at 60 Hz. Although frequency inverters are large and heavy, fixed-wing flights may necessitate their use due to the length of the mission.

This biomedical equipment must also continue to function while patients are transported between aircraft and ground vehicles. Unfortunately, many ground vehicles do not have integral AC power sources. As a result, biomedical equipment used for AE must also have long-lasting batteries. Underestimation of ground transportation time can result in critical battery issues.

Patient Monitoring Equipment

The monitoring standard of care for critically ill patients during transport has been established based on traditional hospital-based practice [26]. The basic tenet is to provide the same physiological monitoring during transport as received in the ICU prior to transfer, if technologically feasible.

The AE environment is a challenging place to monitor patients. Ambient noise in the aircraft cabin significantly impairs the ability of medical personnel to assess patients. This noise also limits the ability of caregivers to detect auditory alarms on ventilators and monitoring systems. This results in almost total reliance on the visual alarms and data presented by on-board medical equipment. Without auditory signals, patient monitoring requires disciplined, continuous visual scanning of alarm lights and displays. Fromm et al. noted that the loss of auditory signals in the flying environment can result in significant delay in observation of visual alarms [12].

The minimal standard for monitoring of a stabilized patient during AE is continuous monitoring of electrocardiogram (ECG) and blood oxygen saturation with pulse oximetry and intermittent measurement of BP, pulse rate, and respiratory rate. In addition, some critically ill patients require continuous monitoring of end-tidal carbon dioxide levels, arterial blood pressure, pulmonary arterial pressure, or intracranial pressures and/or intermittent monitoring of central venous pressure, pulmonary arterial occlusion pressure, or cardiac output.

Blood Pressure Monitoring

In the noisy AE environment, blood pressure cannot be monitored simply with a stethoscope and sphygmomanometer. The noise level typically seen in military rotary and fixed-wing aircraft is approximately 2000 times louder than heart tones and breath sounds [27, 28]. Although commercial aircraft are less noisy, auscultation remains difficult [29]. The use of amplified stethoscopes and monitoring devices has not solved this problem, although new techniques, such as the esophageal stethoscope, may resolve some of these limitations [27, 30, 31].

Alternative methods for the noninvasive assessment of BP include the use of Doppler and pulse oximetry occlusion techniques where systolic BP is calculated by detecting return of blood flow or oximetry waveform following BP cuff release [32]. For critical patients at increased risk for significant hyper- or hypotension during transport, BP can be monitored using an indwelling arterial catheter.

Electrocardiogram

Electrocardiogram (ECG) monitoring is a fundamental requirement for most critical care transport patients. During long-range AE, ECG monitoring is useful for detecting arrhythmias and signs of myocardial ischemia or injury as well as diagnosing pulseless electrical activity. However, ECG monitoring is prone to mechanical and electrical interference.

Oxygen Saturation and Carbon Dioxide Monitoring

Arterial blood oxygen saturation (SO_2) and end-tidal carbon dioxide in exhaled air ($EtCO_2$) are basic indicators of cardiopulmonary function. Because clinical evaluation of patients is difficult in the AE environment, continuous monitoring of SO_2 via pulse oximetry and ETO_2 via capnography has been standard for critically ill patients during AE [5].

Pulse oximetry monitors have been approved for use on USAF AE aircraft for more than two decades. However, not all monitors are suited for use in transport, and some are subject to interference during helicopter transport [16]. To reduce this, some monitors incorporate electrocardiograph synchronization to reduce motion artifacts.

For standard pulse oximetry, a transmissive sensor is placed on a thin part of the body, usually a fingertip or earlobe, and the device passes light at two wavelengths through the body part to a photodetector. Peripheral blood oxygen saturation (SpO_2) is measured as an estimate of SO_2 by comparing the absorbance at the two wavelengths to determine the absorbance due to pulsing arterial blood.

For capnography, a CO_2 sensor) is connected to an oxygen mask or placed in line between the endotracheal tube and the ventilator. Immediately after intubation, the presence of $EtCO_2$ provides evidence of correct positioning of the endotracheal tube; auscultation is not possible in the flight environment. During cardiopulmonary resuscitation, the presence of $EtCO_2$ indicates adequate perfusion, since poor cardiac output results in marked decreased $EtCO_2$.

During AE, stable $EtCO_2$ levels indicate adequate minute ventilation, while dropping levels can indicate endotracheal tube dislodgement and/or a decline in cardiac output.

Temperature Monitoring

Effective temperature management) plays an important role in patient outcome, particularly in the trauma setting. Temperature monitoring can be done via liquid crystalline probes, thermistors, or infrared thermometers at a number of potential monitoring sites including aural, oral, nasopharyngeal, rectal, bladder, skin, and esophagus. The best location depends on available equipment, patient tolerance, and the accuracy required for patient management.

Ventilators

Mechanical ventilation is an essential and important component of critical care transport. This topic is covered in detail in Chap. 18.

Infusion Devices

Infusion therapy is commonly employed in critical care air transport, and adequate infusion pumps are required for safe and effective delivery. A controlled rate of fluid delivery is essential for many infusions delivered in critical care including vasopressors, inotropes, and time-sensitive delivery of potentially lethal agents such as thrombolytic agents.

Infusion devices are the preferred method of delivering both maintenance fluids and emergency medications. This is because passive, flow-controlled IV systems are subject to problems related to decreased pressure at altitude. Any change in IV fluid bag pressure affects delivery rate. Cabin decompression can significantly alter the flow rate and can lead to pressurized bag rupture [25].

Key considerations for selection of a transport infusion device include robustness, operation in multiple orientations, adequate anchorage, extended battery life, pressure-activated occlusion alarms, programming of standard infusions to reduce the risk of medication errors, and a lightweight, compact size.

Laboratory Testing In-Flight

Bedside blood testing during AE flights has become a standard element of critical care air transport. The i-STAT portable clinical analyzer (Abbot, Princeton, NJ) is in widespread use in the civilian air medical transport industry. This unit uses a variety of cartridges and can give reliable results for a number of critical care tests including hematocrit, hemoglobin blood gases, electrolytes, metabolites, and coagulation factors. The current unit has an operating temperature range of 0–40 °C and relative humidity range of 0–90%.

Critical Care Air Transport Team Operational Experience

Since its inception, the CCAT teams have been employed in a broad range of settings. As the program was being established, substantial early experience between 1995 and 2000 came from peacetime movement of critically ill or injured Department of Defense beneficiaries in the continental United States to Wilford Hall Medical Center, Lackland AFB, Texas [19]. These transports allowed the CCATT members to get actual experience working with AE crews and delivering critical care in the air in a relatively controlled environment compared to overseas contingencies. Active duty members who became ill or injured while deployed in the Caribbean, Central America, and South America were also transported in this manner.

The scope of the CCATT program continued to expand to meet the needs of the US military. CCATTs were deployed on a rotating basis to Ramstein AB, Germany, to evacuate casualties from military operations in Bosnia and Kosovo in 1995 [33]. This continued for several years until teams were established in Germany. These teams also evacuated critical casualties from the Khobar Towers bombing in 1996 and performed numerous transports from Germany to the United States.

The CCATT program was developed primarily to support combat operations, and this is where it continues to have its greatest impact. Examination of CCATT experience transporting intra- and inter-theater casualties early in the wars in Iraq and Afghanistan found that 65% of the casualties had a primary trauma diagnosis, and 35% had a medical diagnosis, mostly cardiac [34]. These were high-acuity populations: 60% of the trauma casualties were severely traumatized with average Injury Severity Scores of 15–22. Approximately half were intubated and >10% required treatment with vasopressor infusions. The mean time from injury to evacuation out of Iraq was 28 hours. A modest number of transient physiologic events were recorded, but there were no major complications or deaths related to transport.

The experience from Operation Enduring Freedom and Operation Iraqi Freedom demonstrates that the AE system, with the addition of CCAT teams, is capable of moving unstable casualties on a large scale with a very low rate of complications. This capability allows operational units to rapidly respond to contingencies around the globe, free of the need to deploy large medical teams, which take considerable airlift

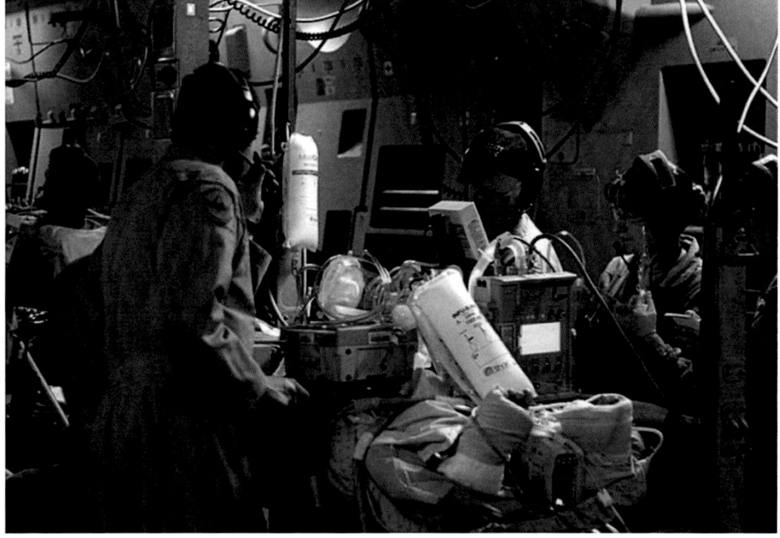

Fig. 9.8 An Air National Guard Critical Care Air Transport Team (CCATT) transports an injured soldier about a C-17 from Balad Air Base, Afghanistan, to Ramstein Air Base. (USAF photo by Daniel Riuley)

resources to transport and time to become operational.

This represents a major paradigm shift in medical support for military operations. Previously military logistic planners would estimate the number of in-theater beds that would be required to support the anticipated number of casualties. With the ability to rapidly evacuate stable and stabilized casualties, logisticians can now plan in terms of the rate at which casualties will need to be evacuated [35].

The CCATT program has also been a great benefit in response to disasters (Fig. 9.8) [36–39]. The teams and their portable equipment are able to enter disaster zones on cargo aircraft without interfering with airlift of relief supplies into the disaster area. After cargo aircrafts have off-loaded their supplies, these same aircraft can be quickly reconfigured to evacuate casualties utilizing AE crews augmented with CCAT teams to provide advanced care for seriously ill or injured casualties. This allows ground medical teams to care for a larger number of lower acuity casualties in the zone.

The CCAT teams have been successfully deployed to respond to both natural and man-made disasters. In 2005 Hurricane Katrina devastated civilian and military medical capability on the US Gulf Coast, and CCATTs were used to evacuate critical casualties from New Orleans [37, 38]. CCATT teams have also been used to evacuate civilian ICUs in advance of hurricanes [22]. The teams transported multiple critical casualties from the terrorist attack on the *USS Cole* [40]. CCAT teams from Wilford Hall Medical Center also evacuated critical casualties following a 747 aircraft crash on Guam that involved a 20-hour flight [41].

References

1. Blumen IJ, Abernathy MK, Dunne MJ. Flight physiology: clinical considerations. Crit Care Clin. 1992;8:597–618.
2. Sheffield PJ, Heimbach RD. Respiratory physiology. In: DeHart RL, editor. Fundamentals of aerospace medicine. 2nd ed. Baltimore: Williams & Wilkins; 1996. p. 69–108.
3. Henry JN, Krenis LJ, Cutting RT. Hypoxemia during aeromedical evacuation. Surg Gynecol Obstet. 1973;16:49–53.
4. Aerospace Medical Association Medical Guidelines Task Force. Medical guidelines for airline travel, 2nd ed. Aviat Space Environ Med. 2003;74(5 Suppl):A1–19.
5. Bendrick GA, Nicolas DK, Krause BA, Castillo CY. Inflight oxygen saturation decrements in aeromedical evacuation patients. Aviat Space Environ Med. 1995;66:40–4.
6. Department of the Air Force. Air Force Instruction 48-307, Volume 1, En route care and aeromedical evacuation medical operations. 9 January 2017. www.e-publishing.af.mil.

7. Majercik S, White TW, Van Boerum DH, Granger S, Bledsoe J, Conner K, Wilson E, Weaver LK. Cleared for takeoff: the effects of hypobaric conditions on traumatic pneumothoraces. J Trauma Acute Care Surg. 2014;77:729–33.
8. Stoner DL, Cooke JP. Intratracheal cuffs and aeromedical evacuation. Anesthesiology. 1974;41:302–6.
9. Thomas G, Brimacombe J. Function of the Dräger Oxylog ventilator at high altitude. Anaesth Intensive Care. 1994;22:276–80.
10. Grissom TE, Papier K, Lawlor D, Farmer JC, Derdak S. Mechanical ventilator performance during aeromedical evacuation. In: Advisory Group for Aerospace Research & Development, editors. Proceedings of aeromedical support issues in contingency operations. London: NATO; 1997;599:34-1–34-7.
11. Cramer D, Ward S, Geddes D. Assessment of oxygen supplementation during air travel. Thorax. 1996;51:202–3.
12. Fromm REJ, Duvall JO. Medical aspects of flight for civilian aeromedical transport. Probl Crit Care Med. 1990;4:495–507.
13. Macnab A, Chen Y, Gagnon F, Bora B, Laszlo C. Vibration and noise in pediatric emergency transport vehicles: A potential cause of morbidity? Aviat Space Environ Med. 1995;66:212–9.
14. Gordon RS, O'Dell KB, Low RB, Blumen IJ. Activity-sensing permanent internal pacemaker dysfunction during helicopter aeromedical transport. Ann Emerg Med. 1990;19:1260–3.
15. Cissik JH, Yockey CC, Byrd RB. Evaluation of the Hewlett-Packard Ear Oximeter for use during routine air transport of patients. Aviat Space Environ Med. 1981;52:312–4.
16. Short L, Hecker RB, Middaugh RE, Menk EJ. A comparison of pulse oximeters during helicopter flight. J Emerg Med. 1989;7:639–43.
17. Low RB, Martin D. Accuracy of blood pressure measurements made aboard helicopters. Ann Emerg Med. 1988;17:604–12.
18. Carlton PK, Jenkins MH. The mobile patient. Crit Care Med. 2008;36(Suppl):S255–7.
19. Johannigman JA. Maintaining the continuum of en route care. Crit Care Med. 2008;36(Suppl):S377–82.
20. Dice WM. The role of military emergency physicians in an assault operation in Panama. Ann Emerg Med. 1992;20:1336–40.
21. Mabry RL, Holcomb JB, Baker AM, Cloonan CC, Uhorchak JM, Perkins DE, Canfield AJ, Hagmann JH. United States Army Rangers in Somalia: an analysis of combat casualties on an urban battlefield. J Trauma. 2000;49:515–29.
22. Beninati W, Meyer MT, Carter TE. The critical care air transport program. Crit Care Med. 2008;36Suppl:S370–6.
23. Critical Care Air Transport Team (CCATT). Air Force tactics, techniques, and procedures 3-42.51. 7 April 2015. www.e-publishing.af.mil.
24. Nish WA, Walsh WF, Land P, Swedenburg M. Effect of electromagnetic interference by neonatal transport equipment on aircraft operation. Aviat Space Environ Med. 1989;60:599–600.
25. Hale JD, Hade E. Safety evaluation of medical equipment before flight certification. Air Med. 1997;3:42–6.
26. McGuire NM. Monitoring in the field. Br J Anaesth. 2006;97(1):46–56.
27. Poulton TJ, Worthington DW, Pasic TR. Physiologic chest sounds and helicopter engine noise. Aviat Space Environ Med. 1994;65:338–40.
28. Patel SB, Callahan TF, Callahan MG, Jones JT, Graber GP, Foster KS, et al. An adaptive noise reduction stethoscope for auscultation in high noise environments. J Acoust Soc Am. 1998;103:2483–91.
29. Bishop LC. Aviation auscultation. JAMA. 1990;263:233.
30. Hunt RC, Bryan DM, Brinkley VS, Whitley TW, Benson NH. Inability to assess breath sounds during air medical transport by helicopter. JAMA. 1991;265:1982–4.
31. Stone CK, Stimson A, Thomas SH, Hume WG, Hunt R, Cassell H, et al. The effectiveness of esophageal stethoscopy in a simulated in-flight setting. Air Med J. 1995;14:219–21.
32. Talke PO. Measurement of systolic blood pressure using pulse oximetry during helicopter flight. Crit Care Med. 1991;19:934–7.
33. Guidelines Committee of the American College of Critical Care Medicine, Society of Critical Care Medicine, and American Association of Critical-Care Nurses Transfer Guidelines Task Force. Guidelines for the transfer of critically ill patients. Crit Care Med. 1993;21:931–7.
34. Mason PE, Eadie JS, Holder AD. Prospective observational study of United States (US) Air Force critical care air transport team operations in Iraq. J Emerg Med. 2011;41:8–13.
35. Snyder D, Chan EW, Burks JJ, Amouzegar MA, Resnick AC. How should Air Force expeditionary medical capabilities be expressed? RAND Project Air Force. https://www.rand.org/content/dam/rand/pubs/monographs/2009/RAND_MG785.pdf.
36. Farmer JC, Carlton PK. Providing critical care during a disaster: the interface between disaster response agencies and hospitals. Crit Care Med. 2006;34(Suppl):56–9.
37. Rice DH, Kotti G, Beninati W. Clinical review: critical care transport and austere critical care. Crit Care. 2008;12:207–14.
38. Beninati W. Evacuation. In: Briggs SM, Brinsfield KH, editors. Advanced disaster medical response. Boston: Harvard Medical International; 2003. p. 15–26.
39. Sariego J. CCATT: A military model for civilian disaster management. Disaster Manag Response. 2006;4:114–7.
40. Alkins SA, Reynolds AJ. Long-distance air evacuation of blast injured sailors from the U.S.S. Cole. Aviat Space Environ Med. 2002;73:677–80.
41. Cancio LC. Airplane crash in Guam, August 6, 1997: the aeromedical evacuation response. J Burn Care Res. 2006;27:642–8.

Part III

The Patients

Aeromedical Evacuation of Patients with Abdominal, Genitourinary, and Soft Tissue Injuries

10

Christopher J. Pickard-Gabriel, Raymond Fang, and Jeremy W. Cannon

Introduction

The mortality rate following combat injuries has steadily declined from a rate of 21% in World War I to 11% today. After arriving at a medical facility, only 2.5% of those with combat injuries die of their wounds. Improvements in the past were made possible in large part because of the advent of antibiotics during World War II and rapid helicopter transport from injury site to medical care during the Korean War. More recent improvements in survival are due to advances in trauma management including damage control resuscitation [1, 2] and damage control surgery [3, 4], which emphasize blood product administration paired with early surgical control of hemorrhage. For soft tissue injuries, negative-pressure wound therapy has greatly simplified the care of large soft tissue defects while also offering the possibility of providing therapeutic infusions directly into the wound [5, 6].

The current standard in the management of combat-related abdominal, genitourinary, and soft tissue injuries is rapid transport to surgical care (within 1 h of a call for medical transport) [7], damage control resuscitation, rapid—often abbreviated—surgical intervention, and transfer to the next echelon of care for ongoing management (Table 10.1). These advances and this new mentality of rapid intervention on only the life-threatening problems early in the course of management significantly impact aeromedical evacuation (AE) crews and Critical Care Air Transport Teams (CCATT) who are now expected to manage severely injured patients within hours of their initial trauma with ongoing resuscitation and surgical care needs (Table 10.2). This chapter will address basic concepts in management of these traumatic injuries. Considerations will be outlined for urgent versus elective evacuation with discussion of the AE requirements for safe transport.

C. J. Pickard-Gabriel
Maj, USAF, MC, Anesthesia Critical Care, Perelman School of Medicine at the University of Pennsylvania, Philadelphia, PA, USA

R. Fang
Col, USAF, MC (ret.), Department of Surgery, Johns Hopkins Bayview Medical Center, Baltimore, MD, USA

J. W. Cannon (✉)
Col, USAFR, MC, Department of Surgery, Penn Presbyterian Medical Center, Perelman School of Medicine at the University of Pennsylvania, Philadelphia, PA, USA

Uniformed Services University of the Health Sciences, Bethesda, MD, USA
e-mail: Jeremy.cannon@uphs.upenn.edu

W. W. Hurd, W. Beninati (eds.), *Aeromedical Evacuation*,
https://doi.org/10.1007/978-3-030-15903-0_10

Table 10.1 Levels of care provided and nomenclature

Care provided	DOD	NATO
Field medic/EMT at point of injury	Echelon I (e.g., self-aid/buddy care)	Role 1 (e.g., self-aid/ buddy care)
General surgeon with limited holding capacity	Echelon II (e.g., Forward Surgical Team)	Role 2 (e.g., Forward Surgical Team)
Limited surgical subspecialties/ ICU	Echelon III (e.g., Craig Joint Theater Hospital)	Role 3 (e.g., Kandahar Airfield Theater Hospital)
Full complement of subspecialties	Echelon IV (e.g., Lanstuhl Medical Center)	Role 4 (allied/home country hospital)
Referral center/ definitive care	Echelon V (e.g., Walter Reed National Medical Center, San Antonio Military Medical Center)	n/a

Abbreviations: *DOD* Department of Defense, *NATO* North Atlantic Treaty Organization, *EMT* emergency medical technician, *ICU* intensive care unit

Table 10.2 US Department of Defense intra-theater transport criteria recommendations

Criteria for transportation
Heart rate < 120 beats/minute
Systolic blood pressure > 90 mmHg
Hematocrit >24%
Platelet count >50/mm^3
INR < 2.0
pH > 7.3
Base deficit <5 mEq/L
Temperature > 35 °C

When any one or more of these criteria are not met, the treating physician should either continue treatment at the current facility or document the limitations at the current facility that compel an urgent, high-risk transfer.

Abdominal Injuries

The universal use of advanced body armor has shifted the burden of combat injuries away from the chest/abdomen toward the pelvis and extremities. However, despite this, abdominal injuries remain common in moderate combat [5].

Hollow Organs: Intestines and Stomach

Intestinal or gastric injuries require evaluation by a surgeon, thus necessitating urgent evacuation to the care of a surgeon in all cases. Hemodynamic stability may lead the surgical team to treat injuries primarily, while instability will drive the team toward damage control surgery. In a combat setting, the vast majority of hollow viscus injuries will have other associated injuries that preclude definitive repair at the initial operation. Thus, many such patients will require further transport with a nasogastric (NG) tube, surgical drains, an open abdominal cavity, and the intestines in discontinuity.

Isolated gastric injuries are rare and should prompt careful exploration for additional injuries. In contrast to the rest of the bowel, most gastric injuries can be repaired primarily with either staples or sutures. Postoperatively, patients will require gastric decompression to avoid stretching the fresh repair. A nasogastric tube placed at the time of surgery is adequate. If a surgical gastrostomy tube is present, this can be placed to gravity for additional venting. Tube dislodgement is a major concern in these patients; so prior to transport, ensure the nasogastric tube is secure with suture, a bridle, or at the very least, fresh tape.

Bowel injuries will be managed differently in the hemodynamically stable versus unstable patient. While the management decision is ultimately up to the surgeon, AE personnel should be aware of the risks with primary repair versus damage control surgery. Patients with primary repairs should be hemodynamically normal. Any subsequent hemodynamic instability in a patient that has been repaired primarily should be re-evaluated and likely re-explored surgically to evaluate for hemorrhage or a source of abdominal sepsis prior to transfer. In contrast, unstable patients are typically managed with damage control surgery. The goal of the expedited damage control surgery is to control intra-abdominal bleeding and then to evacuate and contain contamination (environmental or digestive). This index operation (first operation) is short with the understanding that it is more important to reverse hypocoagulability, hypovolemia, hypotension, and hypothermia—all of which are more difficult intraoperatively—under general anesthesia. Additionally, it is recognized that any repairs in such a compromised patient have a high likelihood of failure prior to full stabilization and resuscitation. Thus, after damage control surgery for intestinal injuries, the bowel is usually left in discontinuity (i.e., the ends of the intestine or colon stapled off at the site of an injury awaiting a safe time to perform a bowel anastomosis).

Urgent Aeromedical Evacuation

Minimal Conditions

After bowel surgery, the minimal conditions that must be met for urgent AE or CCATT transport include no evidence of active hemorrhage, no need for ongoing resuscitation, the ability to provide adequate gas exchange with safe lung-protective ventilator settings, no evidence of evolving abdominal compartment syndrome, adequate urine output, and no life-threatening electrolyte derangements (Table 10.3).

Specific Concerns/Treatment

Most patients will have a nasogastric or orogastric tube in place for AE, especially early after bowel surgery. This tube should be well secured and functioning. If the tube falls out in a patient with recent gastric or duodenal surgery, consider leaving the tube out unless the abdomen is tympanic suggesting gastric distention. In this case, measure out the length of tube insertion externally and do not advance beyond this level. In other cases of intestinal surgery, nasogastric tubes can be readily replaced using standard techniques. If the tube stops suctioning fluid, flush the blue port with air and the clear port with sterile water or saline to clear the occlusion.

Patients with colonic injuries may already have a matured colostomy that will require management in-flight. As air expands at altitude, the ostomy bags risk filling and rupturing or leaking if not frequently attended en route. Patients with bowel injuries are at increased risk for abdominal infections; however, antibiotics for bowel prophylaxis alone should not be continued for more than 24 h after definitive washout [8].

Some patients will have an open abdomen with a temporary closure such as an abdominal negative-pressure wound dressing (Fig. 10.1). Abdominal vacuum-assisted closure should be checked for air-worthiness and accompanied by basic supplies to repair minor leaks and change canisters en route. They may also have abdominal drains that must remain open to atmospheric pressure during AE. If intestinal contents appear in an intraperitoneal drain during AE, this should be noted and communicated to the receiving surgical team. For longer transport times (i.e., >4 h), the capability to monitor bladder pressures and check labs should be available.

Table 10.3 Urgent aeromedical evacuation (AE) considerations: abdomino-pelvic organs and soft tissue injuries

Urgent	Additional criteria for urgent AE	Special needs	Possible complications during transportation
Bowel	–	Nasogastric tube Ostomy care supplies Negative-pressure wound therapy	Hemorrhage Nasogastric tubedislodgement
Spleen	–	Nasogastric tube Vaccines	Hemorrhage
Liver	–	–	Hemorrhage
Pancreas	–	–	Hemorrhage
Genitourinary	–	Bladder catheter	Hemorrhage Oliguria
Soft tissue injury	Contamination controlled	Negative-pressure wound therapy Antibiotics	Wound drainage Negative-pressure wound leak Sepsis

Patients must demonstrate sustained hemodynamic stability prior to urgent AE

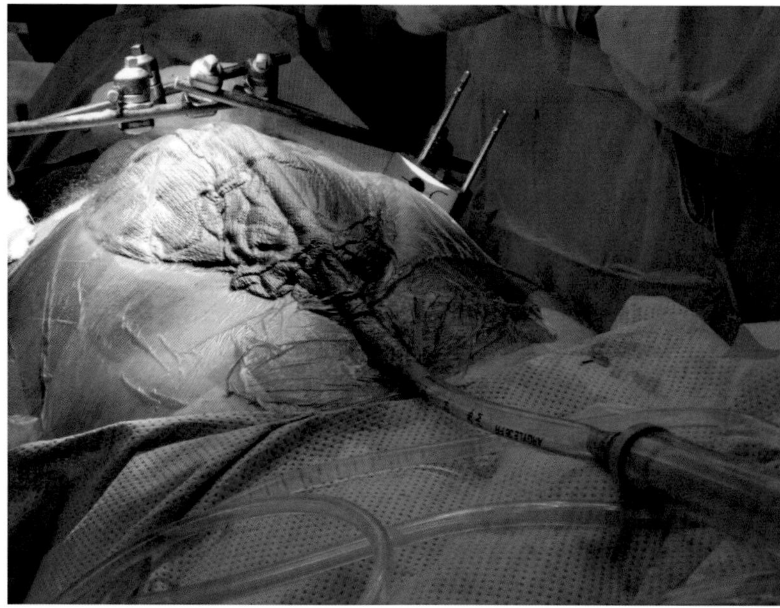

Fig. 10.1 Open abdomen managed with a negative-pressure wound dressing

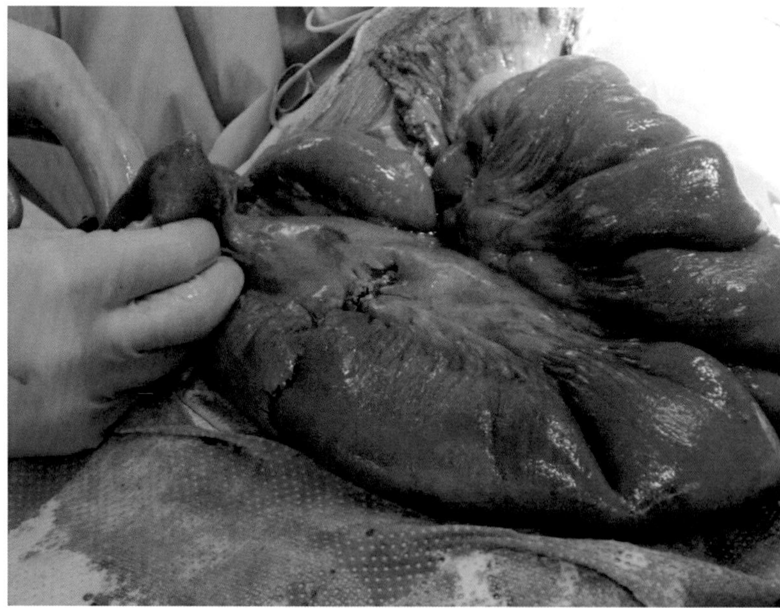

Fig. 10.2 Bowel anastomosis

Elective Aeromedical Evacuation

Minimal Conditions

Patients with hollow viscus injuries can have their intestinal continuity re-established by performing an anastomosis (Fig. 10.2) or a diverting loop or end ostomy can be brought up to the abdominal wall and matured. Once this has been done and there is no evidence of ongoing bleeding, the patient's abdomen can be closed. Sometimes the patient is too edematous or the abdominal wall is too tight to perform abdominal closure. This so-called loss of domain requires a staged reconstruction of the abdominal wall at a later date. In the meanwhile, the open abdomen is typically managed with either negative-pressure wound dressing with or without a Vicryl mesh and an eventual skin graft over the bowel.

Table 10.4 Elective aeromedical evacuation (AE) considerations: abdomino-pelvic organs and soft tissue injuries

Urgent	Additional criteria for urgent AE	Special needs	Possible complications during transportation
Bowel	Bowel continuity re-established Ostomy functioning	Nasogastric tube Ostomy care supplies Negative-pressure wound therapy	Ileus Anastomosis leak Deep space infection
Spleen	–	Nasogastric tube Vaccines	Hemorrhage Sepsis
Liver	–	–	Hemorrhage Bile leak
Pancreas	–	–	Hemorrhage Pancreatic leak
Genitourinary	Reconstruction completed or planned	Bladder catheter	Hemorrhage Urine leak
Soft tissue injury	Infection controlled	Negative-pressure wound therapy Antibiotics	Sepsis

Patients must demonstrate sustained medical stability prior to elective AE

Patients with hollow viscus injuries can be transported electively once they are completely stable with re-established bowel continuity or a functioning ostomy (Table 10.3). Those with an open abdomen can be transported electively with a Vicryl mesh in place to hold the abdominal contents (Table 10.4).

Specific Concerns/Treatment

After bowel injury, patients can have delayed leaks, intra-abdominal infections, surgical site infections, or delayed bowel function (i.e., an ileus). Ideally, these issues should be addressed prior to elective transport. During transport, an ileus can be managed with placement of a nasogastric tube. Leaks and intra-abdominal infections require computed tomography (CT) imaging for confirmation; however, antibiotics can be initiated during AE while awaiting imaging at the receiving location. Surgical site infections can be managed by changing the abdominal wound dressing or removing skin staples/sutures and evacuating fluid that might include an infected seroma, infected hematoma, or frank pus.

Solid Organs: Spleen or Liver/ Pancreas Injuries

Solid organ injuries all require urgent initial evacuation to a surgeon and can then quickly be sorted into hemodynamical stable versus unstable. Stable patients can undergo a trial of nonoperative management with US service members being electively transferred up the echelons of care, while civilians may or may not need transfer to trauma centers. Unstable patients will require exploratory laparotomy and possible damage control surgery depending on the severity of injury. Postoperatively stable US service members can be electively transferred up the echelons of care, while civilians may be monitored locally or transferred to a trauma center. All damage control surgery for US service members should matriculate up the echelons of care urgently, and civilians should be transferred emergently to trauma centers. Specific considerations for AE in various injuries will be discussed below, but all patients, operative and nonoperative, require gastric decompression, and many will have the same drain considerations as previously discussed for hollow viscus injuries.

Spleen

The timing of AE for splenic injuries depends on injury grade and available resources and nonoperative management versus splenectomy. Unstable patients with splenic injuries require emergent splenectomy. For those with normal hemodynamics, the management depends on the injury grade as determined by CT imaging (Table 10.5) [9]. Splenectomy has been the standard for grade III–V

Table 10.5 American Association for the Surgery of Trauma Splenic Injury Grading Scale

Grade	Injury description
I	Subcapsular hematoma, <10% surface area
	Laceration capsular tear, <1 cm parenchymal depth
II	Subcapsular hematoma, 10–50% surface area
	Intraparenchymal hematoma <5 cm diameter
	Laceration 1–3 cm parenchymal depth not involving a parenchymal vessel
III	Subcapsular hematoma, >50% surface area or expanding
	Ruptured subcapsular or parenchymal hematoma
	Intraparenchymal hematoma >5 cm
	Laceration >3 cm parenchymal depth or involving trabecular vessels
IV	Laceration of segmental or hilar vessels producing major devascularization (>25% of spleen)
V	Completely shattered spleen
	Hilar vascular injury which devascularized spleen

Advance one grade for multiple injuries to same organ up to grade III

injuries identified in patients in an austere environment with limited embolization options, very little capacity for intensive care unit (ICU) monitoring, and the concern for delayed hemorrhage during transport. However, a recent retrospective review showed no evidence of delayed hemorrhage or increased mortality in 35 patients with grade III or IV splenic injuries managed with nonoperative management [10].

Regardless of the grade, urgent evacuation to a surgical facility is essential for suspected solid organ injuries. Hemodynamically stable patients and those who respond to resuscitation can undergo CT imaging to further define the injury grade. If the patient remains stable, nonoperative management can be considered for grade I–III injuries. Grade IV and V injuries should be managed with a splenectomy prior to transport. Mature combat theaters often have some angioembolization capabilities that can be used to address a blush in a grade I–III injury being managed with nonoperative management. A follow-up CT at 48 h (and prior to transport out of a Role 3 facility) should be obtained to assess for any interval pseudoaneurysm development or development/increase in any hemoperitoneum. After splenectomy, patients require vaccination against *Streptococcus pneumonia*, *Haemophilus influenzae* type B, and *Neisseria meningitidis*. These should be given in the postoperative period at the first facility with vaccines available.

Liver or Pancreas

Like the spleen, injuries to the liver may be managed either operatively or nonoperatively depending on the patient's stability and injury severity. However, specific indications for intervention based on injury grade are less well defined for liver injuries. Nevertheless, management of liver injuries regardless of severity requires transfer to surgical capability. The surgical approach to patients with severe liver injuries generally involves liver packing with or without resection of devitalized tissue (Fig. 10.3). These patients generally require a massive resuscitation and typically are managed with damage control surgery. Postoperative angioembolization is sometimes also performed to achieve definitive hemostasis. Nonoperative management, in contrast, is reserved for hemodynamically normal patients. Angioembolization may be performed if a blush is seen on CT. Patients are monitored in the ICU for several days to ensure stability, with higher grade liver injuries managed with nonoperative management.

Pancreatic injuries are rarely isolated. They are typically associated with injuries to major vessels and other organs including the duodenum, stomach, spleen, and kidney. These patients need urgent initial evaluation by a surgeon. Stable patients may benefit from advanced imaging (magnetic resonance cholangiopancreatograph or endoscopic retrograde cholangiopancreatography) to further characterize injury location and associated duct injury; however, these imaging modalities are rarely available in the austere environment of combat [11]. Alternatively, intraoperative ultrasound has recently been described as a useful modality for identifying injuries to the pancreatic duct [12]. For those patients undergoing operative intervention, closed suction drainage is typically the mainstay of management. Destructive injuries of the pancreatic head and duodenum require a Whipple procedure, which can be performed in a staged fashion (i.e., resection initially followed by reconstruction at the next operation). Injuries involving the pancreatic duct within the body or tail of the pancreas are generally managed with a distal pancreatectomy and splenectomy.

Trauma patients are at high risk for development of venous thromboembolism and subsequent complications increasing morbidity and mortality [13, 14]. Venous thromboembolism prophylaxis can be started in hemodynamically stable patients 24–48 h after stabilization from major hemorrhage, including nonoperative management for solid organ injury [15, 16]. In general, venous thromboembolism prophylaxis should be administered prior to AE flights if possible [17]. The preferred regimen is enoxaparin 30 mg subcutaneously (SC) twice daily. For those with renal failure, heparin 5000 SC three times daily is given.

Urgent Aeromedical Evacuation

Minimal Conditions

Patients undergoing splenectomy or operative management of liver or pancreatic injuries should be hemodynamically stable with no ongoing blood product resuscitation requirements prior to transport to the next level of care (Table 10.3). After splenectomy for either a primary splenic injury or an associated pancreatic injury, vaccines should be confirmed as having been given prior to movement from Role 3 and 4 facilities.

Those patients with a splenic injury undergoing nonoperative management should have the grade of injury verified (I–III), and the follow-up CT imaging at 48 h post-injury should be reviewed. If there is evidence of a pseudoaneurysm or new/increased hemoperitoneum, angioembolization or splenectomy should be considered. Nonoperative management of liver or pancreatic injuries is much less common during combat operations. In the rare cases where such patients are evacuated, stability for 24–48 h should be confirmed, and any planned re-imaging of liver injuries should be performed prior to AE.

Specific Concerns/Treatment

Some post-splenectomy and all operative liver/pancreatic injury patients will have closed suction abdominal drains in place. These are to monitor for and control any postoperative leakage from the pancreatic duct (splenectomy with injury to the pancreatic tail; pancreatic injury with ductal involvement) or the intrahepatic bile ducts. These closed suction drains should be allowed to equilibrate to cabin pressure during takeoff and landing. Most of these patients will also have an NG tube early in the postoperative period. This should be managed as described previously. Hemorrhage is the other major concern after splenectomy, liver packing, pancreatic resections, and in the course

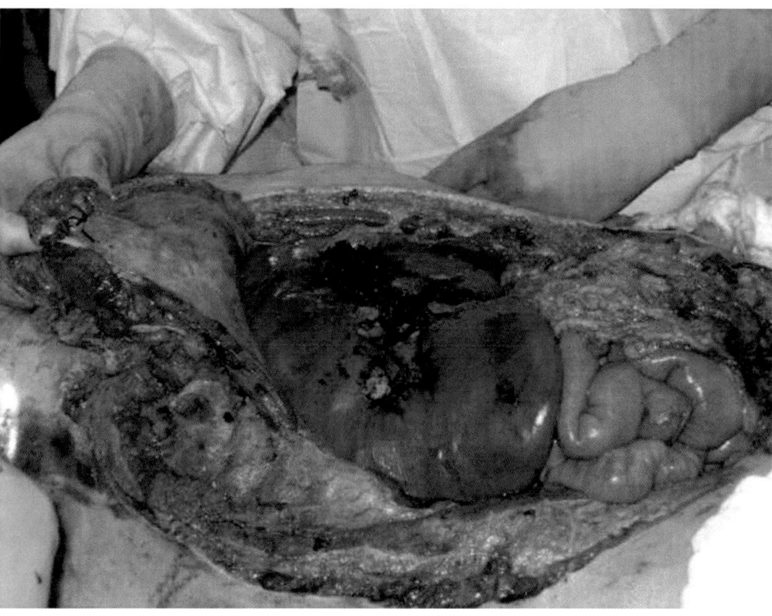

Fig. 10.3 Liver laceration

Table 10.6 Intra-abdominal injury transport checklist

☐ Current fluids (type, rate):______________________

☐ Urine Output

Adequate Urine Output:_______mL/hour

Last Urine Output:______mL/hour _____Date _____Time

☐ Current antibiotics:____________________________

Most recent antibiotic doses:_________________________

Next antibiotic dose due:____________________________

☐ Recent metabolic panel (results, time, date):_______

☐ Nasogastric Tube: Unclamped Y N

☐ Abdominal Vacuum Assisted Closure Device setting:____________

☐ Hollow viscus (Bowel) Injury

Specific injury:_________________

Bowel discontinuity: Y N

Ostomy type/location:_________________________

☐ Spleen Injury

Grade:__________________________

Splenectomy: Y N

Interventions Performed: ______________________

Vaccine(s) given (type, time, date given):__________

☐ Liver Injury

Grade:__________________________

Interventions Performed: ______________________

Management: Packing Nonoperative

of nonoperative management of solid organ injuries. Any change in hemodynamics or frank blood in any abdominal drains should prompt heightened concern for postoperative bleeding, and preparations should be made to provide damage control resuscitation and potentially surgical intervention. After liver injuries, bloody nasogastric tube output can also be a herald of hemobilia. This condition is caused by a traumatic arterial-to-bile duct fistula, typically managed with angioembolization of the arterial source.

Elective Aeromedical Evacuation

Elective AE of patients after operative management of solid organ injuries should occur after all packs have been removed, the abdomen closed, and hemodynamic stability for several days. For those undergoing nonoperative management, complete stability for many days should be documented and any residual concern for delayed bleeding addressed (Table 10.4).

Minimal Conditions

Elective AE of patients with solid organ injuries should be performed only after a prolonged period of stability. Vaccines should have been administered, if indicated, and all follow-up imaging reviewed and acted upon such that the risk of a bleeding complication during transport is minimized.

Specific Concerns/Treatment

Delayed hemorrhage is the greatest concern in patients with a history of solid organ injury managed either operatively or nonoperatively. Management is the same as detailed previously. Using a checklist prior to AE for these patients can be helpful (Table 10.6).

Genitourinary Injuries

Kidney Injuries

Renal injuries are managed by controlling hemorrhage, ensuring adequate renal perfusion, and ensuring adequate urinary drainage. Surgical input from an experienced trauma urologist or trauma surgeon is imperative to preserving renal mass and ultimately adequate renal function. Patients with suspected renal trauma should have a Foley catheter or suprapubic tube placed emergently and then be urgently evacuated to a Role 3 facility. Unstable patients may require partial or total nephrectomy at the time of initial surgical evaluation prior to further evacuation. Prior to performing a nephrectomy, an attempt should be made to confirm the patient has a contralateral kidney—typically by palpation in the operating room (OR). If at all possible, a partial nephrectomy or repair of the renal laceration should be considered before committing the patient to a nephrectomy. However, those patients in shock or with multiple associated injuries should undergo a rapid nephrectomy without hesitation [18]. Nonoperative management of renal injuries may require angioembolization for active extravasation of vascular contrast or placement of a ureteral stent if there is evidence of a collecting system injury. Follow-up imaging with CT is generally recommended to assess the stability of these injuries.

Bladder, Urethra, or Testicles

Bladder, urethral, and testicular injuries are now the predominant genitourinary injury pattern due to the increased use of improvised explosive devices (IEDs). Successful management with preservation of function requires a systematic evaluation to define the injuries, although management of these lower genitourinary track injuries is often superseded by hemorrhage control in critically injured patients. Insertion of a Foley catheter is useful as a diagnostic tool and for future monitoring. A Foley catheter should be placed emergently if the urethra is intact, as verified by lack of blood at the meatus and/or retrograde ureterogram. If an injury is suspected, an experienced provider can still attempt a single-pass Foley placement based on recent guidelines [19]. For destructive injuries and unsuccessful initial Foley insertion, a suprapubic tube is required [18]. Scrotal hemorrhage and exposed testicular tissue can usually be managed with direct pressure initially followed by operative exploration. Postoperative dressings should be non-constricted to allow for subsequent swelling.

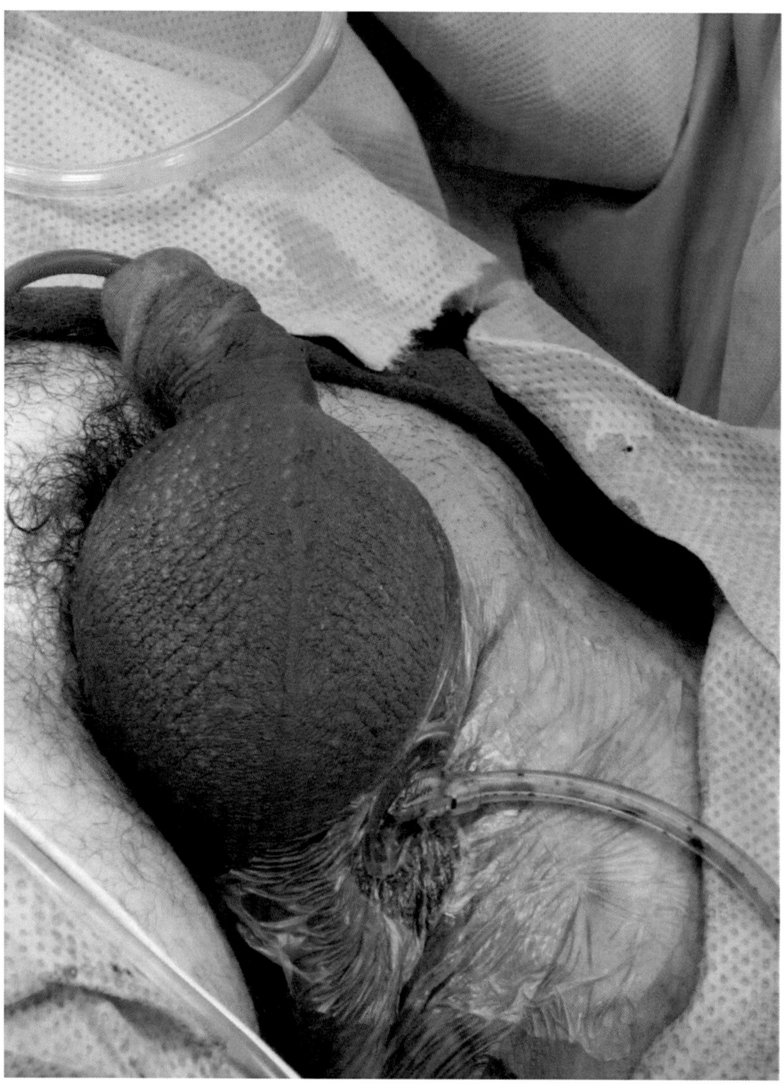

Fig. 10.4 Negative-pressure wound dressing for a perineal soft tissue injury

Negative-pressure wound dressings can be placed on the external genitalia for management of large soft tissue defects (Fig. 10.4).

Urgent Aeromedical Evacuation

Minimal Conditions

Patients with genitourinary injuries should be hemodynamically normal with no evidence of ongoing blood product resuscitation. Electrolytes, especially potassium, should be normal, and any anticipated need for acute renal therapy dialysis should be addressed proactively prior to transport (Table 10.3). The two most common forms of acute renal therapy dialysis used to treat the critically ill after acute kidney injury are (1) continuous renal replacement therapy and (2) therapeutic plasma exchange.

Patients undergoing nonoperative management for renal injuries should have a documented period of stability with no evidence of contrast extravasation on follow-up imaging. Any urine extravasation on imaging should also be addressed prior to transport. Bladder drainage in the form of a Foley or suprapubic catheter should be present. If bladder irrigation is required, a clear plan for the volume of irrigation and duration of irrigation should be detailed. If frequent catheter manipulations are required due to urinary clot formation, transport should be delayed. If an external urinary drain is present (e.g., percutaneous nephrostomy or ureteral catheter), it should be well secured and should be working reliably. Scrotal dressings should be intact and confirmed as loose, and any negative-pressure wound dressings should be functional.

Specific Concerns/Treatment

Hyperkalemia is a completely avoidable complication during transport as continuous renal replacement therapy is now available routinely at Role 3 facilities [20]. However, if it occurs, the usual treatments of insulin/glucose, bicarbonate, calcium, and diuresis should be given. The receiving facility should also be alerted to the likely need for emergent continuous renal replacement therapy. Most patients will not be stable enough for intermittent hemodialysis and thus require continuous renal replacement therapy. Foley or suprapubic tube occlusion is a concern during transport of these patients. If the patient demonstrates new oliguria or anuria, a gentle flush of these catheters should relieve the obstruction. Many of these patients will also have closed suction drains that should be managed as described earlier.

Elective Aeromedical Evacuation

Timing

Patients with genitourinary injuries can be transported electively after a period of demonstrated stability. Ideally, these patients should have most or all of their tubes/lines/drains removed before elective AE (Table 10.4). At most, some patients may have either a Foley or a suprapubic tube for bladder drainage.

Minimal Conditions

At a minimum, a patient should have stable renal function with the ability to urinate or with intact/patient bladder drainage. If renal replacement is required, the patient should be stable on intermittent hemodialysis.

Specific Concerns/Treatment

Electrolyte abnormalities and catheter obstruction should be anticipated and addressed as outlined previously. Using a checklist prior to AE for these patients can be helpful (Table 10.7).

Table 10.7 Genitourinary injury transport checklist

☐ Current fluids (type, rate):____________________

☐ Urine Output

  Adequate Urine Output:_______mL/hour

  Last Urine Output:______mL/hour _____Date _____Time

☐ Current antibiotics:_________________________

  Most recent antibiotic doses:______________________

  Next antibiotic dose due:_________________________

☐ Recent metabolic panel (results, time, date):_______

☐ Renal Injury

  Location: Right Left

  Grade:______________

  Nephrectomy: Y N

  Interventions Performed: __________ ___________

  Drain purpose/location:____________________

☐ Scrotal Dressing: Non-Constricting: Y N

Soft Tissue Injuries

Soft tissue injuries are ubiquitous in combat and are often accompanied by vascular, nerve, and orthopedic injuries [21]. Consequently, anything more than the most trivial wound requires surgical evaluation. After triage and evacuation to an echelon II or rural hospital, these injuries may or may not require surgical intervention. Nonsurgical soft tissue injuries may be managed locally, although US service members may require elective evacuation to a military facility with adequate patient holding capacity (Roles 3–5). Amputations and vascular injuries necessitating tourniquet use require emergent exploration with the goal of washing out the wound and re-establishing perfusion to whatever degree is possible. The majority of these injuries will require serial washouts and complex closure at a Role 4–5 facility. At the initial and early washouts, dead tissue should be debrided but maximal viable tissue should be retained for future closure. Surgeons may place a negative-pressure wound dressing on these wounds as detailed previously.

Urgent Aeromedical Evacuation

Minimal Conditions

Indications for urgent evacuation include vascular shunting or tenuous repairs and other life-threatening injuries. Shunts should be replaced and definitive vascular reconstruction performed prior to evacuation out of a Role 3 facility [22]. Any concern for a possible extremity compartment syndrome should also be addressed prior to AE. All devitalized tissue should be debrided and a healthy wound bed confirmed. Invasive fungal infections are a major concern with destructive injuries. For at-risk patients, soft tissue wounds should be dressed with 1/4 strength Dakin solution [23].

Specific Concerns/Treatment

For patients with negative-pressure wound dressings, AE crews should have available both new canisters and basic supplies to patch small leaks (Table 10.3). For extremity wounds, constricting dressings should be avoided, as swelling is likely to occur post injury and be exacerbated at altitude.

Elective Aeromedical Evacuation

Timing

Patients with soft tissue injuries are generally eligible for elective AE once they are stable between dressing changes (Table 10.4). Definitive closure is not necessary for AE.

Minimal Conditions

Patients should have no ongoing soft tissue necrosis or concern for occult invasive fungal infection and no at-risk extremities with concern for compartment syndrome.

Specific Concerns/Treatment

As detailed above, negative-pressure wound therapy devices should be functional. If wounds have been closed over closed suction drains, they should be patent and managed as described previously. Extremity dressings should be non-constricting to avoid the risk of compartment syndrome at altitude. Using a checklist prior to AE for these patients can be helpful (Table 10.8).

Table 10.8 Soft tissue injury transport checklist

- ☐ Current fluids (type, rate):____________________
- ☐ Urine Output
  - Adequate Urine Output:_______mL/hour
  - Last Urine Output:______mL/hour _____Date _____Time
- ☐ Current antibiotics:_________________________
  - Most recent antibiotic doses:____________________
  - Next antibiotic dose due:_______________________
- ☐ Recent metabolic panel (results, time, date):_______
- ☐ Open Wounds
  - Locations:______________________
  - Last Debridement (time, date):________________
- ☐ Drain purpose/location:______________________
- ☐ Extremities needing compartment checks:_________
- ☐ Abdominal Vacuum Assisted Closure Device
  - Setting:____________
  - Instil lation (location, setting, irrigate):_________
  - Supplies (canisters, sticky drapes)
- ☐ Tourniquets available

Dismounted Complex Blast Injury

One of the signature injury patterns of recent combat operations is the so-called dismounted complex blast injury (Fig. 10.5) [24–26]. This injury pattern includes traumatic amputations with large soft tissue defects, genitourinary injuries, anorectal trauma, and orthopedic injuries. Thus, this extreme form of trauma encompasses many of thc concepts discussed in this chapter, integrated into a single patient. Although these injuries are seen in military personnel traveling by foot, civilian terrorist attacks, major crush injuries, and high-speed motorcycle or motor vehicle crashes can produce a similar injury pattern. The management of these severely injured individuals is therefore instructive as a point of reference.

At their core, dismounted complex blast injuries represent the ultimate polytrauma injury complex, largely directed at the lower body, pelvis, and arms. Many of these injuries are nonsurvivable, with patients dying prior to or immediately upon arrival to Role 2 or 3 facilities. For those patients who arrive at a surgical facility alive, the cumulative nature of the injuries resulting in shock, coagulopathy, systemic inflammatory response, and later sepsis is the greatest threat to life. The original blast typically causes at least one lower extremity traumatic amputation. Limbs that are not lost at the time of the blast are often mangled and require either primary surgical amputation or extreme limb salvage measures. Anatomically higher leg amputations correlate with a greater likelihood of pelvic injuries. Pelvic injuries may include a

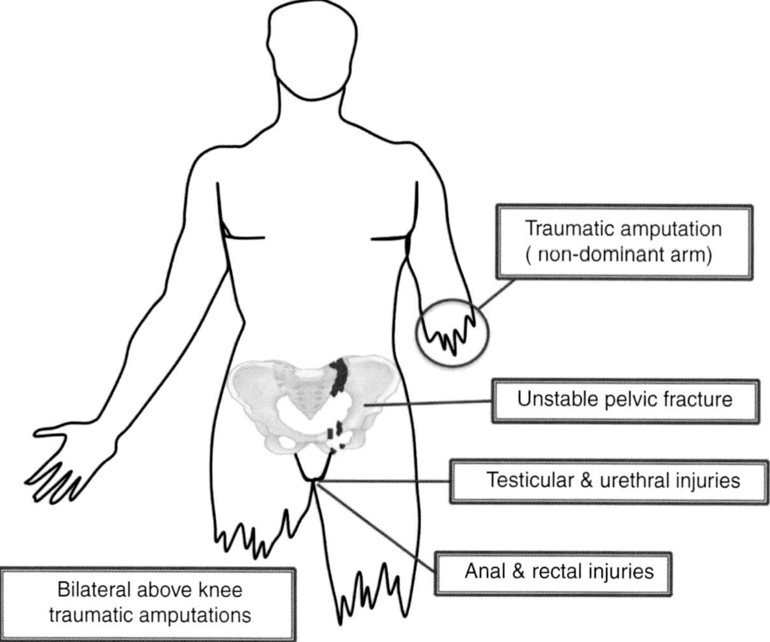

Fig. 10.5 Dismounted complex blast injury. (Reprinted from Cannon et al. [29], with permission of the American College of Surgeons)

combination of unstable pelvic fractures and soft tissue injury to major nerves and blood vessels, genitourinary structures, and colon/rectum/anus.

Traumatic amputations should be managed with aggressive hemorrhage control to include liberal use of tourniquets at the point of injury. Splinting of the mangled extremity will help to control bleeding and pain as well. Tourniquets can remain in place for 2–4 h with little risk of extremity morbidity. Once the patient has reached a surgical facility (Role 2 or higher), tourniquets should be evaluated by a surgeon.

Colorectal injuries sustained as part of a dismounted complex blast injury will most likely require a treatment approach as outlined earlier. In the hemodynamically stable patient, a CT with rectal contrast and/or proctoscopy are indicated. Diverting colostomy for anorectal injuries has been shown to reduce mortality in patients with massive trauma as seen in dismounted complex blast injuries. The descending colon can be stapled off at the index operation and then subsequently matured at a later date when the patient is more stable.

Genitourinary injuries should be managed as described earlier, but with an eye to the likely necessity for a dismounted complex blast injury treatment and abbreviated operative times. These injuries will become more complicated in the face of unstable pelvic fractures that may require working around pelvic binders or external fixators. Pelvic fracture increases the risk of a urethral and bladder injury. Placement of a Foley catheter should be performed as detailed previously. In cases of a failed Foley insertion or a destructive urethral or bladder injury, a suprapubic tube may be required. Penetrating scrotal injuries should be explored, any devitalized testicular tissue debrided, and the dartos fascia closed.

Pelvic stabilization is an integral part of the initial management of dismounted complex blast injuries, and pelvic fractures are discussed in Chap. 11. Stabilization is performed with a pelvic binder initially with early transition to external fixation. Pelvic fractures occurring with dismounted complex blast injuries are generally considered open and contaminated by the associated anorectal and genitourinary injuries. In addition, the original blast often inoculates the tissue planes with local microbes—both bacterial and fungal [27].

Beyond bleeding control, soft tissue injuries with or without associated amputation require early debridement of grossly contaminated and devitalized tissue [21]. In unstable patients requiring damage control surgery, a second surgical team may elect to wash out extremity wounds, while the primary team attempts to achieve hemostasis. Operative times should not be prolonged or evacuation delayed for extremity washouts in unstable patients [26].

Additional considerations in patients with dismounted complex blast injuries include early activation of the massive transfusion protocol and appropriate antibiotic coverage. Cefazolin for skin flora and metronidazole for colonic injuries are indicated with early re-dosing for blood loss and continued prophylaxis dosing while in transit [8].

Urgent Aeromedical Evacuation

Minimal Conditions

These patients are incredibly complex and typically require ongoing resuscitation during their initial course of management. They can quickly outstrip the blood bank and surgical resources of smaller facilities (e.g., split or even full Role 2). Thus, AE is likely to be complicated by ongoing resuscitation and hemodynamic instability.

Specific Concerns/Treatment

Ongoing bleeding and early sepsis are the greatest concerns in these very complex patients. Early on, any hemodynamic instability should be presumed to be caused by bleeding and should primarily be managed with blood product infusion and rapid transport to the nearest surgical facility. After several days, infectious complications start to predominate. In these cases, again, thorough surgical debridement, use of appropriate antibiotic coverage, and even placement of antibiotic-containing cement beads are all important to addressing the bacterial, fungal, and mold infections that develop in these patients. Most dismounted complex blast injury patients will also have at least one if not multiple negative-pressure wound therapy devices, and some may have the ability to instill antibiotic solutions into the wound. These dressings must be carefully and meticulously maintained to avoid loss of suction leading to accumulation of infected effluent under an occlusive dressing.

Elective Aeromedical Evacuation

Timing

These patients will only be eligible for elective transport after multiple surgical procedures. They should have no ongoing soft tissue necrosis or infections. The pelvis should be stabilized. Their colostomy should be functioning. The amputation sites should be definitively closed and the perineal and genitourinary injuries stabilized and in a long-term management phase.

Minimal Conditions

As described previously, these patients should be completely stable and either definitively repaired or at a point of chronic long-term management awaiting definitive repair before being electively transported.

Specific Concerns/Treatment

The specific problems that may arise during elective transport of these patients are detailed in the individual organ system sections above.

Special Aeromedical Evacuation Challenges

Complex Line, Tube, and Drain Management

Combat-injured patients, particularly those with abdominal, genitourinary, and soft tissue trauma, are likely to have numerous tubes, lines, and/or drains. Understanding what each of these tubes, lines, and/or drains are doing and ensuring that they are not displaced represents one of the core imperatives and challenges for AE crews. The transport team must know the course from origin to container for each device present. The team must also know what type and volume of drainage to expect, as well as the implications of changes in consistency and rate. This information is integral to allowing the transport team to assess the patient en route. Additionally, a thorough understanding will help the transport team in managing the inevitable complications from obstruction to dislodgment. Finally, the receiving team will need information about each tube, line, and drain as well.

Considering the importance and complexity of tubes, lines, and drains, each should be directly labeled if possible. Replacements should be available for common devices such as nasogastric tubes, Foley catheters, arterial lines, and venous lines. Extra canisters are a necessity for all vacuum-assisted closure devices and drainage reservoirs. Additional dressings to reinforce bleeding dressings or leaking vacuum-assisted closure device dressings are a requirement as well. Knowledge of prior tubes, lines, and drains may be helpful as well, particularly if they were associated with a complication (e.g., infiltrated intravenous [IV], occluding arterial line) or could become associated with a complication (previously dislodged drain, not replaced).

Oliguria

Managing urine output during AE is complex but integral to the good care of patients. Ideally, all post-surgical and most solid organ nonoperative management patients should have a Foley and/or suprapubic tube to allow for monitoring of urine output. Urine output can be difficult to calculate when there are additional genitourinary tubes or injuries controlled with either closed suction drains. A decrease in urine output can signal hypoperfusion, hypovolemia, obstruction, or acute kidney injury.

AE crews should generally give a fluid challenge for decreased urinary output. However, discriminate fluid boluses should not be given reflexively during long transports in light of the nonspecificity of oliguria. Particularly in the face of normal blood pressure or stable vasopressor requirement, repeated boluses are unlikely to be helpful. Knowledge of the patient's current anatomy post-surgery and pre-flight labs can help guide management [28]. Efforts should be made to assess the patient's intravascular volume (e.g., with abdominal/cardiac ultrasound); determine the patient's fluid responsiveness; check all tubes, lines, and drains for obstruction or malfunction; and re-assess the recorded output for clerical errors.

Disclaimer The opinions expressed in this document are solely those of the authors and do not represent an endorsement by or the views of the US Air Force, the Department of Defense, or the US government.

References

1. Cannon JW, Khan MA, Raja AS, Cohen MJ, Como JJ, Cotton BA, et al. Damage control resuscitation in patients with severe traumatic hemorrhage: a practice management guideline from the Eastern Association for the Surgery of Trauma. J Trauma Acute Care Surg. 2017;82:605–17.
2. Holcomb JB, Jenkins D, Rhee P, Johannigman J, Mahoney P, Mehta S, et al. Damage control resuscitation: directly addressing the early coagulopathy of trauma. J Trauma. 2007;62:307–10.
3. Chovanes J, Cannon JW, Nunez TC. The evolution of damage control surgery. Surg Clin North Am. 2012;92:859–75.
4. Rotondo MF, Schwab CW, McGonigal MD, Phillips GR 3rd, Fruchterman TM, Kauder DR, et al. "Damage control": an approach for improved survival in exsanguinating penetrating abdominal injury. J Trauma. 1993;35:373–5.
5. Fang R, Dorlac WC, Flaherty SF, Tuman C, Cain SM, Popey TL, et al. Feasibility of negative pressure wound therapy during intercontinental aeromedical evacuation of combat casualties. J Trauma. 2010;69(Suppl 1):S140–5.
6. Huang C, Leavitt T, Bayer LR, Orgill DP. Effect of negative pressure wound therapy on wound healing. Curr Probl Surg. 2014;51:301–31.
7. Kotwal RS, Howard JT, Orman JA, Tarpey BW, Bailey JA, Champion HR, et al. The effect of a golden hour policy on the morbidity and mortality of combat casualties. JAMA Surg. 2016;151:15–24.
8. Saeed O, Tribble D, Biever K, Kavanaugh M, Crouch H. Joint trauma system clinical practice guideline: infection prevention in combat-related injuries (CPG ID: 24), 2016. http://jts.amedd.army.mil/assets/docs/cpgs/JTS_Clinical_Practice_Guidelines_(CPGs)/Infection_Prevention_in_Combat-Related_Injuries_08_Aug_2016_ID24.pdf.
9. Stockinger Z, Grabo D, Benov AVI, Tien H, Seery J, Humphries A. Joint trauma system clinical practice guideline: blunt abdominal trauma, splenectomy, and post-splenectomy vaccination (CPG ID: 09), 2016. http://jts.amedd.army.mil/assets/docs/cpgs/JTS_Clinical_Practice_Guidelines_(CPGs)/Blunt_Abdominal_Trauma_Splenectomy_PostSplenectomy_Vaccination_12_Aug_2016_ID09.pdf.
10. Zonies D, Eastridge B. Combat management of splenic injury: trends during a decade of conflict. J Trauma Acute Care Surg. 2012;73:S71–4.
11. Biffl WL, Moore EE, Croce M, Davis JW, Coimbra R, Karmy-Jones R, et al. Western trauma association crit-

ical decisions in trauma: management of pancreatic injuries. J Trauma Acute Care Surg. 2013;75:941–6.
12. Hofmann LJ, Learn PA, Cannon JW. Intraoperative ultrasound to assess for pancreatic duct injuries. J Trauma Acute Care Surg. 2015;78:888–91.
13. Holley AB, Petteys S, Mitchell JD, Holley PR, Collen JF. Thromboprophylaxis and VTE rates in soldiers wounded in operation enduring freedom and operation Iraqi freedom. Chest. 2013;144:966–73.
14. Geerts WH, Code KI, Jay RM, Chen E, Szalai JP. A prospective study of venous thromboembolism after major trauma. N Engl J Med. 1994;331:1601–6.
15. Eberle BM, Schnüriger B, Inaba K, Cestero R, Kobayashi L, Barmparas G, et al. Thromboembolic prophylaxis with low-molecular-weight heparin in patients with blunt solid abdominal organ injuries undergoing nonoperative management: current practice and outcomes. J Trauma. 2011;70:141–6.. discussion 147
16. Nathens AB, McMurray MK, Cuschieri J, Durr EA, Moore EE, Bankey PE, et al. The practice of venous thromboembolism prophylaxis in the major trauma patient. J Trauma. 2007;62:557–62; discussion 562–563
17. Grabo D, Seery J, Bradley M, Zakaluzny S, Kearns M, Fernandez N, Tadlock M. Joint trauma system clinical practice guideline: the prevention of deep venous thrombosis – inferior vena cava filter (CPG ID: 36), 2016. http://jts.amedd.army.mil/assets/docs/cpgs/JTS_Clinical_Practice_Guidelines_(CPGs)/Deep_Venous_Thrombosis_Inferior_Vena_Filter_02_Aug_2016_ID36.pdf.
18. Jezoir J, Hudak S, Walters J, Stockinger Z, Waxman S. Joint trauma system clinical practice guideline: urologic trauma management (CPG ID: 42). 2017. http://jts.amedd.army.mil/assets/docs/cpgs/JTS_Clinical_Practice_Guidelines_(CPGs)/Urologic_Trauma_Management_01_Nov_2017_ID42.pdf.
19. Morey AF, Brandes S, Dugi DD 3rd, Armstrong JH, Breyer BN, Broghammer JA, et al. American urological association. Urotrauma: AUA guideline. J Urol. 2014;192:327–35.
20. Zonies D, DuBose J, Elterman J, Bruno T, Benjamin C, Cannon J, et al. Early implementation of continuous renal replacement therapy optimizes casualty evacuation for combat-related acute kidney injury. J Trauma Acute Care Surg. 2013;75:S210–4.
21. Joint Trauma System Clinical Practice Guideline: Initial management of war wounds: wound debridement and irrigation. 2012. http://jts.amedd.army.mil/assets/docs/cpgs/JTS_Clinical_Practice_Guidelines_(CPGs)/War_Wounds_Debridement_Irrigation_25_Apr_12_ID31.pdf.
22. Rasmussen T, Stockinger Z, Antevil J, White C, Fernandez N, White J, et al. Joint trauma system clinical practice guideline: vascular injury (CPG ID: 46), 2016. http://jts.amedd.army.mil/assets/docs/cpgs/JTS_Clinical_Practice_Guidelines_(CPGs)/Vascular_Injury_12_Aug_2016_ID46.pdf.
23. Rodriguez CJ, Tribble DR, Murray CK, Jessie EM, Khan M, Fleming ME, et al. Joint trauma system clinical practice guideline: invasive fungal infection in war wounds (CPG: 28). 2016. http://jts.amedd.army.mil/assets/docs/cpgs/JTS_Clinical_Practice_Guidelines_(CPGs)/Invasive_Fungal_Infection_in_War_Wounds_04_Aug_2016_ID28.pdf.
24. Cannon JW, Hofmann LJ, Glasgow SC, Potter BK, Rodriguez CJ, Cancio LC, et al. Dismounted complex blast injuries: a comprehensive review of the modern combat experience. J Am Coll Surg. 2016;223:652–64.
25. Ficke JR, Eastridge BJ, Butler FK, Alvarez J, Brown T, Pasquina P, et al. Dismounted complex blast injury report of the Army dismounted complex blast injury task force. J Trauma Acute Care Surg. 2012;73:S520–34.
26. Gordon W, Talbot M, Fleming M, Shero J, Potter B, Stockinger Z. Joint trauma system clinical practice guideline: high bilateral amputations and dismounted complex blast injury (CPG ID: 22), 2016. http://jts.amedd.army.mil/assets/docs/cpgs/JTS_Clinical_Practice_Guidelines_(CPGs)/High_Bilateral_Amputations_Dismnted_Cmplex_Blast_Injury_01_Aug_2016_ID22.pdf.
27. Gordon W, Fleming M, Johnson A, Gurney J, Shackelford S, Stockinger Z. Joint trauma system clinical practice guideline: pelvic fracture care (CPG ID: 34). 2017. http://jts.amedd.army.mil/assets/docs/cpgs/JTS_Clinical_Practice_Guidelines_(CPGs)/Pelvic_Fracture_Care_15_Mar_2017_ID34.pdf.
28. Goren O, Matot I. Perioperative acute kidney injury. Br J Anaesth. 2015;115(Suppl 2):ii3–14.
29. Cannon JW, Hofmann LJ, Glasgow SC, Potter BK, Rodriguez CJ, Cancio LC, et al. Dismounted complex blast injuries: a comprehensive review of the modern combat experience. J Am Coll Surg. 2016;223:652–64.

11 Orthopedic Patients

Russell K. Stewart, Steven L. Oreck, Lucas Teske, and Brian R. Waterman

Introduction

Isolated or combined musculoskeletal trauma comprises a significant percentage of all injuries, both in the civilian population and during military operations. The use of modern personal protective equipment by both civilians and military members has continued to reduce the severity and overall rate of wounding and fatalities yet paradoxically increases the percentage of orthopedic injuries [1–4]. This is because both civilian restraints (e.g., airbags, safety harnesses) and military body armor protect vital central nervous system and visceral structures but do little to protect the peripheral extremities, which remain exposed.

While classically associated with fractures and dislocations, orthopedic injuries may encompass a broad range of soft-tissue injuries, including tendon, volumetric muscle loss, and neurovascular injuries. This unique constellation of trauma is best treated by a multi-disciplinary team of different orthopedic, trauma, general, vascular, and plastic surgeons. The exact composition of the surgical team depends upon several factors, including the setting of the injury, the training of the individuals involved, and the organization of the medical system where they are treated. This chapter will cover these multi-tissue injuries as well as fractures and dislocations.

This chapter will begin with a brief description of the pathophysiology of orthopedic injuries followed by a discussion of treatment and implications for the aeromedical evacuation (AE) of these patients. It will end with a discussion of the preparation for and contraindications of AE.

R. K. Stewart
Wake Forest School of Medicine, Winston-Salem, NC, USA

S. L. Oreck
CAPT, MC, USN (FMF) (ret.), Department of History, University of Wisconsin-Madison, Madison, WI, USA

L. Teske
Department of Orthopedic Surgery, Wake Forest Baptist Health, Winston Salem, NC, USA

B. R. Waterman (✉)
Department of Orthopaedic Surgery, Wake Forest Baptist Health, Winston Salem, NC, USA
e-mail: Bwaterma@wakehealth.edu

Pathophysiology of Orthopedic Injuries

Fractures of the bone result in three immediate and distinctive pathologic responses that can have grave sequelae: pain, bleeding, and the release of "injury amines." Pain is related to both the interruption of the overlying periosteum and the energy and sharp fracture fragments that can inflict damage on adjacent nerves, vessels, and local soft tissue envelope. Pain and deformity can typically be provisionally treated with a combi-

W. W. Hurd, W. Beninati (eds.), *Aeromedical Evacuation*, https://doi.org/10.1007/978-3-030-15903-0_11

nation of immobilization of the fracture, elevation of the limb, and pain medication, as discussed below.

Likewise, potentially massive bleeding originates from both the fracture itself and any associated soft-tissue and vessel injuries. The formation of a fracture hematoma usually controls the bleeding. If left undisturbed, the hematoma will become fibrous and stable. Limb movement related to inadequate splintage can result in hematoma disruption and renewed bleeding. This has obvious implications for AE both in terms of movement techniques and patient monitoring.

The final pathologic response to fracture is the local release of injury amines and other inflammatory mediators. These include histamine, bradykinin, various prostaglandins, and others—with more mediators being elucidated on a regular basis. The predictable consequence is substantial tissue edema that results from local changes in capillary permeability. This can be minimized by both elevation and splintage of the fractured limb.

Flight Edema

Fluid shifts have been noted to occur during altitude exposure in-flight due to reduced barometric pressures [5–9]. This phenomenon, known as "flight edema," has the potential to affect outcomes for orthopedic patients in the AE setting. The extent of that impact, however, has been debated in recent literature. Iblher et al. [10] examined changes in tibia and forehead tissue thickness to assess fluid shifts during 8 hours of simulated air and ground transport in the seated position. Increases in tibial edema were the same in both settings, while increases in forehead tissue thickness were much greater in conditions simulating in-flight altitudes. Although the authors concluded that an upright, seated position might have a much stronger influence on leg edema formation than that exerted by changes in barometric pressure, the observed increase in forehead tissue thickness indicates that fluid shifts due to altitude exposure can still be significant. Such shifts have potential to worsen edema due to orthopedic injury and thus increase risk of complication in-flight.

Fat Embolism Syndrome

A unique and potentially fatal condition that can occur after any significant fracture is fat embolism syndrome. It has long been assumed that this syndrome is caused by the release of marrow fat into the circulation as a direct result of trauma to the bone. A more recent hypothesis is that fat embolism syndrome is caused by the release of injury amines that induce the release of marrow fat, and together they cause damage to capillary beds. This proposed pathogenesis helps explain manifestations in parts of the body beyond pulmonary capillaries (such as the brain and skin) as well as instances of fat embolism syndrome not associated with fracture. Furthermore, the cascade of events may explain the 24- to 72-hour delay in presentation that is classically observed in fat embolism syndrome following a fracture [11]. Regardless of the pathogenesis, it follows that disruption of a fracture hematoma in-flight can result in further release of injury amines or marrow fat, thus increasing risk for fat embolism syndrome.

The Danger Zone

After initial pre-hospital stabilization during "the Golden Hour" [12], the most vulnerable period for immediate orthopedic complications is the first 72 hours after fracture or any major bone surgeries, especially long-bone manipulation. During this period, injury-related edema becomes maximal. In addition, during this period patients are at greatest risk for fat embolism syndrome, manifesting most commonly by acute respiratory distress [3, 11, 13].

Treatment of Orthopedic Casualties

There are several important considerations for the care of orthopedic casualties and recognition of complications in a timely fashion as they occur. Key among these are adequate splintage and elevation of the injured limb, monitoring of general vital signs, and frequent checks of the neurovascular status of the affected limb.

Splinting

After initial reduction or re-alignment of a fracture or dislocation, splinting or immobilization is the single most crucial aspect of orthopedic casualty treatment [1, 14–21]. Stable splinting of orthopedic injuries reduces pain and edema and prevents further damage to the limb by preventing sharp bone ends from lacerating soft-tissue structures. In addition, splinting reduces bleeding by allowing clotting to occur and the fracture hematoma to stabilize. Given the significant bleeding that can occur from long-bone and pelvic fractures, this is an important consideration.

Splintage can be as rudimentary as a rifle strapped around a leg or as complex as an internal fixation device. It also includes casts, traction, and external fixators. For medical evacuation (MEDEVAC), orthopedic injuries with fracture or dislocation need to be splinted using whatever is available. Although the details of splintage are beyond the scope of this chapter, it is important to realize that many orthopedic devices that work well in a hospital setting are incompatible with AE, as discussed below.

Elevation of the Injured Limbs

An important aspect of care of the orthopedic casualty is elevation of the injured limb. This deceptively simple maneuver decreases pain, bleeding, and edema, probably as a result of decreasing venous capillary pressure. Judicious maintenance of elevation during transportation is well worth the small effort required.

Monitoring of Vital Signs

Once the fracture is reduced and the patient's pain is well controlled, the risk of serious complications appears to be decreased. However, the risk of complications remains significant for the first 72 hours. Many of the most serious complications discussed below start with subtle signs and symptoms. Because effective treatment depends on early recognition, careful monitoring of vital signs in the apparently stable orthopedic casualty is essential.

Neurovascular Status Checks

Continued reassessment of limb status is vital during the 72-hour danger zone after fracture and until definitive treatment, as patients continue to be at heightened risk of limb edema and other causes of neurovascular compromise until stable. The standard of care requires thorough documentation of normal neurovascular function before, during, and after AE.

Implications for Aeromedical Evacuation

Orthopedic casualties present specific challenges to both the civilian and military AE system. Due to lack of mobility and potentially bulky and heavy splinting and traction devices, these patients frequently represent both a nursing and transport challenge. Orthopedic emergencies that threaten life or limb are rare during AE but are often difficult to recognize and treat in-flight. For this reason, the cornerstone of the safe AE of orthopedic casualties is adequate preparation and stabilization.

Fortunately, orthopedic injuries are rarely life-threatening, and complications are uncommon after initial stabilization. Notable exceptions to this are patients with significant pelvic fractures (especially posterior) or multiple long-bone fractures. Conversely, the most common complications that may develop in orthopedic casualties during AE are generally beyond the capability of the aeromedical crew to treat and usually require expedient surgical treatment. An understanding of the potential complications and when they might occur will help avoid elective AE of orthopedic casualties during the periods when they are at highest risk for devastating complications. Appropriate planning is crucial to achieve an ideal outcome for all patients.

Table 11.1 Contraindications to elective aeromedical evacuation

Less than 72 hours following major orthopedic trauma or surgery in an otherwise stable patient
Less than 7 days following microvascular reattachment of a limb or digit
Unreduced long-bone fractures or major joint dislocations
Unstable long-bone or pelvic fractures
An anticoagulated patient prior to definitive fracture fixation
Untreated acute compartment syndrome
Gas gangrene

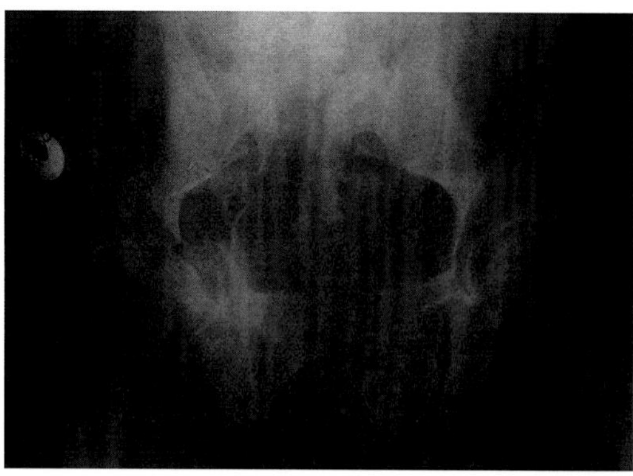

Fig. 11.1 Unstable pelvic/acetabular fracture. Patients with unstable symphysis diastasis and acetabular injuries must at least have provisional external fixation prior to AE to avoid significant problems

Orthopedic Contraindications for Elective Aeromedical Evacuation

There are several orthopedic conditions that are contraindications to elective AE (Table 11.1). While acute, life- or limb-threatening trauma should be escalated to the next higher echelon of care, elective AE should be delayed or deferred for 3 days (72 hours) to avoid the danger zone after major orthopedic surgery. If the injury required microvascular reattachment of a limb or digit, AE should be delayed until 7 days after surgery. Because of the risk of further damage to surrounding tissue, AE should be delayed until fractures are reduced and, if necessary, fixed or provisionally stabilized for transportation. This is especially important if the patient is anticoagulated. Patients with compartment syndrome should be treated prior to AE because the occurrence of any flight edema will only worsen the problem.

Urgent Aeromedical Evacuation

If urgent AE is required relatively soon after major orthopedic injury or surgery, several important precautions should be taken. Above all, the aeromedical crew should be advised of the increased risk patients are at during the 72-hour danger zone following orthopedic injury or surgery. When safe and practical, sea-level cabin pressure restriction might benefit patients who have undergone microvascular reattachment of a limb or digit. Patients who are suspected or known to have gas gangrene require emergent surgical debridement. If this is not available at the origination facility, further tissue damage might be lessened by a sea-level cabin altitude restriction as they are being transported to surgical care; however, this should not be attempted if it delays transporting the patient to surgical care. There are no altitude or cabin pressure restrictions for patients with treated compartment syndrome.

The greatest possible care must be taken when moving patients with unreduced or unstable fractures to minimize damage to surrounding tissue and the associated pain (Fig. 11.1). Serial monitoring of the neurovascular status of the affected limb is required during AE for early detection of developing problems.

Preparation of the Orthopedic Patient for Aeromedical Evacuation

Splintage

The most important consideration for AE is selection and preparation of splintage. Some splints are difficult or impossible to use during AE and others have potential complications. Free weight traction should not be used during AE, even in a sophisticated air ambulance, because of the adverse effect of movement and G-forces on these systems. Both United States and North Atlantic Treaty Organization (NATO) doctrines specifically forbid free weight traction.

Military anti-shock trousers (MAST), a type of pneumatic splint sometimes used for pelvic fractures, is also inappropriate for AE [15, 18]. The amount of pressure exerted by these inflatable trousers will vary with cabin pressure. The resultant excess pressure on the lower extremities can be dangerous when MAST trousers are used for prolonged periods during an AE flight, potentially contributing to soft-tissue compromise and necrosis. Likewise, air splints are relatively contraindicated for AE because splint expansion related to reduced cabin pressure can constrict circulation to the limb [5, 14, 18, 19].

Air splints are acceptable for MEDEVAC, as the altitudes flown will not induce significant expansion of a properly inflated air splint. All splints—whether inflatable or attached with elastic bandages—must be checked before, during, and after any AE flight to ensure they are not too tight.

Circumferential casts, as opposed to splints, present several unique challenges to AE. A rigid cast that fits well on the ground may become dangerously tight during flight because of flight edema or other changes in the patient's condition. For this reason, all casts must be *bivalved down both sides* to accommodate increased tissue edema prior to AE (Fig. 11.2). The underlying cast padding should be divided as well, and the cast held together with an elastic bandage. In some cases, windows must be cut to allow adequate monitoring of neurovascular status. These windows must have plaster covers that can be replaced after every check. If a windowed area is left uncovered, soft-tissue swelling can result in an artificial "hernia."

Negative-Pressure Wound Therapy

Negative-pressure wound therapy (NPWT) is a commonly used method for coverage and drainage of traumatic soft-tissue wounds. NPWT has been shown to reduce edema, aid in the removal of wound exudates, and stimulate growth factors that promote angiogenesis at the site of injury.

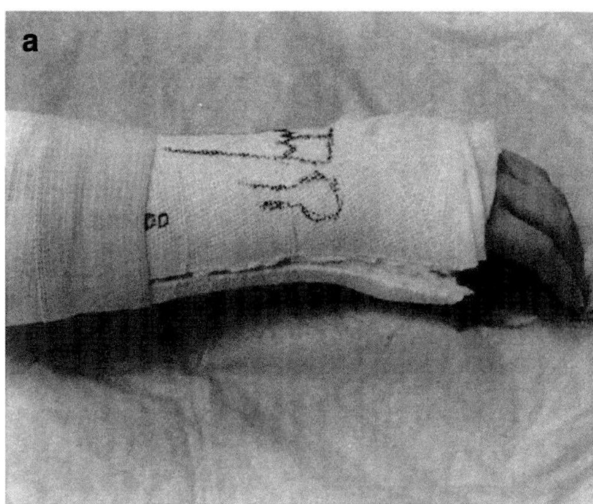

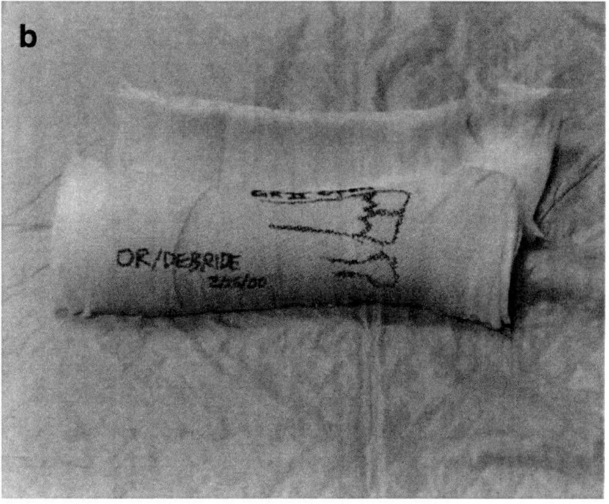

Fig. 11.2 Properly bivalved cast. (**a**) A bivalved cast should also have the padding split and be partially wrapped with an elastic bandage. (**b**) The cast is removed to illustrate the complete split-down both sides. A sketch of the injury and other data should be written on the cast with a marker

Additionally, NPWT enhances granulation tissue formation and decreases wound gapping to improve chances of delayed primary wound closure. Early attempts to utilize NPWT principles with noncommercial, improvised systems in the setting of AE resulted in device failures that limited its in-flight use. However, as NPWT device design and user familiarity have advanced, studies have demonstrated that NPWT has become a reliable option for wound stabilization in various stages of AE [22–24].

Combat-related wounds frequently carry high risk of infection due to extensive necrosis and contamination. In addition, definitive management is often delayed until evacuation to a higher level facility. For these reasons, it is crucial to optimize wound care prior to transport so that dressing changes will not be necessary during flight, thus protecting the wound from further contamination. One advantage of NPWT is that dressing changes can be performed less frequently compared to traditional dressings, thus decreasing risk of infection, improving patient comfort, and decreasing wound care requirements for the air crew [22–24].

Preflight Checklists

There are several steps that should be taken prior to AE to minimize the chance of complications during flight (Table 11.2). Above all, it should be ensured that the medical records are complete and appropriate radiographs accompany the patient. If possible, the fracture should be drawn on the cast, as well as a list of any procedure done. This will guarantee that this important information is available to both the caregivers during the flight and the accepting physicians. If AE is required within the 72-hour danger zone following injury or surgery, the aeromedical crew must be made aware of higher risks for this patient. A flow sheet should be provided to record continuing neurovascular monitoring of the patient during flight. If the patient has undergone microvascular reattachment of a limb or digit within 7 days or has gas gangrene, flight altitude should be restricted to maintain sea-level cabin pressure if it does not delay transporting the patient to surgical care.

Clinically, the most important preparation for AE involves careful examination of any cast or traction devices (Table 11.3). First, it must be verified that no free weight traction, MAST trousers, or air splints are being used. Next, all casts should be examined to ensure they are in good condition and both the plaster and underlying cast padding have been completely bivalved. The entire cast should be held together with an elastic bandage. All windowed areas that have been cut in the cast should have corresponding plaster covers in place to avoid localized soft-tissue swelling. Finally, all spring traction device settings should be checked.

Prior to take-off, it should be confirmed that all required equipment is on board. This should include a spare blanket or pillow to elevate the injured limb during flight, a large paramedic-type scissors capable of cutting cast padding, a cast

Table 11.2 Administrative preflight checklist

Ensure complete medical records and radiographs accompany the patient
If urgent aeromedical evacuation is required during the 72-hour danger zone following injury or surgery, alert the aeromedical crew to increased risk
Consider altitude restriction to maintain sea-level cabin pressure for patients
Within 7 days of microvascular reattachment of a limb or digit
With gas gangrene if it does not delay patient transport
Provide a neurovascular monitoring flow sheet for the patient
Draw on the cast the patient's fracture and a list of any procedures done. In the event that paperwork becomes unavailable, this information will be invaluable to both the in-flight caregivers and the receiving physician

Table 11.3 Clinical preflight checklist

Verify that no free weight traction, military anti-shock trousers (MAST), or air splints are being used
Ensure all casts have been completely bivalved (not just split down one side). Even the underlying cast padding should be cut, and the entire cast held together with an elastic bandage
Ensure all windowed areas cut in the cast have corresponding plaster covers. An uncovered window area will result in localized soft-tissue swelling forming a hernia
Ensure all casts are in good condition. Soft, or soggy, or otherwise "beat-up" casts should be replaced or reinforced
Ensure the availability of a spare blanket or pillow to elevate the injured limb during flight
Check all spring traction device settings
Ensure that normal neurovascular status of any fractured limb has been clearly documented
Ensure the following supplies are available on the aircraft:
Extra elastic bandages
Large paramedic-type scissors capable of cutting cast padding
Cast saw
Standard dressings

saw, extra elastic bandages, and standard dressings. The final clinical step prior to AE is to assure that normal neurovascular status of any fractured limb is present and has been clearly documented.

In-Flight Care

General nursing care for orthopedic patients during AE is straightforward. Adequate patient monitoring and documenting of vital signs and limb neurovascular status should be carried out at regular intervals. This interval may vary from every 1–4 hours and needs to be specified by the referring physician in the preflight orders. If a cast or dressing impedes the caregiver's ability to palpate distal pulses, a small cast "window" may be created and the capillary refill of nailbeds should be evaluated to confirm adequate limb perfusion. If motor testing of distal extremities is difficult to evaluate because of pain, the response to touch may be used as a simple guide. The results of each exam should be recorded with the dates and times.

Potential In-Flight Emergencies

Patients with orthopedic injuries may suffer from all of the problems common to other trauma patients, including infection, external hemorrhage, pulmonary embolism, and dehiscence of surgical wounds at high altitudes, as trapped gas expands at lower barometric pressure. Additionally, gravitational forces (i.e., G-forces) during take-off and landing can result in pooling of blood in the extremities, depending on patient orientation. Whereas hemodynamically stable patients should mount compensatory sympathetic responses to distribute blood volume, those with impaired autonomic function may be unable to do so [25]. This can potentially compromise the integrity of recent microvascular reattachments or surgical wounds.

There are several complications that are relatively unique to orthopedic injuries, many of which are often "hidden." Vascular and neurological complications—especially common with military orthopedic injuries—can be obvious and thus repaired prior to entrance to the AE system. Alternatively, more subtle neurovascular compromise can subsequently occur as a result of progressive intimal tears or the failure of a vascular repair. Concealed hemorrhage, significant enough to result in shock, is a risk for any patient with long-bone or pelvic fractures. Two complications relatively unique to orthopedic injuries are compartment syndrome and fat embolism syndrome. Two other complications for which a patient is at increased risk after orthopedic injuries are gangrene and crush syndrome. Each of these complications is considered below.

Neurovascular Compromise

Neurovascular compromise is always at the top of the list of problems associated with orthopedic injuries. Injuries to nerves or blood vessels can be on the same basis as the fracture (e.g., projectile or crushing injury). A partial vessel injury, such as an intimal tear, can be completely asymptomatic immediately after injury but progress to complete vessel occlusion during transport. The irregular, sharp ends of unstable fractures can impede or injure nerve or vessel function as a result of inadequate splintage. Partially impeded circulation can become further compromised due to edema or the pressure of compartment syndrome.

Vascular compromise from any cause (including compartment syndrome, discussed below) presents with acute loss of distal pulses, a cold extremity, or bleeding through dressings or casts due to the failure of a vascular repair. In-flight management of acute vascular compromise of a limb is limited to supportive measures such as oxygen supplementation and diversion to an appropriate medical facility.

Shock

Shock is both an acute and delayed risk in an apparently stable orthopedic casualty. Absence of external bleeding can lead to a false sense of security in a patient with long-bone or pelvic fractures. The risk of continued bleeding is especially great in patients with unreduced or unstable fractures. These casualties can lose significant amounts of blood into a thigh or pelvis with none of the dramatic distension associated with intra-abdominal bleeding. Transfusion coagulopathy also becomes a risk if large amounts of blood replacement are required.

Compartment Syndrome

A compartment is an anatomic area of the body that is incapable of significant expansion due to rigid bony or fascial boundaries. With increasing edema or bleeding in a rigid compartment, the intramural pressure in the compartment rises. Once the pressure in the compartment exceeds *capillary perfusion pressure*, approximately 30–35 mm Hg or within 30 mm Hg of the diastolic blood pressure (Δ[Delta]P), blood flow at the cellular level to the tissues in the compartment ceases [26]. This is most important to the skeletal muscle because it is the most metabolically active tissue [13, 27, 28]. The resultant ischemic muscle swells further and becomes extremely painful in what is known as compartment syndrome.

Compartments most at risk for this syndrome with an orthopedic injury are the anterior, posterior, and lateral leg compartments and the volar compartment of the forearm. An artificial "compartment" is created whenever a rigid cast is placed around an extremity. If a cast is not bivalved properly so that it does not allow adequate room for edema, iatrogenic compartment syndrome can result.

It is important to note that the compartment pressure at which capillary perfusion of the muscle ceases is well below mean arterial pressure. Therefore, full-blown compartment syndrome can occur even in the presence of an excellent palpable distal pulse. Once compartment syndrome develops, the problem must be treated (i.e., fasciotomy) within 2 hours, or permanent damage, including limb loss, is likely to occur [13, 26, 28]. Swelling of a limb inside an improperly bivalved cast over a prolonged flight has necessitated subsequent amputation [18].

During flight, the diagnosis of possible compartment syndrome is made on clinical grounds in patients at high risk. Both increasing limb pain and pain upon passive stretch of the compartment (elicited by extending the fingers or toes) indicate compartment syndrome until proven otherwise. Loss of distal pulses or neurological changes can be late signs.

For patients with diminished capacity to respond to a clinical exam for compartment syndrome (e.g., decreased consciousness due to central nervous system injury), direct measurement of compartment pressure may be necessary. However, only experienced personnel should place in-dwelling monitoring devices. Commercially available compartment measuring devices not much larger than a hypodermic syringe can be utilized, even in the noisiest AE environment. On the ground or in the relatively quiet environment of modern dedicated AE aircraft, compartment pressure can also be measured with a simple in-dwelling catheter hooked to an arterial pressure monitor [29].

The first step in the treatment of evolving compartment syndrome is loosening of a properly bivalved cast. However, continued symptoms will require diversion to the nearest medical facility because definitive treatment, surgical fasciotomy, should be performed within 2 hours [13, 26, 29–31]. When fasciotomy for acute compartment syndrome release is performed prior to AE, negative-pressure wound therapy may be utilized in the management of fasciotomy wounds during subsequent transport [22, 32].

Fat Embolism Syndrome

Another complication unique to orthopedic injuries is fat embolism syndrome. This is most typically seen in long-bone fractures, such as femur fractures, but can be seen in patients with pelvic fractures or multiple fractures of smaller bones. This complication is most common in the 24–72 hours after orthopedic injury or surgery. Probably the highest-risk surgery for this complication is the placement of an intramedullary rod into the femur with reaming [33]. Postmortem examination of patients who die from this syndrome reveals widespread fat emboli in the microvasculature of the lungs, brain, and sometimes other organs [34].

The clinical presentation of fat embolism syndrome is the rapid development of progressive respiratory distress syndrome in a patient at risk.

Severity ranges from a mild hypoxia with a mild tachypnea to a profound respiratory distress requiring intubation and mechanical ventilatory support. Other clinical signs include progressive tachypnea, confusion secondary to hypoxia, and a distinctive petechial rash on the chest and neck, which is pathognomonic when present [3, 11, 13].

In-flight treatment of fat embolism syndrome consists of supplemental oxygen and diversion to a medical facility if symptoms warrant. Intubation and assisted ventilation may be required in severe cases.

Deep Vein Thrombosis and Pulmonary Thromboembolism

Not limited to the first few days following injury, thromboembolism remains one of the relatively more common complications after orthopedic injury [13]. The symptoms, while commonly respiratory in nature, differ from those of fat embolism in two key ways. First, pulmonary thromboembolism usually presents with acute onset, as opposed to the frequently more insidious onset of fat embolism. This can vary from moderate respiratory distress and pleuritic chest pain to cardiac arrest. Second, jugular venous distension may be seen in some cases of pulmonary thromboembolism, but this would be a very uncommon finding in fat embolism syndrome.

In-flight treatment of pulmonary thromboembolism consists of supplemental oxygen and ventilatory support as needed. Depending on the severity of symptoms, diversion may be necessary to a facility that can initiate immediate anticoagulation, thrombectomy, or, rarely, insertion of an inferior vena cava filter if the patient has an absolute contraindication to anticoagulation.

Gas Gangrene

A particular complication of a contaminated or infected extremity injury—especially with delayed or inadequate debridement—is clostridial myonecrosis, commonly known as gas gangrene. Patients with gas gangrene may require urgent AE to a facility with a hyperbaric chamber to assist in the treatment of this condition.

These patients should be administered supplemental oxygen during AE. An AE-specific management action for these patients is altitude restriction to maintain the aircraft at sea-level air pressure because any reduction in oxygen tension will result in a worsening of this condition [9, 18]. This must be weighed against the potential delay in transport to definitive surgical care. Achieving a cabin altitude restriction generally causes the aircraft to fly at a lower speed and to consume more fuel, and landing for a fuel stop can induce a major delay.

Crush Syndrome

One final complication that is seen in orthopedic casualties is "crush syndrome." Casualties who have crushing injuries of an extremity associated with a significant period of limb hypoxia may develop crush syndrome. Casualties who have been pinned for any length of time in a structure or vehicle are at risk for this syndrome, even in the face of a relatively benign-looking limb. The etiology of this syndrome is muscle ischemia resulting in necrosis. The elements of crush syndrome include compartment syndrome symptoms (which may be delayed) and myoglobinuria, sometimes severe enough to result in acute renal failure.

The cornerstone of therapy for patients with crush syndrome is early and vigorous fluid replacement to minimize the risk of acute renal failure [35]. If symptoms of crush syndrome develop during AE, the treatment is limited to supplemental oxygen, aggressive intravenous volume infusion to treat the myoglobinuria, and diversion for emergency surgical treatment of compartment syndrome.

References

1. Demartines N, Scheidigger D, Harder F. Helikopter und Notarzt an der Unfallstelle. Helv Chir Acta. 1991;58:223–7.
2. Oreck SL. Orthopaedics in the combat zone. Mil Med. 1996;161:458–61.
3. De Tullio A. Problemi aeromedici nel polifrat-turato. Minerva Med. 1977;68:4101–8.
4. White MS, Chubb RM, Rossing RG, Murphy JE. Results of early aeromedical evacuation of Vietnam casualties. Aerosp Med. 1971;43:780–4.
5. Charbanne JP, Sourd JC. Les evacuations sanitaires aeriennes. Soins. 1984;432:35–41.

6. Evard E. Le transport aerienne de maladies et blesses. Bruxell Med. 1970;50:339–59.
7. Pats B. Le transport aerien sanitaire collectif des blesses de guerre. Cahiers Anesthesiol. 1991;39:337–44.
8. Pensiton-Feliciano H. Aeromedical transport. Del Med J. 1995;67:340–5.
9. Unsworth IP. Gas gangrene and air evacuation. Med J Austr. 1974;1:240–1.
10. Iblher P, Paarmann H, Stuckert K, Werner A, Klotz FK, Eichler W. Interstitial fluid shifts in simulated long-haul flights monitored by a miniature ultrasound device. Aviat Space Environ Med. 2013;84(5):486–90.
11. Kwiatt ME, Seamon MJ. Fat embolism syndrome. Int J Crit Illn Inj Sci. 2013;3(1):64–8.
12. Howard JT, Kotwal RS, Santos-Lazada AR, Martin MJ, Stockinger ZT. Reexamination of a battlefield trauma golden hour policy. J Trauma Acute Care Surg. 2018;84(1):11–8.
13. Epps CH Jr, editor. Complications in orthopedic surgery. 3rd ed. Philadelphia: J.B. Lippincott; 1994.
14. Andersen CA. Preparing patients for aeromedical transport. J Emerg Nurs. 1987;13:229–31.
15. Bowen TE, Bellamy RF, editors. NATO handbook: emergency war surgery. Washington, DC: US Government Printing Office; 1988.
16. Hansen PJ. Air transport of the man who needs everything. Aviat Space Environ Med. 1980;51:725–8.
17. Johnson A Jr. Treatise on aeromedical evacuation: II. Some surgical considerations. Aviat Space Environ Med. 1977;48:550–4.
18. Parsons CJ, Bobechko WP. Aeromedical transport: its hidden problems. Can Med Assoc J. 1982;126:337–44.
19. Schwartz DS. Articulating tactical traction splint use on pulseless forearm fracture. J Spec Oper Med. 2014;14(1):6–8.
20. Weichenthal L, Spano S, Horan B, Miss J. Improvised traction splints: a wilderness medicine tool or hindrance? Wilderness Environ Med. 2012;23(1):61–4.
21. Rowlands TK, Clasper J. The Thomas splint--a necessary tool in the management of battlefield injuries. J R Army Med Corps. 2003;149(4):291–3.
22. Streubel PN, Stinner DJ, Obremskey WT. Use of negative-pressure wound therapy in orthopaedic trauma. J Am Acad Orthop Surg. 2012;20(9):564–74.
23. Fang R, Dorlac WC, Flaherty SF, Tuman C, Cain SM, Popey TL, et al. Feasibility of negative pressure wound therapy during intercontinental aeromedical evacuation of combat casualties. J Trauma. 2010;69(Suppl 1):S140–5.
24. Pollak AN, Powell ET, Fang R, Cooper EO, Ficke JR, Flaherty SF. Use of negative pressure wound therapy during aeromedical evacuation of patients with combat-related blast injuries. J Surg Orthop Adv. 2010;19(1):44–8.
25. Joshi M, Sharma R. Aero-medical Considerations in Casualty Air Evacuation (CASAEVAC). Med J Armed Forces India. 2010;66(1):63–5.
26. Collinge CA, Attum B, Lebus GF, Tornetta P 3rd, Obremskey W, Ahn J, et al; Orthopaedic Trauma Association's Evidence-based Quality and Value Committee. Acute compartment syndrome: an expert survey of Orthopaedic Trauma Association Members. J Orthop Trauma. 2018;32(5):e181–e184.
27. Hansen PJ. Safe practice for our aeromedical evacuation patients. Mil Med. 1987;152:281–3.
28. Matsen FA III. Compartmental syndromes. New York: Grune & Stratton; 1980.
29. Tian S, Lu Y, Liu J, Zhu Y, Cui Y, Lu J. Comparison of 2 available methods with Bland-Altman analysis for measuring intracompartmental pressure. Am J Emerg Med. 2016;34(9):1765–71.
30. Yamaguchi S, Viegas SF. Causes of upper extremity compartment syndrome. Hand Clin. 1998;14:365–70.
31. Garlin SR, Mubarak SJ, Evans KL, Hargens AR, Akeson WH. Quantification of intracompartmental pressure and volume under plaster casts. J Bone Joint Surg. 1981;63(3):449–53.
32. Yang CC, Chang DS, Webb LX. Vacuum-assisted closure for fasciotomy wounds following compartment syndrome of the leg. J Surg Orthop Adv. 2006;15(1):19–23.
33. Giannoudis PV, Tzioupis C, Pape HC. Fat embolism: the reaming controversy. Injury. 2006 Oct;37 Suppl 4:S50-8. Review. Erratum in: Injury. 2007t;38(10):1224.
34. Miller P, Prahlow JA. Autopsy diagnosis of fat embolism syndrome. Am J Forensic Med Pathol. 2011;32(3):291–9.
35. Gunal AI, Celiker H, Dogukan A, Ozalp G, Kirciman E, Simsekli H, et al. Early and vigorous fluid resuscitation prevents acute renal failure in the crush victims of catastrophic earthquakes. J Am Soc Nephrol. 2004;15(7):1862–7.

12 Aeromedical Evacuation of the Neurosurgical Patient

Daniel J. Donovan, Matthew A. Borgman, Rose M. Leary-Wojcik, and Mick J. Perez-Cruet

Introduction

Patients with head or spine injury or disease are at high risk for life-altering disability and death. To minimize this risk, it is essential that they receive proper initial management and stabilization, appropriate and timely surgical care, and transport to and from facilities where this care is available. Transport becomes an even more important component of this care when patients are ill or injured in far-distant environments without comprehensive medical facilities, such as a combat theater or natural disaster. Initial life-sustaining medical and surgical care in deployed combat hospitals or other local facilities is critical. However, patients with neurologic injuries often cannot receive definitive care in these locations and must undergo long-range aeromedical evacuation (AE) to have the best chance of survival and functional recovery.

During AE, most clinical priorities for patients with neurologic injuries are similar to those of other patients. However, complications from problems with airway, ventilation, and hemodynamic functions often have even greater consequence for these patients. In addition, there are a number of specific clinical issues for patients with brain and spinal cord injuries that are important when caring for them during AE.

US military medical systems have developed a staged treatment and transport of these patients from the location of injury to definitive care at home in the United States, with increasing expertise at each level for the care of patients with traumatic brain injury (TBI) or spinal cord injury [1]. Medical capabilities during AE have become progressively more advanced over the last decade with continued developments in portable ventilation and monitoring systems. Remarkable outcomes have been achieved through the coordinated efforts of battlefield surgeons, flight surgeons, Critical Care Air Transport Team (CCATT) members and medical personnel at the definitive care hospitals at home [2, 3].

D. J. Donovan (✉)
COL, MC, USAR, Department of Surgery, University of Hawaii John A. Burns School of Medicine, Honolulu, HI, USA

M. A. Borgman
LTC, MC, USA, Pediatric Critical Care Services, Brook Army Medical Center Simulation Center, Joint Base San Antonio - Fort Sam Houston, San Antonio, TX, USA

Department of Pediatrics, F. Edward Hebert School of Medicine - Uniformed Services University, Bethesda, MD, USA

R. M. Leary-Wojcik
Col, USAF, MC (ret.), Oral & Maxillofacial Surgery, Good Samaritan Clinic, DeLand, FL, USA

M. J. Perez-Cruet
Department of Neurosurgery, Oakland University William Beaumont School of Medicine, Royal Oak, MI, USA

W. W. Hurd, W. Beninati (eds.), *Aeromedical Evacuation*, https://doi.org/10.1007/978-3-030-15903-0_12

Despite these advances, AE remains a relatively hostile environment for patients with neurologic injuries. Monitoring is more difficult, and intervention options are limited compared to a hospital setting. Available interventions are limited to the fundamental concerns of airway, ventilation, and circulatory support and avoidance of in-flight disasters. Planning and preparation are essential, and constant vigilance is required during transport. To provide the best clinical outcomes for these patients, aeromedical personnel must be thoroughly familiar with these fundamental skills and should also have a working knowledge of neurosurgical treatment and monitoring devices in common use, as well as a conceptual framework for the pathophysiology of the nervous system.

Military AE continues to be the primary source for aeromedical experience and resultant advances that help decrease patient risks during long-distance air transport. The majority of this experience was obtained from AE of seriously injured military members during the ongoing armed conflicts in the Middle East. Additional experience has been derived from AE support for regional conflicts and natural disaster relief. It has become clear that the most important factors to consider in the AE process include the duration and altitude of the flight, the type of airframe, the number and experience of the aeromedical personnel, and availability of medical equipment at both the sending and receiving stations.

The medical care and transportation processes in these diverse military and civilian scenarios are often very different. A US military member injured in a combat zone may endure one or more tactical transports, receive interim medical care at one or two facilities within the theater of conflict, and then undergo two or more long-distance AE flights before arriving at a continental US (CONUS) hospital. They expect to receive the best possible medical care that can be offered anywhere in the world, even during some of the longest AE journeys in history. Peacetime missions may involve shorter AE flights but may have insufficient or uncertain resources available at the receiving facility, especially in developing nations. The risk of AE may thus extend well beyond the actual time in the air, and this should be considered carefully prior to transport.

This chapter will focus primarily on the care for patients with neurologic diseases and injuries during long-distance AE. The care for AE patients begins with preflight assessment and stabilization and continues with in-flight monitoring and complication avoidance. Specific interventions for adverse developments that may occur during AE will also be covered. In addition, this chapter will briefly discuss concerns for short-distance (tactical or intratheater) transport of these patients.

Traumatic Brain Injury

More than 40% of patients undergoing AE during the recent conflicts in Iraq and Afghanistan have had injuries or diseases of the head, neck, face, or spine, and traumatic brain injury (TBI) patients comprise a large number of those cared for by CCATT members [4–6]. During AE, these patients have many clinical issues that are similar to those of other patients, but some issues have even greater consequences for TBI patients.

Common Head Injuries

Skull Fractures

A skull fracture is a break in one or more of the relatively strong bones of the skull that protect the brain, which is relatively common in head injury [7, 8].

Non-displaced skull fractures involve the full thickness of the skull without displacement of the fractured segments. Although the fracture itself will likely heal without clinically significant problems they can be associated with damage to underlying structures, causing such problems as traumatic brain injury or epidural hematomas.

Open skull fractures are those with a disruption of the overlying scalp. If the fracture is non-displaced, there is no additional risk to the brain. Depressed skull fractures are defined as those with the outer table displaced inward at least as far as the inner table (usually about 10 mm) and are often depressed much more than that, which can result in disruption of the dura and even bone fragments impacted into the brain. An open

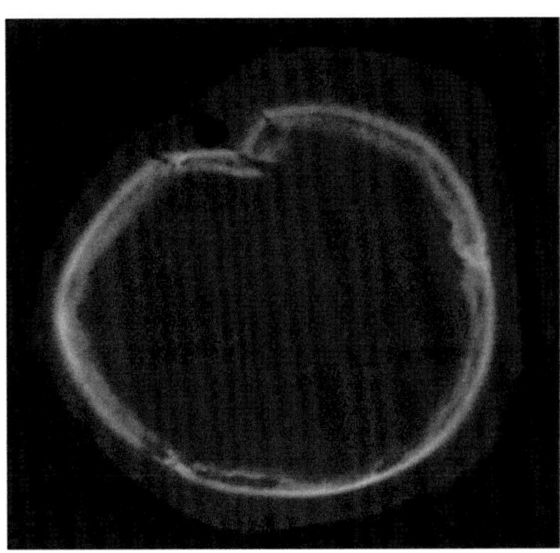

Fig. 12.1 Bone-windowed axial head computed tomography showing depressed skull fracture. Note the outer table of the skull is displaced to a level within the inner table

depressed skull fracture therefore allows direct communication of the brain with the external environment and may also be directly contaminated with bacteria during the trauma. This can result in bacterial brain abscess or meningitis.

Depending on the amount of depression, the location in the skull, the time interval since injury and severity of contamination, surgery is often needed to elevate the bone fragments from the brain, debride the contaminated brain and repair the dura (Fig. 12.1).

Basilar skull fractures occur in the bottom (or base) of the skull. They can result in cerebrospinal fluid (CSF) leakage from the nose if the fracture extends through a paranasal air sinus or from the ear or nose if it extends through the petrous temporal bone near the middle ear or ear canal. These cases can be complicated by pneumocephalus, which may expand at altitude during AE (see pneumocephalus section below). A basilar skull fracture involves a high-risk area around the posterior nasopharynx and is a contraindication to placement of a nasogastric tube.

Intracranial Space-Occupying Mass Lesions

Intracranial space-occupying mass lesions include intracranial hematomas, cerebral contusions with edema, tumors, and abscesses. The most common mass lesions in adults are post-traumatic hematomas [9]. They occupy a portion of the fixed intracranial volume, in turn causing the rise of intracranial pressure (ICP) and displacement of the normal brain against the brainstem, leading to brainstem dysfunction and coma or death. Mass effect can be assessed by imaging techniques as the amount of midline shift of brain structures and/or downward displacement of the brain. Progressive shift results in cerebral herniation.

Surgery is often indicated to remove such a mass, decompress the brainstem, and allow the ICP curve to shift back toward normal. The decision to proceed with surgery depends on the size, volume, and location of the mass, the amount of brain shifting it causes, and the likelihood it will continue to expand.

Epidural Hematoma

An epidural hematoma is located between the inner table of the skull and the dura and is essentially always a post-traumatic injury. It is commonly associated with skull fracture and most commonly results from arterial bleeding from bone fracture or a torn dural blood vessel—most commonly the middle meningeal artery. The hemorrhage must strip the dura away from the skull as it enlarges, and so it is often thicker in the middle or lenticular shaped (Fig. 12.2) but can be any shape. Venous epidural hematomas account for only 10% of all epidural hematomas and are more common in the posterior cranial fossa [10].

Epidural hematomas are usually caused by a relatively low-velocity impact to the head, such as a low-level fall, bicycle accident, or a blow to the head, but any injury resulting in skull fracture can cause one. Clinical presentation is usually a progressive decline in the level of consciousness from the time of injury, and less than half of patients with epidural hematomas have a lucid interval between the injury and the onset of symptoms [10].

Diagnosis

Computed tomography (CT) scanning will reveal that 85–95% of epidural hematomas have an adjacent skull fracture identified, which is far more common than with subdural hematoma. Therefore any clot determined to be located outside the brain and underlying a skull fracture is most likely an epidural hematoma [11].

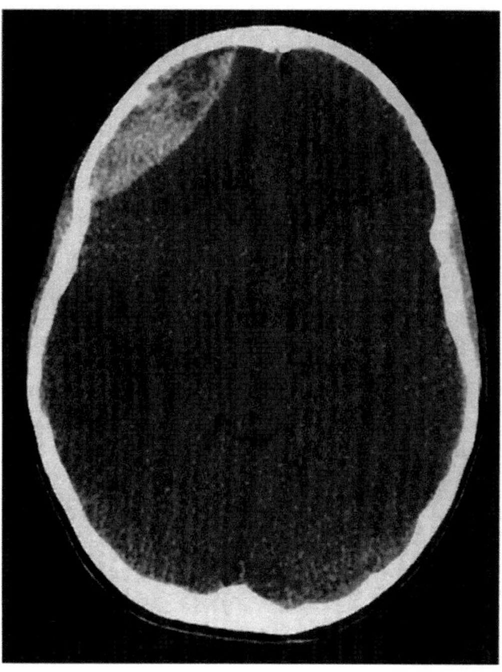

Fig. 12.2 Axial head computed tomography of right frontal acute epidural hematoma

There is usually relatively little energy delivered to the brain itself compared to injuries that result in subdural hemorrhage, so outcome is determined more by timing of evacuation and volume of the expanding blood clot than by the initial brain injury itself.

Treatment and Prognosis

Mortality increases from 1% when the patient is conscious when taken for surgery to 27% if they are in coma, and pre-operative neurological state is the most predictive factor in outcome [10]. The rate of expansion of the blood clot is variable and unpredictable, and there are guidelines to help determine when surgery should be performed, based on size and mass effect of the epidural hematoma [12]. If nonoperative management is chosen, the patient must be carefully observed for any neurologic worsening, as delayed expansion of the clot can occur in about 10% of patients—usually within the first 24 hours [13]. Surgery for acute epidural hematoma requires craniotomy for successful evacuation, and a burr hole alone is usually not effective [12].

Subdural Hematoma

Subdural hematoma results from high-energy impact to the head. It often involves an acceleration-deceleration movement of the head and is usually associated with a much more severe primary injury to the brain than that with epidural hematomas. It often involves laceration of the bridging cortical veins over the surface of the brain, which are anchored to the dural venous sinus on one end and to the more mobile brain surface on the other, resulting in stretching and tearing when the brain moves in relation to the skull and dura.

Patients commonly present with a depressed level of consciousness and focal motor deficits. CT imaging most often shows a crescent-shaped clot over the surface of the brain that is restricted by the dural partitions (Fig. 12.3), but it can occur anywhere, including the posterior cranial fossa [11].

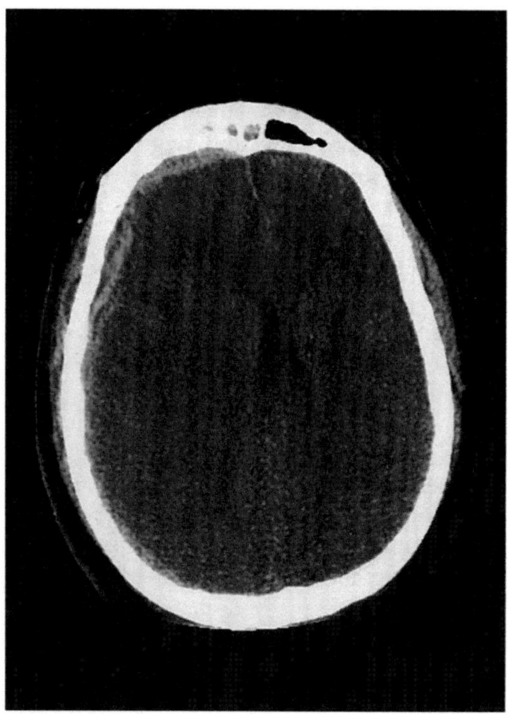

Fig. 12.3 Axial head computed tomography showing right subdural hematoma. Note the shift in ventricles from right to left

Treatment

Surgery is indicated if the hematoma meets criteria based on size and mass effect [12], but the mortality is much higher than with epidural hematoma because the primary problem is the associated brain injury and not as much the clot itself. Timing of surgical evacuation is therefore not as important a prognostic factor as is pre-operative neurologic function [14, 15].

Prognosis

Historically reported mortality has been as high as 30–60% [15, 16]. More recent series have shown much lower mortality of 16–18% but still with as much as 34% severe disability in the survivors [17, 18]. Mortality and morbidity are much higher in patients over 65–75 years old and for those taking anticoagulant medication [19, 20]. The most significant factors affecting outcome for patients with acute subdural hematoma are pre-operative neurologic function/Glasgow Coma Scale (GCS) score, mechanism of injury, age greater than 65 years, and post-operative ICP [14–20].

Cerebral Contusions and Delayed Traumatic Intracerebral Hemorrhage

Brain contusions disrupt the normal microvasculature and often produce surrounding edema. A "coup injury" can occur at the point of impact on the head during a fall or percussive injury, most commonly in areas adjacent to prominences of the bone at the base of the skull. These injuries can produce microhemorrhages that can coalesce over several days into intracerebral hematomas, referred to as delayed traumatic intracerebral hemorrhages. They may be quite large but generally produce less mass effect than either epidural or subdural hematoma. At the same time, a "contrecoup injury" can occur on the contralateral side as the injury energy travels across the brain in a three-dimensional sense and can be larger and have more mass effect than the coup injury. A common scenario is a backward fall resulting in an occipital skull fracture with subsequent development of a massive bilateral frontal lobe delayed traumatic intracerebral hemorrhage.

Treatment and Prognosis

Small contusions can result in a variable amount of white matter injury (i.e., diffuse axonal injury) without hemorrhage or mass effect, and these do not require surgery. Widespread injury, however, can cause severe cognitive and motor disability.

More severe injuries with delayed traumatic intracerebral hemorrhage can sometimes be treated medically with hyperosmolar solutions to limit edema. However, large, multifocal hemorrhages, especially those in the anterior temporal lobe, often require decompressive craniectomy to prevent further brainstem injury. Rapidly developing and massive contusions that involve both hemispheres have a poor prognosis for recovery.

Subarachnoid Hemorrhage

Subarachnoid hemorrhage, bleeding into the subarachnoid space between the arachnoid membrane and the pia mater surrounding the brain, occurs in 30–40% of patients with moderate to severe TBI [22]. It usually occurs over the top of the cerebral hemispheres but can occur in the Sylvian fissure, around the tentorium, and just about anywhere within the skull. It has a relatively low risk of symptomatic vasospasm, as well as hydrocephalus. Non-traumatic subarachnoid hemorrhage is most commonly caused by a ruptured aneurysm, is more often located in the basal subarachnoid cisterns, and has a much higher risk of both vasospasm and hydrocephalus.

Treatment and Prognosis

Subarachnoid hemorrhages tend to occur in more severe TBIs. Fortunately, this type of hemorrhage does not result in a space-occupying hematoma and does not require acute surgical intervention, but the thickness of the hemorrhage may have some correlation with the mortality rate [22]. Hydrocephalus can develop in survivors, requiring a ventricular catheter.

Head Injury Complications

Post-traumatic Seizures

Post-traumatic seizures occur in approximately 10% of patients after TBI [28]. Early seizures—

defined as those ocurring within the first week after injury—have not been shown to affect outcomes overall, but can temporarily exacerbate ICP in critically ill patients. In contrast, status epilepticus severely elevates the cerebral metabolic rate of oxygen, causing neuronal death, leading to worsened brain injury or death.

Seizure prophylaxis with phenytoin or levetiracetam is commonly used in TBI patients for the first 7 days after injury to reduce the incidence of early seizures [29]. Levetiracetam is perhaps more commonly used for this purpose because, in contrast to phenytoin, serum levels do not have to be monitored. This prophylaxis is usually stopped after 7 days because it does not reduce the incidence of late seizures [24].

Decompressive Craniectomy

Decompressive craniectomy refers to the intentional surgical removal of a portion of the skull bone. The removed section is large, at least 12 cm in diameter; the dura is opened widely and left open; and the scalp is closed. The most common indication for this procedure is increased ICP that is refractory to all other forms of therapy, which occurs primarily in patients with TBI and those with large area brain infarction [25].

Unfortunately, decompressive craniectomy has been shown to be of limited value for improving clinical outcomes. Although it reduces ICP and decreases the mortality rate, a greater number of the survivors are severely disabled as a result of the primary brain injury [26].

Aeromedical Evacuation Implications

Decompressive craniectomy does not appear to predispose patients to additional major risks related to AE. Many such patients have been evacuated over long distances after decompressive craniectomy in the recent conflicts overseas, without obvious problems related to it [27].

Cerebral Herniation

The intracranial space is divided into subcompartments by the two major dural partitions: the falx cerebri and the tentorium cerebelli. These relatively fixed structures restrict the free movement of the brain if it is shifted by an intracranial mass lesion. The large volume of the cortical and subcortical structures in the supratentorial compartment cannot expand outward in a patient with an intact skull, so they are forced downward and toward the center. The dural partitions restrict movement even more, and herniation of the brain is concentrated against the brainstem.

Central (i.e., trans-tentorial) herniation is the most common form of cerebral herniation and occurs when the brain is forced downward through the opening between the two sides of the tentorium. An uncal herniation occurs when a mass lesion in the anterior temporal lobe causes the uncus in the medial temporal lobe to move medially, directly against the brainstem. In either type, pressure on the adjacent cerebral peduncle containing the corticospinal pathway and the third cranial nerve (which mediates the pupillary reflex) results in typical clinical presentation.

Clinical signs of cerebral herniation include an ipsilateral third cranial nerve palsy (dilation and loss of reactivity in the pupil, with or without ophthalmoplegia) and contralateral muscular weakness. In about 10–15% of cases, muscular weakness will be ipsilateral to the third nerve palsy [28]. Further herniation leads to a decreasing level of consciousness, flexor posturing, extensor posturing, and progression to brain death. Late findings related to cerebral herniation include hypertension, bradycardia, and breathing abnormalities—referred to as Cushing's triad. Once signs of cerebral herniation are observed, more than three-quarters of patients die and the remainder will have severe permanent disabilities [28].

Pneumocephalus

Pneumocephalus is air within the intracranial compartment. It is most commonly located within the subarachnoid space, displacing CSF. It occurs very commonly following cranial surgery, at least in small amounts, because the skull is open to the air [29]. It can also occur from open skull fractures or fractures through the skull base resulting in a CSF leak through the paranasal air sinuses, which can allow entrainment of air through the same opening. Simple pneumocephalus is intracranial air that is not under pressure, similar to a simple pneumothorax, and almost all pneumocephalus is simple. In contrast, tension pneumocephalus is intracranial air under pressure, which is a very rare event. In such an instance, it probably occurs from a "ball valve" effect, where air is entrained in through the dura, but cannot escape because the dural flap then covers the opening, similar to how a tension pneumothorax may develop from a sucking chest wound. Standard aircraft cabin pressurization is only the equivalent of about 6,000 to 8,000 feet, so the volume of any gas can expand as much as 30% during flight [30, 31], and this theoretical concern has been informed by practical experience involving tension pneumothorax. Unfortunately, the classic CT imaging finding described as being characteristic of tension pneumocephalus (the "Mount Fuji" sign), almost always occurs from intracranial hypotension and brain collapse instead, and so is unreliable in assessing this diagnosis prior to AE.

Aeromedical Evacuation Implications

In the past there has been great theoretical concern for this possible complication of AE [30, 31], but in practice there are only very rare case reports describing tension pneumocephalus occurring during or immediately after air travel, associated with risk factors such as an osseous sinus tumor or barotrauma to the ears [32]. Tension pneumocephalus has not been observed during the high volumes of AE in the recent military conflicts in Iraq and Afghanistan. Donovan et al. have reported the only clinical series to date, with 21 patients who underwent AE with pneumocephalus following craniotomy or head injury during Operation Iraqi Freedom, and none developed tension pneumocephalus [2]. This complication probably occurs so rarely because of compensatory mechanisms that dampen its effect, such as displacement of CSF into the spinal subarachnoid space or scalp in post-surgical patients. It seems likely that only a continuous entrainment of air could overcome these compensatory mechanisms, such as an active CSF leak during flight or external CSF drainage catheter that could allow air in, especially one in the lumbar subarachnoid space. Simple pneumocephalus seen on CT scan is therefore not a contraindication to AE by itself, but CSF catheters must be managed carefully during flight and active CSF leak may be a contraindication. As in tension pneumothorax, the diagnosis is suspected on clinical findings, when all other causes of increased intracranial pressure have been ruled out. It is confirmed by placing a needle through a post-operative burr hole or other opening in the skull (if possible), which results in a rush of escaping air under pressure.

In Flight Treatment

If there is a clinical or monitoring change during AE that suggests increasing ICP, tension pneumocephalus is the least likely culprit, and AE medical crew should re-evaluate the clinical situation in a stepwise manner, focusing on airway, breathing, perfusion, head position, CSF drainage catheter function, medical therapy, etc, before considering tension pneumocephalus as the cause. As in tension pneumothorax, the diagnosis is suspected on clinical findings, when all other causes of increased intracranial pressure have been ruled out. It is confirmed by placing a needle through a burr hole or other opening in the skull (if possible) [33], which results in a rush of escaping air under pressure. This is not recommended for AE crew inexperienced with this maneuver, and the only other solution is to reduce altitude if possible.

Monitoring for Traumatic Brain Injury Patients

Blood Pressure Monitoring

In healthy patients, cerebral autoregulation provides reflex protection against marked changes in cerebral blood flow that could otherwise result from normal physiologic changes in blood pressure (BP). In some TBI patients, autoregulation is impaired and cerebral vascular resistance is decreased. As a result, increasing blood pressure will result in increases in cerebral blood volume and ICP, and decreasing blood pressure will result in the opposite.

Unfortunately, increasing cerebral blood volume (and thus oxygen delivery) to the brain as a whole may not result in additional oxygen in the injured areas where it is needed most [34]. This is especially true if there is post-traumatic vasospasm of the cerebral vasculature, a phenomenon thought to be somewhat rare, except in TBI related to blast injury [35].

In TBI patients where ICP is not being monitored, blood pressure is the only variable that can be used to estimate the adequacy of cerebral blood flow. For these patients, it is recommended that systolic blood pressure be maintained ≥110 mmHg for patients 15–50 years old and > 100 mmHg for patients over 50 years old [36]. If vasopressor support is required, continuous monitoring with an arterial line pressure monitor is standard.

Blood pressure is routinely expressed as mean arterial pressure (MAP). Although MAP can be calculated from peripheral blood pressure readings, it is routinely electronically calculated by monitoring equipment. For critical patients, an indwelling arterial line is commonly used to continuously monitor MAP. Ideally, in TBI patients, both MAP and ICP are continuously monitored and used to estimate cerebral perfusion pressure (CPP) as discussed below.

Intracranial Pressure Monitoring

Control of elevated ICP decreases mortality in the early phase of brain injury [37] It has thus become common practice to monitor ICP continuously, but its effect on patient outcomes remains controversial [38] ICP monitoring is most often used for patients with Glasgow Coma Scale (GCS) between 3 and 8, because increases in ICP may not be observed clinically in these patients. Treatment with osmotic or other medical therapy is recommended [36].

ICP monitoring devices fall into two main categories depending on the location of the catheter tip: intraparenchymal catheters (IPCs) and intraventricular catheters (IVCs). Both are inserted at the bedside under local anesthesia.

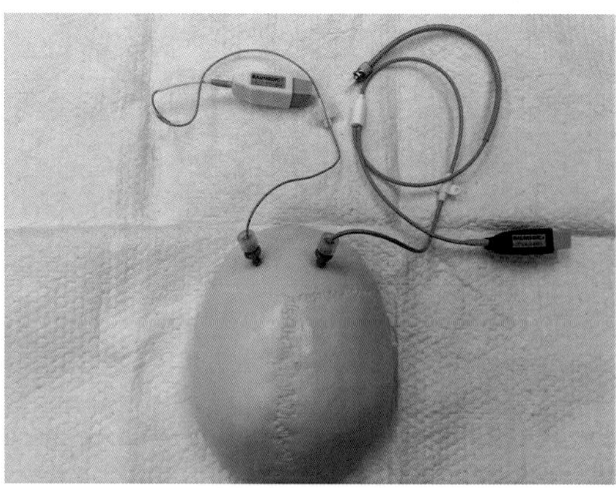

Fig. 12.4 Intraparenchymal ICP monitors (left ICP only, right dual catheter ICP and brain tissue oxygen monitor) inserted through a skull bolt

Intraparenchymal Catheter

An IPC is placed by drilling a small hole through the skull, through which a small fiber-optic wire lead with a pressure transducer at the tip is inserted approximately 1 cm into the brain (Fig. 12.4). The catheter is secured with a locking mechanism at the insertion site and attached to a monitor that displays a continuous wave form and a mean pressure reading. Patients can undergo CT scans with this device in place, but should not undergo magnetic resonance imaging (MRI), since the magnetic field may induce an electric current in the lead. An IPC device is simpler to use than an IVC and has a low complication risk of 3% [39]. However, it cannot be used for CSF removal.

Intraventricular Catheters

An IVC is inserted by drilling a slightly larger hole through the skull through which the catheter is advanced through the parenchyma into a ventricle, usually a distance of at least 5 or 6 cm and the catheter sutured to the scalp. The main advantage of IVC compared to IPC is that in addition to monitoring ICP, therapeutic removal of CSF is possible [40]. The disadvantage is a complication risk as high as 14%, including hemorrhage, infection, malposition, and clogging [39, 40].

The IVC system can be best understood by remembering the simple concept that water runs downhill; that is, the CSF in the brain will flow through the system from higher hydrostatic pres-

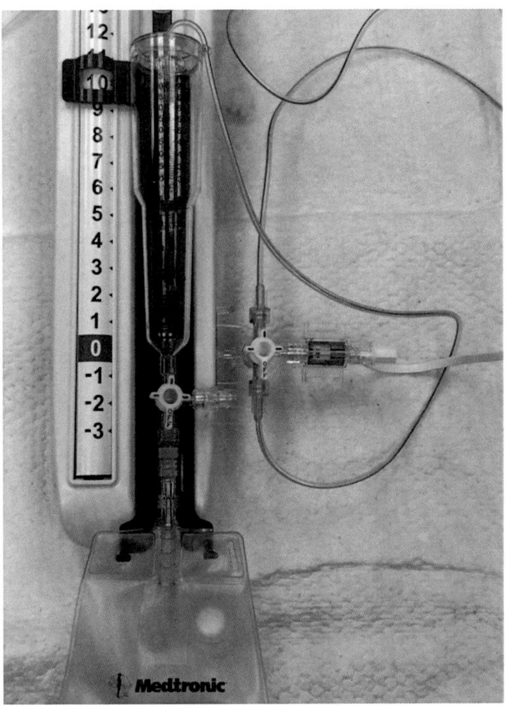

Fig. 12.5 IVC drainage collection system. The pressure transducer is set at the zero level and the "popoff" is set at 10 mm Hg. The stopcock is set to "off" for both drainage and pressure monitoring

sure to lower pressure in the collection bag. The CSF within the head is at approximately the pressure of the ICP (normally 5–15 mmHg), which does not usually change rapidly. The amount of flow is determined by the height of the collection system relative to the center of the head: When the system is lowered relative to the head, the hydrostatic pressure gradient between the two becomes greater, and CSF flow increases. When the collection system is higher than the patient's head, flow is reduced.

For IVC systems, the external drainage collection bag is marked with a 0 reference point, which should be positioned at the level of the external auditory meatus (Fig. 12.5). It is critical to maintain the zero reference point of the external CSF collection system at the level of the patient's auditory canal throughout AE flight (Fig. 12.6). Positioning the collection system too low can result in catastrophic CSF over-drainage, collapse of the brain, stretching and tearing of bridging cortical veins, and subdural hematoma formation.

The IVC is connected to the monitor and collecting system via a stopcock. If continuous CSF drainage is desired, the stopcock is often left opened to the collection system and closed to the

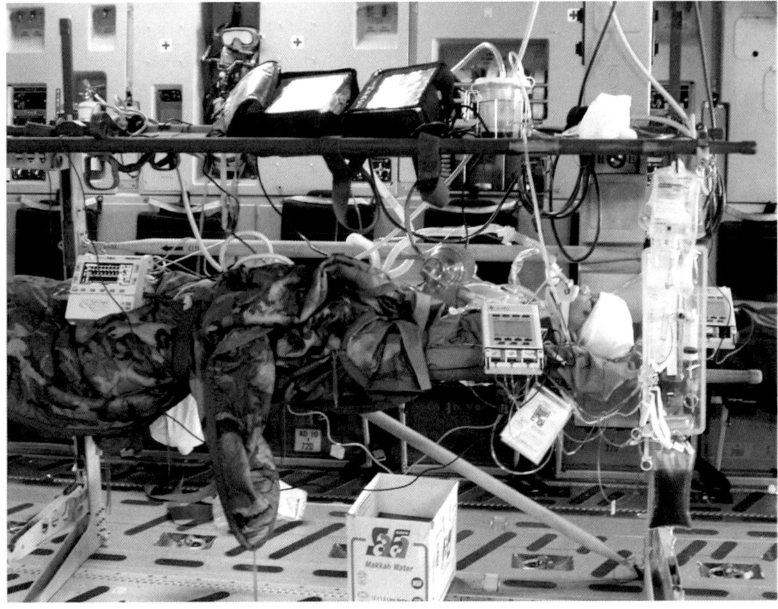

Fig. 12.6 IVC drainage collection system (to the right of the patient's head) used during AE transport from Kuwait to Germany of a patient with brain injury. Note the reference level is set to the height of the patient's ear, and is open to drainage

transducer. Continuous monitoring of ICP requires that the stopcock be open to the transducer and closed to the collection system (the most accurate configuration) or open to both the transducer and the collecting system. In this latter configuration, the stopcock should be periodically closed to the collecting system to allow the most accurate readings [40]. However, forgetting to reopen the stopcock to allow CSF drainage after a pressure check is perhaps the most common cause of increased ICP in these patients.

Implications for Aeromedical Evacuation

Great diligence is required to avoid displacing an ICP catheter and collection system during patient movement since catheter displacement of more than a few millimeters can greatly affect pressure accuracy. IPC catheters are most commonly secured with a gentle locking device and can be easily dislodged during transport. IVC catheters are usually sutured to the scalp but are still susceptible to displacement or inadvertent removal during transport. Reinsertion during transport is difficult even for trained personnel and is not advised for those who are not experienced with this procedure.

The AE crew should keep in mind that ICP monitors are prone to malfunction, particularly in the austere AE environment. In addition, some neurologic conditions, such as a temporal lobe mass lesion, can result in uncal herniation and brainstem compression without appreciably elevated ICP. For these reasons, it is important to remember that treatment should be initiated in response to significant neurologic change, e.g., a new focal deficit such as a new asymmetry of the pupils or new hemiparesis, even in the absence of ICP change.

Troubleshooting of Intracranial Pressure Monitors

ICP monitor malfunction can manifest as either loss of the normal ICP waveform display or inappropriate (or quickly changing) ICP measurements. IVC catheters that also serve as CSF drainage devices can also experience cessation of CSF flow, as discussed below.

Loss of the normal triphasic ICP waveform is often the first indication that the system is no longer functioning properly. The first things to check are monitor display settings. The scale and range of observed ICP can be changed by the user. If either appears too great or too small, the ICP pressure wave will not be visible. The monitor display should be appropriately set prior to transport, but AE personnel should be familiarized with the ICP system in use.

Table 12.1 Stepwise troubleshooting of an intraventricular catheter (IVC) system

1. Check the stopcock to assure the system is open to the monitor, open to drainage, or both, as appropriate
2. Verify that the drainage collection bag reference point is at the height of the external auditory meatus
3. Check the catheter for proper placement and kinking or suture occlusion
4. Flush the distal catheter between the stopcock and the monitor and/or storage bag with preservative-free saline
5. If the system appears to be intact and small ventricles have been documented by computed tomography (CT), wait for 15 minutes for spontaneous return of cerebrospinal fluid (CSF) flow
6. Gently flush the proximal catheter between the stopcock and the ventricle with no more than 2 cc of preservative - free saline. Caution: This risky procedure should only be done by a physician or by physician order. Avoid excessive force
7. If cerebrospinal fluid flow through an IVC catheter cannot be restored, the intracranial pressure monitor is unlikely to be accurate and should not be used to determine the need for therapeutic interventions

Occasionally, the normal ICP waveform suddenly will be altered or disappear, or the serial ICP readings will suddenly be dramatically different. In these cases, the system should be checked for fiber-optic cable dislodgement or fracture or disconnection of some other system component. When the ICP system is not functioning properly, extreme caution should be used when considering clinical intervention based on the ICP readings alone.

Sudden cessation of CSF flow has multiple possible causes, including a closed stopcock, catheter displacement, catheter blockage by choroid plexus in the brain, and ventricle collapse. Collapse of ventricle walls as a result of CSF over-drainage or drainage from compressed ventricles may occlude flow through the very small catheter opening. This can result in cessation of

CSF flow and a false elevation of the recorded ICP, until CSF builds up and the fluid column is re-established through the catheter. A previous finding of small ventricles on CT is an important clue to this possibility.

When an IVC system is not functioning normally, troubleshooting should proceed in a stepwise fashion (Table 12.1). The first steps are to verify that the IVC stopcock is in the proper position and the drainage collection bag reference point is at the level of the external auditory meatus. Sometimes the ICP is simply not high enough to generate flow of CSF through the catheter. In this situation, patency can be confirmed by briefly lowering the collection bag as much as 12 inches below the patient's head. If CSF flow returns, the system is patent and the ICP is simply not high enough to drain CSF. Make sure to return the collection bag to its appropriate height.

The next step is to carefully examine IVC external to the scalp for proper placement. Verify that the catheter has not been dislodged from the patient's head. Make sure that there are no visible catheter kinks and the scalp suture is not so tight that it is occluding the catheter.

If no other cause is found for IVC malfunction, an obstruction within the IVC by blood or debris is likely. The distal catheter between the stopcock and the monitor and/or storage bag can be safely flushed with preservative-free saline injected through the stopcock port. If the system appears to be intact and this point and small ventricles have been documented by CT, it is reasonable to wait for 15 minutes to see if spontaneous CFS flow returns.

The final, relatively risky step is to flush the proximal catheter between the stopcock and the ventricle. This procedure should only be done by a physician or under physician orders. This is done by gently flushing the catheter toward the brain with no more than 2 mL of preservative-free saline. If resistance is met, the attempt should be terminated, since excessive force is unlikely to be successful and may be dangerous.

If CSF flow through the catheter cannot be restored, the ICP monitor is unlikely to be accurate. In this situation, ICP measurements should not be used to determine the need for therapeutic interventions.

Cerebral Perfusion Pressure

Cerebral blood flow is a critical factor in recovery from brain injury, but it cannot be measured directly in a clinical setting. Marked increases in cerebral blood flow can raise ICP, which can independently worsen brain injury, and decreases in perfusion may render inadequate oxygen delivery to the injured brain, causing ischemic changes and worsened cellular damage [41, 42].

Clinically, cerebral perfusion pressure (CPP) is used as a reasonable estimate of cerebral blood flow. CPP is the pressure gradient that drives cerebral blood flow necessary for oxygen and metabolite delivery to the brain. CPP is calculated as the difference in the cerebral vascular system between the arterial side (MAP) and the venous side, which is approximated by ICP:

$$\mathrm{CPP} = \mathrm{MAP} - \mathrm{ICP}$$

For adult patients with TBI, the recommended range to maintain CPP is 60–70 mmHg [36]. For children 6 to 17 years old, CPP above 50 mm Hg is recommended, and above 40 mm Hg in children 5 years old or younger [40]. Aggressive attempts to elevate CPP >70 mmHg should be avoided because this has been associated with an increased risk of acute respiratory distress syndrome (ARDS) [43].

New Monitoring Techniques

Brain Tissue Oxygen Monitoring

Brain tissue oxygen (PbO_2) monitoring is another method in addition to CPP that is used to estimate the adequacy of cerebral blood flow in the injured patient's brain, to detect alterations in the normal coupling of cerebral blood flow and cerebral metabolic rate of oxygen caused by the injury. This technique has been found to be useful in intensive care settings for patients with TBI, even when CPP and ICP are maintained within thresholds [44]. Its use during AE has not yet been reported.

Automated Pupillometry

Automated pupillometry is portable and reliable and has become an indispensable tool in many neurocritical care units, although its use during AE has not yet been reported. It reduces subjectivity in assessing this critical reflex and can provide an ultra-early noninvasive warning about increasing ICP and even impending brain herniation [45].

Aeromedical Evacuation Considerations for Traumatic Brain Injury Patients

Prognosis for survival and good functional outcome after TBI involves many factors that cannot be changed after presentation, such as mechanism and severity of injury and patient age [46]. However, the quality of subsequent medical care plays an extremely important role in preventing or limiting the amount of secondary injury to the brain—primarily by preventing increased intracranial pressure and assuring adequate brain tissue oxygenation and perfusion. Post-injury care can make the difference for the individual patient between death or severe disability and a successful, productive life. The complexity of this care mandates a systematized approach to preflight evaluation and continued monitoring and treatment during AE.

Timing

In the past, long-distance AE of patients with TBI was routinely delayed for a matter of weeks. During World War II, the conflicts in Korea and Vietnam, the regional conflicts of the 1980s or 1990s, and even during the Persian Gulf War, the rationale was to allow time for the intracranial pressure to return to normal and the resolution of any pneumocephalus. The concern was that decreased cabin pressure during AE would increase ICP, decrease cerebral perfusion, and result in expansion of pneumocephalus, all of which could potentially result in brain compression. These concerns were based on theoretical models, since there was virtually no clinical experience on which to support them [32, 47].

Since the beginning of the wars in Iraq and Afghanistan, stable and stabilized TBI patients have been routinely transported via long-distance AE to medical facilities equipped and staffed to care for such patients. Dramatic improvements in AE equipment, routine availability of CCAT teams, and advances in aircraft technology have allowed the safe AE of these patients relatively soon after their injuries from the theaters of conflict to higher levels of care thousands of miles away.

After almost two decades of experience, it has become well established that patients with TBI can undergo AE relatively soon after their injury with reasonable safety with proper attention to risk factors for neurologic deterioration during flight. The handful of published experiences and anecdotal AE experiences involving hundreds of neurosurgical patients suggest that significant in-flight complications, such as exacerbation of increased ICP or episodes of hypoxia and hypotension, are rare with appropriate precautions [2, 48, 49].

Preflight Assessment for Traumatic Brain Injury patients

The patient's diagnosis, ongoing treatments, and documentation should be reviewed with the team handing off the patient. Specific information should be obtained regarding monitoring devices and CSF drains and other important details such as size and depth of endotracheal or tracheostomy tubes, ventilator setting, oxygen requirements, baseline blood pressures, and previous response to fluids or medications.

The preflight physical examination should include a careful neurologic examination, including level of consciousness; notation and severity of focal motor weakness or sensory abnormalities; baseline alterations in pupil size, symmetry, and reaction; and assessment of the level of consciousness.

Glasgow Coma Scale

The Glasgow Coma Scale score is a useful tool to assess the level of consciousness and has become the standard for monitoring it over the course of treatment, especially in the acute period (Table 12.2) [50]. The post-resuscitation GCS can be used to stratify TBI patients into three categories: mild (GCS 14 and 15), moderate (GCS 9–13), and severe (GCS 3–8). Confounding factors that can influence the GCS include pupillary dysfunction, hypoxia or hypotension, and the presence of multiple traumatic injuries. A significant decline in the level of consciousness, defined as a decrease in the GCS of ≥2 points, should prompt immediate reassessment to identify and

Table 12.2 Glasgow Coma Scale (GCS) [50]

	1	2	3	4	5	6
Eye	Does not open eyes	Opens eyes in response to *painful stimuli*	Opens eyes in response to voice	Opens eyes spontaneously	N/A	N/A
Verbal	Makes no sounds	Incomprehensible sounds	Utters incoherent words	Confused, disoriented	Oriented, converses normally	N/A
Motor	Makes no movements	Extension to painful stimuli (*decerebrate response*)	Abnormal flexion to painful stimuli (*decorticate response*)	Flexion/withdrawal to painful stimuli	Localizes to painful stimuli	Obeys commands

potentially treat the source of the neurologic decline prior to AE [51].

The GCS score is calculated by adding the score from three standard subcategories: eye opening (E), motor response (M), and verbal response (V) (Table 12.2). If there is a difference in motor response between the left and right sides, the higher of the two scores is used. The maximum score is 15 and the minimum is 3. The score is best described by documenting all three of the subcategories, as well as the total score (e.g., GCS = E3V1M5 = 9 T). The eye scale is the most straightforward for most examiners. The verbal and motor scales are more prone to disagreement between examiners.

The most common difficulty when assigning the GCS verbal score is determining the difference between "disoriented" (4 points) and "confused" (3 points). As a general statement, a disoriented patient will appropriately respond to most questions, but will not be certain of their location, the date, or, possibly, even their identity. In contrast, a confused patient will have a generalized inability to participate in a conversation or answer questions appropriately. Language barriers must be accounted for, particularly when a translator is unavailable. When documenting the verbal score in an intubated patient, a "T" or "I" is often used next to the score of V1 to indicate this, since they cannot speak.

The GCS motor score is most often the greatest source of disagreement among examiners but also an important predictor of prognosis. Accuracy in determining the motor score depends in part on the experience of the examiner and the type of stimulation used for patients with lower scores. Verbal commands are tried first.

Complex movements are the most reliable indicator of following commands, such as holding up two fingers or moving the toes. Hand grasp is often not as reliable, since it is reflexive in many cases. Even patients who are intubated or paralyzed from spinal cord injuries can potentially follow commands, such as blinking their eyes when directed or protruding their tongue. If there is no response to a verbal request, a noxious stimulus (e.g., sternal rub) is applied centrally, and depending on the response, a peripheral stimulus may need to be applied. If weak elbow flexion is observed at first, the examiner may not know if it represents localization to pain (M5) or just flexion (M3). Stimulation in a different area, such as the lower torso or leg, may allow distinction between the two, since the patient will need to extend the elbow to reach downward.

Positioning During Takeoff and Landing

The proper way to position TBI patients with increased ICP during takeoff and landing of AE aircraft has long been debated: head versus feet forward. When the patient is in a supine position, acceleration during takeoff and deceleration during landing can increase gravitational forces (G) being transmitted to the brain. However, such changes are only slightly greater than 1.0 G in the direction away from acceleration or toward deceleration. Because the brain is somewhat mobile in the cranio-caudal direction, the top of the brain could be compressed against the skull. The clinical significance of these changes is difficult to study.

To date, there is no evidence of significantly prolonged exacerbations of ICP with takeoff or landing in either position and no obvious clinical difference in outcomes [2]. Civilian aeromedical services most often position the patient with the head forward and the feet aft [52] but are not subject to tactical takeoffs that sometimes involve steep ascent. Some flight surgeons even change patient positioning during flight, but there is no compelling evidence currently to mandate one position or the other.

Elevating the head of the bed so that the patient's head is above the heart is the most important aspect of preventing exacerbations of ICP, since it promotes venous drainage and is known to decrease ICP. Special back supports are available to raise the patient's head while lying on a litter or gurney. When patients are immobilized for spine fractures, the litter can be secured in a modest degree on reverse Trendelenburg position if there is a concomitant TBI [53].

Oxygen Therapy

The risk of hypoxia is increased during AE because increasing altitude results in decreased ambient pressure and partial pressure of oxygen in the atmosphere [54]. This risk is lessened, but not eliminated, by pressurization since aircraft cabin pressure is maintained equivalent to an altitude of <8000 feet above sea level [54].

Although mild hypoxia can be tolerated by healthy travelers, it can have severe consequences for TBI patients. This is because of the unique control mechanism of blood flow to the brain related to blood vessel diameter and capillary and regional differences in oxygen delivery, uptake, and use of injured brain tissue [55]. When TBI patients are properly screened and treated, the incidence of hypoxic insults during AE are very unlikely [47].

It is recommended that all TBI patients undergoing AE receive supplemental inspired oxygen at a minimum [48]. The goal for TBI patients is to maintain peripheral oxygen saturation at ≥90% and ideally >95%. Arterial PaO_2 should be kept at ≥60 mmHg and ideally >90 mmHg [56]. If the preflight assessment reveals difficulty maintaining these parameters, the patient is at increased risk of secondary brain injury during flight due to hypoxia. Restricting the cabin altitude can also decrease the incidence of hypoxia-related complications and is being used more often as a prevention strategy when feasible.

In patients who are breathing spontaneously and not intubated, oxygen levels can be continuously monitored using standard transcutaneous pulse oximetry. However, documentation of adequate peripheral oxygen saturation does not guarantee adequate oxygen delivery to injured brain tissue, and alterations in peripheral oxygenation can occur as a relatively late finding with respiratory compromise. For this reason, advanced systems for monitoring of oxygen delivery to the brain have been developed for TBI patients during AE and are described in more detail in the section on monitoring.

Intravenous Fluids and Osmotic Therapy

Intravenous fluid therapy is needed for most patients with moderate or severe TBI. The ideal fluid state for these patients is slightly hyperosmolar and euvolemic. Dehydration should be assiduously avoided, to preserve adequate circulation and prevent hypotension. Intravenous fluids containing glucose or dextrose should be used with caution since hyperglycemia can exacerbate secondary brain injury and hypotonic solutions exacerbate brain edema [57].

Osmotic therapy for TBI patients has been used for many years to remove fluid from the injured, edematous brain. Both mannitol and hypertonic saline have been used, and there is little evidence to recommend a preference for one over the other [58]. Either can be given as a bolus for patients with elevated ICP or with obvious clinical signs of brain herniation [36].

When central venous access is available, either mannitol (0.25–1.0 g/kg) or hypertonic saline (10–20 cc) can be given as a bolus. If only a peripheral intravenous line is available, mannitol can be given slowly through a large bore catheter. A Foley catheter is essential for these patients, as they will immediately begin diuresis. Neither should be given at large enough doses to result in hypotension secondary to intravascular depletion. Neither should be given by continuous infusion for long periods of time, and they should not be used to drive serum sodium levels up to extreme levels [59].

Intubation and Ventilation Management

Endotracheal intubation and ventilation support should be considered for TBI patients with a GCS score ≤ 8 [60]. However, a secure airway and/or ventilation assistance might be required in some patients with GCS >8 based on other factors such as compromised respiratory capacity. For example, a patient with a cervical spinal cord injury may require ventilation support because of weakness of the thoracic cage musculature or the diaphragm despite a GCS score of 15. Severe facial trauma or smoke inhalation may compromise the airway and require intubation or tracheostomy.

Delivering the correct amount of ventilation to TBI patients is essential, both to avoid increasing intracranial pressure and to prevent hypoxic injury. The cerebral vasculature is unique for several reasons, with properties that directly affect the risk of secondary brain injury. The vessels undergo reflex changes in size in reaction to changes in blood flow, a phenomenon known as autoregulation (described below), but also in relation to tissue oxygen and carbon dioxide levels.

Arterial carbon dioxide level ($PaCO_2$) is the most important factor affecting the size of the cerebral arterioles, with a directly and linearly proportional relationship. With decreased ventilation, the cerebral vessels dilate as $PaCO_2$ rises, resulting in increased cerebral blood flow, which in turn increases the ICP. Increased ICP may further exacerbate brain injury, so hyperventilation was used in the past to lower cerebral blood flow and ICP in TBI patients [61]. However, hyperventilation is no longer used for these patients because the effect is short lived and the reduction in cerebral blood flow results in lower oxygen delivery to the injured brain [62, 63].

In TBI patients who are intubated and mechanically ventilated, end-tidal CO_2 should be monitored closely, to ensure it is within the normal range. The goal for ventilation is to keep the $PaCO_2$ at normal levels: 35–45 mmHg. Correlation of ventilation with the clinical neurologic exam and monitoring feedback (ICP and/or brain tissue oxygen) may help to ensure the proper amount.

Special care should be taken if on-demand ventilator settings are used (e.g., pressure support or assist/control) since any decrease in respiratory drive sedation is not automatically compensated for and hypoventilation can occur over the course of a long flight. Mandatory ventilation settings will prevent this, but close monitoring is needed to avoid the adverse effects of overventilation.

Blood Pressure Management

Cerebral perfusion pressure in patients with TBI is likely to decrease whenever MAP decreases or ICP increases. This is in contrast to healthy individuals, whose normal cerebral blood flow is maintained by cerebral autoregulation over the range of normal blood pressures. In TBI patients, even short periods of systemic hypotension can have a significant impact on cerebral blood flow.

The most important principle to keep in mind for blood pressure management in TBI patients is to avoid hypotension. Systemic hypotension lasting more than a few minutes in most TBI patients is associated with worsened neurologic outcomes, and if both hypotension and hypoxia are present, the risk of poor neurologic outcome and death is very high [64].

For TBI patients, it is recommended that systolic blood pressure be >110 mmHg for patients 15–50 years old and > 100 mmHg for ages 50–69 years old [36]. It is recommended that MAP be maintained at >90 mmHg. In an effort to avoid hypotension in TBI patients, AE crews should assure continuous intravenous fluid administration and avoid overtreatment with intravenous pain or sedative medications.

Sedation and Neuromuscular Blockade

Sedation is often used for TBI patients to minimize discomfort and agitation associated with an endotracheal tube or the cognitive effects of the brain injury, for control of seizures, and for control of increased ICP [65]. Although many drugs have been used for this purpose, perhaps the three most common drugs used today are propofol, midazolam, and ketamine.

Propofol is a commonly used drug for this purpose because it has the advantage of being rapidly metabolized so that periodic neurologic exams can be performed within minutes of interrupting the infusion. At doses less than 4 mg/kg/hour, propofol preserves cerebrovascular reactivity, brain oxygenation, and coupling of cerebral blood flow and the cerebral metabolic rate of oxygen. At doses above 5 mg/kg/hour, it can induce electroencephalography (EEG) burst suppression to reduce the cerebral metabolic rate of oxygen and cerebral blood flow and is an effective treatment of status epilepticus.

Propofol infusion syndrome is a rare complication of this therapy, particularly at infusion rates >4 mg/hour for >48 hours of duration. It is characterized by acute refractory bradycardia (which can lead to asystole) associated with one or more of the following: metabolic acidosis (base deficit >10 mmol/L), rhabdomyolysis, hyperlipidemia, or fatty liver.

Midazolam, a benzodiazepine, is also commonly used at a maintenance dose of 0.01–0.2 mg/kg/hour. Its disadvantages include accumulation of metabolites, increasing tolerance with prolonged infusions, and an increased chance of delirium. It is not as quickly reversible as propofol for neurologic examinations.

Ketamine has also been used for TBI patients. It provides excellent sedation, does not inhibit respiratory drive so it can be used in non-intubated patients, and has some analgesic effect as well—potentially lowering the need for narcotic pain medications [65]. It has had the reputation for many years of causing increases in ICP, but this has clearly been demonstrated to be false, and it may even reduce ICP in some cases [66]. It is usually given as an infusion at a rate of 1–5 mg/kg/hour.

Neuromuscular Blockade

Neuromuscular blockade is used for patients during endotracheal intubation and also for patients on ventilators who demonstrate coughing, shivering, or dyssynchronous breathing, since these issues can impair venous return and exacerbate ICP elevation.

Clinical neurologic examination, other than pupillary reflex, can no longer be used in the presence of neuromuscular blockage as an early sign of cerebral herniation. For this reason, it is rarely used for TBI patients who do not have an ICP monitor in place, or for any patients at high risk of herniation such as those with a known intracranial mass.

Spinal Cord Injuries

Spinal injuries are relatively common in armed conflict and represented more than 8% of total injury admissions among US army soldiers deployed to Iraq and Afghanistan [67]. These spinal injuries are almost always traumatic, although non-traumatic (primarily infectious) injuries can also occur. In combat, spinal cord injuries are most commonly blast injuries, which are more severe and more likely to involve multiple levels of the spine than noncombat injuries [68].

The primary injury is related to displacement or fracture of spinal vertebrae. Secondary spinal cord injury occurs primarily as a result of ischemia or edema. Injuries are classified as cervical C1–C8, thoracic T1–T12, lumbar L1–L5, or sacral S1–S5 based on the lowest level of full sensation and function. The essential responsibility of the AE team is to prevent or minimize secondary damage or non-neurologic complications during transport.

Spinal cord injuries are further classified as complete or incomplete. Patients with complete spinal cord injury have a poor chance of regaining ambulation or other significant function. Those with incomplete spinal cord injury have some preservation of function below the level of the injury and have a greater chance of neurologic recovery. The severity of symptoms in survivors can range from very mild paresthesia and muscle weakness to paraplegia and quadriplegia, depending on the level of the injury. Complete injuries are life-altering conditions and place the patient at higher risk of significant complications and mortality.

Prehospital Patient Movement

The care of patients with suspected spinal cord injuries starts at the scene of the injury with immobilization and examination. Using standard prehospital trauma treatment protocols, the cervical spine is protected from movement throughout the primary survey, including during intubation if needed, prior to performing a detailed neurologic exam [69, 70].

A cervical collar is applied if there is any possibility of a cervical spine fracture, and the entire

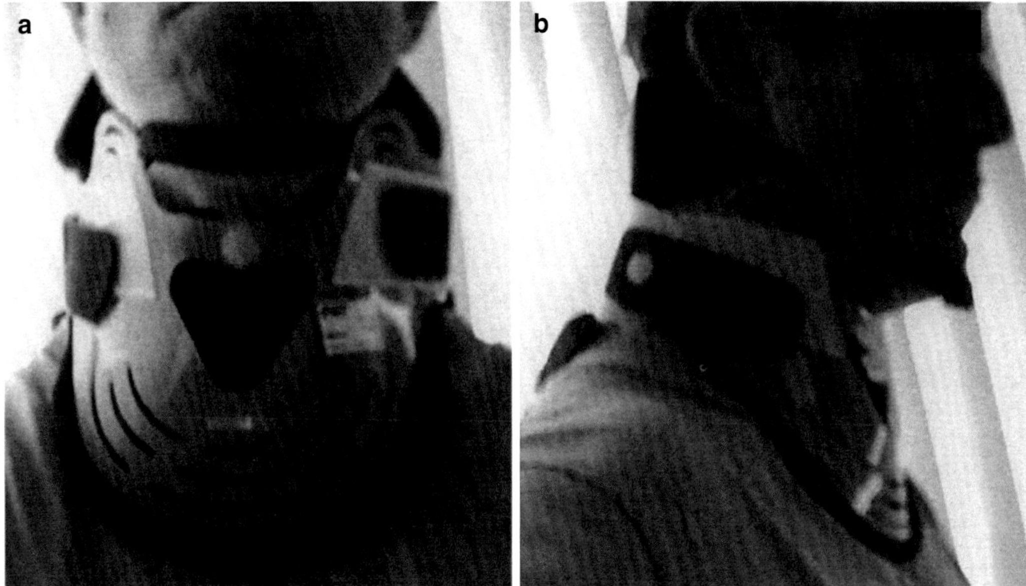

Fig. 12.7 Correct placement of cervical collar: anteroposterior (**a**) and lateral (**b**) views

head, neck, and shoulders are immobilized. Even when applied correctly, cervical collars allow a surprising amount of motion, but as long as the patient is supine, they are reasonably well protected from further spinal cord damage (Fig. 12.7). If there is head injury and the patient is confused or agitated, additional support with straps, tape, or other devices may be needed, and sedation also may be required.

If the patient has an obvious deformity of the spine and complains of worsened pain with attempted placement of a collar, they should not be forced into a more neutral position in order to apply it, since they may be protecting their spinal cord in that position and worsened compression could occur with forced movement.

Special attention should be directed toward assuring adequate ventilation, since patients with spinal cord injury are at risk for decreased ventilation. Airway compromise in these patients often requires urgent intubation, which can be difficult in patients immobilized to avoid movement of the spine.

If injury to the thoracic or lumbar spine is possible, the patient's entire spine is immobilized on a long transport board. The patient is logrolled in a standard fashion, with one person immobilizing the head, neck, and shoulders and another rolling them as one unit, while a third person applies the board under them. Patients should be carefully transferred to a soft mattress as soon as possible after reaching a medical facility, since transport boards pose a high risk of causing decubitus ulcers.

Spinal Cord Injury Treatment

Spinal Surgery

After careful examination and imaging, spinal surgery is sometimes required to decompress the spinal cord, remove bone or disk fragments or foreign objects, and stabilize the spine. Internal or external fixation devices are often used to prevent spinal cord damage during fracture healing. Following surgery, a brace is used to support the spine until the damaged area is again stable.

Medical Therapy

Medical therapy consists primarily of supportive care, including ventilatory assistance if needed and blood pressure support. Immobilized patients are given prophylaxis for deep venous thrombosis and decubitus ulcers. Steroids, which were

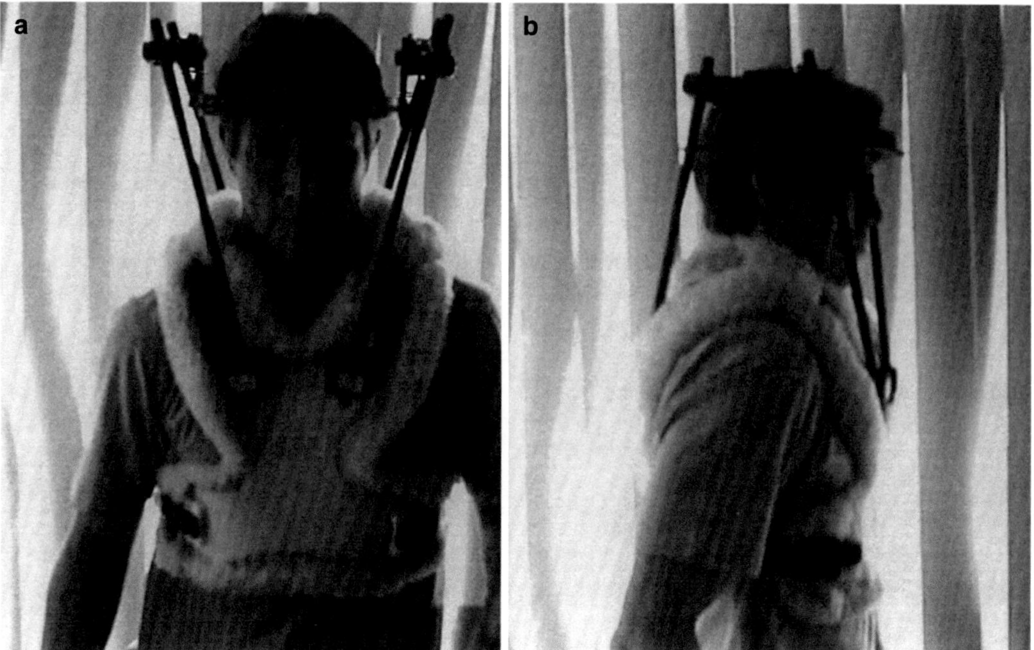

Fig. 12.8 Correct placement of halo vest: anteroposterior (**a**) and lateral (**b**) views

used for decades to treat patients with spinal cord injuries, are no longer recommended [71].

Systolic pressure should be corrected to >90 mmHg as soon as possible and then maintenance of MAP between 85 and 90 mmHg for the first 7 days after injury. Hypotension is treated with norepinephrine, which is preferred to dopamine especially in patients over 55 years old; there is some risk of cardiogenic complications with both [72]. Vasopressor use is not recommended for penetrating spinal cord injury [73].

Craniocervical Traction

Patients with fracture-subluxation injuries of the cervical spine often benefit from rapid reduction of the deformity to remove pressure from the spinal cord and restore vascular circulation. This is accomplished by the neurosurgeon with craniocervical traction, using either a halo device (Fig. 12.8) with a traction bail or by applying Gardner-Wells skull tongs (Fig. 12.9). This procedure can be performed rapidly by a trained and experienced surgeon under local anesthesia if a traction setup is available, or else field expedient systems can be devised when it is not, using a simple rope and any weighted objects.

Radiographic visualization is mandatory after placement of a traction device to determine if the deformity has been reduced and to avoid overtraction, which can result in spinal cord injury. Post-reduction neurologic exam must be performed. If there is neurologic deterioration, traction should be removed and the patient reassessed. Worsened neurologic dysfunction can be the result of over-distraction, hypotension, or when traction is applied when there is an immobile compressive lesion present, such as a traumatic disk herniation or epidural hematoma. After reduction is performed, a cervical collar or halo vest is applied.

Thoracolumbar-Sacral Orthosis Brace

Thoracolumbar fractures most commonly occur at the thoracolumbar junction. This is the transition point where the relatively immobile thoracic spine with its kyphotic curve meets the more mobile lumbar spine with its lordotic curve. Fractures at this location are immobilized with a thoracolumbar-sacral orthosis

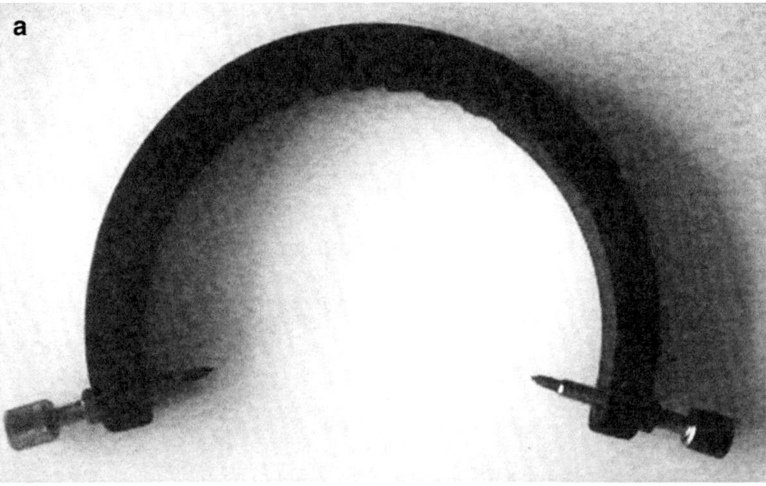

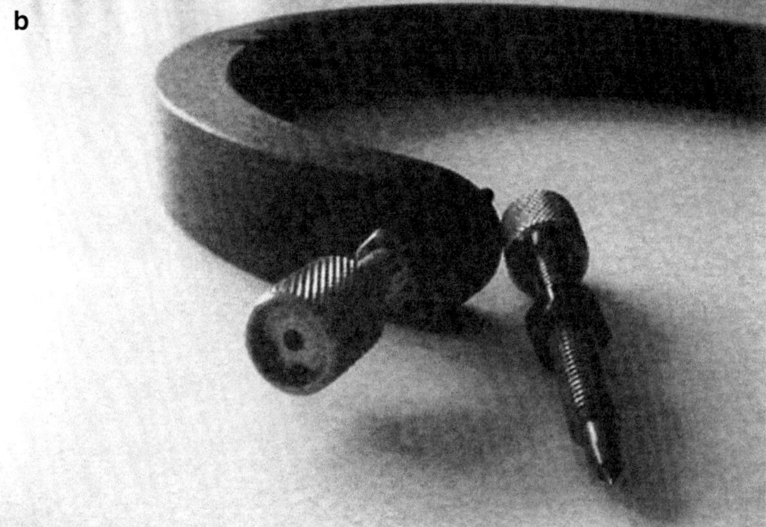

Fig. 12.9 Gardner-Wells skull tongs (**a**), with a close-up view of the pins that are inserted into the scalp (**b**)

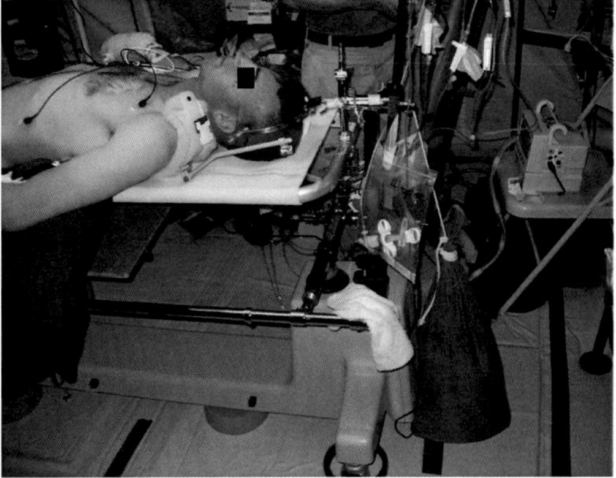

Fig. 12.10 Craniocervical traction setup for a patient with cervical spine fracture-dislocation and spinal cord injury in a combat support hospital, using Gardner-Wells traction tongs and a sand bag for field expedient weight

brace that extends from the upper torso to the pelvis.

Aeromedical Evacuation Considerations for Spinal Cord Injury Patients

Spinal fractures can pose risk for compression and injury during later transport, even if there was no spinal cord or nerve root injury at the time of the initial trauma. The presence of an unstable spinal fracture should be determined by a neurosurgeon or spinal surgeon since imaging reports alone are not sufficient to make this determination.

Traction and Braces

Prior to AE, unstable spinal fractures should be stabilized surgically or using external orthosis or traction devices. The AE crew should be made aware of any unstable or potentially unstable fractures prior to the flight.

Some spinal cord injury patients will need to be transported while still in craniocervical traction. If so, the gurney and traction assembly must be securely fastened to avoid movement during takeoff and landing or with turbulence. Even so, these patients require side-to-side repositioning at least every 2 hours to avoid decubitus ulcers.

Patients transferred in thoracolumbar-sacral orthosis braces are generally at low risk of subsequent spinal cord damage. It should be determined prior to AE whether or not the treating surgeon approves removal of the brace for comfort during transport while the patient remains supine. In all cases, the brace should be re-applied before the patient is moved.

Blood Pressure Support

Patients with spinal cord injuries may develop hypotension from dysfunction of the sympathetic system pathways. Acutely, systolic blood pressure should be maintained at ≥90 mmHg [74].

Current clinical guidelines for these patients recommend using vasopressors to elevate the MAP in an effort to increase spinal cord perfusion. Although a number of vasopressors are commonly used for this purpose, norepinephrine might be the best at restoring blood flow and oxygenation. MAP should be maintained between 85 and 90 mmHg for the first 7 days.

Decubitus Ulcer Prevention

The prevention of decubitus ulcers is an important consideration for spinal cord injury patients who cannot feel the discomfort of prolonged pressure on their body from lying supine. A decubitus ulcer can form in as little as 2 hours if prolonged pressure prevents adequate blood flow to the skin and subcutaneous tissues, resulting in ischemia and necrosis.

To prevent decubitus ulcers, all pressure points should be carefully padded, especially overlying bony prominences. Patients should be gently turned from one side to the other every 2 hours, using rolled blankets or other soft supportive materials to keep them on their side. Periodic patient rolling is essential for any transport longer than about an hour, including on the bus or ambulance to and from the airfield, even for patients in traction and braces.

Other Prophylactic Measures

Patients with spinal cord injuries require a number of prophylactic treatment regimens, which should be established prior to AE. All of these patients should be given histamine H2 receptor blockers for gastric ulcer prophylaxis, and pneumatic compression hose or thrombo-embolic deterrent (TED) hose stockings for deep vein thrombosis (DVT) prophylaxis. A nasogastric tube should be placed to prevent expansion of gastric and intestinal air during flight, since paralytic ileus is common in these patients. A bladder catheter should be placed for spinal cord injury patients who are not neurologically intact or unable to use a urinal or bedpan while supine. Finally, these patients will require adequate blankets, since they are at increased risk of thermal instability secondary to sympathetic dysfunction and vasodilation.

Stroke Patients

The term stroke refers to brain tissue death secondary to hypoxia resulting from sudden loss of blood flow to that area of the brain. An ischemic stroke occurs when a clot obstructs a brain blood vessel. A hemorrhagic stroke is the result of a ruptured brain blood vessel or aneurysm and is often the result of hypertension. A related condition is a subarachnoid hemorrhage related to a ruptured aneurysm.

Blood Pressure Monitoring

For patients with non-traumatic intracranial conditions, such as stroke or hypertensive intracerebral hemorrhage, blood pressure monitoring is standard. Neither ICP nor CPP monitoring is routinely recommended for these patients.

For acute stroke patients, moderate blood pressure reduction is recommended [75, 76]. Patients with BP >220/120 mmHg should have their BP decreased to approximately 190/105. If the patient is a candidate for thrombolytic therapy, BP should be lowered to <180/105 mmHg. Pre-stroke antihypertensive therapy is often restarted, and no specific antihypertensive medications have been shown to be advantageous.

For patients with subarachnoid hemorrhage from a ruptured aneurysm, blood pressure goals depend on whether or not the aneurysm has been secured. If the aneurysm has not been secured, systolic BP <160 mmHg is a reasonable goal [77].

After an aneurysm has been secured by either microsurgical clipping or endovascular obliteration, vasospasm is the primary concern. For vasospasm prophylaxis, most of these patients are treated with nimodipine for 2–3 weeks after the hemorrhage. Prior to AE, specific BP goals for these patients should be delineated by the neurosurgeon or other treating physician. The target BP to prevent or treat vasospasm is often moderately higher than the BP target for those with unsecured aneurysms.

References

1. Reno J. Military aeromedical evacuation, with special emphasis on craniospinal trauma. Neurosurg Focus. 2010;28(5):E12.
2. Donovan DJ, Iskandar JI, Dunn CJ, King JA. Aeromedical evacuation of patients with pneumocephalus: outcomes in 21 cases. Aviat Space Environ Med. 2008;79(1):30–5.
3. Hoffman C, Falzone E, Dagain A, Cirodde A, Leclerc T, Lenoir B. Successful management of a severe combat penetrating brain injury. J R Army Med Corps. 2014;160(3):251–4.
4. Butler WP, Steinkraus LW, Fouts BL, Serres JL. A retrospective cohort analysis of battle injury versus disease, non-battle injury – two validating flight surgeons' experience. Mil Med. 2017;182:155–61.
5. Goodman MD, Makley AT, Lentsch AB, Barnes SL, Dorlac GR, Dorlac WC, Johannigman JA, Pritts TA. Traumatic brain injury and aeromedical evacuation: when is the brain fit to fly? J Surg Res. 2010;164(2):286–93.
6. Fang R, Dorlac GR, Allan PF, Dorlac WC. Intercontinental aeromedical evacuation of patients with traumatic brain injuries during Operations Iraqi Freedom and Enduring Freedom. Neurosurg Focus. 2010;28(5):E11.
7. White IK, Pestereva E, Shaikh KA, Fulkerson DH. Transfer of children with isolated linear skull fractures: is it worth the cost? J Neurosurg Pediatr. 2016;17:602–6.
8. Bonfield CM, Naran S, Adetayo OA, Pollack IF, Losee JE. Pediatric skull fractures: the need for surgical intervention, characteristics, complications and outcomes. J Neurosurg Pediatr. 2014;14:205–11.
9. Sumas M, Narayan RK. Head trauma. In: Grossman RG, Loftus CM, editors. Principles of neurosurgery. 2nd ed. Philadelphia: Lippincott Raven; 1999. p. 117–72.
10. Rivas JJ, Lobato RD, Sarabia R, Cordobes F, Cabrera A, Gomez P. Extradural hematoma: analysis of factors influencing the courses of 161 patients. Neurosurgery. 1988;23:44–51.
11. Osborn AG, Blaser SI, Salzman KL, Katzman GL, Provenzale J, Castillo M, Hedlund GL, Illner A, Harnsberger HR, Cooper JA, Jones BV, Hamilton BE, editors. Diagnostic imaging: brain. Salt Lake City: Amirsys; 2007.
12. Bullock MR, Chesnut R, Ghajar J, Gordon D, Hartl R, Newell DW, Servadei F, Walters BC, Wilberger JE. Guidelines for the surgical management of traumatic brain injury. Neurosurgery. 2006;58(3):S2-1–3.
13. Piepmeier JM, Wagner FC. Delayed post-traumatic extracerebral hematoma. J Trauma. 1982;22:455–60.
14. Wilberger JE, Harris M, Diamond DL. Acute subdural hematoma: morbidity, mortality and operative timing. J Neurosurg. 1991;74:212–8.
15. Dent DL, Croce MA, Menke PG, Young BH, Hinson MS, Kudsk KA. Prognostic factors after acute subdural hematoma. J Trauma. 1995;39:36–43.
16. Zumkeller M, Behrmann R, Heissler HE, Dietz H. Computed tomographic criteria and survival rate for patients with acute subdural hematoma. Neurosurgery. 1996;39:708–13.
17. Lee JJ, Segar DJ, Morrison JF, Mangham WM, Lee S, Asaad WF. Subdural hematoma as a major determinant of short-term outcomes in traumatic brain injury. J Neurosurg. 2018;128:236–49.
18. Lukasiewicz AM, Grant RA, Basques BA, Webb ML, Samuel AM, Grauer JN. Patient factors associated with 30-day morbidity, mortality and length of stay after surgery for subdural hematoma: a study of the American College of Surgeons National Surgical Quality Improvement Program. J Neurosurg. 2016;124:760–6.
19. Taussky P, Hidalgo ET, Landolt H, Fandino J. Age and salvageability: analysis of outcome of patients older than 65 years undergoing craniotomy for acute traumatic subdural hematoma. World Neurosurg. 2012;78:306–11.
20. Raj R, Mikkonen ED, Kivisaari R, Skrifvars MB, Korja M, Siironen J. Mortality in elderly patients operated for an acute subdural hematoma: a surgical case series. World Neurosurg. 2016;88:592–7.
21. Wong GK, Yeung JHH, Graham CA, Zhu X, Rainer TH, Poon WS. Neurological outcome in patients with traumatic brain injury and its relationship with com-

puted tomography patterns of traumatic subarachnoid hemorrhage. J Neurosurg. 2011;114:1510–5.
22. Pagni CA, Zenga F. Posttraumatic epilepsy with special emphasis on prophylaxis and prevention. Acta Neurochir Suppl. 2005;93:27–34.
23. Khan NR, VanLandingham MA, Fierst TM, Hymel C, Hoes K, Evans LT, Mayer R, Barker F, Klimo P Jr. Should levetiracetam or phenytoin be used for post-traumatic seizure prophylaxis? A systematic review of the literature and meta-analysis. Neurosurgery. 2016;79:775–82.
24. Temkin NR, Dikmen SS, Wilensky AJ, Keihm J, Chabal S, Winn HR. A randomized, double-blind study of phenytoin for the prevention of post-traumatic seizures. NEJM. 1990;323(8):497–502.
25. Hutchinson PJ, Kolias AG, Timofeev IS, Corteen EA, Czosnyka M, Timothy J, Anderson I, Bulters DO, Belli A, Eynon CA, Wadley J, Mendelow AD, Mitchell PM, Wilson MH, Critchley G, Sahuquillo J, Unterberg A, Servadei F, Teasdale GM, Pickard JD, Menon DK, Murray GD, Kirkpatrick PJ, RESCUEicp Trial Collaborators. Trial of decompressive craniectomy for traumatic intracranial hypertension. N Engl J Med. 2016;375(12):1119–30.
26. Cooper DJ, Rosenfeld JV, Murray L, Arabi YM, Davies AR, D'Urso P, Kossmann T, Ponsford J, Seppelt I, Reilly P, Wolfe R, DECRA Trial Investigators, Australian and New Zealand Intensive Care Society Clinical Trials Group. Decompressive craniectomy in diffuse traumatic brain injury. NEJM. 2011;21(364):1493–502.
27. Roberts SA, Toman E, Belli A, Midwinter MJ. Decompressive craniectomy and cranioplasty: experience and outcomes in deployed UK military personnel. Br J Neurosurg. 2016;30(5):529–35.
28. Andrews BT, Pitts LH. Functional recovery after traumatic transtentorial herniation. Neurosurgery. 1991;29:227–31.
29. Reasoner DK, Todd MM, Scamman FL, Warner DS. The incidence of pneumocephalus after supratentorial craniotomy. Observations on the disappearance of intracranial air. Anesthesiology. 1994;80:1008–12.
30. Brandstrom H, Sundelin A, Hoseaseon D, Sundstrom N, Birgander R, Johansson G, Winso O, Koskinen LO, Haney M. Risk for intracranial pressure increase related to enclosed air in post-craniotomy patients during air ambulance transport: a retrospective cohort study with simulation. Scand J Trauma Resusc Emerg Med. 2017;25(1):50.
31. Andersson N, Grip H, Lindvall P, Lars-Owe DK, Brandstorm H, Malm J, Eklund A. Air transport of patients with intracranial air: computer model of pressure effects. Aviat Space Environ Med. 2003;74(2):138–44.
32. Huh J. Barotrauma-induced pneumocephalus experienced by a high risk patient after commercial air travel. J Korean Neurosurg Soc. 2013;54(2):142–4.
33. Donovan DJ, Moquin RR, Ecklund JM. Cranial burr holes and emergency craniotomy: review of indications and technique. Mil Med. 2006;171(1):12–9.
34. Stiefel MF, Udoetuk JD, Spiotta AM, Gracias VH, Goldberg A, Maloney-Wilensky E, Bloom S, Le Roux PD. Conventional neurocritical care and cerebral oxygenation after traumatic brain injury. J Neurosurg. 2006;105:568–75.
35. Duckworth JL, Grimes J, Ling GSF. Pathophysiology of battlefield associated traumatic brain injury. Pathophysiology. 2013;20(1):23–30.
36. Carney N, Totten AM, O'Reilly CO, Ullman JS, Hawryluk GWJ, Bell MJ, Bratton SL, Chesnut R, Harris OA, Kissoon N, Rubiano AM, Shutter L, Tasker RC, Vavilala MS, Wilberger J, Wright DM, Ghajar J. Guidelines for the management of severe traumatic brain injury, 4th ed. Neurosurgery. 2017; 80(1):6–15.
37. Talving P, Karamanos E, Teixeira PG, Skiada D, Lam L, Belzberg H, Inaba K, Demetriades D. Intracranial pressure monitoring in severe head injury: compliance with Brain Trauma Foundation guidelines and effect on outcomes: a prospective study. J Neurosurg. 2013;119(5):1248–54.
38. Chaswt RM, Temkin N, Caracy N, Dikmen S, Rondina C, Videtha W, Petrani G, Lujan S, Pridgeon J, Barber J, Machamer J, Chaddock K, Celix JM, Churner M, Hendrix T. A trial of intracranial-pressure monitoring in traumatic brain injury. NEJM. 2012;367(26):2471–81.
39. Liu H, Wang W, Cheng F, Yuan Q, Yang J, Hu J, Ren G. External ventricular drains versus intraparenchymal intracranial pressure monitors in traumatic brain injury: a prospective observational study. World Neurosurg. 2015;83(5):794–800.
40. Nwachuku EL, Puccio AM, Fetzick A. Intermittent versus continuous cerebrospinal fluid drainage management in adult severe traumatic brain injury: assessment of intracranial pressure burden. Neurocrit Care. 2013;20(1):49–53.
41. Juul N, Morris GF, Marshall SB, Marshall LF. Intracranial hypertension and cerebral perfusion pressure: influence on neurological deterioration and outcome in severe head injury. J Neurosurg. 2000;92(1):1–6.
42. Allen BB, Chiu YL, Gerber LM, Ghajar J, Greenfield JP. Age-specific cerebral perfusion pressure thresholds and survival in children and adolescents with severe traumatic brain injury. Pediatr Crit Care Med. 2014;15(1):62–70.
43. Contant CF, Valadka AB, Gopinath SP, Hannay HJ, Robertson CS. Adult respiratory distress syndrome: a complication of induced hypertension after severe head injury. J Neurosurg. 2001;95(4):560–8.
44. Narotam PK, Morrison JF, Nathoo N. Brain tissue oxygen monitoring in traumatic brain injury and major trauma: outcome analysis of a brain tissue oxygen-directed therapy. J Neurosurg. 2009;111:672–82.

45. Jahns F-P, Miroz JP, Messerer M, Daniel RT, Taccone FS, Eckert P, Oddo M. Quantitative pupillometry for the monitoring of intracranial hypertension in patients with severe traumatic brain injury. Critical Care. 2019;23:155.
46. Jagannathan J, Okonkwo DO, Yeoh HK, Dumont AS, Saulle D, Haizlip J, Barth JT, Jane JA Sr, Jane JA Jr. Long term outcomes and prognostic factors in pediatric patients with severe traumatic brain injury and elevated intracranial pressure. J Neurosurg Pediatr. 2008;2:240–9.
47. Macmillan AJF. The effects of pressure change on body cavities containing gas. In: Ernsting J, Nicholson AN, Rainford DJ, editors. Aviation medicine. 3rd ed. Oxford: Reed Educational and Professional Publishing Ltd; 1999. p. 13–9.
48. Dukes SF, Bridges E, Johantgen M. Occurrence of secondary insults of traumatic brain injury in patients transported by critical care air transport teams from Iraq/Afghanistan: 2003-2006. Mil Med. 2013;178(1):11–7.
49. Butler WP, Steinkraus LW, Burlingame EE, Fouts BL, Serres JL. Complication rates in latitude restricted patients following aeromedical evacuation. Mil Med. 2016;87(4):352–9.
50. Teasdale G, Jennett B. Assessment of coma and impaired consciousness: a practical scale. Lancet. 1974;2:81–4.
51. American College of Surgeons Committee on Trauma. Advanced trauma life support. 10th ed. Chicago American College of Surgeons; 2018.
52. U.S. Air Ambulance website. http://www.usairambulance.net/effects-of-altitude.php. Accessed 3 Aug 2018.
53. Hart KR. The passenger and the patient in flight. In: DeHart RL, editor. Fundamentals of aerospace medicine. 2nd ed. Baltimore: Williams & Wilkins; 1996. p. 667–83.
54. Macmillan AJF. The pressure cabin. In: Ernsting J, Nicholson AN, Rainford DJ, editors. Aviation medicine. 3rd ed. Oxford: Reed Educational and Professional Publishing Ltd; 1999. p. 112–27.
55. McHugh GS, Engel DC, Butcher I, Steyerberg EW, Lu J, Mushkudiani N, Hernández AV, Marmarou A, Maas AIR, Murray GD. Prognostic value of secondary insults in traumatic brain injury: results from the IMPACT study. J Neurotrauma. 2007;24(2):287–93.
56. American College of Surgeons, Committee on Trauma. Trauma quality improvement program: best practices in the management of traumatic brain injury. Chicago: American College of Surgeons; 2015.
57. DeSalles AAF, Muizelarr JP, Youn HF. Hyperglycemia, cerebrospinal fluid lactic acidosis, and cerebral blood flow in severely head-injured patients. Neurosurgery. 1987;21:45–50.
58. Mortazavi MM, Romeo AK, Deep A, Griessenauer CJ, Shoja MM, Tubbs RS, Fisher W. Hypertonic saline for treating raised intracranial pressure: a literature review with meta-analysis. J Neurosurg. 2012;116:210–21.
59. Hawryluk GWJ. Editorial: sodium values and the use of hyperosmolar therapy following traumatic brain injury. Neurosurg Focus. 2017;43(5):E3(1–3).
60. McKhann GM, Copass MK, Winn HR. Prehospital care of the head-injured patient. In: Narayan RK, Wilberger JE, Povlishock JT, editors. Neurotrauma. New York: McGraw-Hill; 1999. p. 103–17.
61. Bouma GJ, Muizelaar JP. Cerebral blood flow in severe clinical head injury. New Horiz. 1995;3(3):384–94.
62. Muizelaar JP, Marmarou A, Ward JD, Kontos HA, Choi SC, Becker DP, Gruemer H, Young HF. Adverse effects of prolonged hyperventilation in patients with severe head injury: a randomized clinical trial. J Neurosurg. 1991;75:731–9.
63. Liu S, Wan X, Wang S, Zhu M, Zhang S, Liu X, Xiao Q, Gan C, Li C, Shu K, Lei T. Posttraumatic cerebral infarction in severe traumatic brain injury: characteristics, risk factors and potential mechanisms. Acta Neurochir. 2015;157(10):1697–704.
64. Robertson CS, Contant CF, Gokaslan ZL, Narayan RK, Grossman RG. Cerebral blood flow, arteriovenous oxygen difference, and outcome in head-injured patients. J Neurol Neurosurg Psychiatry. 1992;55:594.
65. Oddo M, Crippa IA, Mehta S, Menon D, Payen J-F, Taccone FS, Citerio G. Optimizing sedation in patients with acute brain injury. Crit Care. 2016;20:128.
66. Zeiler FA, Teitelbaum J, West M, Gillman LM. The ketamine effect on ICP in traumatic brain injury. Neurocrit Care. 2014;21(1):163–73.
67. Wojcik BE, Curley KC, Szeszel-Fedorowicz W, Stein CR, Humphrey RJ. Spinal injury hospitalizations among U.S. Army soldiers deployed to Iraq and Afghanistan. Mil Med. 2015;180(2):216–23.
68. Szuflita NS, Neal CJ, Rosner MK, Frankowski RF, Grossman RG. Spine injuries sustained by U.S. military personnel in combat are different from non-combat spine injuries. Mil Med. 2016;181(10):1314–23.
69. Brain Trauma Foundation. Guidelines for prehospital management of traumatic brain injury. 2nd ed. New Rochelle: Mary Ann Liebert. New York; 2007.
70. Brain Trauma Foundation. Guidelines for the field management of combat-related head trauma. New Rochelle: Mary Ann Liebert. New York; 2005.
71. Hurlbert RJ, Hadley MN, Walters BC, Aarabi B, Dhall SS, Gelb DE, Rozzelle CJ, Ryken TC, Theodore N. Guidelines for the management of acute cervical spine and spinal cord injuries, chapter 8: Pharmacological therapy for acute spinal cord injury. Neurosurgery. 2013;72:93–105.
72. Readdy WJ, Whetstone WD, Ferguson AR, Talbott JF, Inoue T, Saigal R, Bresnahan JC, Beattie MS, Pan JZ, Manley GT, Dhall SS. Complications and outcomes of vasopressor usage in acute traumatic central cord syndrome. J Neurosurg Spine. 2015;23:574–80.

73. Readdy WJ, Saigal R, Whetstone WD, Mefford AN, Ferguson AR, Talbott JF, Inoue T, Bresnahan JC, Beattie MS, Pan J, Manley GT, Dhall SS. Failure of mean arterial pressure goals to improve outcomes following penetrating spinal cord injury. Neurosurgery. 2016;79(5):708–14.
74. Saadeh YS, Smith BW, Joseph JR, Jaffer SY, Buckingham MJ, Oppenlander ME, Szerlip NJ, Park P. The impact of blood pressure management after spinal cord injury: a systematic review of the literature. Neurosurg Focus. 2017;43(5):E20.
75. Ryken TC, Hurlbert RJ, Hadley MN, Aarabi B, Dhall SS, Gelb DE, Rozzelle CJ, Theodore N, Walters BC. Guidelines for the management of acute cervical spine and spinal cord injuries, chapter 7: The acute cardiopulmonary management of patients with cervical spinal cord injuries. Neurosurgery. 2013;72:84–92.
76. Powers WJ, Rabinstein AA, Ackerson T, Adeoye OM, Bambakidis NC, Becker K, Biller J, Brown M, Demaerschalk BM, Hoh B, Jauch EC, Kidwell CS, Leslie-Mazwi TM, Ovbiagele B, Scott PA, Sheth KN, Southerland AM, Summers DV, Tirschwell DL. On behalf of the American Heart Association Stroke Council. 2018 guidelines for the early management of patients with acute ischemic stroke: a guideline for healthcare professionals from the American Heart Association/American Stroke Association. Stroke. 2018;49:E1–E244.
77. Connolly ES Jr, Rabinstein AA, Carhuapoma JR, Derdeyn CP, Dion J, Higashida RT, Hoh BL, Kirkness CJ, Naidech AM, Ogilvy CS, Patel AB, Thompson GB, Vespa P. Association for healthcare professionals from the American Heart Association/American Stroke Guidelines for the management of aneurysmal subarachnoid hemorrhage: a guideline. Stroke. 2012;43(6):1711–37.

13 Otorhinolaryngology Head and Neck Surgery Patients

Skyler W. Nielsen, David G. Schall, Joseph A. Brennan, and John R. Bennett

Introduction

In the field of otorhinolaryngology, head and neck surgery is strongly interwoven with the fields of flight medicine and aeromedical evacuation (AE). Successful flying requires the proper function of the middle ear spaces and sinuses. An intact and functioning audiovestibular system is also highly desirable for passengers in aircraft and is required for those controlling aircraft. Otorhinolaryngology has had a long and close relationship with aviation.

The environment of flight posed many physiological challenges that were recognized during the earliest human flights. The first ear block was described by J. A. C. Charles in 1783 when he experienced sharp ear pain upon descent in a balloon [1]. A decade later, Benjamin Rush noted problems with epistaxis in a French balloonist. The first physician assigned as a "flight surgeon" to the US Army Signal Corps (1917) was an otorhinolaryngologist from Philadelphia by the name of Robert J. Hunter [2]. This close relationship has continued to this day.

The transport of postoperative, wounded, or ill patients by aeromedical evacuation introduces another level of complexity in the physical response to flight. The anatomy and physiology of the head and neck is complex. When this anatomy is disrupted, the potential for troublesome or even disastrous complications is significant. An understanding of normal anatomy and function, and how this has been altered in the AE patient, is the key to safe and successful transport of these patients.

This chapter will begin with a discussion of specific otorhinolaryngologic problems of flight. Next, it will address the aeromedical evacuation concerns regarding the movement of patients who have relevant otorhinolaryngologic diseases, have sustained trauma to the head and neck, or have undergone recent otorhinolaryngologic surgery.

S. W. Nielsen
Capt, USAF USARMY MEDCOM BAMC, Department of Otolaryngology, San Antonio Military Medical Center, Fort Sam Houston, TX, USA

D. G. Schall
Col, USAF, MC, CFS (ret.), Formerly Otolaryngology Head & Neck Surgery Consultant to the USAF Surgeon General, Regional Flight Surgery/Aerospace Neurology, Office of Aerospace Medicine, Federal Aviation Administration, Des Plaines, IL, USA

J. A. Brennan
Col, USAF, MC (ret.), Clinical Operations, Department of Surgery, Uniformed Services University of the Health Sciences, Annapolis, MD, USA

J. R. Bennett (✉)
Ear Nose & Throat Center of Utah, Salt Lake City, UT, USA
e-mail: jrb@entcenterslc.com

W. W. Hurd, W. Beninati (eds.), *Aeromedical Evacuation*,
https://doi.org/10.1007/978-3-030-15903-0_13

Flight-Associated Otorhinolaryngology Problems

Ear Block

The most common otorhinolaryngologic symptom associated with flight is middle ear barotrauma, the commonest of which is often referred to as "ear block." Middle ear barotrauma occurs in approximately 20% of adults and 55% of children in a single flight, while 10% of adults and 22% of children have otoscopic evidence of damage to the ear drum [3]. During ascent, atmospheric pressure decreases and causes gases in the middle ear to expand in accordance with Boyle's law. Most passengers do not experience problems as gas expansion in the middle ear forces open the normally closed Eustachian tube at approximately 15 mm Hg of pressure differential, thus releasing the pressure [1].

In contrast, upon descent the atmospheric pressure increases, and the gas in the middle ear contracts. The Eustachian tube must be actively opened by chewing, swallowing, yawning, or performing the Valsalva maneuver. When the differential pressure becomes 60 mm Hg, discomfort starts to occur. If the pressure is not equilibrated before 80 mm Hg, the Eustachian tube may become locked, referred to as "ear block," and there may be inability to equalize the pressure. If the pressure differential rises above 100 mm Hg, there is an increasing risk of tympanic membrane (TM) perforation [1].

A Danish study showed that 46% of adults and 33% of children who experienced pain from middle ear barotrauma were able to clear their ears using the Valsalva maneuver. A majority of the remaining adults and children who were unable to clear their ears were found to have signs of barotrauma (e.g., tympanic membrane redness, retraction, clear fluid in the middle ear, or hemotympanum), but none had ruptured ear drums [4].

Passengers with upper respiratory infections, allergic rhinitis, or abnormal nasal cavity anatomy are at increased risk of middle ear barotrauma due to edematous Eustachian tubes and mucus membranes, which makes equilibrating the pressure on both sides of the ear drum more difficult. Symptoms associated with this include ear pain, dizziness, sensation of fullness, and muffled hearing [5].

Ear Block Prevention

To decrease the risk of ear block, sleeping passengers should be awakened before descent to begin attempting to equilibrate the pressure. If all else fails and if the circumstances permit, symptoms also can be controlled by returning the aircraft to an altitude above the point at which symptoms developed. Descent can then be attempted again at a slower rate while the person attempts to equalize the pressure in the middle ear.

In those individuals who are known to have a history of Eustachian tube dysfunction and middle ear barotrauma, other options may be available in addition to performing a Valsalva maneuver. Patients are encouraged to try yawning, chewing gum, or swallowing throughout the flight. Other medical management consists of oral/topical nasal decongestants, topical steroids, and oral/topical antihistamines [5]. Topical decongestants such as oxymetazoline (Afrin®) may be used as follows: spray in the both nostrils, and wait for 3–5 minutes, and then spray a second time to decongest the posterior portion of the nose and Eustachian tube.

Ear Block Treatment

Several methods can be used to treat ear block. The Valsalva maneuver is performed by occluding both nares and exhaling against a closed mouth, thus forcing air into the nasopharynx to open the Eustachian tubes [2].

In severe cases, a Politzer bag can be used to apply pressure to the nasopharynx (Fig. 13.1a). To use this device, the mouth is closed along with one nostril, the Politzer tip is placed in the other nostril, and the patient is instructed to swallow while pressure is applied with the bag.

Another method used to dilate the Eustachian tube is a nasal balloon inflation device; this is used for those persons who cannot perform the Valsalva maneuver or for children. One nostril is occluded while the device is placed to the other and the patient tries to blow up the balloon by breathing out through their nose. This causes an

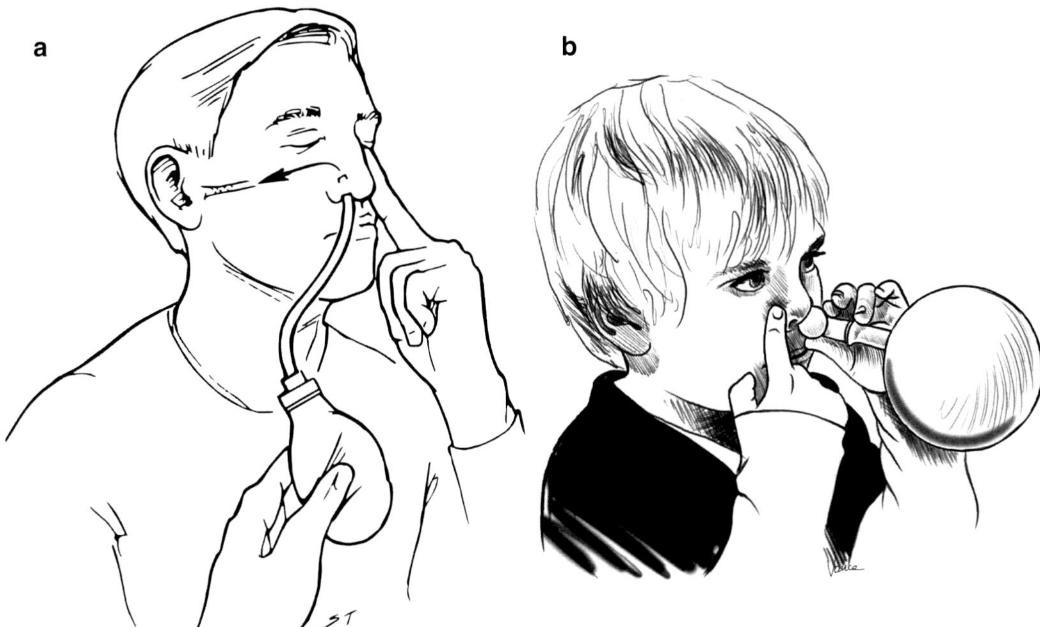

Fig. 13.1 (**a**) A Politzer bag is used by having the patient close their mouth and occlude one nostril while the doctor places the tip in the opposite nostril and applies brisk pressure to the bag to open the Eustachian tube. (**b**) A nasal balloon insufflation device is used by placing the balloon up to one nostril and occlusion of the other forcefully exhaling out nose to blow up balloon

increasing pressure within the nose to open the Eustachian tube (Fig. 13.1b).

In the event of a perforation of the tympanic membrane related to barotrauma, observation is the typical plan of care. Perforations will typically heal spontaneously as long as infection does not occur and water is kept out of the ear. The patient with an acute tympanic membrane perforation will not experience further barotrauma in that ear as long as the perforation remains; however, repeated flying can delay closure of the perforation. The patient should not fly until the tympanic membrane perforation heals, which may take several weeks or more.

Delayed Otic Barotrauma

Patients who are transported on 100% oxygen by mask will have the middle ear cavity filled with oxygen. The oxygen is easily absorbed by the middle ear mucosa, which then results in a negative middle ear pressure and pain. If frequent Valsalva maneuvers are not performed, the negative pressure may lead to serous otitis media, frequently seen with bubbles behind the TM. This condition is further exacerbated by sleeping when swallowing and Valsalva maneuver are infrequent [6].

Alternobaric Vertigo

Alternobaric vertigo is another form of middle ear barotrauma that results in vertigo, thought to be induced by unequal pressure between the left and right middle ear. The vertigo is self-limiting and resolves with clearing of the pressure differential [5]. Obviously, this can have disastrous consequences if it occurs in pilots while they are taking off or landing an aircraft.

Inner Ear Barotrauma

Inner ear barotrauma can occur from air travel, nose blowing, diving, or any other phenomena that cause a middle ear overpressure. The most common damage to the inner ear is rupture of either the round or oval window membranes, which results in the loss of perilymph fluid from the otic capsule and injury to the hair cells of the auditory vestibular system. The clinical results can include sensorineural hearing loss and vertigo. Patients typically present with a "flat" hearing loss upon audiometric testing (all frequencies equally affected). In one study, only 15% of patients presented with vertigo or dizziness [7].

The effects of inner ear barotrauma may be permanent. However, if patients present for treatment within 2 weeks of their injury, approximately 70% will have marked or almost complete improvement [7]. Treatment consists of bed rest with the head of the bed elevated to 30–40 degrees, stool softeners, and vestibular suppressants [8]. Patients who have no improvement or worsening of their auditory or vestibular symptoms after 2 weeks of treatment may have a perilymph fistula. Exploratory tympanotomy and repair of the fistula will usually improve their vertigo; however, in some patients hearing will not improve [1, 7].

Inner Ear Decompression Sickness

Decompression sickness (DCS also known as the "bends") occurs when nitrogen bubbles form in various tissues following a deep saturation underwater dive. During descent, inert gases dissolve in the blood according to Henry's law. Upon ascent, a reverse reaction occurs, and the inert gas can form bubbles within the labyrinthine or cochlear artery resulting in ischemia. These patients will typically experience hearing loss, tinnitus, vertigo, nausea, vomiting, and nystagmus [9, 10].

Scuba divers and individuals involved in military special operations should be aware that flying within 24 hours of diving significantly increases their risk of developing decompression sickness [10]. For those patients who experience sudden sensorineural hearing loss, the mainstays of treatment include corticosteroids, antivirals, vasodilators, and vasoactive substances. More recently, hyperbaric oxygen therapy has been used with efficacy in up to 80% of patients. Overall, approximately 65% of patients experience some improvement with no treatment [9]. Patients with suspected DCS may be moved inside portal hyperbaric chambers, such as the Hyperlite®, which have been used on pressurized AE aircrafts.

Sinus Barotrauma

Sinus barotrauma results when pressure cannot equalize, most commonly in the frontal or maxillary sinuses, and can be severely painful or even potentially disabling (Fig. 13.2). This typically occurs due to narrowed sinus ostia. Typical etiologies include sinus or upper respiratory infections, allergies, nasal polyps, and enlarged

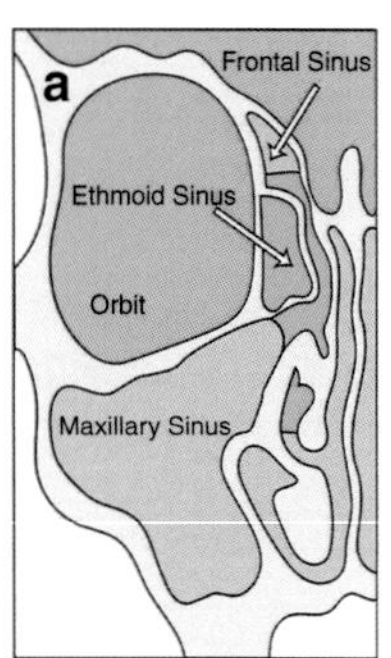

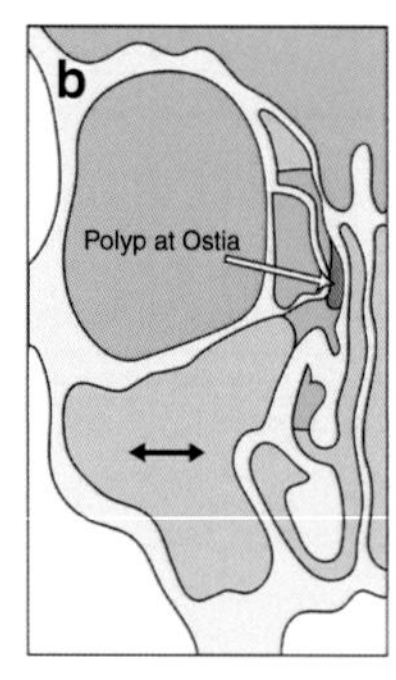

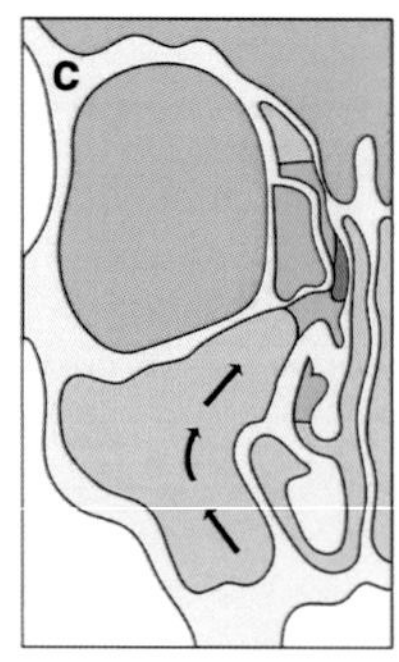

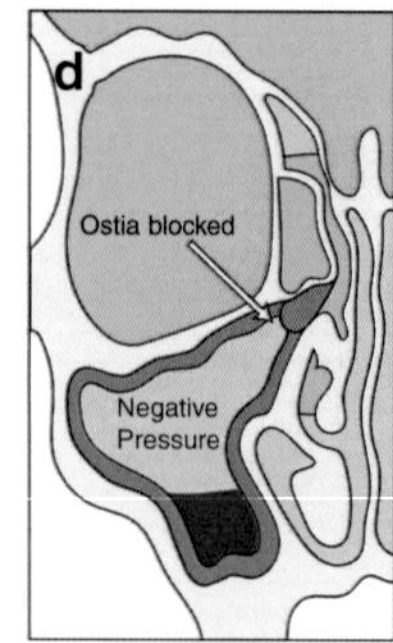

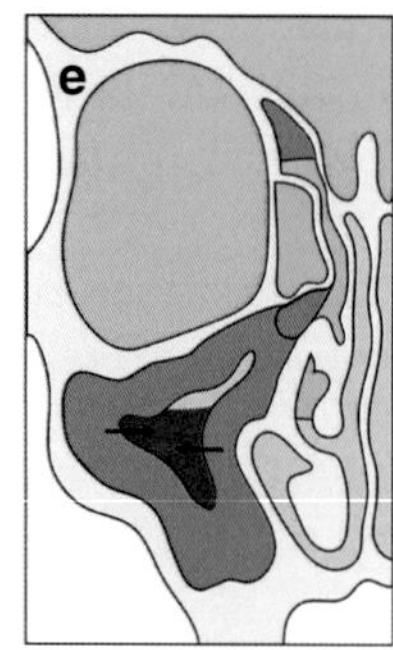

Fig. 13.2 Sinus barotrauma caused by a nasal polyp depicted in right-sided coronal slices through sinus cavities. (**a**) The osteomeatal complex is a critical area where obstruction can cause blockage to the maxillary, ethmoids, and frontal sinuses. The osteomeatal complex (green area) is depicted with the three sinuses involved in drainage to this area. (**b**) The pressure within the sinus is equilibrated with ambient air. (**c**) During ascent the polyp is displaced as air flows out of the sinus to equilibrate with the lower pressure. (**d**) Upon descent the polyp is pushed into the ostia, blocking the sinus and preventing equilibration. The pressure within the sinus can only be reduced by hemorrhage and dehiscence of the lining. (**e**) At the conclusion of the flight, sinus pressure re-equilibrates with continued hemorrhage and lining dehiscence

turbinates [5]. Symptoms include facial pain, headache, dental pain, and occasional epistaxis and can occur during either ascent or descent, with descent occurring more frequently.

Treatment is similar to those patients with middle ear barotrauma and includes both Valsalva maneuvers as well as medical management with topical and oral decongestants and antihistamines. Recurrent sinus barotrauma may require surgical intervention, as described later in the chapter.

Barodontalgia

Barodontalgia, also known as tooth squeeze, is tooth pain caused by a change in ambient pressure. It can occur when increases in pressure causes gas expansion in fillings, caps, crowns, root canals, or inflamed pulp. It is a relatively infrequent condition with a 0.26% incidence in patients who fly at high altitudes, as noted in a recent German study [5]. The differential diagnosis of tooth pain during flight includes sinus barotrauma because sinus pain may be referred to the teeth.

It is generally recommended that those who fly frequently, such as pilots, should undergo at least annual dental examinations. In addition, persons who have had a recent procedure should avoid flying for at least 24 hours [5].

Epistaxis

Epistaxis may be controlled by a number of methods, including pinching the nose, cautery, anterior packing, and, on occasion, posterior packing for persistent bleeds. Rarely is ligation or embolization required. Posterior packing has by tradition been accomplished with placement of a bulb catheter, such as a Foley catheter, through the nares and inflated with saline after positioning in the nasopharynx. This is followed by placement of multiple layers of Vaseline-soaked gauze to form the anterior pack and then placement of a c-clamp, taking care not to put pressure on the nasal alae.

Specially designed catheters can be used specifically to stop epistaxis if they are readily available. If the bleeding is felt to be coming from an anterior source, a catheter such as a Rapid Rhino Balloon® (Smith & Nephew, London, England) can be inserted (Fig. 13.3a). This balloon is

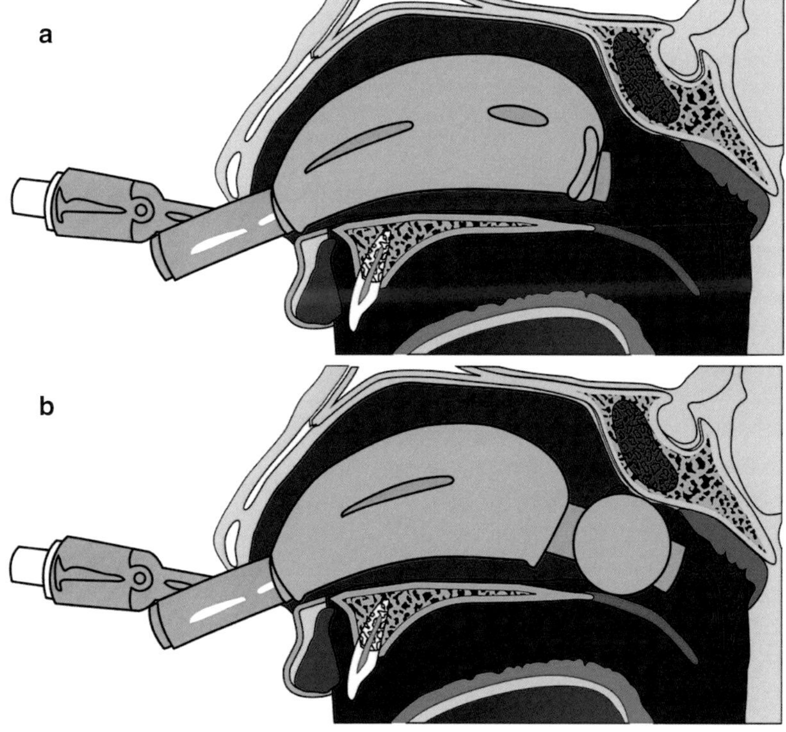

Fig. 13.3 (**a**) Epistaxis not responding to conservative measures can be treated with single-balloon catheter. (**b**) If this fails, a double-balloon catheter with both anterior and posterior balloons can be used

designed to be filled with air. For AE, the balloon pressure should be closely monitored, since flight-related pressure changes will greatly increase the volume of the balloon.

If the bleeding continues, a two-balloon catheter system with post-anterior and posterior balloons should be placed, such as the Epistat (Medtronic, Minneapolis, Minnesota) or Storz T3100 (Bausch + Lomb, Bridgewater, New Jersey) (Fig. 13.3b). This catheter is designed to be filled with water or saline, which is ideal for AE as flight-related pressure changes will not appreciably change the volume of the balloons.

Patients with occluded nares will need increased humidification and hydration during the flight because these patients must breathe through their mouths. Usually blood has filled the lower sinuses (maxillary and sphenoid), resulting in few barometric pressure sinus symptoms. Patients with posterior packs must be closely monitored as the complication rate averages 17% and include alar necrosis, sepsis, aspiration, and even cardiac arrhythmias and death [11]. Elderly patients are especially at risk for the aforementioned complications.

Otorhinolaryngologic Trauma

Epidemiology

Maxillofacial trauma constitutes a significant proportion of the trauma treated in civilian trauma centers and may be initially overlooked in patients with multiple organ system trauma. An Israeli study of prehospital diagnoses performed by flight surgeons found that 10% of trauma patients had facial injury, 3% had soft-tissue neck trauma, and 22% had cranial head injuries [12]. Approximately 26% of the potentially identifiable facial trauma diagnoses were missed, compared to only 8% of the soft-tissue neck trauma and 7% of the head trauma. An Australian study found that 33% of facial injuries (primarily fractures) of head-injured patients seen in the emergency department were missed [13].

During armed conflicts, the types of maxillofacial traumas have changed throughout the years, based on the changes in types of combat. During World War II, the massive application of artillery and bombing resulted in 75% of facial injuries from shrapnel, while only 10% were from gunshot wounds [14]. During the Vietnam War, close combat and in particular guerilla warfare were more common, and thus 58% of the maxillofacial trauma was secondary to bullet wounds, only 30% from artillery, with the remaining 12% resulting from accidents [15].

More recently, from the armed conflicts in Iraq and Afghanistan, approximately 26% of injuries were categorized as craniomaxillofacial (CMF) in origin. The primary mechanism of injury in 84% of cases involved improvised explosive devices (IEDs), with gunshot wounds making up 8%. Penetrating soft-tissue injuries and facial fractures accounted for the majority of CMF injuries at 58% and 27%, respectively [16]. It appears that the incidence of CMF injuries is increasing due to the effective use of body armor that protects the chest and abdomen but leaves the face and neck exposed [17].

There are four mechanisms by which IEDs can produce complex injuries: primary, secondary, tertiary, and quaternary [18]. The primary injury is caused from sudden increase in air pressure after an explosion and affects the air-filled bones in the maxillofacial region. Secondary blast injuries are caused from penetrating fragments. Tertiary blast injury occurs when the casualty is thrown into other objects. Lastly, quaternary blast injuries are related to thermal effects of the explosion and cause burn and inhalational injuries.

Midface Trauma

Facial fractures are often overlooked in the field, even in the presence of facial lacerations. Fortunately, fractures of the sinus cavities are unlikely to cause sinus barotrauma during flight because the sinus is no longer a fixed-wall cavity and thus allows expansion of gas into the nose or surrounding tissue (cutaneous emphysema).

Skull Base Fracture

If a skull base fracture is suspected in a patient, pneumocephalus must be considered and ruled out if possible prior to AE. A patient with an unrecognized pneumocephalus may suffer increased cerebral pressure or brain stem herniation due to expanding gases as the aircraft ascends. If a patient with a documented or suspected pneumocephalus must be transported (i.e., urgent or contingency AE), the cabin should remain pressurized at the altitude of the departure facility. In helicopters and smaller transport aircrafts where this is not possible, the lowest possible altitudes should be flown.

All head-injured patients should be placed headfirst in the aircraft (i.e., head toward the front) to lessen the risk of increased cerebral pressures (pooling of blood in the head) during the take-off acceleration and climb [19]. Drugs to manage potential cerebral complications should be available if possible, as discussed elsewhere in this book.

In those patients who have a known pneumocephalus, delayed transfer is recommended. There have been rare case reports of tension pneumocephalus in the early twentieth century, with none recently largely due to pressurized cabins. There have been several case studies in recent years showing overall safe aeromedical transport for patients with pneumocephalus in pressurized cabins [20].

Temporal Bone Trauma

Temporal bone trauma may manifest as Battle's sign (postauricular ecchymosis), tympanic membrane rupture, facial nerve paralysis, or hearing loss. If the middle ear is filled with blood, barotrauma during flight does not occur. In some cases, temporal bone fractures can breach the cranial vault, resulting in leakage of cerebrospinal fluid (CSF) and a potential pneumocephalus. A delayed complication is meningitis, as nasopharyngeal organisms contaminate the CSF.

Airway Management AFTER After Maxillofacial Trauma

Airway control is crucial to victims of maxillofacial trauma, whether the trauma is to the face or neck, penetrating or blunt, and a bony injury or strictly a soft-tissue injury. Airway control is in particular important for unconscious patients and those with cranial vault trauma, facial trauma, or inhalation burns. In the most recent war efforts in Iraq and Afghanistan, approximately 51% of patients with CMF injuries required intubation with approximately 19% eventually requiring a tracheostomy [17].

Any patient who is reasonably likely to need intubation should have an orotracheal or nasotracheal tube placed prior to AE. It is far better to intubate a patient in a controlled environment on the ground than in an emergency situation in the turbulent and cramped environment of an aircraft.

Orotracheal Versus Nasotracheal Intubation

A definitive airway can be obtained by insertion of either an orotracheal or nasotracheal tube. Orotracheal intubation has the disadvantage of requiring cervical spine manipulation and direct visualization of the trachea, which can be difficult with massive trauma and bleeding of the lower face or oral cavity. Because victims of maxillofacial trauma are at increased risk of coexisting cervical spine trauma, orotracheal intubation should be performed cautiously with in-line cervical spine immobilization in these patients. The advantages of nasotracheal intubation are that it can be done blindly with a high degree of success and is better tolerated by conscious patients [21]. However, nasotracheal intubation is contraindicated in apneic patients. It is also contraindicated in patients suspected of having a skull base fracture, as there is a risk that the endotracheal tube could pass through the cribriform plate into the cranial vault. Evidence of a possible skull base fracture includes midface and cranial instability or deformity and hemotympanum.

Orotracheal and nasotracheal intubation should be performed with caution in patients presenting with blunt anterior neck trauma (e.g., "clothesline" injuries) because laryngotracheal separation or severe laryngeal fracture may have occurred. A tracheotomy is a safer approach to securing the airway with these devastating injuries. Blunt passage of the endotracheal tube into a partially separated larynx and trachea could sever any remaining soft-tissue attachments, thus causing the trachea to partially retract into the chest with resultant loss of the airway.

Blind Insertion Airway Device

A Combitube, also known as an esophageal tracheal double-lumen airway, can be blindly passed in the field to stabilize an airway when directed endotracheal intubation is not an option (Fig. 13.4). With blind passage, these devices most commonly enter the esophagus, or, less commonly, the trachea is intubated. With insufflation of one or both of the balloons depending on location, adequate ventilation is possible.

Upon insertion of a Combitube, the distal balloon is inflated first. If the tube is confirmed to be within the trachea by verifying airflow via lung auscultation, the second balloon stays deflated and the circuit is maintained on the #2 lumen. Lack of airflow after inflating the first balloon indicates that the distal tip is within the esophagus. The second balloon, which will be at the level of the larynx, is inflated to prevent air backflow. The circuit is transferred to the #1 lumen, and perforations between the two balloons allow air to be forced through the vocal cords and into the lungs. A Combitube should be converted to an endotracheal tube as soon as possible and certainly prior to AE, for a more stable airway.

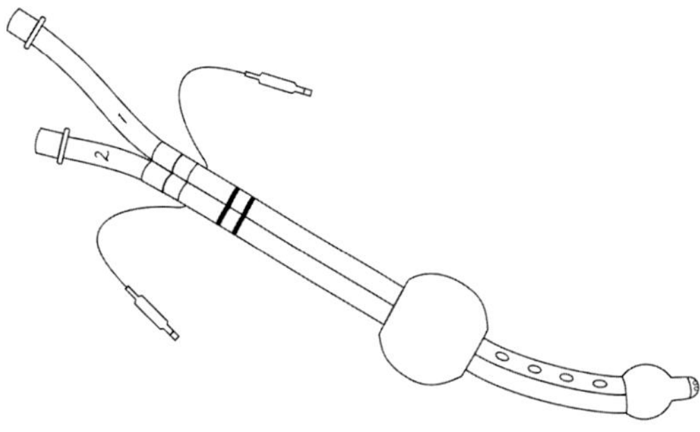

Fig. 13.4 The Combitube blind insertion airway device

Needle Cricothyrotomy

Needle cricothyrotomy is useful to rapidly provide limited and temporary airway access in any trauma scenario where the trachea cannot be readily intubated. A large-caliber angiocatheter is placed through the cricothyroid membrane into the trachea. This should be a 12- or 14-gauge catheter in an adult or a 16- or 18-gauge catheter in a child. The cannula should then be connected to oxygen at 15 L/minute at 40–50 psi via tubing with either a Y-connector or with a side hole cut in the tubing. Intermittent insufflation, 1 second on and 4 seconds off, can be achieved by placing a thumb over the Y-connector or hole in the tube. Patients can be maintained with this technique for 30 to 45 minutes, assuming they previously had normal pulmonary function and have no significant chest injury.

Needle cricothyroidotomy allows oxygenation and not ventilation. Carbon dioxide will build up, which will limit the usefulness of this technique in head-injured patients. Caution must also be used if there is complete airway obstruction at the glottic level; and if such obstruction occurs, the flow should be lowered to 5–7 L/minute. A more definitive airway should be obtained before considering AE transport.

Surgical Cricothyrotomy

Surgical cricothyrotomy is safer and more dependable than needle cricothyrotomy and allows appropriate ventilation through a larger endotracheal tube. Multiple studies have demonstrated the efficacy and safety of this procedure in the hands of appropriately trained caregivers in field conditions [22–24]. The technique consists of making either a horizontal or preferably a vertical skin incision and then a horizontal incision through the cricothyroid membrane, dilating the opening with a curved hemostat or the blunt end of a scalpel, and inserting a 5- to 7-mm endotracheal tube or tracheostomy tube. Surgical cricothyrotomy should not be performed in children under the age of 12 due to the risk of damage to the cricoid cartilage. It also should not be performed in patients who have trauma to the larynx and trachea, with possible tracheal disruption. Both needle and surgical cricothyrotomy must be converted to tracheostomy when the patient has reached a surgical facility to minimize the long-term risk of subglottic stenosis.

Aeromedical Evacuation Implications of Specific Conditions and Diagnoses

Tracheal Tube Cuff Pressure Management

AE patients traveling with either an endotracheal tube or a cuffed tracheostomy tube should have adequate cuff pressure management. During ascent, the cuff pressure increases and if unchecked can reach as high as 385 torr leading to damage to the tracheal mucosa. During descent, cuff pressure reductions may lead to aspiration, which has been implicated in ventilator-associated pneumonia, as well as inefficient ventilation due to low tidal volumes from cuff leaks [25, 26].

It is a simple matter to check the cuff pressure with a cufflator upon reaching cruising altitude, every 30 minutes during the flight, and again during descent. Self-regulating cuffs are now also readily available, which adjust the pressure in the cuff automatically throughout the flight. If the number of aeromedical personnel available is not sufficient to satisfactorily perform cuff pressure monitoring or an automated cuff regulator is not available, replacement of the air with saline remains a reasonable alternative [25, 27]. The current recommendation, however, is to leave air in the tracheostomy tube cuff because the use of fluid causes difficulty in monitoring cuff pressure and leakage. It could also cause damage to the cuff valve, requiring premature changing of the tube [27].

Tracheostomy Tubes

There are many types of tracheostomy tubes, but the typical tube consists of an inner cannula with an outer sleeve (Fig. 13.5). This inner cannula can be readily removed for cleaning, while the outer sleeve maintains the patency of the tracheostomy. The cuff is inflated to isolate the trachea from the larynx and secretions above and allow for a seal during ventilator use. When the patient is spontaneously breathing, this cuff may be deflated to allow passage of air through the mouth. The patient may be able to speak if the cuff is deflated

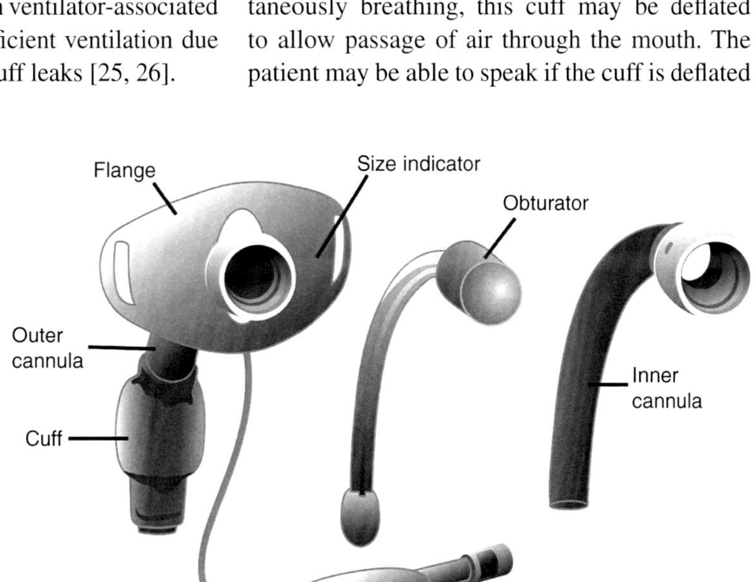

Fig. 13.5 The typical tracheostomy tube is made up of three parts: the outer sleeve, inner cannula, and obturator used to place the tracheostomy tube

and the tube is occluded on exhalation, thus allowing air to pass through the larynx.

To facilitate speech, the patient may use a custom tube that is cuffless and typically is of a smaller size, or is fenestrated. Fenestrated tubes have a hole on the outer curve (posterior) of the tube to allow passage of air through the mouth. A fenestrated inner cannula must be used in conjunction with the fenestrated outer sleeve. The fenestrated tube has fallen into some disfavor because of possible irritation against the posterior trachea leading to infection and possibly subglottic stenosis.

Foam-filled cuffs are available that have a lower pressure against the tracheal mucosa. The foam cuff is collapsed through an external valve in the same fashion that air-filled cuffs are. Also commonly seen are customized and irregularly shaped tracheostomy tubes that may have only a single lumen.

Several principles apply to the use of all tracheostomy tubes. Tracheostomy tubes should be frequently cleaned and inspected. Spares should be available. Suction should also be readily available. Either air or oxygen, if required, should be humidified and applied to the tracheostomy tube rather than to the mouth or nose.

If a tracheostomy tube is dislodged, the inner cannula should be removed and replaced by an obturator that allows smooth reintroduction of the outer cannula of the tracheostomy tube into the airway passage. The obturator is then removed and the inner cannula is reinserted. The tracheostomy tube with obturator should be lubricated or moistened prior to introduction, and this should be done with the patient's neck extended under good lighting. For this reason, the obturator should be secured in an obvious place prior to AE, such as on the front of the patient's chart or on the head of the bed. Replacement of the tracheotomy tube within 5 days of placement and before the surgical tract has matured is potentially very dangerous and should be performed, if possible, in the operating room.

Patients who have tracheostomies are ready to fly as soon as they have recovered from their operation and preferably have undergone their first tracheostomy tube change—usually after the fifth postoperative day. However, in the combat zone, aeromedical evacuation typically occurs within 24 hours of tracheotomy tube placement. Consequently, the tracheotomy tube should be adequately secured using techniques such as silk sutures securing the tube collar to the skin, a safety suture around the cricoid cartilage, and an inferior-based Bjork flap [28]. The tracheostomy provides an excellent airway and should be kept free of secretions and crusts. Humidification should be provided due to the low relative humidity of cabin air.

Postoperative Otorhinolaryngologic Patients

The AE of patients after otorhinolaryngologic procedures poses unique challenges in maintaining the comfort and safety of these patients. This can be disconcerting to the aeromedical flight crew if they are unfamiliar with the particular procedure performed or if written details of the operation are lacking. Familiarizing oneself with these procedures, as well as good communication with the otorhinolaryngologist, should alleviate concerns.

Tonsillectomy

Patients who have undergone a tonsillectomy, with or without adenoidectomy or uvulopalatopharyngoplasty, are at risk of hemorrhage at two different times during the postoperative period. The time of greatest risk is the first several hours after surgery. A postoperative tonsillectomy hemorrhage that can be controlled in an emergency department or operating room might be fatal in an aircraft. For this reason, elective aeromedical evacuation of these patients should be delayed until 14 days after surgery (Table 13.1).

The second period of increased risk of hemorrhage is approximately 7–14 days after surgery, when the eschar separates from the tonsillar fossa. For this reason, elective AE should be delayed until 2 weeks after tonsillectomy or after the eschars in the tonsillar fossa separate (Table 13.2).

Table 13.1 Contraindications to aeromedical evacuation (AE) for otorhinolaryngologic patients

Absolute (contraindication to elective, urgent, and contingency AE)
Unstable airway Decompression sickness (DCS)[a] Skull fracture with intracranial air[a]
Relative (contraindication to elective AE)
Within 14 days after tonsillectomy, tympanoplasty, or neck surgery Within 24 hours after rhinoplasty, septoplasty, or sinus surgery

[a]Stabilized patients can be moved in aircraft capable of pressurization to the elevation of the departure site if the arrival site is not at a higher elevation. DCS patients may be moved with a portable hyperbaric chamber in a pressurized AE aircraft

Table 13.2 Aeromedical evacuation checklist for otorhinolaryngologic patients

Hearing protection for all patients (ear plugs or muffs) where required
Patients at risk for hypoxia (e.g., anemia <8.5 g Hg, sickle cell anemia) Oxygen supplementation given
Tracheostomy patients Humidified air or oxygen used to avoid airway irritation Obturator readily available Spare tracheostomy tube
Unconscious patients Eyes protected (ophthalmic ointment and taped shut) Flashlight available to check pupils
Intubated patients Tube position and security confirmed Steps taken to avoid cuff overpressure if using air Monitor cuffs for incorrect pressure Upon ascent until cruise altitude reached Every 30 minutes during flight On descent **Or** *fill cuffs with saline* Spare tube and functioning laryngoscope, suction available Appropriate ventilator and Ambu bag available Oxygen supply is adequate for the anticipated trip length
Patients with nasogastric or feeding tubes Anticipate a possible sinus block on tubed side
Trauma patients Wire cutters readily available for patients with maxillomandibular fixation Head-injured patients on litters are placed with head toward the front of the aircraft Pneumocephalus ruled out with temporal bone, orbital, or LeFort fractures Air in globe ruled out with ophthalmic trauma

If urgent or contingency AE is required sooner than 2 weeks, the risk of bleeding may be decreased by giving the patient humidified air and ensuring adequate fluid intake en route to counteract the dry atmosphere. If significant bleeding occurs, diversion to the nearest medical facility is required.

Rhinoplasty and Septoplasty

Patients who have undergone rhinoplasty or septoplasty are able to undergo AE after the nasal passage has been cleared of splints and packing, which typically occurs within 1 week from surgery. The majority of patients will be able to breathe better through their noses after septoplasty. However, for several weeks after surgery, residual edema of the turbinates and mucosa may predispose the patient to sinus blockage. Patients should be treated with a nasal decongestant spray before and during flight if AE is required within the first few weeks postoperatively.

Endoscopic Sinus Surgery

Conditions that put patients at increased risk for sinus barotrauma are often treated surgically. Endoscopic sinus surgery is used to enlarge natural sinus openings for patients with chronic infections, tenacious mucus, or congenital bony abnormalities and remove obstructing pathology such as sinonasal polyps and tumors.

Aviators who have undergone functional endoscopic sinus surgery have significantly fewer or no episodes of sinus barotrauma postoperatively. A study at Wilford Hall Medical Center of 54 aviators who had undergone this procedure found that 98% had returned to active flight duty [29]. Aviators who have undergone endoscopic sinus surgery should be preflight tested in an altitude chamber prior to returning to flying status.

In general, patients who have undergone such surgery have few problems with air travel [30]. However, elective AE should be delayed for at least 24 hours to allow resolution of any postoperative edema. Patients who require AE sooner should be treated with nasal decongestants and frequent Valsalva maneuvers to minimize the risk of sinus block. Patients should be cautioned that vigorous Valsalva maneuvers after some types of ethmoid surgeries (e.g., involving the lamina papyracea, cribriform plate, or fovea ethmoidalis) may result in orbital emphysema or pneumocephalus. Sinus surgery itself can cause pneumocephalus or orbital emphysema, which may be unknown after surgery if the skull base or lamina papyracea is violated. These patients should be treated similarly as those with pneumocephalus from other causes, such as trauma, with delayed transport unless medically necessary. If transport is required, this must be done in a pressurized cabin [31].

If a sinus block occurs during flight in a patient post-sinus surgery, the aircraft should ideally climb back to the altitude where the sinus block developed. Decongestants should be administered if available and descent then can be resumed at a more gradual rate with regular Valsalva maneuvers. Analgesics may be administered if the patient is not in control of the aircraft. Sinus barotrauma may result in an episode of epistaxis that is usually self-limiting and easily controlled.

Pressure Equalization Tubes

Patients with patent pressure equalization (PE) tubes in their tympanic membranes should have no difficulty with ear blocks. These patients may fly as soon as they have recovered from surgery. The patency of these tubes can usually be determined with direct otoscopy and insufflation. If patency cannot be determined by direct visualization, formal tympanography is another option. A patent tube on tympanography will show a flat or type B appearance of the pressure curve with a high external auditory canal volume. A type B tympanogram with low volume indicates either a plugged PE tube with middle ear effusion or one that has extruded and the tympanic membrane has since sealed, with the development of serous otitis media. A fluid-filled middle ear is not affected by altitude change because fluid does not expand and contract as gases do at altitude.

Stapedotomy/Stapedectomy

Otosclerosis is a disease that causes fixation of the stapes to surrounding bone, causing a conductive hearing loss. This can be treated with hearing aids or surgically corrected by stapedotomy. This procedure involves removing the stapes suprastructure over the stapes footplate, drilling or lasing a small hole through the footplate, and placing a piston-like prosthesis into the hole, which is then directly connected to the incus. This restores ossicular mobility, resulting in improved hearing. A stapedectomy is a similar procedure; however, the entire footplate is removed and replaced with fascia/vein or perichondrium. Theoretically, these patients are at a higher risk of perilymph fistula. Patients who have undergone stapes surgery are allowed to fly in commercial aircraft after they have recovered from the anesthetic and are symptom free. If the patient had a perilymphatic fluid leak during the surgery, it would be best to wait until symptoms of vertigo are resolved plus an additional 2 weeks to ensure no further inner ear trauma that may be caused from altitude changes.

Tympanoplasty/Mastoidectomy

Tympanoplasty encompasses a variety of operations that may involve the removal of middle ear pathology, repair of ossicles, or reconstruction of the eardrum. Mastoidectomy is the removal of diseased mastoid air cells. A variety of materials may be used to repair the tympanic membrane and ossicles. A patient who has undergone recent tympanoplasty or even a tympanoplasty associated with some form of mastoid surgery should be able to fly as soon as recovered from the effects of the anesthetic and demonstrates no otologic complications. Typically after surgery, the middle ear space is filled with fluid and absorbent surgical packing that dissolves in about 3 weeks.

Not every otologic surgery involves middle ear packing. In the absence of packing, an ossicular reconstruction or tympanic membrane graft should be allowed to heal in place for at least 2 weeks before being subjected to barotrauma and Valsalva maneuvers. Movement of the tympanic membrane flap during pressure changes may dislodge grafts or prostheses. Prior to taking a flight after healing, these patients should begin performing frequent Eustachian tube clearing maneuvers, including gentle Valsalva maneuvers, chewing, yawning, and swallowing [32].

Placement of some types of ossicular prostheses creates a small but serious risk of perilymphatic fistula, regardless of the time since surgery. A prosthesis such as a total ossicular replacement prosthesis (TORP) lacks the natural lever action of the ossicle that it replaces. Excessive tympanic membrane motion transmitted directly to the footplate of the stapes may acutely create a perilymphatic fistula [33]. This can rarely occur while the patient is trying to clear an ear block with forceful Valsalva maneuvers or during abrupt changes in cabin pressure (i.e., explosive decompression). Symptoms can include sudden vertigo, nausea, vomiting, and a sensorineural hearing loss. Treatment is supportive, with immediate follow-up by a specialist after scheduled landing.

Vestibular Nerve Schwannoma and Cerebellar Pontine Angle Surgery

Vestibular nerve schwannoma is a benign slow-growing lesion that causes compression of the contents of the internal auditory canal and ultimately grows into the cerebellopontine angle. These lesions can be treated with surgery, stereotactic radiation, or observation. The surgical accesses most commonly used include the translabyrinthine, retrosigmoid, and middle fossa approaches. Depending on the approach, the patient has a 9–29% risk of developing a CSF leak within the first few postoperative days [34].

If a CSF leak develops after surgery, patients should not undergo elective AE for 2 weeks after any leakage has resolved. In the past, it was considered safe to fly immediately after a CSF leak resolved. However, there are reports of patients who flew immediately after the leakage resolved (following a translabyrinthine approach) and developed bacterial meningitis within hours of landing [34]. The hypothesis is that during descent the relative negative pressure that develops within the middle ear and Eustachian tube allows nasopharyngeal pathogens to reflux back into the middle ear and come into contact with CSF, resulting in meningitis.

Laryngectomy

Patients who have undergone total laryngectomy have had the larynx removed and the trachea brought out through the anterior neck. They may have a short single lumen tube similar to that of a tracheostomy tube that fits within the trachea and helps prevent contracture at the tracheostoma site. Patients who have undergone a total laryngectomy may have a small tracheoesophageal prosthetic one-way valve inserted on the posterior wall of their trachea and into the pharynx that allows oral speech when the tracheostoma opening is occluded with their thumb. There are no problems associated with this condition during flight other than excessive drying. One pilot was reported to return to flying as pilot in command after his total laryngectomy [35].

Mandible Fractures

Patients with mandible fractures will usually require maxillomandibular fixation (i.e., their jaws are wired shut). For this type of fixation, arch bars are wired to the mandibular and maxillary teeth and then wired to each other, typically with four wire loops.

Patients with maxillomandibular fixation are at risk of aspiration if they vomit with the wire fixation in place. If patients have a tendency toward motion sickness, they should be given antiemetics and placed on their side with the head down. In high-risk patients, the fixation wires should be removed (can be temporarily replaced with rubber bands during the flight) [36]. If wires are left in place, wire cutters should be worn around the neck for the rapid release from fixation in the case of vomiting (Fig. 13.6). It is only necessary to cut and remove the wire loops spanning between the maxillary and mandibular bars (Fig. 13.7). Trauma patients with maxilloman-

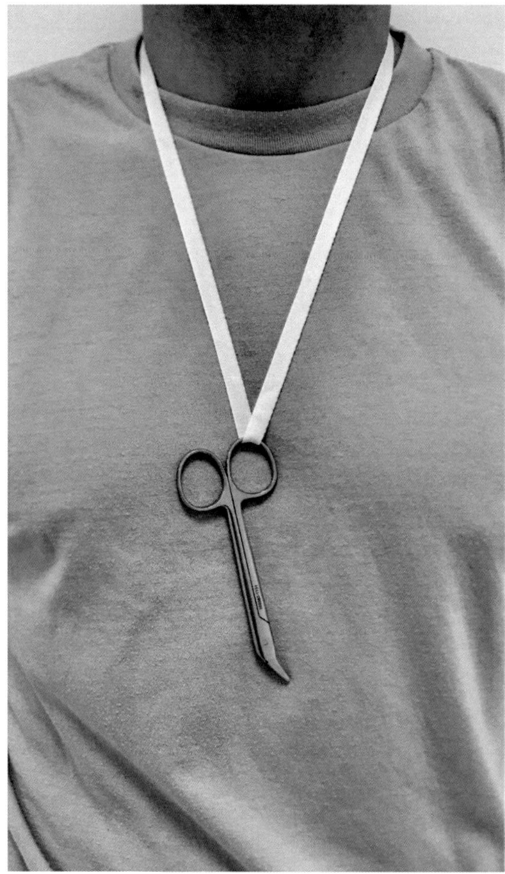

Fig. 13.6 Wire cutters should be attached to a lanyard around the necks of patients with maxillomandibular fixation who are undergoing AE for rapid release from fixation in the case of vomiting

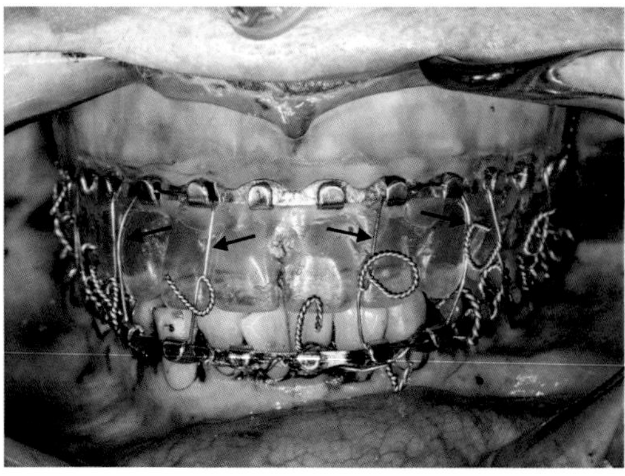

Fig. 13.7 Maxillomandibular fixation because the patient no longer had maxillary teeth, and a splint was made to act as her upper denture. Arrows show wire cut sites for emergency release of maxillomandibular fixation, which would be standard in any patient

dibular fixation and mental status changes should have a tracheotomy placed prior to flying due to their high risk of airway compromise.

Neck Dissection/Thyroidectomy/Free and Pedicled Flaps

Patients who have undergone a neck dissection, thyroidectomy, or free or pedicled flap should ideally be moved by elective AE after 2 weeks and after all drains have been removed, no fistula exists, and the flaps are viable. Earlier movement may predispose patients to cutaneous emphysema or pneumopericardium. However, recent studies in the combat zones have demonstrated the safety of immediately moving patients after extensive neck surgery with passive (Penrose) drains in place [37].

References

1. Mirza S, Richardson H. Otic barotrauma from air travel. J Laryngol Otol. 2005;119(5):366–70.
2. Randel H, editor. Anonymous. Aerospace medicine. 2nd ed. Baltimore: Williams & Wilkins; 1971.
3. Zhang Q, Banks C, Choroomi S, Kertesz T. A novel technique of otic barotrauma management using modified intravenous cannulae. Eur Arch Otorhinolaryngol. 2013;270(10):2627–30.
4. Stangerup SE, Tjernström O, Klokker M, Harcourt J, Stokholm J. Point prevalence of barotitis in children and adults after flight, and effect of autoinflation. Aviat Space Environ Med. 1998;69(1):45–9.
5. Lynch JH, Deaton TG. Barotrauma with extreme pressures in sport: From scuba to skydiving. Curr Sports Med Rep. 2014;13(2):107–12.
6. Landolfi A, Autore A, Torchia F, Ciniglio Appiani M, Morgagni F, Ciniglio AG. Ear pain after breathing oxygen at altitude: prevalence and prevention of delayed barotrauma. Aviat Space Environ Med. 2010;81(2):130–2.
7. Kozuka M, Nakashima T, Fukuta S, Yanagita N. Inner ear disorders due to pressure change. Clin Otolaryngol Allied Sci. 1997;22(2):106–10.
8. Elliott EJ, Smart DR. The assessment and management of inner ear barotrauma in divers and recommendations for returning to diving. Diving Hyperb Med. 2014;44(4):208–22.
9. Van Der Wal AW, Van Ooij PJ, De Ru JA. Hyperbaric oxygen therapy for sudden sensorineural hearing loss in divers. J Laryngol Otol. 2016;130(11):1039–47.

10. Alberti P. Otologic medicine and surgery. New York, NY: Churchill Livingstone; 1988.
11. Gluckman J. Renewal of certification study guide in otolaryngology-head and neck surgery. Dubuque: Kendall/Hunt; 1988.
12. Linn S, Knoller N, Giligan CG, Dreifus U. The sky is a limit: errors in prehospital diagnosis by flight physicians. Am J Emerg Med. 1997;15(3):316–20.
13. Tulloh BR. Diagnostic accuracy in head-injured patients: an emergency department audit. Injury. 1994;25(4):231–4.
14. Rowe N, Killey H. Fractures of the facial skeleton. E&S Livingstone Ltd: Edinburgh; 1955.
15. Andrews JL. Maxillofacial trauma in Vietnam. J Oral Surg. 1968;26(7):457–62.
16. Lew TA, Walker JA, Wenke JC, Blackbourne LH, Hale RG. Characterization of craniomaxillofacial battle injuries sustained by United States service members in the current conflicts of Iraq and Afghanistan. J Oral Maxillofac Surg. 2010;68(1):3–7.
17. Keller MW, Han PP, Galarneau MR, Brigger MT. Airway management in severe combat maxillofacial trauma. Otolaryngol Head Neck Surg. 2015;153(4):532–7.
18. Stevens JR, Brennan J. Management and reconstruction of blast wounds of the head and neck. Curr Opin Otolaryngol Head Neck Surg. 2016;24(5):426–32.
19. Reddick EJ. Aeromedical evacuation. Am Fam Physician. 1977;16(4):154–60.
20. Donovan DJ, Iskandar JI, Dunn CJ, King JA. Aeromedical evacuation of patients with pneumocephalus: outcomes in 21 cases. Aviat Space Environ Med. 2008;79(1):30–5.
21. O'Brien DJ, Danzl DF, Sowers MB, Hooker EA. Airway management of aeromedically transported trauma patients. J Emerg Med. 1988;6(1):49–54.
22. Boyle MF, Hatton D, Sheets C. Surgical cricothyrotomy performed by air ambulance flight nurses: A 5-year experience. J Emerg Med. 1993;11(1):41–5.
23. Xeropotamos NS, Coats TJ, Wilson AW. Prehospital surgical airway management: 1 year's experience from the helicopter emergency medical service. Injury. 1993;24(4):222–4.
24. Miklus RM, Elliott C, Snow N. Surgical cricothyrotomy in the field: experience of a helicopter transport team. J Trauma. 1989;29(4):506–8.
25. Blakeman T, Rodriquez D, Woods J, Cox D, Elterman J, Branson R. Automated control of endotracheal tube cuff pressure during simulated flight. J Trauma Acute Care Surg. 2016;81(5 Suppl 2 Proceedings of the 2015 Military Health System Research Symposium):S116–20.
26. Stoner DL, Cooke JP. Intratracheal cuffs and aeromedical evacuation. Anesthesiology. 1974;41(3):302–6.
27. Britton T, Blakeman TC, Eggert J, Rodriquez D, Ortiz H, Branson RD. Managing endotracheal tube cuff pressure at altitude: a comparison of four methods. J Trauma Acute Care Surg. 2014;77(3 Suppl 2):S240–4.
28. Brennan J, Gibbons MD, Lopez M, Hayes D, Faulkner J, Eller RL, et al. Traumatic airway management in operation iraqi freedom. Otolaryngol Head Neck Surg. 2011;144(3):376–80.
29. Parsons DS, Chambers DW, Boyd EM. Long-term follow-up of aviators after functional endoscopic sinus surgery for sinus barotrauma. Aviat Space Environ Med. 1997;68(11):1029–34.
30. Bolger WE, Parsons DS, Matson RE. Functional endoscopic sinus surgery in aviators with recurrent sinus barotrauma. Aviat Space Environ Med. 1990;61(2):148–56.
31. Willson TJ, Grady C, Braxton E, Weitzel E. Air travel with known pneumocephalus following outpatient sinus surgery. Aviat Space Environ Med. 2014;85(1):75–7.
32. Syms CA. Flying after otologic surgery. Am J Otol. 1991;12(3):162.
33. Moser M. Fitness of civil aviation passengers to fly after ear surgery. Aviat Space Environ Med. 1990;61(8):735–7.
34. Callanan V, O'Connor AF, King TT. Air travel induced meningitis following vestibular schwannoma (acoustic neuroma) surgery. J Laryngol Otol. 1996;110(3):258–60.
35. Stoll W, Delank W. Fitness for flying despite laryngectomy. Laryngorhinootologie. 1994;73(12):654–5.
36. Sanger A, Stoner P. Air force flight surgeon's manual. U.S. Department of the Air Force; 1976.
37. Brennan J, Lopez M, Gibbons MD, Hayes D, Faulkner J, Dorlac WC, et al. Penetrating neck trauma in operation iraqi freedom. Otolaryngol Head Neck Surg. 2011;144(2):180–5.

Care of Ophthalmic Casualties

14

Nathan Aschel Jordan, Robert A. Mazzoli, Bryan Propes, and Jo Ann Egan

Introduction

"Life, Limb, and Sight" are well-accepted medical priorities for emergency care. However, patients often reprioritize this list as "Life, Sight, and Limb" because of the importance of eyesight as the most precious sense. Indeed, loss of sight is one of society's greatest fears [1]. Military ophthalmologists who treat combat casualties report being told "Doc, you can have my other leg if you can give me back my sight."

The unfortunate reality, however, is that the eye is often overlooked in trauma patients such that "Life, Limb, and Sight" becomes shortened to "Life and Limb." One study documented that only 4% of obvious combat eye injuries were properly treated with rigid eye shields placed prior to ophthalmic care [2]. In the Boston Marathon bombing, ophthalmologists found no eye shields placed in the 22 eye casualties treated, and in the West Texas explosion, only one eye shield was placed in the 14 casualties referred for ophthalmic consultation [3].

Many factors contribute to this: Life-threatening injuries must always take precedence to the eye; in the chaos of combat, other nonlethal wounds may be more visible or gruesome and attract more immediate attention; and it may be difficult to recognize an eye injury in the presence of debris, blood, coagulum, and other contamination.

In addition, many non-ophthalmic medical providers are uncomfortable when dealing with eye injuries.

During aeromedical evacuation (AE), appropriate medical care of ocular casualties is essential. The goal is to prevent further eye injury while providing rapid and efficient transportation to an appropriate facility capable of providing the required ophthalmologic care. This could be a medical treatment facility (MTF) either intra-theater or a continent away.

N. A. Jordan (✉)
MAJ, MC, USA, Department of Surgery, Tripler Army Medical Center, Uniformed Services University of the Health Sciences, Honolulu, HI, USA
e-mail: nathan.a.jordan6.mil@mail.mil

R. A. Mazzoli
COL, MC, USA (ret.), Department of Ophthalmology, Ophthalmic Plastic, Reconstructive, and Orbital Surgery, Madigan Army Medical Center, Tacoma, WA, USA

Uniformed Services University of the Health Sciences, Bethesda, MD, USA

Former Consultant to the US Army Surgeon General, DoD-VA Vision Center of Excellence, Bethesda, MD, USA

B. Propes
CDR, MC, USN, Department of Ophthalmology, Naval Medical Center San Diego, San Diego, CA, USA

J. A. Egan
Department of Ophthalmology, Madigan Army Medical Center, Tacoma, WA, USA

DoD-VA Vision Center of Excellence, Bethesda, MD, USA

W. W. Hurd, W. Beninati (eds.), *Aeromedical Evacuation*,
https://doi.org/10.1007/978-3-030-15903-0_14

The aim of this chapter is to provide information that will assist AE personnel in providing appropriate and seamless care across the numerous echelons, locations, and transitions of care. This chapter describes the nature and environment of combat eye injuries, clinical evaluation of the eye, and emergency care for ocular injuries. Next, we describe AE patient regulation and other AE considerations for patients with ocular injuries. The chapter concludes with descriptions of common ocular injuries and their AE implications.

Combat Eye Injuries

The modern battlefield is characterized by numerous hazards that increase the risk of eye injuries. Most common in traditional warfare are the conventional gunshot wounds and thermal burns. Modern warfare has seen the increased use of high-energy explosive fragmentary munitions, such as artillery, mortars, hand-thrown and rifle-propelled grenades, fragmentary mines, and improvised explosive devices. High-explosive fragmentary munitions create particularly devastating injuries, the hallmark being systemic polytrauma wherein multiple body organs and regions are injured simultaneously [4]. Likewise, combat ocular injuries themselves represent ocular polytrauma, with multiple ocular structures being involved.

Combat Eye Protection and Eye Injuries

The eye and face are necessarily and preferentially exposed to combat injury. This is because combat is an intensely visual activity with survival in the balance: If you cannot see, you cannot shoot. In fact, despite representing only 0.1% of the total body surface area, eye injuries account for an inordinate and increasing proportion of modern combat injuries [5, 6]. As a result, anti-ballistic eye protection ("eyepro") has become a high priority in the US military.

Modern military anti-ballistic eye protection has greatly decreased the incidence of eye injury, but it has limitations. While it provides significant protection against small fragments and shrapnel, historically the predominant cause of penetrating combat eye injuries, it is not as effective against primary effects of blast overpressure, leading to the potential of significant nonpenetrating injuries [7–10]. Additionally, blasts can dislodge the eye protection, exposing the eye to the secondary debris wind and tertiary and quaternary blast effects. Furthermore, because combatants are understandably reluctant to put anything in front of their eyes that they feel might degrade their vision, compliance with wearing eye protection is not assured. Consequently, eye injuries continue to account for 6–19% of combat injuries [6, 11, 12].

Evaluating Patients With Ocular Injuries

History

A careful history should be obtained from a conscious patient. Important details to determine are:

- What the patient was doing at the time of the injury
- What hit or came into contact with the eye
- Was eye protection worn during the injury
- Any chemicals that might have been involved
- Any treatment given since the injury

Eye Examination

The examination of the eye begins with a visual acuity evaluation, which is the single most important piece of information concerning an ocular injury (Table 14.1). Visual acuity is the vital sign of the eye, and its initial evaluation provides a baseline for further monitoring. It is an accurate indication of the severity of an ocular injury and carries important triage and prognostic implications: The worse the visual acuity, the more profound the injury; the worse the prognosis, and the

Table 14.1 Initial care for patients with ocular injuries

History	Circumstances of injury, including eye protection status Chemical injury Surgical procedures and treatments since injury
Initial examination	Visual acuity is the most important part, the eye's vital sign All caretakers should know how to evaluate vision without an eye chart Do not put any pressure on a potentially open globe injury Close external visual inspection of each eye Pupils (look for retained contact lenses at the same time) Ocular motility Confrontation visual fields Intraocular pressure (do not attempt in open globe)
Shield and ship	Place and maintain a rigid eye shield ("Shield") that vaults cleanly over the injured eye without any dressing underneath (e.g., eye pads or gauze) Transport ("Ship") to the nearest ophthalmologist for evaluation and treatment Patients should see an ophthalmologist within 8–12 hours Continue prescribed medications (See Table 14.2)

Table 14.2 CATS mnemonic for initial treatment of ocular trauma

C	Computerized tomography
A	**A**ntibiotics, **a**ntiemetics, and **a**nalgesics
T	Tetanus
S	Shield

more urgent the need to evacuate the patient to see an ophthalmologist. However, retained visual acuity in the presence of a serious ocular injury does not justify delaying evacuation for immediate ophthalmic attention.

Each eye should be tested separately with occlusion of the opposite eye with the patient wearing any prescribed corrective lenses, if available. It is insufficient to simply document that vision is "normal" after an ocular injury. Reasonably accurate evaluation of visual acuity can be done with a Snellen acuity chart viewed from a distance of 6 feet or a pocket vision screener card held about 14 inches from the face. For patients who do not read English, a chart of symbols, pictures, or a "tumbling E" can be substituted.

Lacking a formal eye chart, the examiner should document visual acuity using the Army Combat Optotype (i.e., military name tapes, rank insignias, patches, emblems, and helmet camouflage bands) (Fig. 14.1) or any printed materials (e.g., newspapers, medical wrappers, and identification [ID] badge print) [13]. Visual acuity should be documented as the smallest readable print and the distance, e.g., "helmet band letters at 3 feet" and "name on ID badge at 2 feet."

If a patient is unable to identify any printed letters or symbols, it remains important to quantify the patient's best vision. Gross tests of vision include (in order of worsening function):

- Count fingers (CF)
- Detect hand motion (HM)
- Light perception with projection (bright light shined from various angles) (LPj)
- Light perception (bright light shined at the affected eye) (LP)
- No light perception (NLP)

Documentation should indicate the best vision obtained and the distance, e.g., "count fingers at 5 feet" and "light perception at 6 inches."

The next part of the examination after testing visual acuity is close visual inspection of each eye. The pupils should be examined for size, shape, and reactivity to light, noting any differences between the two pupils. It should be documented if the pupils are either round and centered or changed in shape, size, or symmetry. A distorted or displaced pupil, particularly if "peaked" or "teardrop" shaped, suggests an open globe injury regardless of visual acuity and constitutes an ophthalmologic emergency.

Eye motility should be assessed by having the patient gaze in different directions. This can be prompted by having the patient follow a finger moved in an H-pattern and noting any restricted movement or diplopia. Visual fields should be

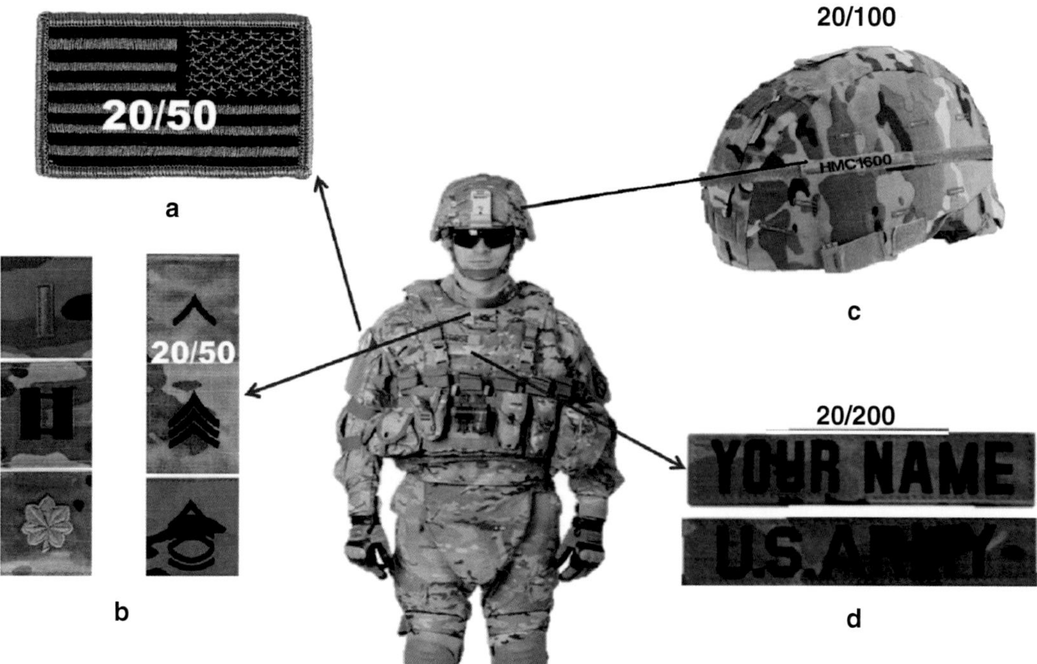

Fig. 14.1 Army combat optotypes for rapid field estimation of visual acuity. The ability to see uniform parts at various distances corresponds to the following visual acuities: (**a**) stripes on a flag arm patch at 3 feet, 20/50; (**b**) chevrons at 2 feet, 20/50; (**c**) helmet band letters at 3 feet, 20/100; (**d**) name tape at 5 feet, 20/200. (Adapted from Ref. [13])

grossly evaluated for each eye by having the patient cover the opposite eye and count the examiner's fingers presented in the four quadrants.

The final component of an initial eye exam is intraocular pressure. However, if there is *any* suspicion of an open globe injury, absolutely *no pressure should be applied* to the eye, and intraocular pressure determination should be deferred to an ophthalmologist after evacuation. Without suspicion of an open globe injury, a tonometer can be used to quantify intraocular pressure. If a tonometer is unavailable, the examiner can gently palpate the closed eye and compare the resistance to the opposite eye.

Eye Glasses and Contact Lenses

During any type of injury and subsequent evacuation, glasses are commonly irreparably damaged or lost. Patients without ocular trauma but with significant baseline visual impairment can be rendered functionally blind without their glasses and might require assistance until replacement glasses can be procured. If such a patient has lost their glasses, this should be documented and passed on to the patient's caregivers so that replacements can be obtained as soon as possible.

Military members are prohibited from wearing contact lenses in a combat zone. However, this does not completely preclude their use. Previously undetected contact lenses will occasionally be discovered in seriously injured patients during pupil exams. These patients are at increased risk of corneal ulcers as described later in this chapter.

When a contact lens is discovered, a gentle attempt at removal may be made. However, if an apparent contact lens resists removal, it should not be forced since a dislocated refractive laser LASIK flap can resemble a contact lens. When a previously undetected contact lens is discovered during an AE flight, the arriving facility should be alerted so that prompt ophthalmic evaluation can be arranged.

Emergency Ocular Injury Care

The care of eye injuries in a combat environment is complicated by several factors. Principally, the eye is notoriously intolerant of both injury and inappropriate treatment thereafter. Second, only ophthalmologists can effectively treat significant eye injuries. Therefore, patients with eye injuries must reach ophthalmic care as soon as possible. Third, there is usually a substantial distance between the point of injury and initial ophthalmic capabilities in theater. Likewise, there are even greater distances to more specialized care at higher echelons. Clearly, it is critical to provide proper care at every level and through every transfer in order to mitigate the injury and enhance the chances of preserving sight.

Initial Evaluation and Treatment

Initial evaluation and treatment should include several items in addition to an eye shield, except in the most austere environments. A "CATS" mnemonic (Table 14.2) can be used to remember the initial evaluation and care that should be delivered prior to transport to definitive ophthalmic care. However, the two most important aspects of emergency care for patients with serious eye injuries are to (1) protect the eye and (2) immediately transport to an ophthalmologist—a dictum often stated as "Shield and Ship" [14, 15].

CATS mnemonic:

- *"C"—Computerized tomography (CT)*—An orbital/facial protocol axial CT scan should be obtained if readily available and all images transferred with the patient. Only reconstructed coronal and sagittal views are recommended, since positioning for true coronal imaging has a high potential for extruding intraocular contents in patients with open globe injuries. All images should be transferred with the patient, even if only plain skull films are performed.
- *"A"—Antibiotics, antiemetics, and analgesics*—Open globe injuries expose the intraocular contents to new environmental pathogens and thus carry a high risk of intraocular infection (i.e., endophthalmitis), particularly in the presence of intraocular foreign bodies. Thus, prophylactic systemic antibiotics should be administered upon suspicion of an open globe injury and continued until the patient has been evaluated by an ophthalmologist. Current clinical practice guidelines recommend initial treatment with systemic fourth-generation fluoroquinolones (e.g., moxifloxacin or levofloxacin) because of their good intravitreal penetration [14, 15]. Cefazolin or vancomycin is also commonly added [16].

  Antiemetics and analgesics should also be administered in an effort to minimize the risk of Valsalva reactions secondary to vomiting, retching, or pain, which could result in expulsion of intraocular contents. Analgesic doses of ketamine, commonly used in the field to treat systemic polytrauma casualties, are not contraindicated in patients with open globe injuries [14, 15].

- *"T"—Tetanus*—The tetanus status of the patient should be confirmed and a booster given if necessary.
- *"S"—Shield*—The goal of an eye shield is to make certain that no direct pressure is applied to the globe in order to reduce the risk of further extrusion of intraocular contents and damage. For this reason, the shield should be applied such that its points of contact are on the bony structures of the orbital rim and the forehead, and not on the globe itself. Standard convex ophthalmic shields have protected edges and are perforated to provide for air circulation (Fig. 14.2, patient's right). No patch, gauze, or dressing of any kind should be placed underneath the shield to avoid applying pressure to the open globe. If a standard ophthalmic shield is not available, a makeshift shield can be fashioned from any rigid, convex structure (Fig. 14.2, patient's left), including the patient's own anti--ballistic polycarbonate eye protection. In cases of concomitant head and/or facial trauma requiring a tight head wrap, rigid eye shields

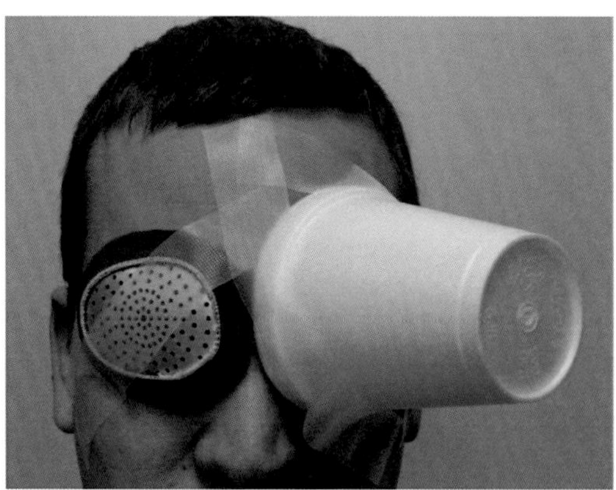

Fig. 14.2 Standard and makeshift eye shields. In the field, injured eyes can be shielded with a standard convex ophthalmic shield (right eye) or any rigid, convex structure (left eye). The patient's own ballistic eye protection can be used primarily as well (see Fig. 14.3). (Photo by Robert A. Mazzoli)

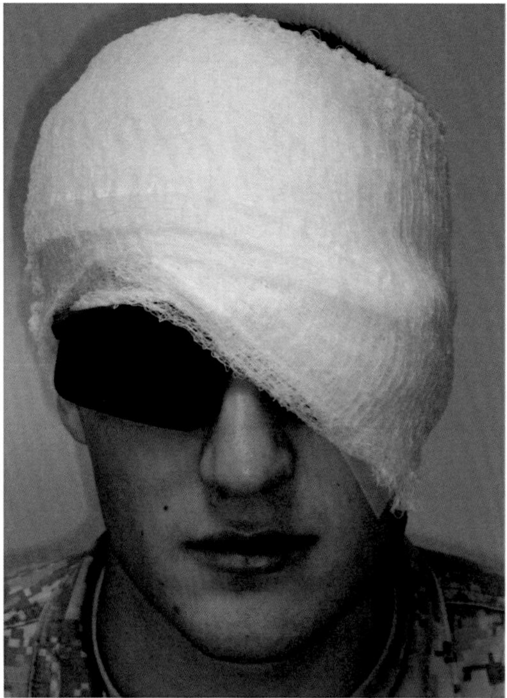

Fig. 14.3 A makeshift eye shield under a head wrap dressing. When a tight head wrap dressing is required for head or facial trauma, rigid eye shields should be placed over the eyes beneath the dressing. (Photo by Robert A. Mazzoli)

should be placed over the eyes beneath the dressings or wraps whether the eye is injured or not (Fig. 14.3).

An eye shield should remain in place throughout the evacuation process and only be removed when examination or eye medication is necessary. The eye shield should be promptly replaced afterward and remain in place until the patient reaches definitive care.

Damage Control Ophthalmology

In-theater ophthalmic care is often limited to damage control ophthalmology. The goal is immediate stabilization of the globe and setting a foundation for further revisions and interventions at more sophisticated facilities outside the theater of operations. The immediate objectives are watertight closure of an open globe, properly managing herniating intraocular tissues, providing adequate corneal coverage, and preventing subsequent intraocular infection. This is followed by Urgent AE to an ophthalmologist at a higher echelon of care.

Damage control ophthalmology principles also apply when time for intervention is limited, such as in the setting of mass casualties; during expeditionary, insertion, or high-movement phases of combat, when the fluidity of combat operations demands rapid and limited interventions; or during times of rapid AE evacuation. In other circumstances, such as when casualty arrival or evacuation is delayed or in host national care, the ophthalmologist may find himself doing more extensive and even definitive procedures at the first intent.

Aeromedical Evacuation Considerations for Ocular Casualties

Aeromedical Evacuation Regulation

It is essential that theater medical regulating and AE personnel are made aware of ocular injuries so that these casualties can receive proper and timely attention (Table 14.3). It is imperative not to overlook the ocular diagnosis in a patient with multiple serious injuries. In this regard, even

Table 14.3 Aeromedical evacuation (AE) regulating for patients with ocular injuries

Patients with ocular injuries should be evacuated to a facility with an ophthalmologist
True ocular emergencies should be classified as Urgent:
Retinal tears and detachment
Penetrating ocular trauma
Chemical injuries
Orbital compartment syndrome
Acute glaucoma
When returning to the continental United States:
Serious ocular injuries require treatment by subspecialty-trained ophthalmologists
Patients should be regulated to the regional ophthalmic specialty care center closest to their home station

nonpenetrating injuries must be considered as a potentially severe threat to vision. Remember: Life, Sight, and Limb.

AE regulators should know where various ophthalmic assets are located within theater and their various capabilities, including optometric and spectacle fabrication capabilities [17]. It is important to remember that theater ophthalmic surgical assets are typically very limited and that each service is likely to have its own ophthalmic providers, each with potentially different capabilities. Early consultation with the theater ophthalmic consultant (typically the most senior ophthalmologist in theater) can help ensure the casualty is sent to the most appropriate facility.

Head and Neck Teams

Theater ophthalmic surgical assets are almost always co-located with Head and Neck Teams consisting of an ophthalmologist, otolaryngologist, neurosurgeon, and/or an oral-maxillofacial surgeon [18]. The rationale for these teams is the predictable coexistence of such wounds in modern combat: More than 60% of ocular injuries will have an associated facial, intracranial, or neck injury; 30% of penetrating head injuries are associated with eye injuries; and more than 20% of eye injuries have associated head injuries [19].

Head and Neck Teams are usually deployed as theater-level assets distributed at specified locations within a combat zone. Each service branch follows its own distribution and logistical doctrine to augment basic Role 3 MTFs, although not every Role 3 MTF will have an ophthalmologist. The US Army teams are quickly mobile and sometimes less robustly equipped than other services because they are often deployed early in the conflict, in greater numbers, and in relatively forward locations during the expeditionary and maneuver phases of a conflict. US Air Force and US Navy teams typically deploy their teams later during a conflict to more stable and developed locations. Whereas every Role 3 MTF with ophthalmic capability will be able to take care of a casualty's systemic polytrauma, not every Role 3 MTF capable of handling polytrauma will be prepared to evaluate and treat a serious eye injury. Hence, it is essential that theater medical regulating personnel stay abreast of evolving ocular capabilities and locations.

Theater casualty regulators must also be aware of the full extent of each casualty's injuries, paying particular attention to eye, head, and neck injuries. Special care should be taken to assure that eye injuries do not get overlooked in the list of a patient's polytrauma. Overlooking this may lead to inappropriately sending an eye casualty to an inadequate facility [17, 20]. Therefore, unless immediate life-saving measures dictate otherwise, casualties with known or suspected ocular trauma should preferentially be regulated to the nearest ophthalmic facility (remember: Life, Sight, and Limb). Efforts should be made to minimize transfers, stopovers, treatment delays, and physical movements that have the potential to aggravate the ocular injury and jeopardize prognosis [20].

Ophthalmology Subspecialists and Strategic Regulation

Serious ocular injuries often require specialized care by a collaborative team of ophthalmic subspecialists, often working in close cooperation with other trauma and rehabilitation specialists [21]. A serious ocular injury may require the simultaneous and collaborative efforts of a cornea specialist, a retina specialist, a glaucoma specialist, an oculoplastic/orbit/reconstructive specialist, a neuro-ophthalmologist, *and* a strabismologist, in addition to specialty optometrists and appropriate vision rehabilitation specialists. At least nine ophthalmologic subspecialties are currently recognized today.

The supply of these subspecialists is exceptionally limited in the US Department of Defense (DoD). As a result, knowing that a facility has *an* ophthalmologist on staff does not guarantee that the facility has *the correct* ophthalmologist. A facility with specialty ophthalmologists can care for non-specialty eye conditions, but a facility without specialty ophthalmologists cannot care for specialty needs.

At overseas facilities, the limited supply of military subspecialists limits the predictable ability to provide ophthalmologic care. Most Role 4 MTFs can provide definitive surgery and medical care for most combat-related injuries, but for eye injuries, these facilities usually provide only pass-through care. These facilities are typically neither staffed nor equipped to perform definitive eye surgeries required of ocular polytrauma. When urgent complex ocular surgery is required, these casualties are either referred to local civilian facilities for acute specialty intervention or rapidly returned to an appropriate military ocular specialty care center in the continental United States. For these patients, every effort must be made to avoid en route delays in the AE system (i.e., re-routings, diversions, overnight stays, etc.) since these can adversely affect the ultimate outcome of serious eye injuries.

When casualties with eye injuries return to the continental United States, every attempt should be made to regulate them to their home region as soon as possible. Fortunately, regional military ocular specialty care centers are geographically distributed across the country, and each has virtually identical fundamental capabilities. These ocular specialty care centers and the specialty ophthalmologists assigned there are almost exclusively found at the military MTFs with ophthalmic residency programs, which are invariably located at academic military medical centers. This is because residency accreditation is contingent on robust subspecialty staffing and because residencies require ancillary support of medical, surgical, specialty optometric, and blind rehabilitation services, as well as advanced neurodiagnostics, pathology, and research support.

US military ocular specialty care centers are currently located at four locations:

- Walter Reed National Military Medical Center in Bethesda, Maryland
- San Antonio Military Medical Center in San Antonio, Texas
- Naval Medical Center San Diego in San Diego, California
- Madigan Army Medical Center in Tacoma, Washington.

Aeromedical Evacuation Precedence for Ocular Injury Patients

Each patient is assigned a movement precedence category by AE personnel based on their condition and associated medical needs. Each patient's precedence category allows AE planners to assure that patients are moved in an appropriately timely fashion with the appropriate personnel and equipment. The three standard precedence categories are (1) Routine, AE on the next scheduled flight; (2) Priority, AE within 24 hours; and (3) Urgent, AE as soon as possible to save life, limb, or eyesight [22].

It is incumbent on the clinician to communicate clearly the needed casualty arrival window to AE regulating personnel. Patients with true ocular emergencies should be given an Urgent precedence category. These include retinal tears and detachment, penetrating ocular trauma, chemical injuries, orbital compartment syndrome, and acute glaucoma, which can result from ocular trauma. Patients with less serious ocular injuries can be categorized as Priority.

Patients with ocular injuries should not be categorized as "Routine." AE patients with Routine precedence often do not reach their final destination for a number of days because of the multiple requirements of the global AE system. A Routine patient scheduled for a relatively short AE flight might not depart for several days, and the mission might involve a multiday transit with several overnight stays along the way.

Enplaning and Deplaning Considerations

Patients with serious ocular injuries require special considerations during AE that might not be as obvious as for major trauma patients. A thorough understanding of the needs of these patients will decrease the chance of permanent loss of vision for these patients (Table 14.4).

Ocular injury patients with bilateral vision impairment and those with serious unilateral ocular injuries may require physical assistance to board the aircraft and should be transported as litter patients. Ocular casualties (as well as patients with poor vision who have lost their glasses) are at a physical disadvantage. If vision is lost in only one eye, the loss of stereo vision limits depth perception and increases fall hazards. Some patients will require assistance with eating and toilet functions. Assistive fact sheets and instructions for both outpatient and inpatient care of visually impaired patients are available online [23, 24].

Patients with serious ocular injuries should avoid any activity that would cause them to use Valsalva maneuver, including lifting, sitting up unassisted, or straining. Ambulatory ocular casualties, including those who are recently postoperative or have nonpenetrating trauma, should not be allowed to carry luggage or strain. Similarly, medical personnel should avoid procedures that might induce increased central venous pressure, gagging, or retching, such as intubation or orogastric suctioning while awake.

Table 14.4 Enplaning and deplaning of patients with ocular injuries

Minimize movements and straining:
  Transport as litter patients when possible
  Do not let ambulatory patients with ocular injuries lift baggage

Patients with ocular injuries or lost glasses are visually impaired:
  Ambulatory will need assistance navigating aircraft obstacles
  Be familiar with sighted guide techniques
  Patients may need assistance with eating and bodily functions, especially if litter

Patient Medications and Monitoring

Important considerations for caring for patients with ocular injuries include ocular medications and monitoring for signs and symptoms of ocular deterioration (Table 14.5). Ocular medications should be administered as prescribed and documented. Self-administration of medications should be avoided for patients with ocular injuries. If necessary, patients should be closely monitored and compliance documented.

AE personnel should be familiar with signs and symptoms of ocular deterioration. Concerning symptoms include decreasing vision,

Table 14.5 In-flight care for ocular injuries

Patient monitoring	Postoperative patients: ocular shields are usually not removed during aeromedical evacuation Remove and replace shields to administer ocular medications en route as ordered Self-administration of ocular medications is discouraged Periodic ocular examinations as ordered
Signs of an ocular emergency	Sudden increase in ocular pain Headache Nausea/vomiting Decreasing vision Diplopia Increasing proptosis Abnormal pupillary reaction to light Increased intraocular pressure Flashing lights, new "floaters," or "curtain" visual field defect

Management of sudden onset of severe pain	Treat pain
	Examine the eye, including visual acuity
	Differential diagnosis:
	  Orbital compartment syndrome
	  Acute glaucoma
	Obtain en route ophthalmologic consultation
	Consider increasing cabin pressure or descent if air/gas expansion is suspected
	Divert to nearest medical treatment facility with ophthalmologic care if necessary

ocular pain or headache, nausea/vomiting, diplopia, flashing lights with new onset floaters, or a "curtain" visual field defect. New onset of any of these signs or symptoms should prompt an examination of the eye, and overlooking them can impact outcome. Physical findings that are concerning for a worsening ocular condition and possibly increased intraocular pressure include decreased or asymmetric pupillary reaction to light, increased pain, increasing eye protrusion (proptosis), or increased firmness of an eye.

In-Flight Emergencies

True ocular emergencies require prompt recognition and urgent care by an ophthalmologist to maximize the chance of preserving vision (Table 14.5). Emergencies that might first become apparent during an AE flight include orbital compartment syndrome and acute glaucoma, both of which are relatively common after serious ocular trauma. When either is suspected, in-flight ophthalmologic consultation should be obtained and flight diversion to the nearest facility with ophthalmologic care should be considered. The symptoms and findings of these conditions can overlap and are described in the following section.

Specific Ocular Injuries and Conditions

Open Globe Injuries

Open globe injuries (also referred to as penetrating ocular trauma) are among the most devastating ocular injuries. The eye is a watertight structure and is the most forward extension of the brain, with no ability to regenerate. Anytime the integrity of the globe is compromised, the consequences can be severe.

The final visual outcome can vary widely, depending on the ocular tissue disrupted: The lid and cornea may mend; the retina will not. Because combat trauma usually represents ocular polytrauma with more than one ocular structure involved, the prognosis for combat-related open globe injury remains grim. In Operations Iraqi Freedom and Enduring Freedom in Afghanistan, 75% of open globe injuries resulted in a best-corrected visual acuity of 20/200 or worse [25].

Most commonly, open globe injuries result from penetrating lacerations of the cornea or sclera or both (an "outside-in" injury) with or without a retained foreign body. However, significant blunt force trauma can also rupture the globe (an "inside-out" injury). Defects may affect either the anterior or posterior segments of the globe, or both. Thus, open globe injuries must be excluded regardless of the apparent mechanism of injury.

Open globe injuries represent the most dire ocular condition and must be treated emergently by skilled ophthalmologists. Unlike injuries elsewhere, an inviolable guiding dictum in treating open globe injuries is "there is no such thing as delayed primary closure of an open globe" [20]. Optimally, closure should be accomplished within 8–12 hours for the best outcome.

Aeromedical Evacuation Considerations

An open globe injury is an ophthalmologic emergency and should be given an AE precedence classification of Urgent, regardless of etiology. While the prognosis for any open globe injury is guarded, the patient will have the best chance of an optimal outcome if they reach definitive ophthalmic care quickly after the injury.

AE personnel should ensure that no eye casualty is transported without an eye shield. Patients with open globe injuries, regardless of level of consciousness, should be transported as litter patients, since even minor additional trauma to the affected eye could have devastating consequences. These patients should be transported in a semi-recumbent position with the head elevated at least 15–30°. Trendelenburg position (head-down) should be avoided.

Aircraft cabin altitude restriction is not routinely required for patients with open globe injuries. An exception is the rare instance in which imaging or examination demonstrates air within the globe, in which case maintaining cabin altitude pressure near sea level (or the highest airport altitude) is a reasonable precaution, if feasible. This subject is considered further below (see sections "Orbital Compartment Syndrome" and "Intraocular Gas").

During transport, every effort should be made to minimize the risk of increased intraocular pressure that could lead to extrusion of intraocular contents. Conscious patients can close both eyes for comfort and to reduce the pressure on the globe from the extraocular muscles, but there is no need to shield both eyes if only one is injured.

Nausea and pain in these patients should be aggressively treated with antiemetics and analgesics. Intubated patients with open globe injuries should be deeply sedated to avoid dyssynchrony with the ventilator (i.e., bucking) since this increases the risk of extruding intraocular contents.

Chemical Eye Injuries

Chemical eye injuries are common in both military and civilian environments. Common agents include acids, alkalis, solvents, fuels, and industrial detergents. While all are toxic and can cause significant injuries, alkalis are typically the most harmful.

Treatment for any chemical exposure of the eyes is immediate copious irrigation with the cleanest water available. Irrigation should take precedence over all other aspects of eye care, with "dilution being the solution to pollution." No attempt should be made to neutralize the chemical agent.

The preferred irrigation technique utilizes liters of electrolyte solutions, e.g., normal saline or lactated Ringers. However, any clean, nontoxic fluid will suffice. A topical anesthetic, if available, should be applied first because of the extended times required for irrigation. The process can be simplified by using an irrigating contact lens (Morgan lens) or nasal prongs placed over the nasal root and directed toward the eyes (Fig. 14.4). Irrigation should be continued for 30 minutes or longer, until the pH of the injured eye determined by urine test strips returns to approximately 7.4, or similar to the contralateral eye.

After extensive irrigation, the eyes should be inspected thoroughly, and any remaining particulate debris swept away with moistened cotton-tipped applicators. Ophthalmic antibiotic ointment should be instilled into the affected eyes and eye shields applied. Pain should be treated with oral analgesics. The patient should be immediately transported to an ophthalmologist.

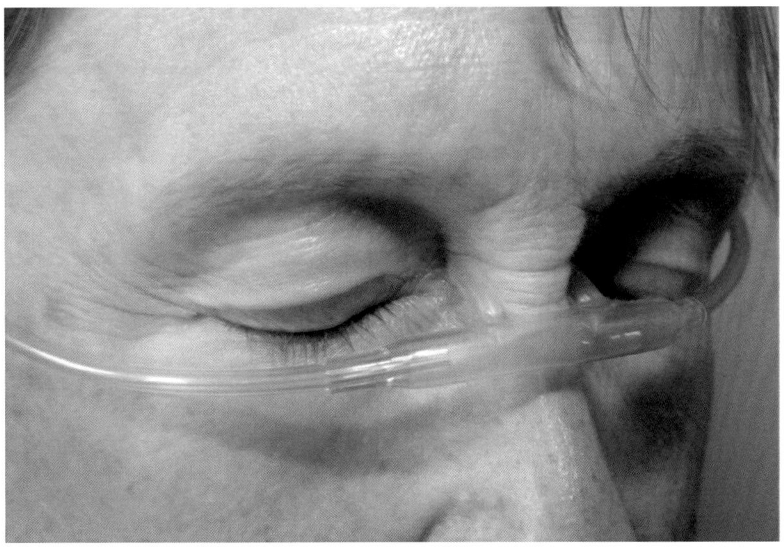

Fig. 14.4 Ocular irrigation. Nasal prongs placed over the nasal root and directed to the medial eye canthi can be used for eye irrigation after chemical exposure. (Photo by Robert A. Mazzoli)

Aeromedical Evacuation Considerations

Eye irrigation for patients with chemical exposure of the eyes should be finished prior to long-distance AE. Rarely, eye irrigation will have to be continued during transport. In either case, these patients should be given an AE precedence classification of Urgent. Those with bilateral eye involvement will be functionally blind and require litter transportation. Most patients with unilateral eye involvement can be transported as ambulatory patients unless loss of stereo vision has resulted in depth perception problems. An adequate supply of pain medication should be available to keep the patient comfortable during transport.

Orbital Compartment Syndrome

Orbital compartment syndrome is a vision-threatening condition caused by acute elevation of intraorbital pressure within the confined bony orbit—the eye socket of the skull. The orbit, like the abdomen and extremities, is a compartment, with expansion limited by the rigid bony walls posteriorly and the inelastic orbital septum and eyelids anteriorly [26]. Orbital compartment syndrome ensues when the pressure in the orbit exceeds ocular perfusion pressure. The result is retinal ischemia and rapid development of ischemic optic neuropathy. Without intervention within 60–90 minutes, the outcome is permanent blindness.

Orbital compartment syndrome most commonly occurs after either blunt or penetrating orbital/facial trauma resulting in a traumatic retrobulbar hematoma, particularly in patients who are on anticoagulants. Less common etiologies include third spacing of fluid after a massive resuscitation, particularly after a burn injury [26], compressive pneumo-orbita from air expansion after sino-orbital fracture or other pneumatic injury [27], hyper- and hypobaric exposure, and orbital cellulitis with subperiosteal abscess. Drainage pathways provided by orbital fracture and sino-orbital communication do not protect against hemorrhagic orbital compartment syndrome.

The diagnosis of orbital compartment syndrome is purely clinical and based on the findings of acute pain; tense eye protrusion (proptosis); profoundly decreasing vision; conjunctival edema (chemosis), which is usually hemorrhagic; increased intraocular pressure; decreased light-induced pupillary constriction (afferent pupillary defect); and decreased extraocular motility. Intense ocular pain is often accompanied by nausea and vomiting. Gentle palpation of the lids and orbit discloses a "rock hard" orbit. It should be noted that this is one of the few times it is acceptable to palpate a traumatized eye.

When orbital compartment syndrome is diagnosed, the required treatment is immediate lateral canthotomy and inferior cantholysis [28]. This bedside procedure decompresses the orbital compartment by releasing the lower lid and opening the septum. It is the ocular equivalent of a decompressive fasciotomy and, when completed properly, will immediately reduce the intraorbital pressure and restore retinal and optic nerve perfusion. Steps include making a 1 cm full-thickness scissors cut across the lateral canthus to the lateral bony orbital rim (canthotomy), then turning the scissors inferiorly to make a 1 cm full-thickness cut across the lateral eyelid and septum, directed toward the corner of the mouth or nasal ala (cantholysis). This procedure must be performed within 60–90 minutes of diagnosis and should not be delayed for imaging or transfer to an ophthalmologist. However, this procedure should not be attempted by personnel who have not received hands-on training in the technique.

Aeromedical Evacuation Implications

When orbital compartment syndrome occurs prior to AE, the patient should have already undergone a lateral canthotomy and inferior cantholysis. These patients should be given an AE precedence classification of Urgent and transported by litter.

A greater AE concern is patients with facial trauma who develop orbital compartment syndrome during an AE flight. It is important for AE personnel to recognize the signs and symptoms of this condition when transporting patients after significant eye trauma or who have recently received massive fluid resuscitation. These patients should be examined closely for visual acuity, orbital pressure, and, if possible, intraocular pressure while in the AE system. If orbital compartment syndrome is suspected, immediate en route consultation is recommended, with consideration for diversion to an emergency facility with the ability to perform a lateral canthotomy and inferior cantholysis. If suspected to be secondary to compressive pneumo-orbita, descent or increasing cabin altitude pressure may be therapeutic.

Acute Glaucoma

Glaucoma refers to increased intraocular pressure and can result in permanent loss of sight. Acute glaucoma (i.e., acute angle-closure glaucoma) is a painful, suddenly increased pressure in the eye secondary to acute blockage of the normal circulation and outflow of aqueous fluid. As a result, normal intraocular pressures of 10–20 mm Hg rise acutely to 40–60 mm Hg. This is in contrast to chronic glaucoma (i.e., primary open-angle glaucoma)—a painless, age-related condition characterized by slowly increasing intraocular pressure to levels of 25–30 mm Hg. While chronic glaucoma usually affects both eyes, acute glaucoma is more likely monocular.

Acute glaucoma can be the result of eye trauma, although it usually occurs spontaneously. Either penetrating or blunt ocular trauma can result in acute glaucoma by disrupting the pressure-regulating mechanism of the eye (the trabecular meshwork), which resides in the "angle" of the anterior chamber. These patients can have delayed angle blockage secondary to intraocular hemorrhage from either hyphema or vitreous hemorrhage or from blood cell casts (i.e., "ghost cells").

The hallmark of acute glaucoma is intense ocular pain, often described as an intense headache, "brow ache," or "eye ache" [29]. This pain can become so intense that it results in nausea and vomiting. Signs of acute glaucoma include eye redness; decreasing vision, often associated with halos around lights; visible corneal edema and cloudiness; mid-dilated and nonreactive pupil; and dramatically elevated intraocular pressures. When a tonometer is not available, this increased pressure can be detected by gentle digital palpation of the eyes. The affected eye will feel much more tense and tender compared to the contralateral eye.

Aeromedical Evacuation Implications

Acute glaucoma can occur any time after significant eye trauma and may occur during AE en route to an ophthalmologist [30]. AE personnel should be aware that sudden onset of extreme ocular pain may be a sign of acute glaucoma. Most eye injury pain, even postoperative, is well controlled by normal pain medications and does not abruptly increase. Therefore, an acute increase in eye pain in these patients is a cause for increased concern, especially when associated with nausea, vomiting, and decreasing vision. Rather than simply treating the pain, these patients should be evaluated for acute glaucoma and en route consultation obtained if symptoms persist.

If acute glaucoma is suspected during an AE flight, the only en route treatment available is pain medication. It is imperative that the patient be evaluated by an ophthalmologist as soon as possible after landing at the next scheduled stop. For this reason, it is important to alert the receiving medical personnel about the situation prior to landing. Flight diversion should be considered if there are no ophthalmologic resources available at the scheduled stop.

Retinal Tears and Detachment

A retinal tear is a rip in the retina without separation of the retina from the underlying tissue. Retinal tears create a pathway for vitreous fluid to enter the subretinal space and are at significant risk of quickly progressing to retinal detachment, where the retina pulls away from the underlying retinal pigment epithelium. Both tears and detachments are common in the general population but are also common consequences of blunt and penetrating eye trauma. Both are often associated with significant vitreous hemorrhage. They are considered true ocular and medical emergencies since retinal detachment can result in permanent loss of vision. Consequently, patients being transferred with either diagnosis should receive an Urgent AE precedence.

Symptoms include flashing lights, the sudden onset of multiple small black "floaters" in one eye, the sensation of a curtain or veil coming over the vision, or loss of visual acuity. However, retinal detachment cannot be definitively diagnosed by symptoms alone but requires detailed ophthalmic examination, which should be done promptly after the onset of suggestive symptoms.

Once a retinal tear or detachment has been diagnosed, multiple surgical treatment options exist and are successful in restoring vision to some degree in 90% of patients. Specific treatments are tailored to the individual patient but can include laser or cryotherapy retinopexy, extraocular scleral buckling, intraocular vitrectomy with infusion of a variety of surgical gasses or fluids, or a combination of all. The selection of procedure can dramatically impact (and can be impacted by) eventual AE requirements.

The primary factors affecting prognosis include visual acuity, the cause and nature of the detachment, and the anatomic extent. Prompt treatment maximizes visual outcome; however, delay can allow progression of a limited retinal detachment (with an excellent prognosis) to a detachment that includes the macula, requiring more extensive surgery and most likely poorer vision after treatment.

Aeromedical Evacuation Implications

Patients with symptoms consistent with retinal tear or detachment should be given an Urgent AE precedence classification since expedient diagnosis and treatment by an ophthalmologist are necessary to preserve vision. A baseline visual evaluation should be documented prior to AE by the sending medical team so that the receiving ophthalmologist can judge progression. This should include visual acuity and confrontation visual fields checked for each eye separately prior to departure and rechecked during any layover.

AE patients with suspected retinal detachments should be transported as litter patients so that the patient can remain as immobile as possible during the flight. Minimizing rapid eye movements by avoiding activities such as reading, operating a smart phone, and playing video games may decrease the movement of fluid into the subretinal space and reduce the risk of extension, while promoting spontaneous absorption.

Intraocular Gas

Expansile surgical gasses are often used to treat retinal detachments. In addition, intraocular air can result after open globe injury or ocular surgery. It is well appreciated that the intraocular gasses most commonly used to treat retinal detachments expand to approximately two to four times their original volumes within 2 days after surgery depending on the type of gas used. Decreased cabin pressure at cruise altitude will increase the volume of any gas by an additional 33%. This expansion at altitude can cause a dramatic rise in intraocular pressure and ultimately affect retinal perfusion. Additionally, the increased volume can cause gas to extrude through any surgical incisions or traumatic wounds into the orbit and cause pneumo-orbital compartment syndrome [27] (see section "Orbital Compartment Syndrome"). For these reasons, expansile gasses are unlikely to be used in a combat theater. However, a discussion of AE implications is nevertheless indicated, as casualties can be transferred after subsequent reconstructive surgeries.

Aeromedical Evacuation Implications

Therapeutic gasses injected into the eye to treat retinal detachments present a difficult problem when considering AE, since their reabsorption rates are much slower compared to air and depend on the type of gas and the volume injected (Table 14.6). According to Aerospace Medical Association guidelines regarding routine air travel following intraocular surgery, flight is contraindicated until any injected gas bubble

Table 14.6 Reabsorption rates for intraocular gasses used to treat retinal detachment

Type of gas	Reabsorption time (1 cc of injected gas)
Air	7 days
Sulfur hexafluoride (SF_6)	10–14 days
Perfluorocarbon gasses (C_3F_8)	10–65 days

decreases to less than 30% of the volume of the vitreous [31, 32]. In the case of sulfur hexafluoride (SF6), this will take approximately 2 weeks and approximately 6 weeks in the case of perfluoropropane (C3F8) [32, 33].

Elective AE should be delayed after intraocular injection of therapeutic gasses until the gas bubble has decreased in size to <30% of the volume of the vitreous. If urgent AE is required prior to this time, an altitude restriction should be requested to maintain a cabin pressure equivalent to ≤2000 feet above sea level or equivalent to the higher altitude of the departure or arrival airfields if higher than this altitude [31–33].

All patients with open globe injuries or recent ocular surgery are at risk for an intraocular air bubble, but repaired globes are at higher risk of consequences than unrepaired open globes. Most studies indicate that a gas bubble ≤10% of the volume of the vitreous can be safely transported without altitude restrictions, though larger volumes of intraocular gas are more likely to be problematic [34–36]. When intraocular air is detected after ocular surgery prior to AE, elective AE should be delayed until little or no intraocular gas is visible. When urgent AE to the next echelon of care is required with greater amounts of intraocular air, cabin altitude restriction should be requested.

An undetected intraocular air bubble is a possibility in any patient with an open globe injury or recent ocular surgery. If a postsurgical patient experiences sudden, severe eye pain and decreased vision during AE, an expanding intraocular air bubble flight should be considered (see also section "Acute Glaucoma", above). Even small amounts of intraocular gas (as little as 0.25 cc of air) can expand significantly at altitude resulting in increased intraocular pressure and decreased retinal perfusion [32–34].

The first step in these patients is to check visual acuity compared to baseline. Reviewing surgical records and operative notes should reveal if gas was infused. Examining the eye may reveal gas in the anterior chamber. Intraocular pressure should be checked with a portable tonometer; if the eye has been surgically repaired (i.e., no open globe) and no tonometer is available, the orbit could be gently palpated through the lid to detect increased firmness suggestive of increased intraocular pressure (no pressure should be put on an open globe). En route consultation with the operating surgeon or available ophthalmologist should be attempted and consideration given to diverting to a location with ophthalmic capability. Next, if increased intraocular pressure secondary to expanding gas is suspected, a request should be made to descend as soon as practicable to the altitude necessary to maintain a cabin altitude equivalent to ≤2000 feet above sea level [31, 32]. Vision must be monitored closely. Personnel at the receiving medical facility should be made aware of the situation so that an ophthalmologic evaluation immediately after landing can be arranged.

Blunt Ocular Trauma

Ocular injury should be considered in all patients with head, face, or neck trauma, particularly related to a blast injury [5, 6, 10–12, 14, 15, 19]. Once open globe injuries and intraocular foreign bodies have been excluded, the goal is to determine if blunt ocular trauma was substantial enough to put the patient at risk for permanent vision loss. A worrisome consequence of blunt ocular trauma is intraocular bleeding in either the anterior chamber (hyphema) or into the posterior segment of the eye, involving the vitreous cavity (vitreous hemorrhage), one of the layers of the retina (intraretinal hemorrhage), or the space beneath the retina (subretinal hemorrhage). Intraocular hemorrhage of any kind is manifest evidence of significant ocular injury and requires prompt evaluation by an ophthalmologist; lack of it, however, does not indicate the absence of serious injury.

Hyphema

Blunt ocular trauma can tear fragile intraocular tissues, resulting in bleeding into the anterior chamber of the eye, referred to as a hyphema. A hyphema can cause acute glaucoma and result in permanent vision loss. Patients require Urgent evacuation for ophthalmologic evaluation and may require emergent surgical intervention.

Symptoms of hyphema can include pain, decreased vision, or light sensitivity. Examination will reveal visible blood in the front of the eye, which can partially or completely fill the anterior chamber—the latter of which is referred to as a total (or "8-ball") hyphema. However, blood is not always visible if the hyphema is small.

Immediate treatment for a patient with a hyphema consists of eye protection (shield), rest in a recumbent or supine position with the head elevated, and serial monitoring. Elevating the head 15–30° may allow the blood to settle inferiorly and clear the visual axis. Monitoring consists of documenting any changes in vision, the amount of intraocular blood, and intraocular pressure, when possible. Topical ocular steroids and cycloplegic drops (e.g., atropine or homatropine) are commonly prescribed and should be maintained en route. Medications that increase bleeding risk should be avoided if possible, including anticoagulants and medications that decrease platelet function such as nonsteroidal anti-inflammatory drugs (NSAIDs). Caretakers should remember that treatment with cycloplegic drops will cause the pupil to dilate and become nonreactive, an important consideration if transporting a polytrauma or head-injured patient.

Posterior Segment Hemorrhages

The nature of a posterior vitreoretinal segment hemorrhage depends on which tissues were injured and can be a vitreous hemorrhage (into the vitreous cavity), an intraretinal hemorrhage (into any of the layers of the retina), or a subretinal hemorrhage (into the subretinal space). Visual symptoms will vary depending on the location of the blood, as will the treatment.

Vitreous hemorrhage symptoms can include blurred vision, new floaters, a reddish tint to vision, or brief flashes of light in the peripheral vision (i.e., photopsia, indicating a potential serious retinal injury). Large vitreous hemorrhages and intra- and subretinal hemorrhages can result in decreased visual acuity, decreased visual field, and/or distortion or a blind spot in an otherwise normal visual field (i.e., metamorphopsia or scotoma). Diagnosis requires a detailed fundus examination.

Vitreous hemorrhage can be the result of retinal tears and detachments, which are ophthalmologic emergencies. Treatment will vary depending on the location of the bleed and associated pathology. Patients suspected of having an intraocular bleed in any location should be immediately referred for ophthalmologic evaluation.

Aeromedical Evacuation Implications

Due to the potential need for emergent surgical intervention for hyphema, and the inability to rule out retinal tear or detachment in the presence of a new vitreous hemorrhage, patients with blunt ocular trauma and intraocular hemorrhage should be given an AE precedence classification of Urgent and transported via litter with the head elevated 15–30°. The eye should be shielded and ocular movement discouraged. This will allow the blood to settle inferiorly and in some cases clear the visual axis. Hyphema medications should be administered as ordered, but en route treatment of vitreous hemorrhages is otherwise largely supportive.

Patients are at high risk of a rebleed within the first 3–7 days after the initial trauma. These patients should be evaluated for baseline and re-evaluated periodically. Particular attention should be paid to the intubated and sedated polytrauma patient whose eyes will be closed and whose condition precludes them from exhibiting symptoms related to increased ocular pressure (i.e., pain, nausea, vomiting, complaint of decreased vision). Patients at the highest risk of rebleed are those treated with prophylactic anticoagulants to prevent venous thromboembolism.

Thermal Burns

Thermal burns involving the eyes are uncommon because of protective reflexes to avoid the source of a burn including the blink reflex, Bell's phenomenon (upward and outward movement of the eyes), and reflex movements of the head and arms. However, facial burns involving the eyelids occur frequently and can lead to lid scarring, cicatricial lid retraction, and the inability to close the eyelids completely (lagophthalmos). This can result in severe corneal desiccation and scarring, which in turn can result in permanent loss of vision, or corneal perforation and loss of the eye. Even a small amount of lagophthalmos and eyelid retraction can create severe and permanent problems.

Eyelid burns can also result in eyelid margin malpositions, most commonly turning inward (entropion) putting the patient at risk for corneal abrasions from singed eyelash stubs. Short-term treatment is aggressive lubrication with ophthalmic ointments, whereas long-term treatment is usually surgical.

Aeromedical Evacuation Implications

The cornerstone of treatment for patients with facial burns involving the eyelids is keeping the corneas moist before and during AE. This is particularly important during AE because of low cabin humidity. The corneas can be kept moist by frequent application of ophthalmic ointment or the placement of moisture chambers, which are plastic chambers that resemble swimming goggles. They are held over the affected eye(s) by an elastic band to keep the eye moist. Alternatives include transparent film dressings (e.g., Tegaderm®, Opsite®, etc.) placed over a well-lubricated eye. Ophthalmologists will also aggressively rely on temporary suture tarsorrhaphy (suturing the eyelids shut) in worrisome cases.

Another concern for burn patients is the possibility of orbital compartment syndrome from orbital fluid third spacing during burn resuscitation [26]. When patients develop chemosis (conjunctival edema) and/or proptosis, orbital compartment syndrome must be considered and treated appropriately (see section "Orbital Compartment Syndrome").

Corneal Abrasion

Corneal abrasion occurs any time the epithelial layer is disrupted and can vary from superficial, involving only the epithelium, to deep, with the potential for corneal scarring. The causes of corneal abrasions are multiple and include inadvertent eye trauma from a hard object (e.g., fingernail, pen, makeup brush, tree branch, shell casing) or a foreign body in the eye (e.g., sand, soil, sawdust, ash, rotor wash). The risk of corneal abrasions can be minimized by proper use of protective eyewear.

Corneal abrasions are unlikely to be the sole indication for AE but can be a secondary diagnosis in AE patients with other more serious injuries. Corneal abrasions can be painful, and these patients should be treated with topical antibiotic drops or ointment to reduce the risk of infection and a cycloplegic agent to improve comfort. The affected eye may be patched to improve comfort for the duration of symptoms, typically 1–2 days. However, a patch should never be applied if the eye is at increased risk for infection or ulcer, since it can further increase that risk (see section "Corneal Ulcers"). Topical anesthetic drops should never be prescribed or administered routinely for eye pain since they slow healing and can lead to permanent corneal scarring [37, 38].

Corneal Ulcers

Corneal ulcers are infected corneal abrasions and pose an immediate risk to losing the eye. Treatment requires aggressive therapy, often including hourly (or more frequent) eye drops around the clock, and may require evacuation from operational areas. The most common causal factor for this condition is contact lens wear, especially extended or prolonged wear. Although contact lenses are prohibited in deployed settings, the prohibition is often ignored. Contact lens-associated ulcers may have a worse prognosis in the deployed environment [39]. While abrasions usually heal inconsequentially, corneal ulcers can lead to scarring and permanent vision loss, and even corneal perforation and loss of the eye, so it is essential to differentiate an abrasion from an ulcer and to treat accordingly.

Aeromedical Evacuation Implications

Corneal abrasion patients should be treated with topical antibiotic drops and can be sent for ophthalmologic evaluation in a Priority AE precedence category. Corneal ulcer patients, on the other hand, may require Urgent evacuation to ensure expeditious arrival at a facility prepared for delivering the intense treatments often needed. Those with unilateral eye involvement can be transported as ambulatory patients. If visual acuity and eye pain worsen despite antibiotic treatment, AE precedence should be upgraded to Urgent. Direct communication with the sending and receiving ophthalmologists is imperative to clearly communicate travel routes and arrival times of ulcer patients; stopovers should be avoided.

It is critical that the eye drops be administered as prescribed throughout the AE process, even during stopovers, since the consequences of missed medications are so significant. Intense dosing schedules will tax in-flight crews, especially if flying with other critically ill patients. When administering multiple medications via eye drops, caregivers should wait at least a minute between drops so that the second medication does not wash out the first. Accurate documentation of eye drop administration and en route eye exams is important information for the accepting ophthalmologist.

References

1. Scott AW, Bressler NM, Ffolkes S, Wittenborn JS, Jorkasky J. Public attitudes about eye and vision health. JAMA Ophthalmol. 2016;134(10):1111–8.
2. Mazzoli RA, Gross KR, Butler FK. The use of rigid eye shields (Fox shields) at the point of injury for ocular trauma in Afghanistan. J Trauma Acute Care Surg. 2014;77:S156–62.
3. Yonekawa Y, Hacker HD, Lehman RE, Beal CH, Veldman PB, Vyas NM, et al. Ocular blast injuries in mass-casualty incidents: the marathon bombing in Boston, Massachusetts, and the fertilizer plant explosion in West Texas. Ophthalmology. 2014;121:1670–6.
4. Ficke JR, Eastridge BJ, Butler FK, Alvarez J, Brown T, Pasquina P, Stoneman P, Caravalho J. Dismounted complex blast injury report of the army dismounted complex blast injury task force. J Trauma Acute Care Surg. 2012;73(6 SUPPL 5).
5. Scott RAH, Blanch RJ, Morgan-Warren PJ. Aspects of ocular war injuries. Trauma. 2015;17:83–92.
6. Scott R. The injured eye. Philos Trans R Soc Lond Ser B Biol Sci. 2011;366(1562):251–60.
7. Williams ST, Harding TH, Statz JK, Martin JS. Blast wave dynamics at the cornea as a function of eye protection form and fit. Military Med. 2017;182:226–9.
8. Cockerham GC, Rice TA, Hewes EH, Cockerham KP, Lemke S, Wang G, et al. Closed-eye ocular injuries in the Iraq and Afghanistan Wars. N Engl J Med. 2011;364:2172–3.
9. Cockerham GC, Lemke S, Rice TA, Wang G, Glynn-Milley C, Zumhagen L, et al. Closed-globe injuries of the ocular surface associated with combat blast exposure. Ophthalmology. 2014;121:2165–72.
10. Vlasof A, Ryan DS, Ludlow S, Weichel ED, Colyer MH. Causes of combat ocular trauma-related blindness from Operation Iraqi Freedom and Enduring Freedom. J Trauma Acute Care Surg. 2015;79:S210–5.
11. Wade AL, Dye JL, Mohrle CR, Galarneau MR. Head, face, and neck injuries during Operation Iraqi Freedom II: results from the US navy-marine corps combat trauma registry. J Trauma. 2007;63:836–40.
12. Thomas R, McManus JG, Johnson A, Mayer P, Wade C, Holcomb JB. Ocular injury reduction from ocular protection use in current combat operations. J Trauma. 2009;66:S99–103.
13. Godbole NJ, Seefeldt ES, Raymond WR, Karesh JW, Morgenstern A, Egan JA, Colyer MH, Mazzoli RA. Simplified method for rapid field assessment of visual acuity by first responders after ocular injury. Mil Med. 2018 Mar 1;183(suppl_1):219–23.
14. Joint Trauma System Clinical Practice Guideline. Initial care of ocular and adnexal injuries by non-ophthalmologists at Role 1, Role 2, and non-ophthalmic Role 3 facilities. San Antonio: Institute of Surgical Research, Joint Base San Antonio; 2014.
15. Committee on Tactical Combat Casualty Care. Tactical combat casualty care guidelines for medical personnel. San Antonio: Institute of Surgical Research, Joint Base San Antonio; 2018.
16. Gerstenblith AT, Rabinowitz MP, editors. The Wills Eye Manual. 6th ed. Philadelphia: Lippincott, Williams & Wilkins; 2012. p. 46.
17. Stallard HB. The eye department in a middle east general hospital. Br J Ophthalmol. 1946;28:261–75.

18. Greenwood A. Ophthalmology in the American Expeditionary Forces. In: Ireland MW, editor. Medical Department of the United States Army in the World War. Vol 11, Part 2. Washington, DC: War Department, Government Printing Office; 1924. p. 659–728.
19. Cho RI, Bakken HE, Reynolds ME, Schlifka BA, Powers DB. Concomitant cranial and ocular combat injuries during Operation Iraqi Freedom. J Trauma. 2009;6:516–20.
20. La Piana FG, Mader TH. Lessons learned. In: Thach AB, editor. Ophthalmic care of the combat casualty: textbook of military medicine. Washington, DC: Office of The Surgeon General of the United States Army, Borden Press US Government Printing Office; 2003. p. 17–39.
21. Committee on Trauma. Resources for optimal care of the injured patient. Chicago: American College of Surgeons; 2014.
22. Department of the Air Force. Air Force Instruction 48–307. En route care and aeromedical evacuation medical operations. Washington, DC: US Government Printing Office; 2017.
23. Caring for patients who are blind or visually impaired: a fact sheet for the outpatient care team. 2014. DoD-VA Vision Center of Excellence, Bethesda, MD. Available at https://vce.health.mil/Resources/Products. Accessed 15 Oct 2018.
24. Caring for patients who are blind or visually impaired: a fact sheet for the inpatient care team. 2014. DoD-VA Vision Center of Excellence, Bethesda, MD. Available at https://vce.health.mil/Resources/Products. Accessed 15 Oct 2018.
25. Weichel ED, Colyer MH, Ludlow SE, Bower KS, Eiseman AS. Combat ocular trauma visual outcomes during Operations Iraqi and Enduring Freedom. Ophthalmology. 2008;115:2235–45.
26. Sullivan SR, Ahmadi AJ, Singh CN, Sires BS, Engrav LH, Gibran NS, et al. Elevated orbital pressure: another untoward effect of massive resuscitation after burn injury. J Trauma. 2006;60:72–6.
27. Rodriguez-Cabrera L, Rodrigues-Loaiza JL, Tovilla-Canales JL, Zuazo F. Orbital emphysema as a rare complication of retinal surgery. Ophthal Plast Reconstr Surg. 2017;33:e141–2.
28. Reynolds ME, Hoover C, Riesberg JC, Mazzoli RA, Colyer M, Barnes S, Calvano CJ, et al. Evaluation and treatment of ocular injuries and vision-threatening conditions in Prolonged Field Care. J Spec Opns Med. 2017 Winter;17(4):115–26.
29. Emanuel ME, Parrish RK 2nd, Gedde SJ. Evidence-based management of primary angle closure glaucoma. Curr Opin Ophthalmol. 2014;25(2):89–92.
30. Turnbull AM, Smith M, Ramchandani M. Angle-closure glaucoma on long-haul flights. JAMA Ophthalmol. 2014;132:1474–5.
31. Ivan DJ. Ophthalmic patients. In: Hurd WW, Jernigan JG, editors. Aeromedical evacuation: Management of Acute and Stabilized Patients. New York, NY: Springer-Verlag; 2003. p. 215–24.
32. Aerospace Medical Association Medical Guidelines Task Force. Medical Guidelines for Airline Travel, 2nd ed. Aviat Space Environ Med. 2003;74(5Suppl):A1–19.
33. Chang S. Retina, vol. 3. chapter 131,. Philadelphia: Mosby; 1994. p. 2115–29.
34. Dieckert JP, O'Connor PS, Schacklett DE, Tredici TJ, Lambert HM, Fanton JW, et al. Air travel and intraocular gas. Ophthalmology. 1986;93:642–5.
35. Lincoff H, Weinberger D, Reppucci V, Lincoff A. Air travel and intraocular gas. I. The mechanisms for compensation. Arch Ophthalmol. 1989;107:902–6.
36. Mills MD, Devenyi RG, Lam WC, Berger AR, Beijer CD, Lam SR. An assessment of intraocular pressure rise in patients with gas-filled eyes during simulated air flight. Ophthalmology. 2001;108:40–4.
37. Rosenwasser GO, Holland S, Pflugfelder SC, Lugo M, Heidemann DG, Culbertson WW, Kattan H. Topical anesthetic abuse. Ophthalmology. 1990;97(8):967–72.
38. Wu H, Hu Y, Shi XR, Xu F, Jiang CY, Huang R, Jia H. Keratopathy due to ophthalmic drug abuse with corneal melting and perforation presenting as Mooren-like ulcer: a case report. Exp Ther Med. 2016;12(1):343–6.
39. Musa F, Tailor R, Gao A, Hutley E, Rauz S, Scott RA. Contact lens-related microbial keratitis in deployed British military personnel. Br J Ophthalmol. 2010;94:988–93.

Peripheral Vascular Casualties

15

Ryan E. Earnest, Anthony J. Hayes, and Amy T. Makley

Introduction

Knowledge of the comprehensive diagnosis and treatment of vascular injuries is essential to trauma care in both times of war and peace. The appropriate management of vascular injuries is important in the proper execution of aeromedical evacuation (AE) of wounded casualties and has evolved over the past century. Historically, the incidence and treatment of vascular injuries were challenging to assess.

Estimates of the incidence of vascular injury during the conflicts of the late nineteenth century through World War II (WWII) ranged from 0.07% to 2.4% [1]. Primary surgical care frequently involved ligation of the bleeding vessel, and limb salvage was not considered as a treatment priority. During WWII, many casualties succumbed due to infection and hemorrhage, and successful vascular repair was restricted by the limitations of the medical evacuation system [1]. During the Korean and Vietnam wars, the advent of rapid evacuation to advanced surgical care allowed for the timely repair of vascular injuries that previously was unachievable. This progression led to the increased reported limb salvage rate of 86.5% during the Vietnam War, primarily attributed to the increased ability to attempt timely revascularization [2].

Traumatic vascular injury treatment further evolved as a direct result of improved medical care and processes implemented during the conflicts in Afghanistan and Iraq. The quick response of the AE system allowed for the application of a rapid and organized approach to the treatment of vessel injury. In addition, advanced body armor is considered a leading factor in increasing the frequency and distribution of peripheral vascular injuries to 12% in these engagements, as it protected soldiers from torso injuries but left the extremities relatively at risk. This recent increase in peripheral vascular trauma in modern conflict represents a growth of more than five times that during WWII, Korean War, and Vietnam War [3]. The rapid application of tourniquets and novel hemostatic adjuncts now available to teams at the point of injury has also contributed to increased survival. Casualties previously without access to treatment are receiving point-of-care hemorrhage control and timely evacuation enabling revascularization in patients that previously was not possible [3, 4].

R. E. Earnest
LtCol, USAF, MC, Surgical Critical Care, Department of Trauma and General Surgery, University of Cincinnati Medical Center, Cincinnati, OH, USA

A. J. Hayes
LT, MC, USN, Department of General Surgery, Navy Medical Center Camp Lejeune, Camp Lejeune, NC, USA

A. T. Makley (✉)
Department of Surgery, University of Cincinnati, Cincinnati, OH, USA
e-mail: makleyat@ucmail.uc.edu

W. W. Hurd, W. Beninati (eds.), *Aeromedical Evacuation*,
https://doi.org/10.1007/978-3-030-15903-0_15

Both the increase in frequency of extremity injury and the recent increase in successful treatment underline the importance of a rapid, available AE system that is advanced and equipped to manage peripheral vascular casualties. The key principles in the management of these injuries include hemorrhage control, balanced and hemostatic resuscitation, damage control surgery, and timely evacuation to the appropriate level of care. These principles make AE fundamental to the care of peripheral vascular injury, which ultimately facilitates limb salvage. In this chapter, we will discuss the basic treatment of peripheral vascular injury at the major levels of combat care and civilian equivalents and the considerations for evacuation and the AE provider. Knowledge of these approaches will provide the AE provider with the skills necessary to diagnose, stabilize, and treat peripheral vascular casualties as well as respond to any changes or emergencies in-flight.

Vascular injuries can result from a multitude of mechanisms of injury, ranging from direct injury via blunt or penetrating trauma or indirect injury due to stretch, blast, or cavitation effects in close proximity to adjacent trauma. A high suspicion of potential vascular injury is necessary to diagnose more minimal nonocclusive injuries including intimal flaps, which can subsequently thrombose or propagate, leading to devastating limb loss. Prompt and efficient management of vascular injuries is necessary and requires special attention. Each major level of combat care, including prior to and during AE, has unique priorities regarding the management and treatment of peripheral vascular casualties.

Roles of Care

Timely and appropriate staging of the care of vascular injuries has contributed to the recent success in improving both survival and limb salvage. US Army doctrine recently introduced "roles of care" as a new terminology to describe the various levels of medical capabilities and resources previously referred to as "echelons." Each role of care is uniquely equipped to diagnose and treat vascular injury, with varying resources available to providers. Ultimately, staging the management of vascular injuries can move initial, temporizing measures far forward to the time of injury. After stabilization, the definitive surgical treatment of vascular injuries can be delayed to other levels of care after transport to centers with increased resources. Central to this process is an efficient and widely available medical evacuation (MEDEVAC) and AE system.

Role 1, or Point of Injury Intervention

Role 1 care most commonly involves a combat lifesaver or combat medic [5]. Key to the treatment of peripheral vascular injury in this setting is first and foremost hemorrhage control. Tactical Combat Casualty Care (TCCC) has evolved to focus on specific, lifesaving adjuncts. These have resulted in newfound success in the treatment of exsanguinating hemorrhage, especially from extremity injury. Tourniquets, hemostatic agents, and basic hemostatic maneuvers are now commonplace on the battlefield and are moving into civilian prehospital care [6].

MEDEVAC from this level is most commonly casualty evacuation (CASEVAC) as defined in Chap. 5. However, urgent evacuation to a higher role of care has evolved to incorporate higher-level providers and resources closer to the point of injury: Tactical Critical Care Evacuation Team (TCCET) and Tactical Critical Care Evacuation Team–Enhanced (TCCT-E). As an AE provider, it is imperative to be familiar with this evolution, as treatment of vascular injuries in a timely manner with hemorrhage control is thought to lead to better outcomes and is an evolving field [5].

Role 2, or Level II/III Civilian Trauma Center

Key to the treatment of vascular injury is rapid transport from the point of injury to surgical intervention. The first point of access to surgical care in theater is a Role 2 facility. In a mature conflict zone, such as was present during the height of operations during Operation Iraqi

Freedom (OIF) and Operation Enduring Freedom (OEF), evacuation times occurred within 60 minutes. The nomenclature and organization of Role 2 facilities are service dependent, and while there is no exact civilian equivalent, it is similar to a level 3 trauma facility or a rural facility with a skilled general surgeon.

Role 2 care should be centered on damage control surgery. There is no capability for extended and complicated postoperative monitoring, and sub-specialist vascular care is not available. In the context of peripheral vascular injuries, surgical care at a Role 2 facility typically involves the use of temporary vascular shunts to restore distal perfusion in anticipation of evacuation to a higher-level facility for definitive management. Transfer to a Role 3 facility is typically accomplished by fixed-wing or rotary-wing aircraft with appropriate MEDEVAC personnel based on the patient's degree of injury.

Casualties at a Role 2 facility are evaluated according to standard trauma patient evaluations, with airway, breathing, and circulation (ABC) being addressed in a systematic manner. Damage control, or balanced resuscitation, is key to treatment of exsanguinating hemorrhage and correcting hemodynamic deficits. Evaluation for extremity peripheral vascular injuries should be a part of the secondary survey. If the casualty is stable, any previously placed tourniquets can be removed under observation to evaluate for continued hemorrhage and initial injury assessment based on the location of the injury.

If the surgeon determines a peripheral vascular injury is present, this is best managed at a Role 2 facility by use of a temporary vascular shunt [4, 7, 8]. Following hemorrhage control, damage control surgery (temporary vascular shunt), and hemodynamic stabilization, the patient should be rapidly transferred to the Role 3 facility or next civilian level of care.

Role 3/Level 1 Trauma Center

Transfer to a high level of care in the civilian setting is likely the nearest level 1 trauma center, and within the military theater, this is the Role 3 center. At this level, definitive vascular repair should be planned [7].

A Role 3 facility or level 1 trauma facility should have a surgeon available to provide definitive limb salvage intervention. The surgeon should begin to address the need for repair of the vascular injury by determining if attempted limb salvage is an appropriate course of action. The surgeon will need to take concomitant soft tissue and orthopedic injuries into account, and the opinion of an orthopedic colleague, if available, is invaluable.

In the civilian theater, level 1 is the highest level of care and the definitive treatment center. For military casualties, following Role 3 care, the patient often undergoes long-distance AE during transfer to the continental United States for treatment at a Role 4 facility.

Management of Vascular Injuries

Treatment of vascular injuries can be focused to specific goals by targeting management appropriate to each role of care. The details of each of these treatment modalities including hemorrhage control, resuscitation, diagnosis of vascular injuries, and both temporizing and definitive surgical care must be explored.

Hemorrhage Control

Both the patterns and mechanisms of injury on the modern battlefield have changed substantially, and many factors contribute to this evolution. Understanding these new mechanisms has led to emphasis on implementing strategies for hemorrhage control close to the point of injury. These mechanisms of injury now include improvised explosive devices (IEDs) with novel patterns of devastating tissue loss and vascular injury. The advent of better protective devices such as modern body armor to protect against lethal truncal injuries leaves the extremities relatively vulnerable.

Regardless of these evolutions, hemorrhage control at the point of injury has repeatedly been demonstrated to be vitally important to survival in extremity injuries. The Joint Theater Trauma Registry and the Armed Forces Medical Examiner system demonstrated the importance of rapid control of bleeding during both OIF and OEF [9]. These data revealed that of nearly 4600 combat deaths, 25% were potentially survivable. Of these, approximately 91% were attributed to hemorrhage and 13.5% were secondary to peripheral extremity hemorrhage. The widely cited report published by the National Academy of Sciences, Engineering, and Medicine in 2016 tasked the integration of military and civilian health care systems to achieve a goal of zero preventable deaths after injury. Targeting the potentially survivable early deaths from hemorrhage using the following strategies will be instrumental in achieving this goal.

Tourniquets

Treatment of hemorrhage at the point of injury (Role of Care 1) is essential in severe peripheral vascular injury. Intervention changed substantially throughout the course of OIF and OEF. The use of tourniquets as the primary modality to control extremity hemorrhage, with the use of hemostatic dressings as an adjunct, has been the most substantial changes.

Tourniquets are considered to be the standard first line of care for controlling life-threatening extremity hemorrhage at the point of injury (Fig. 15.1). In the past, tourniquets were considered a method of last resort for hemorrhage control because of concerns about prolonged tourniquet application inducing ischemic injury and increasing the risk of subsequent amputation. These concerns have been disproven and are secondary to the need to halt life-threatening hemorrhage.

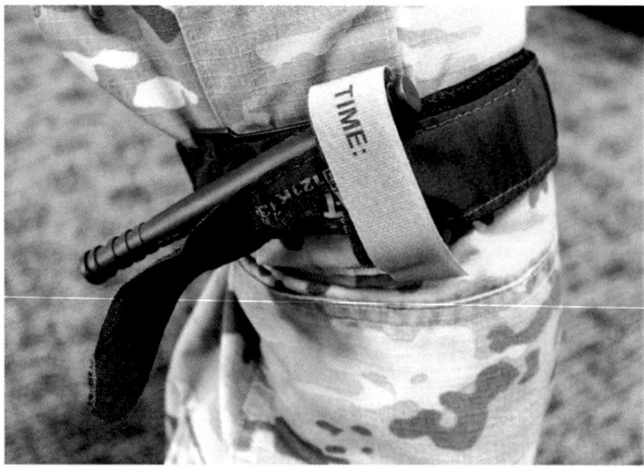

Fig. 15.1 Combat Application Tourniquet (CAT) Generation 7 (North American Rescue, Greer, South Carolina) applied to a soldier's leg. (US Army photo by Ellen Crown)

This change in paradigm has filtered into the care of civilian trauma patients in the United States as well. Emergency medical service personnel as well as civilians are now being trained in the use and application of tourniquets and hemostatic dressings. The US Department of Homeland Security, with the support of organizations such as the American College of Surgeons, has initiated a public education campaign, Stop the Bleed, with the goal of educating the public in the use of tourniquets and hemostatic dressings during mass casualty events and as bystanders who encounter trauma victims with extremity hemorrhage.

This approach to early control of hemorrhage from vascular injuries is supported by data from OIF and the Israel Defense Forces in Operation Protective Edge [10–12]. This analysis showed that tourniquet use was associated with better hemorrhage control, increased survival in extremity injury, and low rates of complications. Though there was a high rate (20%–40%) of non-therapeutic tourniquet use, the low complication rate supports few negative outcomes from tourniquet use. In additional supportive evidence, Kragh et al. found that the use of tourniquets by US military personnel increased from 4% to 40% from 2001 to 2010, with an associated increase in survival while controlling for similar injuries [6].

Early tourniquet use is recommended with the suspicion for major extremity vascular injury, as patients in hemorrhagic shock may have vascular injuries without obvious pulsatile bleeding due to hypoperfusion. Proper tourniquet placement should include appropriate positioning above the area of injury but placement as distal as possible on the extremity to avoid additional ischemic injury. After tightening to the point of hemorrhage control, the time of placement should be noted and recorded on the tourniquet itself if possible to ensure communication to future providers.

Hemostatic Adjuncts

Adjuncts for hemorrhage control include hemostatic dressings and direct manual pressure. While novel hemostatic dressings are constantly changing, there is no substitute for direct manual pressure. There are currently multiple commercial hemostatic agents for control of peripheral/extremity hemorrhage. These products include QuikClot (Z-Medica, LLC, Wallingford, CT), CELOX gauze (Medtrade Products, Ltd., Crewe, United Kingdom), ChitoGauze (Rescue Essentials, Salida, CO), and XSTAT (Revolutionary Medical Technologies, Wilsonville, OR). QuikClot, CELOX gauze, and ChitoGauze are products that are applied to wounds with direct pressure to assist in hemostasis.

XSTAT is a product that is used with an injector applicator. Multiple small sponges are able to be injected into a wound tract and will expand to accommodate the space. Hemostatic dressings should be placed with manual pressure and held in place for 3 minutes for hemorrhage control. If hemorrhage continues, a second hemostatic dressing can replace the first. XSTAT dressings should not be removed in the field.

The specific hemostatic dressing available for use will be dependent on the particular unit of the casualty, but these different products all demonstrate similar efficacy in animal models [13]. Shina et al. reported on the efficacy of hemorrhage control using hemostatic dressings by Israel Defense Force. They concluded the dressings were approximately 89% and 92% successful in control of junctional and peripheral extremity hemorrhage, respectively, and recommended that hemostatic dressings are an appropriate second-line option for control of peripheral extremity hemorrhage [14]. The use of new hemostatic products is an area of continued research that requires up-to-date knowledge of the latest advances. Regardless, manual pressure and use of tourniquets are the current mainstay of treatment of peripheral vascular injuries.

Resuscitation

Patients with peripheral vascular injury are commonly subject to large amounts of blood loss from concomitant injuries in addition to extremity injury. This requires careful resuscitation of the casualty to maximize survival [9, 15]. Resuscitation guidelines have evolved over the past two decades due to data from massive transfusions in OIF and OEF. Evidence now supports hemostatic resuscitation that approximates the transfusion of whole blood. This is typically done with a ratio of packed red blood cells to platelets to plasma of 1:1:1 [15–17] or the transfusion of fresh whole blood itself.

During AE, balanced hemostatic resuscitation should also be continued as necessary. While the patient must be stabilized prior to long-distance AE, it is important to know the current transfusion status prior to transport and whether he or she continues to require blood product resuscitation. If the patient has unforeseen hemorrhage during AE, resuscitation should proceed in a balanced ratio or with whole blood, noting that hemorrhage control remains a priority.

Diagnosis of Peripheral Vascular Injury

Evaluation of peripheral vascular events can often be diagnosed on physical exam. As with all patients who have suffered traumatic injury, the assessment begins with a primary survey following the ABCs of airway, breathing, and circulation. There are adjuncts that can be used for further investigation if the diagnosis is not initially clear. The following gives basic guidelines for the assessment of vascular injury, including hard and soft signs of vascular trauma and diagnostic adjuncts.

Hard Signs of Vascular Injury

During the primary evaluation, evaluation for hard signs of vascular injury should take place, as identification of these signs is highly predictive

Table 15.1 Hard and soft signs of vascular injury

Hard signs	Soft signs
Absent distal pulses	Small expanding, nonpulsatile hematoma
Audible bruit	Peripheral neurologic deficit
Palpable thrill	History of significant hemorrhage at scene
Pulsatile hematoma	Proximity of wound to major artery
Signs of arterial occlusion and ischemia	Abnormal ankle-brachial index (<0.9)
Pallor, paresthesia, pain, paralysis, poikilothermia	

of vascular injury requiring rapid surgical intervention. Hard signs of vascular injury include absent distal pulses; a cold, pale limb; audible bruits or palpable thrills at site of injury; active pulsatile hemorrhage; and the presence of large and expanding or pulsatile hematomas (Table 15.1). Obvious hemorrhage/exsanguination should be addressed rapidly. At later stages of care, signs of controlled hemorrhage including a well-placed tourniquet or hemostatic dressing should be evaluated during initial evaluation and addressed surgically. Distal ischemia is diagnosed as the absence of a Doppler signal in an injured extremity and may represent either a vascular injury or hypoperfusion from hemorrhagic shock. The presence of significant distal ischemia as manifested by pallor, paresthesia, pain, paralysis, or poikilothermia mandates rapid assessment. The patient should be warmed and resuscitated for a true assessment of absent pulses in the extremity in question.

Soft Signs of Vascular Injury

Following the primary survey, the secondary survey should include evaluation for soft signs of vascular injury. Soft signs of vascular injury can include history of significant or arterial hemorrhage at the scene or prior to presentation; a reduced pulse distal to injury; or dislocations, fractures, penetrating wounds, or other hematomas/bruising in an extremity. These signs require evaluation for occult vascular injuries. These range from significant vascular injury to consequences of hemorrhagic shock, but all merit additional exploration with concern for vessel injury. Assessment of any neurologic deficits is vital to the management of extremity trauma.

Doppler Ultrasound

Identification of an injury can be accomplished using a continuous wave Doppler ultrasound. Most commonly, the ankle-brachial index (ABI) or arterial pressure index (API) is used to assess for occult vascular injury. This measurement is accomplished by measuring the pressure at which the Doppler signal returns during deflation of a blood pressure cuff in the injured extremity. The index is achieved by dividing that number by the same measurement in an uninjured extremity; for example, the ankle-brachial index normalizes the pressure of the injured extremity to an uninjured upper extremity. If the result is greater than 0.9, there is low likelihood of vascular injury. If the ABI is <0.9, further investigation with angiography or computed tomography (CT) angiography is required.

Angiography

When vascular injury is suspected, subsequent study using angiography or CT angiography is indicated. However, in the setting of a combat theater, these resources may not be readily available until transport to Role 3/higher levels of care. The AE provider may be transporting a suspected vascular injury to a center of higher care for these evaluations and must be equipped to manage these injuries during transport. During the evacuation of these patients, serial vascular exams are essential to monitor for adequate limb perfusion using Doppler ultrasound.

Surgical Treatment of Vascular Injuries

Applying the philosophy of damage control surgical principles to the treatment of vascular injuries has resulted in the staging of surgical treatment of vascular injuries depending on the resources available at each level of care. With the goal of controlling hemorrhage, preventing contamination, and protection from further ischemic injury, vascular shunting has predominated the initial surgical care of extremity vascular injuries.

Vascular Shunts

In Role 2 facilities, a damage control approach is shown to improve outcomes in vascular trauma as opposed to striving for complete, definitive surgical repair in unstable polytrauma patients. This approach often utilizes the placement of temporary vascular shunts [8]. The use of vascular shunts was shown to have a high patency rate in proximal arterial and venous injuries (86%) upon arrival at Role 3 facilities and did not increase rates of limb loss in multiple studies of the casualties of OIF and OEF [4, 8, 18–20].

There are multiple commercial temporary vascular shunts available, including Argyle shunts (Kendall Healthcare Products, Mansfield, MA), Javid shunts (Bard Peripheral Vascular Inc., Tempe, AZ), and Sundt shunts (Integra, Plainsboro, NJ). These shunts come in varying lengths and diameters, and their use in theater may depend on surgeon preference or availability, ideally sized to the appropriate vessel of injury. Some commercially available shunts, including the Pruitt-Inahara shunt, have a third arm that effectively facilitates the intravascular administration of vasoactive medications (papaverine) and local anticoagulants. If a commercial temporary vascular shunt product is not available, various other silastic products that may be available can be substituted if necessary, including smaller diameter chest tubes and nasogastric tubes.

Operative Principles

Temporary vascular shunt placement should follow damage control principles. Tourniquets controlling hemorrhage are prepped into the operative field. Major thoracoabdominal injuries should be addressed first while tourniquets and/or hemostatic pressure dressings maintain extremity hemorrhage control. Once central injuries are addressed, attention can be turned to the extremities. The surgical principles of obtaining proximal and distal control of the injured vessels should be achieved. If the hemorrhage is being controlled proximally using a tourniquet, the injured vasculature can initially be exposed distally and controlled with placement of vessel loops or atraumatic vascular clamps.

Proximal control of injuries is often best obtained by exposing the proximal vessels in an area outside of the field of injury. In the upper extremity, this may involve exposing the brachial artery and vein or exposing the axillary artery and vein deep to the pectoral muscles proximal to the shoulder. Lower extremity injuries may require exposure of the femoral vessels in the groin or entering the abdomen or retroperitoneum for more proximal injuries. The inguinal ligament is a useful anatomic landmark to obtain proximal control assuming the region is free of hematoma and soft tissue injury. If control of the femoral vessels is not feasible by division of the inguinal ligament, control via the iliac vessels should be considered. The iliac vessels can be approached via laparotomy or by a retroperitoneal approach through an oblique flank incision.

After obtaining proximal and distal control of injured vessels, temporary vascular shunts should be placed using an in-line or loop configuration. Prior to placing a temporary vascular shunt, an embolectomy catheter (Fogerty) should be used to clear the proximal and distal vessel of thrombus. The vessels should also be flushed with heparinized saline if available and back-bleeding should be evaluated. Using the resources at their disposal in the austere environment, the surgeon should place either an in-line or looped temporary vascular shunt of appropriate size (matched approximately to the size of the injured vessel) to restore distal perfusion.

Placing an in-line temporary vascular shunt requires that the proximal and distal vessel have enough length to insert the catheter proximally or distally in order to place the other end within the vessel. If this cannot be done, a looped vascular shunt can be considered. After the shunts are placed, they must be secured on each end. The shunts can be secured with a variety of methods, including heavy silk suture, vessel loops, or Rummel tourniquets. When securing the shunt in place, the surgeon should consider the length of time the shunt is anticipated to be in place, as well as a clear plan for control of hemorrhage should the shunt become dislodged during transport. This plan must be feasible to perform by AE personnel should an emergency occur during evacuation.

When receiving a patient with a temporary vascular shunt in place, the AE provider should ascertain where the shunt is, document the vascular exam, and identify a plan to control hemorrhage should recurrent bleeding or shunt dislodgement occur. These plans should be discussed with the operating surgeon prior to departure. If shunting is not viable, ligation or amputation is an acceptable damage control procedure that can also be performed prior to evacuation.

Limb Salvage/Revascularization/ Primary Repair

At a Role 3 or level 1 trauma center, definitive care of the casualty can take place. In this setting, collaboration with other specialties may be required to appropriately plan the course of action for the patient. With devastating tissue loss or mangled extremity injury, orthopedic surgeons and plastic surgeons may be necessary to determine a multidisciplinary approach to limb salvage. If orthopedic stabilization is required, it is best to leave temporary vascular shunts in place and allow external fixation to proceed. Definitive vascular repair can then follow.

Repair of arteries proximal to the popliteal artery in the lower extremity is essential. The brachial artery and proximal arteries of the upper extremity should be repaired as well. Venous injuries in the same pattern in the upper and lower extremities should be repaired if feasible, particularly in the setting of a combined arterial and venous injury. Veins distal to the brachial artery in the upper extremity and distal to the popliteal artery in the lower extremity can generally be ligated with minimal expected morbidity.

Primary Repair and Bypass

Limb salvage, whether arterial or venous, remains the priority of surgical treatment as originally established in the Korean and Vietnam conflicts [4, 21, 22]. Primary repair can be accomplished if the vascular injury is focal across a short segment of vessel. The injured vessel should be sharply debrided to healthy tissue and the vessel mobilized from the surrounding tissue to allow for a tension-free repair. If this is not possible, repair with autogenous vein is the next repair of choice.

Autogenous vein is harvested from the least injured lower extremity when possible and is most often the greater saphenous vein. The surgeon can also utilize autogenous vein from an amputated extremity if no other option is available. If autogenous vein is not available, prosthetic conduits can be utilized with acceptable short-term results [23]. Replacement with an autogenous vein graft can be accomplished in a delayed fashion following further stabilization and evacuation to a higher level of care. Thrombectomy should be performed at the time of definitive vascular repair, with completion angiography utilized as a diagnostic adjunct to ensure distal perfusion. The surgeon should clearly document and communicate the vascular exam and mark the skin overlying distal pulses prior to leaving the operating room for easy identification and monitoring by ancillary personnel.

Tissue Coverage

Combat-related extremity vascular injuries are often heavily contaminated with debris and clothing and are at exceedingly high risk for future infection. Key principles in the management of concomitant soft tissue injuries include serial debridement, low-pressure or gravity irrigation, and the use of wound vacuum dressings. Early collection of culture data with guided antimicrobial therapy can be beneficial in treating infections common to large blast injuries to the extremity. Continuous negative-pressure vacuum-assisted therapy is beneficial in controlling large open wounds, but caution must be exercised to avoid vacuum therapy adjacent to a site of vascular injury.

All blood vessels, vascular repairs, and vascular grafts including both autogenous and prosthetic grafts require soft tissue coverage to prevent subsequent desiccation and infection with the development of pseudoaneurysms and delayed rupture. While skin or subcutaneous tissue can serve as temporary coverage, fascial and muscular coverage is ideal to prevent late complications. These rotational muscle or tissue flaps often require the advanced microscopic surgical skills of plastic and reconstructive surgeons available at later or higher levels of care. With patterns of injury characterized by devastating tissue loss due to modern explosive devices and concomitant blast effect, it is vitally important to route surgical grafts around the developing zone of injury. Initially viable tissue may become necrotic and require serial debridement in the future due to the adjacent blast effect. Tunneling or routing vascular grafts in nonanatomic positions may be required to achieve viable tissue coverage.

Although many definitions and scoring systems exist, any extremity sustaining a severe injury including vascular, bony, soft tissue, and/or nerve injuries should be considered a mangled extremity (Table 15.2). Following control of active hemorrhage, the bony alignment should be established and vascular continuity restored. Ultimately, preservation of a functional limb is the goal, and multiple scoring systems have attempted to identify the success or failure of limb salvage. In the setting of devastating tissue destruction, these scoring systems—including the Mangled Extremity Severity Score (MESS) and the Predictive Salvage Index (PSI)—all attempt to predict an injury pattern that will ultimately require amputation due to poor functional outcome. Multiple studies have failed to prove validity of each of these scoring systems in large prospective analyses of high-energy extremity injuries. The degree of tissue destruction and need for soft tissue debridement are the main factors that determine the need for early amputation, in addition to failure to control hemorrhage or associated devastating bony injuries. Although the need for amputation and loss of an extremity represent a significant psychological, social, and economic burden to the patient, no attempts at limb salvage should jeopardize life.

Table 15.2 Scoring systems predictive for need of limb amputation

Predictive Salvage Index (PSI)—1987	Factors include extent of vascular, muscle, and bone injury and ischemia time 100% specificity and 78% sensitivity to identify successful limb salvage
Mangled Extremity Severity Score (MESS)—1990	Factors include skeletal/soft tissue injury, limb ischemia, shock, and age Scores doubled for ischemia time of >6 hours MESS ≥7 associated with amputation with 100% accuracy
Nerve injury, ischemia, soft tissue injury, skeletal injury, shock, and age score (NISSA)—1994	Addition of nerve injury component Loss of plantar sensation heavily weighted
Limb Salvage Index (LSI)—1991	Score includes seven variables: arterial, nerve, skeletal, skin, muscle, deep venous injury, and warm ischemia time
Hannover fracture scale—1993	Thirteen characteristics with respective weightage Cumbersome and requires advanced bacterial specimens from the initial wound
Gustilo-Anderson's classification—1976	Designed to identify the need for tissue coverage of extremity fractures Does not specifically address question of salvage Low inter-observer agreement

Compartment Syndrome

Compartment syndrome is a devastating complication of extremity trauma and occurs when the interstitial pressure within a confined fascial compartment in the extremity exceeds its capillary perfusion pressure. This leads to localized tissue ischemia and muscle death. The extremities, including the hands and feet, all contain osteofascial compartments that are surrounded by a relatively inflexible fascial layer. Swelling into these nonexpandable compartments from crush injuries, combined arterial-venous injuries, or severe ischemia-reperfusion injuries are at high risk. In some cases, such as with deep circumferential burns, the skin itself or eschar serves as the restricting membrane responsible for increased compartment pressures as opposed to the deeper fascia.

The urgent diagnosis and treatment of compartment syndrome is necessary to prevent muscle death and nerve injury that can ultimately cause severe functional deficits. Early signs and symptoms of compartment syndrome include swelling, pain with passive movement of the muscles in the at-risk compartment, and sensory loss and paresthesia. Late signs and symptoms include loss of pulses and motor deficits, which both represent prolonged ischemia and may lead to irreversible injury.

If suspicious for compartment syndrome, measurement of compartment pressures or prophylactic fasciotomies are recommended prior to AE. Compartment pressures can easily be measured either with portable pressure monitoring systems (Stryker) or by inserting a needle or intravenous catheter into the compartment in question and transducing pressures. Measured compartment pressures of <15 mmHg effectively excludes the diagnosis of compartment syndrome. Pressures of 20–30 mmHg are concerning for hypertension in the measured compartment, and pressures >30 mmHg require urgent decompression. Alternatively, practitioners can use the "delta-P" method to calculate tissue pressures in patients with systemic hypoperfusion. The compartment pressure is subtracted from the diastolic blood pressure to obtain the "delta-P." If the "delta-P" is <30 mmHg, there is concern for compartment syndrome, and fasciotomies should be performed.

Compartment syndrome is often accompanied by metabolic derangements attributable to rhabdomyolysis with muscle breakdown leading to acidosis, hyperkalemia, renal insufficiency, and cardiac arrhythmia. These conditions must be identified, closely monitored, and rapidly treated, both prior to transport and during AE.

Aeromedical Evacuation Considerations for Peripheral Vascular Trauma

There are unique implications regarding the effect of AE on the care of patients with peripheral vascular trauma. As the in-flight provider during AE could have a background in a variety of specialties, it is important to be familiar with these considerations and have a working knowledge of potentially necessary interventions during transport. Though the casualty is ideally stabilized prior to transfer, continued monitoring to avoid unrecognized decompensation is essential to avoid complications including ischemia, development of compartment syndrome, and recurrent hemorrhage. Thorough preparation prior to transport is required to care for all patients undergoing AE; however, this is vital for patients with peripheral vascular injury.

Hemorrhage

As outlined previously, casualties should have all major hemorrhage controlled prior to AE, whether transport is urgent or elective. The use of tourniquets and their benefits have been outlined above [5, 6, 10–12]. Significant blood loss should be accounted for and blood products appropriately available. Ideally, control of bleeding, appropriate resuscitation, and correction of coagulopathy are attained prior to transport to avoid in-flight complications.

Resuscitation

As mentioned in previous sections, damage control resuscitation with the appropriate ratio of packed red blood cells (pRBCs) to plasma and platelets is shown to improve survival [15–17]. Continued resuscitation may be required during AE. Prior to departure, the appropriate blood products and volume, with contingency products, should be obtained. This will allow for the appropriate resuscitation and treatment of unforeseen hemorrhage.

Compartment Syndrome

All patients with extremity injuries should be evaluated for compartment syndrome and considered for fasciotomies prior to AE. Regardless of the disease process or treatment modality (shunting, ligation, or revascularization), injury, ischemia, and subsequent reperfusion of an ischemic limb can lead to compartment syndrome. Rapid identification or prevention of compartment syndrome in a patient with extremity injury is essential to avoiding long-term morbidity. This is especially true in the AE environment. Casualties who undergo intervention on an extremity have a reported amputation rate of 41% when they develop postoperative compartment syndrome, whereas those who do not develop compartment syndrome have an amputation rate of 6.7% [24].

Historically, approaches have varied from monitoring of compartment pressures, limited prophylactic fasciotomies, and wide preflight fasciotomies. During OIF and OEF, it was noted that delayed fasciotomy or inadequate fasciotomy in patients with extremity injury led to an unacceptable rate of compartment syndrome with late diagnosis [24, 25]. This led to a recommendation of prophylactic skin and fascial incisions with complete openings of all compartments. A robust education program on proper fasciotomies of the extremities with adequate skin and fascia incisions prior to transport led to decreased revisions and improved survival in patients with extremity injuries [25].

In-flight fasciotomies have been proposed in the past but are difficult to perform in the AE environment. Complete release of all compartments can be difficult to achieve with limited lighting and resources and may be fraught with complication. Therefore, if feasible and potentially necessary, fasciotomies should be completed prior to AE.

Monitoring

During transport, it is important to perform serial vascular exams on the effected extremities (Fig. 15.2). There is not an intervention that can be performed in-flight to restore perfusion; however, documentation of the time the exam changed helps determine ischemic time and plan for intervention on arrival at the destination facility. If a Doppler probe is to be used to monitor the extremity, ensure the equipment is secured for the flight, as this equipment is not in the standard allotment.

Conclusion

In the modern era of current military conflict, peripheral vascular injury has become an increasingly common occurrence with good evidence that an aggressive and staged approach can drastically increase overall survival and limb salvage. These approaches are immediate hemorrhage control with tourniquets and other adjuncts, damage control resuscitation, increased use of vascular shunts, and definitive surgical care with limb salvage after transport to the appropriate level of care. As this field continues to evolve, there is promise of using other adjuncts, such as retrograde endovascular balloon occlusion of the aorta, new hemostatic agents, and innovative treatments to improve survival and decrease morbidity. Central to these adjuncts is a robust and efficient AE system that brings the casualty quickly and efficiently to surgical care.

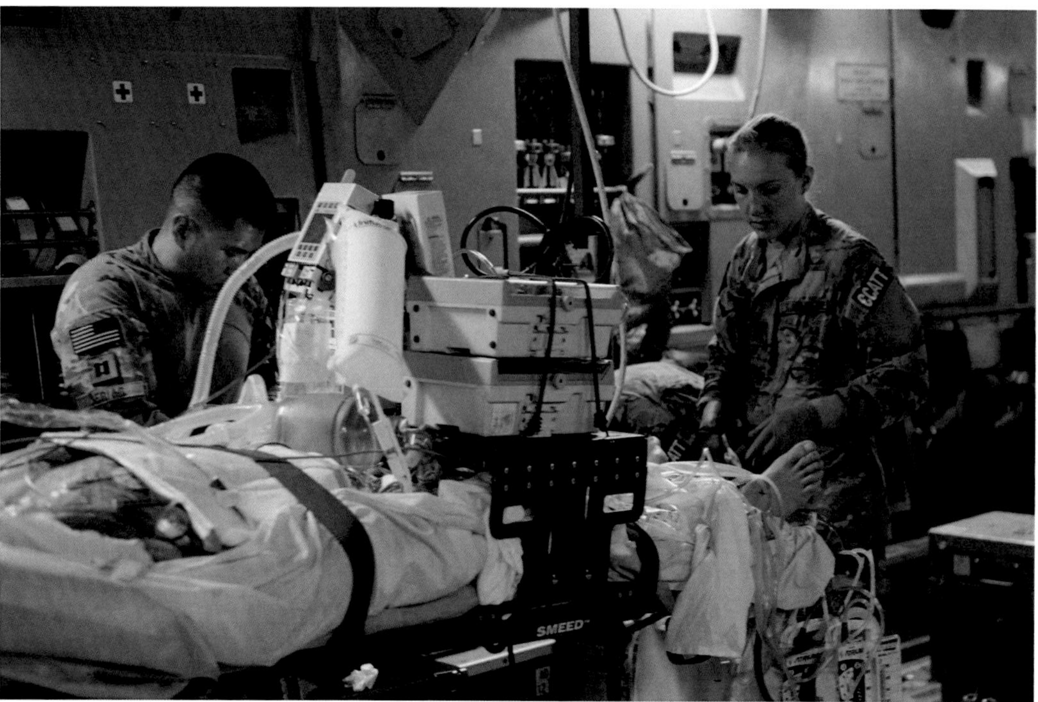

Fig. 15.2 A Critical Care Air Transport Team member monitoring lower extremities while transporting a polytrauma patient from Bagram Airfield, Afghanistan, to Ramstein Air Base, Germany. (US Air Force photo by Maj. Tony Wickman)

References

1. Debakey ME, Simeone FA. Battle injuries of the arteries in world war II: an analysis of 2,471 cases. Ann Surg. 1946;123(4):534–79.
2. Rich NM, Baugh JH, Hughes CW. Acute arterial injuries in vietnam: 1,000 cases. J Trauma. 1970;10(5):359–69.
3. White JM, Stannard A, Burkhardt GE, Eastridge BJ, Blackbourne LH, Rasmussen TE. The epidemiology of vascular injury in the wars in Iraq and Afghanistan. Ann Surg. 2011;253(6):1184–9.
4. Clouse WD, Rasmussen TE, Peck MA, Eliason JL, Cox MW, Bowser AN, et al. In-theater management of vascular injury: 2 years of the Balad vascular registry. J Am Coll Surg. 2007;204(4):625–32.
5. Borden Institute (U.S.). Emergency war surgery. In: Fourth United States revision. Washington, DC: Borden Institute; 2013.
6. Kragh JF Jr, Dubick MA, Aden JK, McKeague AL, Rasmussen TE, Baer DG, et al. U.S. Military use of tourniquets from 2001 to 2010. Prehosp Emerg Care. 2015;19(2):184–90.
7. Rasmussen TE, Clouse WD, Jenkins DH, Peck MA, Eliason JL, Smith DL. Echelons of care and the management of wartime vascular injury: a report from the 332nd emdg/air force theater hospital, Balad air base, Iraq. Perspect Vasc Surg Endovasc Ther. 2006;18(2):91–9.
8. Rasmussen TE, Clouse WD, Jenkins DH, Peck MA, Eliason JL, Smith DL. The use of temporary vascular shunts as a damage control adjunct in the management of wartime vascular injury. J Trauma. 2006;61(1):8–12; discussion 12-15.
9. Eastridge BJ, Mabry RL, Seguin P, Cantrell J, Tops T, Uribe P, et al. Death on the battlefield (2001-2011): implications for the future of combat casualty care. J Trauma Acute Care Surg. 2012;73(6 Suppl 5):S431–7.
10. Beekley AC, Sebesta JA, Blackbourne LH, Herbert GS, Kauvar DS, Baer DG, et al. Prehospital tourniquet use in operation iraqi freedom: effect on hemorrhage control and outcomes. J Trauma. 2008;64(2 Suppl):S28–37; discussion S37.
11. Kragh JF Jr, Littrel ML, Jones JA, Walters TJ, Baer DG, Wade CE, et al. Battle casualty survival with emergency tourniquet use to stop limb bleeding. J Emerg Med. 2011;41(6):590–7.
12. Shlaifer A, Yitzhak A, Baruch EN, Shina A, Satanovsky A, Shovali A, et al. Point of injury tourniquet application during operation protective edge-what do we learn? J Trauma Acute Care Surg. 2017;83(2):278–83.
13. Rall JM, Cox JM, Songer AG, Cestero RF, Ross JD. Comparison of novel hemostatic dressings with quikclot combat gauze in a standardized swine model

of uncontrolled hemorrhage. J Trauma Acute Care Surg. 2013;75(2 Suppl 2):S150–6.
14. Shina A, Lipsky AM, Nadler R, Levi M, Benov A, Ran Y, et al. Prehospital use of hemostatic dressings by the Israel defense forces medical corps: a case series of 122 patients. J Trauma Acute Care Surg. 2015;79(4 Suppl 2):S204–9.
15. Holcomb JB, Jenkins D, Rhee P, Johannigman J, Mahoney P, Mehta S, et al. Damage control resuscitation: directly addressing the early coagulopathy of trauma. J Trauma. 2007;62(2):307–10.
16. Borgman MA, Spinella PC, Perkins JG, Grathwohl KW, Repine T, Beekley AC, et al. The ratio of blood products transfused affects mortality in patients receiving massive transfusions at a combat support hospital. J Trauma. 2007;63(4):805–13.
17. Holcomb JB, Wade CE, Michalek JE, Chisholm GB, Zarzabal LA, Schreiber MA, et al. Increased plasma and platelet to red blood cell ratios improves outcome in 466 massively transfused civilian trauma patients. Ann Surg. 2008;248(3):447–58.
18. Borut LT, Acosta CJ, Tadlock LC, Dye JL, Galarneau M, Elshire CD. The use of temporary vascular shunts in military extremity wounds: a preliminary outcome analysis with 2-year follow-up. J Trauma. 2010;69(1):174–8.
19. Gifford SM, Aidinian G, Clouse WD, Fox CJ, Porras CA, Jones WT, et al. Effect of temporary shunting on extremity vascular injury: an outcome analysis from the global war on terror vascular injury initiative. J Vasc Surg. 2009;50(3):549–55; discussion 555–546.
20. Taller J, Kamdar JP, Greene JA, Morgan RA, Blankenship CL, Dabrowski P, et al. Temporary vascular shunts as initial treatment of proximal extremity vascular injuries during combat operations: the new standard of care at echelon ii facilities? J Trauma. 2008;65(3):595–603.
21. Dua A, Patel B, Kragh JF Jr, Holcomb JB, Fox CJ. Long-term follow-up and amputation-free survival in 497 casualties with combat-related vascular injuries and damage-control resuscitation. J Trauma Acute Care Surg. 2012;73(6):1517–24.
22. Sohn VY, Arthurs ZM, Herbert GS, Beekley AC, Sebesta JA. Demographics, treatment, and early outcomes in penetrating vascular combat trauma. Arch Surg. 2008;143(8):783–7.
23. Vertrees A, Fox CJ, Quan RW, Cox MW, Adams ED, Gillespie DL. The use of prosthetic grafts in complex military vascular trauma: a limb salvage strategy for patients with severely limited autologous conduit. J Trauma. 2009;66(4):980–3.
24. Ritenour AE, Dorlac CW, Fang R, Woods T, Jenkins DH, Flaherty SF, et al. Complications after fasciotomy revision and delayed compartment release in combat patients. J Trauma Acute Care Surg. 2008;64(2):S153–62.
25. Kragh JF, San Antonio J, Simmons JW, Mace JE, Stinner DJ, White CE, et al. Compartment syndrome performance improvement project is associated with increased combat casualty survival. J Trauma Acute Care Surg. 2013;74(1):259.

Aeromedical Evacuation of Cardiothoracic Casualties

16

Michael J. Eppinger and Kenton E. Stephens Jr.

Introduction

Cardiothoracic injuries that occur during combat, natural disasters, or peacetime usually result from dramatically different mechanisms. However, due to their effects on the cardiopulmonary system, the subsequent pathophysiology can be similar. The nature of each type of injury will determine specific care requirements. These injuries can be especially difficult to care for in forward combat or field areas due to the "black box" nature of the injuries; difficulty assessing degree of injury, inability to stop hemorrhage, and lethality of injuries if not rapidly addressed. Even after definitive surgical treatment, patients with cardiothoracic injuries remain relatively unstable for a matter of days. In a combat zone or natural disaster, this dictates the expertise and equipment requirements of the aeromedical evacuation (AE) of these patients. This chapter will address common cardiothoracic injuries, their sequelae, and management during elective and urgent AE.

M. J. Eppinger (✉)
Col, USAF (ret.), Cardiothoracic Surgery, Department of Surgery, South Texas Veterans Health Care System, San Antonio, TX, USA
e-mail: Michael.eppinger@va.gov

K. E. Stephens Jr.
Cardiothoracic Surgery, Denali Cardiac & Thoracic Surgical Group, Anchorage, AK, USA

W. W. Hurd, W. Beninati (eds.), *Aeromedical Evacuation*, https://doi.org/10.1007/978-3-030-15903-0_16

Cardiothoracic Injuries

Severe cardiothoracic injuries are particularly lethal in both civilian and military domains [1]. The mechanisms and resultant pathology of these injuries determine their physiologic effects and clinical courses. The most important factors influencing the patient's condition are:

- Blood loss, which can result in hypoperfusion, hypothermia, acidosis, and coagulopathy
- Direct destruction of organ tissue, e.g., myocardial contusion
- Secondary effects of tissue injury or sepsis on thoracic organ function, e.g., adult respiratory distress syndrome
- Tension effects, e.g., tension pneumothorax or pericardial tamponade

Significant blood loss that often results from cardiothoracic injuries can require massive fluid resuscitation that has detrimental effects on many organ systems. Thus, it comes as no surprise that massive cardiothoracic trauma requiring greater fluid resuscitation volume is associated with a poorer prognosis. Sequelae of massive fluid resuscitation include pulmonary edema with consequent decreased pulmonary compliance, decreased thoracic compliance, increased ventilatory pressures, pulmonary parenchymal barotrauma, pulmonary hypertension and resultant right ventricular dysfunction, increased abdominal compartment pressures, and visceral edema. Over the last several years, there has been a shift away from crystalloid resuscitation in favor of earlier use of blood products when available, and yet the volume of fluid resuscitation in the first 24–48 hours is still a crude marker of the severity of trauma and overall prognosis.

Cardiothoracic injuries are frequently life-threatening. However, the true severity of such injuries is not always initially apparent. Patients, particularly those that are young and otherwise healthy, will partially compensate for severe injuries with tachycardia, vasoconstriction, and anaerobic metabolism. Each of these compensatory mechanisms will eventually be exhausted, resulting in the rapid deterioration of the patient's condition. For this reason, safe AE requires that the aeromedical crew have an accurate understanding of the injury, its variants, natural history, associated risk, and predictable complications. This is especially important when patients are transported early in the course of their recovery. Significant changes in managing combat casualties have occurred as a result of military medical experience in the Afghanistan and Iraq conflicts. As a result, AE crews have been asked to move farther forward and transport less stable patients. This has led to transport of "stabilized" rather than "stable" patients, often with ongoing resuscitation requirements.

Critical Care Air Transport Teams

Significant changes in casualty management have taken place as a result of the conflicts in Afghanistan and Iraq, as well as conflicts in the Middle East and Africa. Surgical teams with smaller footprints are being pushed farther forward in order to decrease the amount of time from injury to surgical stabilization. Many of these teams have little to no holding capacity to manage critically ill patients, in terms of both personnel and materiel resources. The strategic solution has been transporting patients much closer to the time of surgical treatment.

These real-world needs have resulted in major advances in en-route AE care secondary to advances in personnel training, equipment, and techniques inherent to the Critical Care Air Transport Team concept (see Chap. 9). High-level techniques such as renal replacement therapy, complex ventilator strategies, and even extracorporeal life support have been pushed far forward to dramatically improve the survival of once fatal injuries (Fig. 16.1) [2]. A poignant example was successful AE of a combat casualty post-pneumonectomy utilizing extracorporeal life support [3]. These AE advances and innovations have been adapted for use in the civilian air transport system.

Chest Tube

A chest tube, inserted through a lateral thoracostomy, is commonly used to evacuate air, blood, or fluid from the pleural cavity, allowing full expansion of the lung on the affected side. Chest tubes are used to treat a pneumothorax or hemothorax diagnosed by chest X-ray or after the pleural cavity has been entered traumatically or surgically.

In an emergency situation, chest tubes are inserted at the bedside using local anesthesia [4, 5]. The supine patient is slightly rotated and with the ipsilateral arm positioned over the head. A sterile field is created on the lateral chest wall. Local anesthesia is injected and a skin incision is made between the third and fifth intercostal spaces within the "quadrangle of safety" bordered anteriorly by the pectoral groove and posteriorly by the mid-axillary line. The chest wall layers are bluntly dissected and the pleural space is entered bluntly. Chest tube insertion is sometimes done with ultrasound guidance, when available. The chest tube is inserted so that all fenestrated holes are within the pleural space. It is sutured to the skin at the edge of the incision to prevent it from moving and the insertion site is covered with a sterile dressing. Immediately after insertion, a chest X-ray is obtained to assess lung inflation and confirm proper placement.

The chest tube is connected to a collection-drainage system that provides continuous

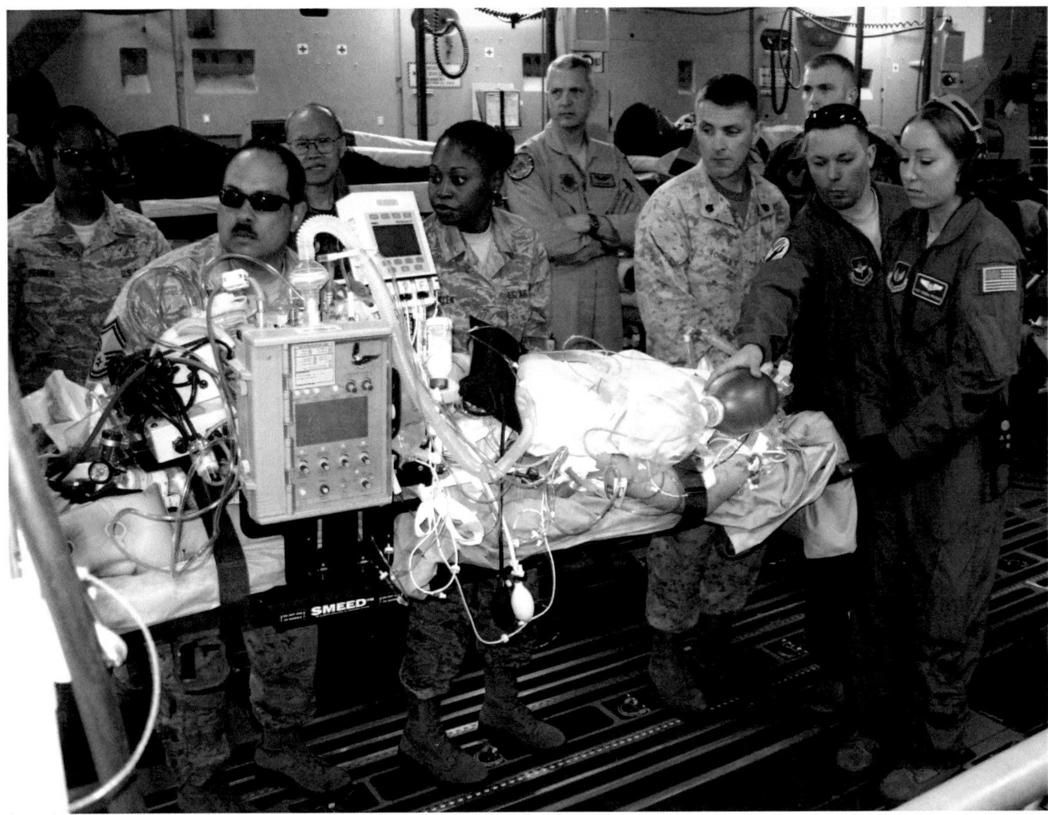

Fig. 16.1 A Critical Care Air Transport Team prepared to transport a critically wounded patient aboard a C-17 from Ramstein Air Base, Germany to Joint Base Andrews, Maryland. (US Air National Guard Photo by Donna Miles)

negative pressure that provides continuous drainage and prevents fluid or air from flowing back into the chest cavity. Traditional systems required a column of water to maintain vacuum and were prone to becoming non-functional if tipped over, and thus are not used during AE. Newer waterless vacuum systems incorporate a valve into the collection system resulting in a safer and less error-prone configuration (Fig. 16.2) [6].

Chest tubes can be associated with a number of early and late occurring complications [4, 5, 7]. Early complications can include:

- Hemothorax – most commonly as a result of intercostal blood vessel laceration. Continued intrapleural bleeding after chest tube placement can require an emergency thoracotomy for treatment.
- Injury to the lung or diaphragm.
- Tube placement outside the pleural cavity, into either the abdomen (with risk of injury to the spleen, stomach, or liver) or the subcutaneous space (Fig. 16.3) [7].
- Pain – which might be more likely if the chest tube is inserted too deeply.
- Accidental drain displacement – best avoided by adequately suturing the chest tube to the skin at the point of the incision.

Late chest tube complications can include:

- Tube blockage – more common with smaller chest tubes
- Incomplete hemothorax drainage
- Infection at the insertion site or within the plural space (empyema)
- Pneumothorax after chest tube removal

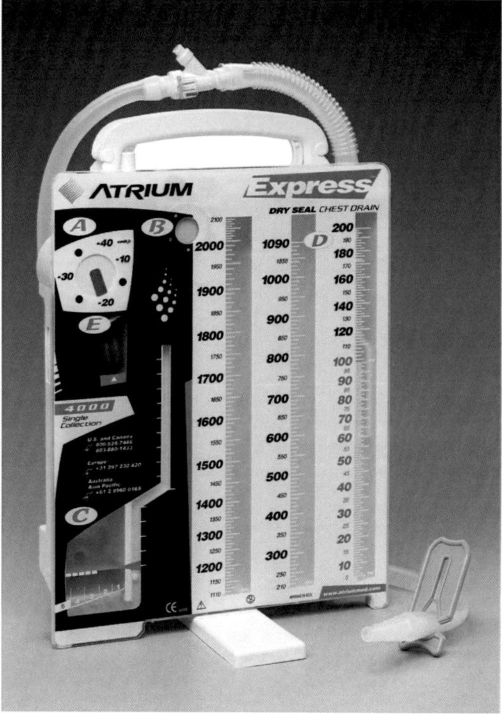

Fig. 16.2 A modern dry suction dry seal chest tube drainage system (Express, Atrium, Inc, Hudson, New Hampshire) approved for use during aeromedical evacuation [6]. (Photo of Atrium Express 4050 Dry Seal Chest Drain courtesy of Atrium Inc, Hudson, New Hampshire)

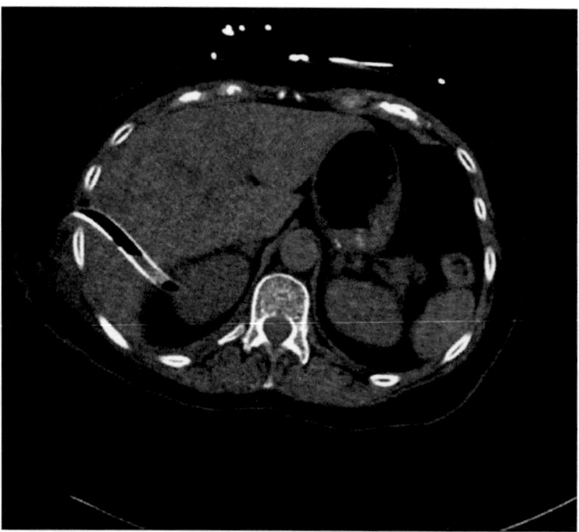

Fig. 16.3 Computerized tomogram image of a chest tube inadvertently placed into the liver parenchyma. (Reprinted with permission from Kwiatt et al. [7])

Table 16.1 Checklist for chest tube management for patients undergoing aeromedical evacuation

Preflight
Proper placement has been verified radiographically
Tube is connected to a drainage apparatus
Adequate oxygenation verified
Tube insertion site inspected for air leaks and secure tube anchor
Therapeutic suction capability available onboard
Supplies for emergency tube replacement verified
Pain control plan prepared and drugs available
In-flight
Tube connected to a collection system
Prophylactic antibiotics
Supplemental oxygen
Pulse oximetry

Aeromedical Evacuation Implications

Medical providers taking care of these patients need an understanding of chest tube design, placement, management, and approaches to troubleshooting (Table 16.1). A tube that is malpositioned, obstructed, too small for the injury, or not properly connected to suction and drainage can create a critical in-flight situation.

Chest tube management includes wound and dressing care to prevent wound infections. Dry dressings are generally preferable, as ointments do little to seal the leak around an inadequately secured tube, but can create a moist anaerobic environment that can encourage bacterial growth. Careful monitoring to ensure continued tube function is mandatory. The chest tube system may malfunction due to chest tube occlusion (e.g., kinking of the tubing, external occlusion, fibrin clots within the tube), detached or leaking connections, or malfunction of the suction sources. A poorly secured tube may partially back out of the thoracic cavity, leaving the most proximal drainage hole outside the chest wall and rendering the tube non-functional.

General Aeromedical Evacuation Considerations for Cardiothoracic Patients

Safe AE of the cardiothoracic patient depends on an adequate understanding of the unique aspects of their injuries and the associated postoperative risks. Although pain control, respiratory hygiene, and fluid management are required for all postoperative patients, post-thoracotomy patients have special concerns that should be recognized.

Pain Control

Effective pain management is essential for optimizing respiratory function in the post-thoracotomy patient. Intermittent narcotics are effective, but have the disadvantage of respiratory depression. Ketorolac is an effective adjunct but should not be used in patients with renal insufficiency, coagulopathy, or a history of gastrointestinal bleeding. When available, a thoracic epidural catheter is an excellent method for providing pain relief without depressing sensorium. However, their use places additional monitoring burdens on the AE crew, and they can be variable in effectiveness. Intercostal nerve blocks with long-acting local anesthetics are an effective adjunct that can provide significant pain relief during critical intervals.

Respiratory Hygiene

It is critical to minimize atelectasis in post-thoracotomy patients. The cornerstone of this effort is effective pain management to allow deep inspiration. Other methods include incentive spirometry, chest physiotherapy, and bronchodilators to aid in clearing secretions. All of these methods must be continued throughout the AE process. Aggressive baseline therapy when the patient appears stable can prevent sudden hypoxia and respiratory distress that can occur when atelectasis or mucous retention reaches a critical level.

Fluid Management

Cardiothoracic trauma can be associated with massive blood loss, which creates the need for fluid resuscitation to restore equilibrium. In addition, pulmonary injury and cardiac failure are both associated with "third spacing" of fluids. In the presence of cardiac dysfunction, it is critical to discriminate between left- and right-sided heart failure. Pulmonary artery catheters can be useful to assess volume status, but may not be available in more austere environments. Normovolemia is the preferred goal to achieve optimum pulmonary and other organ function.

Thromboembolic Prophylaxis

Post-thoracotomy patients are at increased risk of pulmonary embolus due to immobility and hypercoagulability. In addition, compromised respiratory physiology increases the physiologic impact of such events. All such patients should be treated on the ground with at least sequential compression devices on their lower extremities. All postoperative patients who have not achieved full ambulation and are not at risk for active bleeding should also be receiving chemoprophylaxis with either unfractionated or low molecular weight heparin.

Specific Cardiothoracic Conditions

Pneumothorax

Pneumothorax is defined as free air in the pleural space. In a casualty situation, this can occur as a result of blunt or penetrating trauma to the lung, trachea, or chest wall. However, pneumothorax can also occur spontaneously in tall, thin, young men with pre-existing apical blebs or in patients with emphysema or other lung conditions predisposing to bullous disease. Pneumothorax can also occur after pulmonary barotrauma, which creates alveolar over-pressurization and rupture. Common causes of barotrauma include a sudden blow to the chest against a closed glottis, severe bronchospasm as in asthma, or iatrogenic ventilator injuries in an intubated patient.

Traumatic pneumothorax can arise from blunt or penetrating chest injuries. With penetrating injuries, air can be forced into the pleural space through injured lung parenchyma, through the chest wall defect, or both. In blunt trauma, air leak can commonly occur as a result of focal damage to pulmonary parenchyma from fractured ribs, or leak from a large parenchymal tear.

There are essentially three types of pneumothoraces: simple, open, and tension. A simple pneumothorax is just that: air in the pleural space causing incomplete expansion and function of the affected lung. Patients can complain of pain and dyspnea, but especially in the younger, healthier population there is unlikely to be any substantial physiologic distress. A tension pneumothorax results from a physiologic one-way valve that occurs as a result of lung injury; air can get out of the lung into the pleural space, but becomes trapped within the pleural space. As a result, air can accumulate in the pleural space, with resulting increasing intrathoracic pressure that ultimately can compromise venous return to the heart and lead to hemodynamic collapse. An open pneumothorax is the result of a defect in the chest wall such that with inspiration, air enters through the chest wall into the pleural space, rather than ventilating the lungs. This causes ineffective respiratory effort and ultimately hypoxia and collapse.

The immediate remedy for either an open or tension pneumothorax is to convert it to a simple pneumothorax. As mentioned previously, a simple pneumothorax rarely causes an immediate threat to life. An open pneumothorax can be converted by covering the defect and allowing any air under pressure to escape, and a tension pneumothorax can be converted to a simple pneumothorax with needle decompression (see below). After emergency treatment of either a tension or open pneumothorax, a chest tube will ultimately need to be placed for treatment.

Implications for Aeromedical Evacuation

An untreated pneumothorax is a contraindication to AE (Table 16.2). Left untreated, a pneumothorax can severely compromise patient oxygenation and circulation during AE by three methods:

1. The pneumothorax may enlarge due to ongoing air leak from the injured lung or bronchus.

Table 16.2 Cardiothoracic contraindications to long-distance aeromedical evacuation (AE)

Absolute
Untreated pneumothorax
Untreated pneumomediastinum or pneumopericardium
Untreated ruptured diaphragm with herniation into the chest
Active endobronchial bleeding
New or unstable arrhythmias
Deteriorating hemodynamics
Deteriorating respiratory status
Requires Critical Care Air Transport for AE
Within 48 hours of any cardiothoracic surgery
Within 24 hours of repair of ruptured diaphragm
Contraindications to elective AE
Hemothorax with continued chest tube bleeding
Within 48 hours of significant chest wall trauma
Within 14 days of most cardiothoracic surgery
Within 7 days of repair of ruptured diaphragm

2. The decreased cabin pressure associated with flight may cause the volume of a previously stable pneumothorax to increase.
3. The partially collapsed lung on the side of the pneumothorax may cause arterial desaturation from shunting, exacerbating the altitude-related hypoxia [8, 9].

For patients with a very small pneumothorax, elective AE should be delayed until there is radiographic evidence that the pneumothorax has spontaneously resolved. When urgent AE is required for patients with any size pneumothorax, a chest tube should be inserted and verified to be functioning properly.

Prior to AE, all chest tubes need to be connected to a contained suction-collection apparatus. Additional aspects of in-flight management include connection of the collection system to continuous suction, administration of supplemental oxygen if necessary, and verification of adequate oxygenation by pulse oximetry (Table 16.1).

Patients at high risk of developing a pneumothorax (e.g., patients with existing blebs or bullous disease) do not require prophylactic chest tube placement prior to AE. The risk of bleb rupture during flight in a pressurized aircraft is low, and tube placement itself may injure the lung, resulting in an air leak or other complication.

Tension Pneumothorax

A tension pneumothorax can occur in any patient, particularly after polytrauma to the upper body. For this reason, AE crews should be prepared to recognize and treat a tension pneumothorax during any AE flight.

Symptoms of a tension pneumothorax include sudden onset of respiratory distress and chest pain associated with tachycardia. This can progress to hypotension if left untreated. Physical examination will often reveal tracheal deviation away from the affected side and jugular venous distention with or without abdominal distention. The affected hemithorax will be hyperresonant, and auscultation will reveal absent breath sounds on that side.

Needle Thoracostomy

The emergency treatment for tension pneumothorax is needle thoracostomy, whereby a needle is inserted into the pleural space to decompress the tension pneumothorax. In the short term, needle thoracostomy is adequate treatment comparable to placement of a tube thoracostomy [10]. However, ultimately a thoracostomy tube will need to be placed to definitely treat the pneumothorax.

Needle thoracostomy is performed by inserting a 5–8-cm-long 10- to 16-gauge over-the-needle catheter into the pleural space on the side of the affected hemithorax. The correct location is just over the upper edge of the rib that makes up the caudal margin of the second intercostal space in the midclavicular line. After piercing the skin, the needle should be directed cephalad over the rib until the pleura is punctured, which is indicated by a "pop" or sudden decrease in resistance. If the medical condition permits, the patient should be placed in a supine position prior to insertion, and the insertion site prepped with an antiseptic solution.

Hemothorax

Hemothorax is a potentially life-threatening manifestation of a pulmonary parenchymal, chest wall, mediastinal, or thoracic vascular injury. Hemothorax can also occur as a complication of chest tube placement or any thoracic surgery.

Three aspects of a hemothorax put these patients at increased risk for rapid deterioration. First, a significant volume of blood can be lost into the pleural cavity with minimal symptoms. Second, tamponade does not occur as the lung collapses, which is in contrast to bleeding into other confined spaces. Finally, pulmonary function is decreased as the volume of a hemothorax increases, thus exacerbating the physiologic effects. These factors combine to create the high mortality rate for patients with uncontrolled hemothorax.

The objective of hemothorax treatment is to stop the bleeding and to decrease the long-term risk of fibrothorax or empyema as a result of retained clot. The cornerstone of treatment for hemothorax is a chest tube alone and will be adequate therapy for the vast majority of these patients. Most hemothoraces occurring as a result of chest wall or parenchymal bleeding will be treated by evacuating the blood and getting apposition of the lung to the chest wall with a well-placed thoracostomy tube. If the initial amount of blood is greater than 1000 ml, or if the continued blood loss is more than 200 ml/hour, thoracotomy is indicated to stop the bleeding.

Implications for Aeromedical Evacuation

Active bleeding from an intrapleural source after chest tube placement is a contraindication to elective AE. AE for a patient with a residual stable hemothorax is acceptable as long as bleeding has stopped for at least 24 hours. The residual chest tube output should be serosanguinous and the patient should have adequate pulmonary reserve. In addition, the patient must remain hemodynamically stable, with no concern for ongoing bleeding.

Urgent AE may be required during armed conflict or in a mass-casualty situation despite continued intrapleural bleeding. Patients can be moved with a reasonable degree of safety if the chest tube blood loss is less than 100 ml/hour. Greater rates of blood loss put the patient at considerable risk of progressive anemia, hypotension, hypoxia, and dilutional coagulopathy during transport. Urgent AE for patients with >100 ml/hour chest tube blood loss requires a Critical Care Air Transport Team equipped with appropriate blood products, transfusion supplies, and autotransfusion equipment, if available.

For all patients with a chest tube, the amount and type of chest tube output must be closely monitored during AE. Routine chest tube management, as described for pneumothorax, will also be required.

In-Flight Complications

Patients with hemothorax and continued bleeding are at risk for chest tube obstruction by clotted blood. Signs of hemodynamic instability with ineffective chest tube drainage should raise concerns for undetected intrapleural bleeding or a clotted tube. In this situation, every effort should be made to clear the tube, or replace it if necessary.

Effective techniques for clearing an obstructed chest tube can be successfully accomplished even in austere AE environments. The chest tube is first disconnected and then the obstructing clot is removed with either an endotracheal suction catheter or a Fogarty balloon catheter. If increased intrathoracic hemorrhage results in hemodynamic instability, resuscitation with fluids and blood products will be required until the patient can be transported to the nearest medical facility.

Pleural Effusion

A pleural effusion is any collection of fluid in the pleural space and is common in trauma patients. Pleural effusions are described as either transudative or exudative based on the relative concentrations of protein and lactate dehydrogenase in the fluid. Exudative effusions are the most common in the acute trauma patients and have a pleural fluid to serum protein ratio >0.5 and a lactate dehydrogenase ratio >0.6 [11]. Transudative effusions are the result of pre-existing heart failure, cirrhosis, or accumulated third spacing of fluid.

Exudative effusions have a wide variety of causes, such as pneumonia, malignancy, mediastinal or subphrenic abscess, or secondary to injuries to adjacent organs, such as esophagus, pancreas, or chest wall. Conditions that appear to be effusions, such as hemothorax or chylothorax, can be differentiated by diagnostic thoracentesis. Therapy consists of placement of chest tube for diagnosis and drainage. AE management does not depend on the cause of the effusion.

Pneumomediastinum

A pneumomediastinum or pneumopericardium occurs when bronchial air leaks proximally into the mediastinal space rather than into the pleural space (Fig. 16.4) [12]. This is frequently associated with subcutaneous emphysema, and if the air dissects across the diaphragm or retroperitoneum, pneumoperitoneum can develop as well [12].

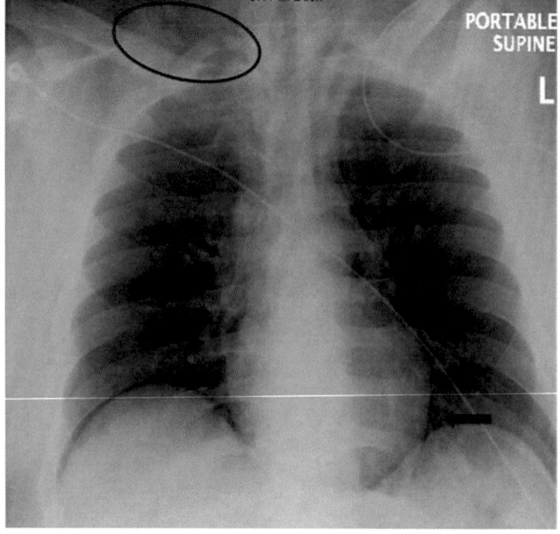

Fig. 16.4 Chest X-ray displaying pneumomediastinum and subcutaneous emphysema at the right base of the neck. (Reprinted with permission from Guzman Rojas et al. [12])

In the trauma patient, the presence of pneumomediastinum or related conditions should prompt a search for an injury to the central airway or esophagus. A large central airway defect will require surgical repair. No specific treatment is necessary for stable patients who do not require air transportation. However, the patient should be observed for the development of pneumothorax, because even a small leak can extend into the pleural space. Similarly, although subcutaneous emphysema can create an alarming appearance, it poses no immediate threat to the patient as long as the pleural cavity is decompressed.

If it is unclear whether a pneumothorax is or is not present, it is safest to place bilateral chest tubes prior to transporting the patient. Very rarely, placement of a tube via the subxiphoid route into the pericardial space is necessary for decompression of tension pneumopericardium.

Implications for Aeromedical Evacuation

Untreated pneumomediastinum is a contraindication to AE because of the risk of subsequent pneumothorax in these patients (Table 16.2). Prior to AE, these patients should have prophylactic chest tubes placed.

Untreated pneumopericardium is a contraindication to AE because expansion of air in the pericardium during flight can result in cardiac tamponade. Although tension pneumopericardium is rare, the results can be disastrous. For this reason, these patients must have adequate pericardial drainage prior to AE, with either a subxiphoid pericardial drain or a pericardial window (Fig. 16.5).

Tracheobronchial Bleeding

Airway bleeding may be the result of a penetrating lung injury, massive blunt chest trauma, inflammation, burns, infection, pulmonary hypertension, foreign bodies, or malignancy. Significant endobronchial bleeding is associated with a high mortality rate.

Emergency treatment begins with endotracheal intubation to secure the airway. The patient should be positioned with the bleeding side, if known, down. Oxygen should be administered and aggressive respiratory care implemented to clear the airway of blood. Coagulopathy should be identified and corrected. If the airway cannot be cleared due to the amount of bleeding, proceed with advancement of the endotracheal tube

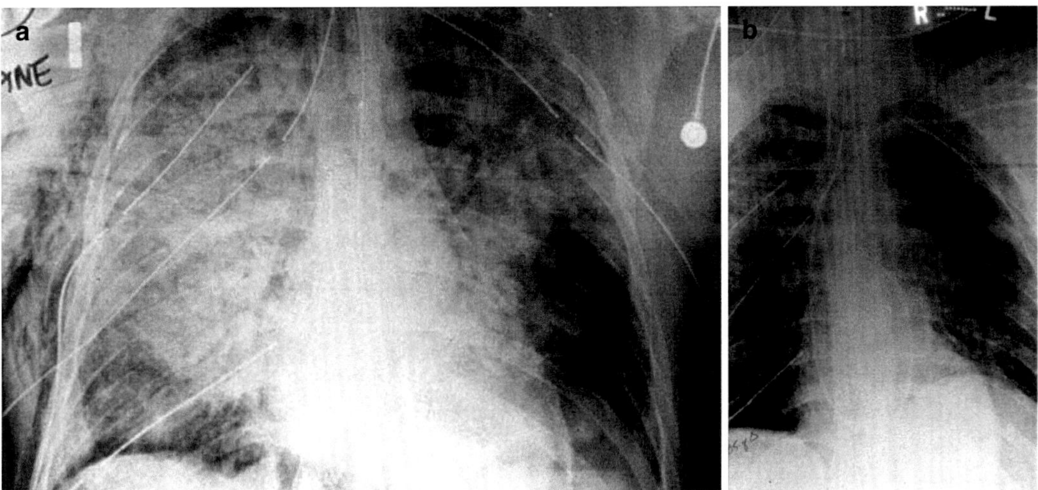

Fig. 16.5 Tension pneumopericardium is demonstrated by chest radiograph (**a**) despite bilateral chest tubes. Clinical signs of cardiac tamponade and the abnormally enlarged cardiac silhouette (**b**) resolved after emergency placement of a subxiphoid pericardial drainage tube

into the mainstem bronchus contralateral to the site of the bleeding. This temporizing maneuver permits "one-lung" ventilation and prevents entry of blood into the ventilated lung.

More definitive temporization involves placement of a double-lumen endotracheal tube. Angiographic localization and embolization can be helpful if available, as the bleeding source is frequently a bronchial branch of the thoracic aorta.

Uncontrolled tracheobronchial bleeding may necessitate emergency thoracotomy with resection of the bleeding segment. These procedures have a significant mortality rate, even in a fully equipped operating room. Radiographic selective embolization of the bronchial or pulmonary artery generally is preferred as a first choice if available.

Implications for Aeromedical Evacuation

Uncontrolled endobronchial bleeding is always a contraindication to AE. Medical evacuation to the nearest appropriate medical facility should only be undertaken after the bleeding has been isolated with mainstem bronchus intubation and any coagulopathy has been corrected.

Air Embolism

Lung injury is a major risk factor for air embolism. Air can pass from injured alveoli into the pulmonary venous circulation, where it is then transported to the left atrium and ejected by the left ventricle into the aortic root. Air naturally rises to the highest point, which in the supine patient is the anterior aortic root, near the ostium of the right coronary artery. The bubbles pass down the right coronary artery and lodge in small vessels or the myocardium. This can create ischemia in the right ventricle, inferior left ventricle, and septum, which can quickly become dysfunctional. This can result in rapid, profound hypotension, right ventricular failure, bradycardia, and cardiac arrest.

The most effective approach to air embolism is prevention. In high-risk patients with parenchymal pulmonary injuries, prophylactic measures include maintenance of low airway pressures and relatively high atrial filling pressures as reflected by central venous pressure and pulmonary capillary wedge pressure.

The most important treatment approach is increasing coronary perfusion pressure by administration of epinephrine or other adrenergic agonists and fluids in an effort to flush air out of the coronary circulation and restore coronary capillary perfusion pressure. Further measures include placing the patient in the left lateral decubitus, Trendelenburg position to direct air away from the aortic root and toward the ventricular apex. Halting further entry of air into the circulation requires an emergency thoracotomy for pulmonary hilar control, repair or resection of the injured lung, and potentially aspiration of the air pockets in the ventricles and great vessels.

Air entering the circulation through intravenous (IV) lines can also be dangerous because a right-sided air embolization can be fatal. A large amount of air (>10–100 mL) can cause right ventricular cavitation and cardiogenic shock. Less commonly, air bubbles in the venous circulation can pass through a patent foramen ovale or atrial septal defect, becoming a left-sided air embolus. These latter two entities are more likely in conditions that increase right-sided cardiac pressures, such a hypoxia, volume overload, acidosis, pulmonary hypertension, or tamponade.

Emergency management of venous air embolism includes halting the ingress of air, fluid resuscitation, inotropic support, and repositioning the patient into the left lateral decubitus, Trendelenburg position to allow the air to accumulate in the apex of the right ventricle. If available, a pulmonary artery catheter can be floated into the right ventricular outflow tract to aspirate air causing the obstruction.

Flail Chest and Pulmonary Contusion

Flail chest refers to chest wall trauma in which one or more ribs are fractured in at least two places, mobilizing a plate of chest wall from the remainder of the thorax. It can be the result of blunt trauma, projectile, or blast shock wave. The paroxysmal, painful inward movement during inhalation limits respiratory excursion and efficiency. Flail chest is almost universally accompanied by pulmonary contusion and commonly by pleural effusion or hemothorax as well. It is generally the underlying contusion that is felt to primarily contribute to the hypoxia that accompanies this condition.

Pulmonary contusion is characterized by interstitial and alveolar hemorrhage with architectural disruption resulting in decreased gas exchange across the capillary-alveolar interface. Severe cases may develop regions of lung necrosis and hemoptysis.

On chest X-ray, pulmonary contusion is generally evident at the time of injury as an area of consolidation. The radiographic lesion will often progress in size and density over the next 24 to 96 hours. The lung injury can be aggravated by massive fluid administration, as may occur in trauma resuscitation.

Respiratory Insufficiency

Significant chest wall trauma can result in respiratory insufficiency, which manifests as hypoxemia with or without hypercapnia. Causes of respiratory insufficiency after significant chest wall trauma include pulmonary contusion, splinting secondary to pain from rib fractures, hemothorax, atelectasis, pneumonia, or deranged respiratory mechanics due to flail chest.

Treatment for respiratory insufficiency in patients with chest wall trauma begins with supplemental oxygen with the addition of adequate pain medication, bronchodilators, and active pulmonary hygiene. Although these steps will maximize chest wall compliance and pulmonary function, these patients need to be closely observed for early signs of deterioration. Endotracheal intubation and ventilator support are often required in patients with significant pulmonary contusions.

Implications for Aeromedical Evacuation

The first 48 hours after significant chest wall trauma is a critical period during which deterioration of pulmonary function is most likely to occur. For this reason, patients with fractured ribs should not be transported by elective AE for the first 48 hours post injury (Table 16.2). Patients transported by AE within 7 days of pulmonary contusion should be given supplemental oxygen.

During a military operation or mass-casualty situation, or if appropriate medical care is not available locally, movement of these patients by urgent AE may be required after little more than initial stabilization. The presence of a pneumothorax will require placement of a chest tube with appropriate drainage including a one-way valve, as discussed above. The presence of untreated hemothorax can be especially dangerous, as discussed above. Pain relief can be provided by oral or parenteral narcotic and non-narcotic drugs, local injection such as intercostal blocks, or regional anesthesia. If a spontaneously breathing patient continues to have severely low oxygen saturation on 100% supplemental oxygen, endotracheal intubation is recommended prior to AE.

Tracheobronchial Injuries

Intrathoracic tracheobronchial injuries can result from penetrating, crush, or severe deceleration injuries. They are associated with significant morbidity and mortality. These injuries can create airway obstruction, pneumothorax or pneumomediastinum, and significant blood loss.

Initial care for tracheobronchial injuries is primarily supportive, and emergent surgery is often required. The operation itself can be technically challenging for both the surgeon and the anesthetist. Associated injuries can cause substantial blood loss with a fatality rate approaching 25% at tertiary care centers. Surgical tracheobronchial repair leaves an anastomotic suture line that is delicate, slow to heal, and vulnerable to barotrauma, tension, ischemia, and infection. Postoperatively, early extubation is indicated to minimize airway pressure and avoid anastomotic erosion from airway catheters.

Implications for Aeromedical Evacuation

Elective AE should be deferred until the convalescent period, usually at least 14 days after surgery. The patient should no longer require chest tubes and be substantially recovered from coexisting injuries.

In an emergency situation, urgent AE should be delayed for 12 hours after definitive surgery to observe for early operative complications (anastomotic disruption or pneumothorax) and fluid resuscitation. These patients will be relatively unstable and require the special expertise of a CCATT team for safe movement so soon after surgery.

Prior to urgent AE, patients should be afebrile and the chest tube output should be <50 ml/hour. Thoracic air leaks often continue for the first 2–5 days postoperatively, and AE during this time will require effective chest tube management with an appropriate collection chamber and continuous suction. For intubated patients, neuromuscular blockade is usually necessary to maximize thoracic compliance and manage the patient effectively.

Patients who have undergone emergency lung resections must be observed for postoperative air leaks from the raw parenchymal surface. These patients may undergo urgent AE 12 hours postoperatively if the air leaks are adequately managed with chest tubes connected to a drainage system and on suction.

Patients with profound injury to one lung may have asymmetric pulmonary compliance. If this is severe enough to cause hypoxia and hypoventilation from shunting through the injured lung and overventilation of the compliant lung, two ventilators may be needed to provide differential lung ventilation during transport. In addition to pulse oximetry, the patient may require central venous and arterial pressure monitoring.

In-Flight Emergencies

Dehiscence of a tracheobronchial anastomosis, although uncommon, can be fatal unless the condition is quickly recognized. Signs of anastomosis dehiscence are massive air leak through the chest tube secondary to pneumothorax and sudden intractable hypoxia. If the patient is mechanically ventilated, lack of air return will accompany air being evacuated out of the chest tube.

The treatment for an anastomosis dehiscence is lung isolation, which refers to single lung ventilation of the contralateral lung. Tracheal anastomosis dehiscence can be treated by advancing a single-lumen endotracheal tube beyond failed anastomosis. More distal anastomosis dehiscence can be treated by advancing a single-lumen endotracheal tube into the mainstem bronchus of the contralateral lung from the bronchial anastomosis. If the expertise (i.e., pulmonologist) and equipment (i.e., bronchoscope) are available, a double-lumen endotracheal tube or bronchial blocker within a single-lumen tube can be placed and positioned to isolate the leak.

Cardiac Trauma

Cardiac trauma may be either blunt or penetrating. Cardiac contusions clinically resemble acute myocardial infarctions in many ways, although the area of tissue damage and dysfunction are more likely to conform to regions of impact rather than anatomic boundaries of coronary perfusion. These patients generally do not require specific medical intervention unless they develop significant dysrhythmias or heart failure symptoms. Implications for AE after such an injury are covered in more depth in Chap. 19: Medical Casualties.

Penetrating cardiac injuries must be treated surgically. Military trauma patients with penetrating cardiac injuries rarely survive to the point of AE unless their injuries are from fragmentation devices and the patients make it to surgical capability early. Patients with more limited injuries may survive after repair through thoracotomy or sternotomy. Their postoperative course will be similar to that of any other post-thoracotomy patient.

Implications for Aeromedical Evacuation

Elective AE should be delayed until well into the convalescent phase of recovery: 7–10 days after surgery like most postoperative cardiothoracic patients. The difficulties encountered when attempting to perform emergency operations in-flight are enormous, and consequently every effort should be made to delay AE until the patient is stable.

Urgent AE can be performed 12 hours after surgery, but will require the assistance of a fully equipped and well-trained CCATT team. The patient must be hemodynamically stabilized with coagulation factors in the normal range. It is imperative that chest tube output be less than 100 ml/hour because patients with greater rates of output are at significant risk of anemia, coagulopathy, and cardiac tamponade – a potentially fatal complication requiring emergency re-exploration.

In-flight care should include monitoring of central venous and arterial pressure as well as pulse oximetry. Blood pressure must be carefully controlled because excessive hypertension can result in the failure of an otherwise secure arterial or cardiac suture line, especially early in the post-operative period.

Complications are common in the first 72 hours after cardiac surgery and may require immediate treatment. Inotropic, vaso-regulatory, and anti-arrhythmic drugs should be available. Because cardiac arrhythmias are common post-operatively, a defibrillator with internal and external paddles and a pacing device compatible with both surgically placed and transvenous temporary pacing wires should be available. An open-chest instrument tray and skilled personnel should be present for the emergency treatment of cardiac tamponade, should it occur. Blood and clotting factors should be available if significant bleeding is a problem. Warming devices are mandatory to keep the patient normothermic.

Blunt Aortic Trauma

Blunt aortic trauma resulting in aortic transection is frequently lethal. In peacetime, almost 90% die at the scene and many more die before diagnostic studies are completed [13]. The diagnosis should be suspected in any patient in hemorrhagic shock after significant blunt chest trauma, especially after sudden deceleration.

Emergency care is limited to airway management and intravascular volume expansion with blood products and fluids. In surviving patients, exsanguination is usually prevented by the formation of an adventitial hematoma. The most important aspect of care prior to repair is to prevent significant hypertension, which may disrupt the hematoma. Hypertension can be managed by the adequate treatment of pain and hypoxia, avoidance of fluid overload, beta-adrenergic antagonist therapy, and if necessary mechanical ventilation and pharmacologic muscular paralysis.

Implications for Aeromedical Evacuation

Patients with aortic trauma who are still alive when they reach a medical facility will often require further transport to a higher level of care for definitive treatment. Cardiopulmonary bypass is often required for surgical repair of this injury, although it has now become commonplace to repair these via transcatheter placement of a stented graft. If the patient does require open surgical repair, the same caveats regarding transport apply as with any other post-thoracotomy patient. Elective AE should be delayed 7–10 days if possible.

Urgent AE will require the assistance of a well-equipped CCATT team and may be initiated approximately 12 hours after surgery, when the patient is hemodynamically stable and coagulation parameters have returned to normal.

A distinct problem related to aortic disruption and surgical repair is visceral ischemia secondary to intraoperative aortic clamping. Within the first 72 hours after surgery, bowel edema and significant third space fluid losses can increase intra-abdominal pressure. If abdominal compartment syndrome is suspected in-flight, diversion to a medical facility for decompressive laparotomy is indicated. Measurement of a decompressed bladder pressure of greater than 30 cm of water is suggestive of this diagnosis. Delayed spinal cord ischemia can also occur after aortic clamping. If this occurs, intrathecal decompression by lumbar drainage of cerebrospinal fluid can be beneficial to increase perfusion. Although the patient stable enough for AE will generally be outside the time window for this complication, the well-prepared AE crew will have the necessary expertise to identify and treat should the patient develop it.

Esophageal Perforation

Esophageal perforation may result from penetrating trauma, blunt trauma, caustic ingestion, barotrauma, impaction of sharp objects, food, or pills, or instrumentation. Penetrating injury to the thoracic esophagus is seen less often because the accompanying injuries to the great vessels or heart are usually fatal. Penetrating injury to the cervical esophagus should be suspected with any deep neck injury, especially in the presence of subcutaneous air. Treatment of associated vascular or tracheal injuries must take precedence over esophageal repair but is generally done in the same setting.

Barotrauma to the esophagus usually is as a result of violent emesis (Boerhaave's syndrome). The most common site of perforation is near the hiatus at the left lateral wall, where the esophagus lies next to the pleural space.

The primary effect of esophageal rupture is mediastinal and pleural contamination with oral and gastric contents resulting in chemical and bacterial contamination and sepsis. Pleural and mediastinal contamination requires surgical repair of the injury, ample drainage of the contaminated area with chest tubes, and antibiotic therapy. Delay in treatment of these injuries results in an exceedingly high mortality rate.

Implications for Aeromedical Evacuation

Time from injury to surgical repair is critical for esophageal perforation because necrotizing mediastinitis will make repair more difficult as time passes. The dramatic fluid shifts that occur due to mediastinal inflammation create more hemodynamic instability with time. Urgent AE should be undertaken as soon as possible after the diagnosis of esophageal perforation is made, assuming the patient is stable with respect to other injuries. Prior to AE, these patients should have nasoesophageal or nasogastric tubes placed to limit contamination and should receive broad-spectrum antibiotics.

Postoperative patients, like other thoracotomy patients, should be allowed to recover for 7–10 days prior to elective AE. After esophageal repair, oral alimentation is generally held for several days until a swallow study demonstrates the integrity of the repair site. Prior to elective AE, the patient should be able to swallow normally and be adequately recovered from any coexisting injuries.

Urgent AE can be carried out after the patient has been allowed to recover for 12 hours postoperatively, assuming the patient has been stabilized with respect to other injuries. The patient will generally require multiple large-bore chest tubes and potentially neck drainage as well. Broad-spectrum antibiotics with good anaerobic coverage are mandatory.

Diaphragmatic Rupture

Diaphragmatic rupture is relatively common in trauma patients and can be difficult to diagnose, especially if the defect is small. At surgery, 19% of patients with penetrating lower thoracic trauma, but without preoperative evidence of visceral herniation, can be found to have diaphragmatic perforation [14]. In blunt trauma, the left hemidiaphragm is more likely to be injured, due to the protective effect of the liver on the right; 85% of diaphragm injuries involve the left, and fewer than 15% occur exclusively on the right [15]. Preoperative imaging modalities remain poor in detecting injuries.

Implications for Aeromedical Evacuation

A ruptured diaphragm with herniation of abdominal contents into the chest is a contraindication to AE prior to surgical repair (Table 16.2). Visceral ischemia and respiratory compromise may worsen as intestinal gas expands during flight. Rupture of the stomach, colon, or small intestine into the pleural space can lead to sepsis and death. Surgical repair of the hernia and nasogastric decompression is mandatory before transport.

Elective AE for patients after surgical repair of a ruptured diaphragm should be delayed for 7 days to minimize the risk of in-flight complications. Urgent AE may be undertaken as soon as the patient demonstrates hemodynamic and respiratory stability postoperatively.

References

1. Pape HC, Remmers D, Rice J, Ebisch M, Krettek C, Tscherne H. Appraisal of early evaluation of blunt chest trauma: development of a standardized scoring system for initial clinical decision making. J Trauma. 2000;49:496–504.
2. Cannon JW, Zonies DH, Benfield RJ, Elster EA, Wanek SM. Advanced en-route critical care during combat operations. Bull Am Coll Surg. 2011;96:21–9.
3. Neff LP, Cannon JW, Stewart IJ, Batchinsky AI, Zonies DH, Pamplin JC, Chung KK. Extracorporeal organ support following trauma: the dawn of a new era in combat casualty critical care. J Trauma Acute Care Surg. 2013;75(2):S120–9.
4. McElnay PJ, Lim E. Modern techniques to insert chest drains. Thorac Surg Clin. 2017;27(1):29–34.
5. McBeth PB, Savage SA. Tube thoracostomy. Atlas Oral Maxillofac Surg Clin North Am. 2015;23(2):151–7.
6. Department of the Air Force. Air Force Instruction 10-2909. Aeromedical Equipment Standards. Washington, DC: US Government Printing Office; 2013.
7. Kwiatt M, Tarbox A, Seamon MJ, Swaroop M, Cipolla J, Allen C, et al. Thoracostomy tubes: a comprehensive review of complications and related topics. Int J Crit Illn Inj Sci. 2014;4(2):143–55.
8. Bendrick GA, Nicolas DK, Krause BA, Castillo CY. Inflight oxygen desaturation decrements in aeromedical evacuation patients. Aviat Space Environ Med. 1995;66:40–4.
9. Henry JN, Krenis LJ, Cutting RT. Hypoxemia during aeromedical evacuation. Surg Gynecol Obstet. 1973;136:49–53.
10. Baron ED, Epperson M, Hoyt DB, Fortlage D, Rosen P. Prehospital needle aspiration and tube thoracostomy in trauma victims: a six year experience with aeromedical crews. J Emerg Med. 1995;13:155–63.
11. Heffner JE, Brown LK, Barbieri CA. Diagnostic value of tests that discriminate between exudative and transudative pleural effusions. Chest. 1997;111:970–80.
12. Guzman Rojas P, Agostinho J, Hanna R, Karasik O. Spontaneous pneumomediastinum as a consequence of severe vomiting in diabetic ketoacidosis. Cureus. 2018;10(5):e2562.
13. Cowley RA, Turney SZ, Hankins JR, Rodriguez A, Attar S, Shankar BS. Rupture of the thoracic aorta caused by blunt trauma. A fifteen year experience. J Thorac Cardiovasc Surg. 1990;100:652–61.
14. Madden MR, Paull DE, Finkelstein JL, Goodwin CW, Marzulli V, Yurt RW, Shires GT. Occult diaphragmatic injury from stab wounds to the lower chest and abdomen. J Trauma. 1989 Mar;29(3):292–8.
15. Brooks JW. Blunt traumatic rupture of the diaphragm. Br J Surg. 1978;26:199–204.

17 Burn Casualties

David J. Barillo, Julie A. Rizzo,
and Kristine P. Broger

Introduction

Since the initial publication of *Aeromedical Evacuation: Management of Acute and Stabilized Patients* in 2003, the US military has been continuously involved in wartime operations. This chapter, based on lectures given by Burn Flight Team members at the Critical Care Air Transport Basic class, will review the basic concepts of in-flight burn care, with emphasis on doctrinal changes and lessons learned as a result of the conflicts in Afghanistan and Iraq. Major improvements in resuscitation, speed of transport, and wound care have occurred. In addition, replacement of older airframes (C-141 Starlifter and C-9 Nightingale) with the C-17 Globemaster has greatly facilitated transcontinental aeromedical evacuation (AE) and allowed the in-flight use of technologies such as high-frequency percussive ventilation (HFPV) and continuous renal replacement therapy.

Tertiary burn care to all branches of the US military is provided on a worldwide basis by the US Army Burn Center, US Army Institute of Surgical Research, located at the San Antonio Military Medical Center in San Antonio, Texas. Since 1951, the Army Burn Center has also operated a burn flight team to provide safe and expeditious transfer of burned patients to the institute. From 1951 until the beginning of Operations Iraqi Freedom and Enduring Freedom (2002/2003), the burn flight team has successfully transported nearly 5000 burn patients over a total distance of approximately eight million miles. In 15 years of continuous wartime operations, more than 900 additional patients have been transported from Iraq and Afghanistan through the combined efforts of US Army and US Air Force (USAF) AE teams, including more than 300 patients with injuries serious enough to require transport by the burn flight team.

In 1994, the USAF developed a new critical care transport capability with the establishment of critical care air transport teams (CCATT). It quickly became apparent that the missions of the CCATT and the burn flight team were complementary rather than competitive, so efforts were made to seamlessly merge missions. Wherever possible, the medical equipment and supplies carried by both teams have been standardized.

D. J. Barillo (✉)
COL, MC, USA (ret.), Former, Clinical Division/Director US Army Burn Center, Former, US Army Burn Flight Team, U.S. Army Institute of Surgical Research, Joint Base San Antonio-Fort Sam Houston, San Antonio, TX, USA

Disaster Response/Critical Care Consultants, LLC, Mount Pleasant, SC, USA

J. A. Rizzo
MAJ, MC, USA, Burn Unit, United States Army Institute of Surgical Research, Fort Sam Houston, TX, USA

K. P. Broger
LTC, NC, USA, US Army Burn Flight Team, Nursing, US Army Medical Department, Guthrie MEDDAC, Fort Drum, NY, USA

W. W. Hurd, W. Beninati (eds.), *Aeromedical Evacuation*,
https://doi.org/10.1007/978-3-030-15903-0_17

During the time that the USAF School of Aerospace Medicine was located in San Antonio, completion of the CCAT course was a training requirement for the entire burn flight team, and several burn flight team members functioned as adjunct faculty for the CCATT basic course.

The respective roles of the CCATT and burn flight team in the aeromedical evacuation of burn patients were further defined in a US Transportation Command memorandum in 2004 [1]. Guidelines for selection of patients for burn flight team transfer include patients with burns of ≥20% body surface area; smoke inhalation injury requiring mechanical ventilation; burn patients with associated severe mechanical trauma; mechanically ventilated burn or inhalation injury patients with acute respiratory distress syndrome (ARDS) (PaO_2-FiO_2 ratio < 200); burn patients with high-voltage (≥1000 V) electrical injury; or any other burn patient whose severity of illness or injury merits, in the view of the attending surgeon, transport by the burn team [1]. More importantly, this memorandum also established that the burn flight team would not normally travel into the Central Command Area of Responsibility. Thus, nearly all burn patients evacuated out of Iraq or Afghanistan to Landstuhl Regional Medical Center in Germany were managed by USAF Air Evac or CCAT teams. Depending on severity of injury, transfer of burn patients from Landstuhl to San Antonio was accomplished by AE crews, CCAT Teams, burn flight teams, or combinations of the three.

Burn flight team members are burn surgeons (usually with trauma experience and additional certification in surgical critical care), burn intensive care unit (ICU) nurses, burn-licensed vocational nurses, and respiratory therapists who are in the full-time practice of burn medicine. In addition, a senior sergeant travels with the team as the Operations and Logistics Noncommissioned Officer. The en route care provided is simply an extension of usual burn center practice, which utilizes the interdisciplinary care team model.

The burn flight team program has been successful due to each team member's clinical expertise, ability to work under suboptimal conditions, and dedication to their patient's survival. Interdisciplinary care teams have been proven to improve patient outcomes within healthcare organizations. This delivery model uses communication and teamwork as its foundation. Members of the burn flight team must rely on each other's knowledge, skills, and expertise during a flight mission. Each member is well versed and confident in not only their own roles and responsibilities but those of their team members. Interdependent collaboration and shared decision-making are the cornerstone to the success of the burn flight team program.

CCAT teams follow a similar interdisciplinary model and consist of an intensive care physician (usually from the specialties of emergency medicine, cardiology, anesthesia, or pulmonary critical care), an intensive care nurse, and a respiratory therapist. Very few CCAT teams are staffed by surgeons, and virtually none have either a burn surgeon or burn nurse. Lack of this surgical subspecialty, coupled with a paucity of useful educational or reference materials on in-flight burn care, makes such missions a challenge.

The majority of available burn textbooks or courses, such as the Advanced Burn Life Support and Advanced Trauma Life Support programs, concentrate on civilian burn care—an arena in which injury severity is usually lower, burns associated with multiple injuries are uncommon, and long-range transportation is unnecessary. Similarly, military references such as the *North Atlantic Treaty Organization (NATO) War Surgery Handbook* [2] concentrate on initial, austere, or surgical management. This is of limited utility to a transport team, which will first encounter a burn patient a few hours preflight, with resuscitation well underway, and possibly after one or more surgical procedures have already been performed.

Burn Epidemiology

In civilian practice in the United States, annually there are 486,000 burn injuries that require medical treatment and approximately 3275 fire or smoke inhalation-related deaths [3]. Forty thousand patients are admitted to hospitals,

Table 17.1 American burn association burn center referral criteria

1. Partial-thickness burns greater than 10% total body surface area
2. Burns that involve the face, hands, feet, genitalia, perineum, or major joints
3. Third-degree burns in any age group
4. Electrical burns including lightning injury
5. Chemical burns
6. Inhalation injury
7. Burn injury in patients with pre-existing medical disorders that could complicate management, prolong recovery, or affect mortality
8. Any patient with burns and concomitant trauma (such as fractures) in which the burn injury poses the greatest risk of morbidity or mortality. In such cases, if the trauma poses greater immediate risk, the patient may be initially stabilized in a trauma center before being transferred to a burn center. Physician judgment will be necessary in such situations and should be in concert with the regional medical control plan and triage protocols
9. Burned children in hospitals without qualified personnel or equipment for the care of children
10. Burn injury in patients who will require special social, emotional, or rehabilitative intervention

Reprinted with permission from American Burn Association/American College of Surgeons [5]

including 30,000 who are admitted to specialized burn care facilities [3]. Specialized burn care is delivered by a network of 123 burn centers located in 42 states and the District of Columbia, comprising approximately 1800 beds [4]. The American Burn Association (ABA) is the professional organization of burn care providers and consists of more than 2000 burn surgeons, nurses, therapists, firefighters, and prevention specialists. The American Burn Association provides an Advanced Burn Life Support course, maintains a national burn registry, and establishes criteria for referral to specialized burn care facilities (Table 17.1) [5].

Military service is associated with an increased risk of burn injury during both armed conflict and peacetime because of proximity to weapons systems, munitions, explosives, aviation fuel, steam pipes on ships, and field heating and cooking devices [6]. The wartime incidence of burns is usually quoted as 10% of all battle injuries. This is based on data collected during the Vietnam War by the Wound Data and Munitions Effectiveness Team showing that thermal injury or other major soft tissue injuries requiring operative debridement will be present in 10% of combat casualties [6, 7]. Others estimate a war burn incidence of between 5% and 20% [8]. Burn injury was present in 4.6% of Israeli casualties from the Six-Day War in 1967 [9], 10.5% of injuries in the 1973 Yom Kippur War [8, 10], approximately 8% of casualties from the Lebanon war of 1982, [8, 9, 11], 7.9% of injuries from Operation Desert Storm [8, 12], and 18% of British casualties from the Falklands War [6, 9, 13]. These statistics are somewhat misleading as the presence of a burn injury is not synonymous with the need to aeromedically evacuate a burn patient back to the United States.

A more meaningful dataset is the number of patients admitted to the Army Burn Center from recent conflicts. From the Vietnam War, there were 1162 burn patients flown back to the United States and admitted to the Army Burn Center between the years 1965 and 1972. During Operations Desert Shield/Desert Storm, there were a total of approximately 75 burn injuries treated, including 35 service members requiring aeromedical evacuation to the Army Burn Center. From the beginning of Operations Enduring Freedom and Iraqi Freedom until the end of 2016, more than 900 US service members have been aeromedically evacuated to the Army Burn Center from Iraq or Afghanistan. More than 300 with severe injuries were transported by the burn flight team with the remainder transported by USAF CCAT and AE teams.

Burn Care Systems

Burn care is resource- and personnel-intensive. Experienced burn nurses are a rare commodity, and it is not unusual for a burn ICU patient to constantly require two nurses at bedside. Daily wound care takes hours to perform and requires both dressing supplies and a clean environment in which to work. Our current practice is to excise and skin graft all deep burn injuries in one operative case within 72 hours of burn center admission. This requires experienced burn surgeons and burn anesthesiologists, robust blood bank capabilities, and 7-day-a-week availability of an operating room. Burn care is inherently multidisciplinary, with physical and occupational therapists, psychiatric nurses, rehabilitation medicine physicians, dietitians, pharmacists, and case managers integral to the burn team and involved in care from the first day of admission.

Many US states have specialized burn care facilities. However, even in those that do not, regionalization makes burn care available to all patients within hours of injury, and most civilian burn care courses or protocols assume the availability of a specialized facility within a reasonable timeframe.

Prehospital care and transfer usually involves ground or rotary wing air transportation, although contract fixed-wing services are available in some areas. The transport distances are usually much shorter than that seen in military practice. Most transport teams are staffed by paramedics or nurses, and physicians are rarely involved in civilian prehospital transportation or care. The majority of patients in civilian burn practice have isolated burn injuries or burn injuries combined with smoke inhalation. Burn injury complicated by multiple trauma is uncommon, and the combined burn/blast/overpressure/multiple trauma injuries so frequently seen in Iraq and Afghanistan are seldom encountered.

Within the US Department of Defense, the US Army Institute of Surgical Research Burn Center (i.e., the Army Burn Center) is the only specialized burn care center anywhere in the world. The Army Burn Center has a normal capacity of 16 ICU beds and 24 step-down beds. Each of the step-down beds is equipped with ICU monitors, oxygen, and suction and can function as an intensive care bed in the event of a mass casualty incident. By utilizing other floors at the San Antonio Military Medical Center for step-down patients, the Army Burn Center can expand to become either an 80-bed or 200-bed burn center on short notice.

During the medical planning for Operation Iraqi Freedom, guidance from the US Army Surgeon General specified that the burn care of injured service members would meet or exceed US civilian standards. This requirement cannot be met by in-theater burn care because of logistical and personnel requirements. The Joint Trauma System Burn Clinical Practice guideline states that "the mortality for burn casualties who cannot be evacuated out of theater is significantly higher than that experienced in CONUS facilities." [14]. For these reasons, burn patients have been flown back to the United States in both present and previous conflicts. A major difference, however, is the efficiency of transport currently achieved.

Stable Versus Stabilized Patients

In World War I, World War II, the Korean War, and the Vietnam War, aeromedical doctrine emphasized the transportation of the ***stable*** patient. Experience in Operations Just Cause and Desert Storm showed that earlier transport was feasible, and current doctrine emphasizes transport of the ***stabilized*** patient [15]. As an example, the 1162 patients flown to the Army Burn Center from the Vietnam conflict arrived an average of 18 days postinjury. During Operation Desert Storm, burned service members arrived at an average of 11.8 days postinjury. In Operations Enduring Freedom and Iraqi Freedom, burned service members requiring either burn flight team or CCAT transport are arriving at the Army Burn Center at an average of 3–5 days postinjury [16].

Dermal Burns

Pathophysiology

In addition to the obvious effects on skin, burn injury produces profound derangement in most organ systems. These changes are proportional to the size of the burn and dramatically increase at a burn size of approximately 20% total body surface area (TBSA). At the burn site, capillary integrity is lost and large protein molecules leak out of the circulation [17]. For burns of approximately 25% TBSA or larger, capillary leak becomes generalized, and capillary beds remote to the injury site also leak [18, 19], resulting in generalized edema, intravascular hypovolemia, and shock requiring fluid resuscitation.

The hypovolemic shock of burn injury is different from the hemorrhagic shock seen in traumatic injury. Hypovolemic shock in trauma results from disruption of large blood vessels. This is corrected by vessel ligation, tourniquet placement, damage-control laparotomy, fracture stabilization, or similar procedures. Once the "hole" has been plugged, fluids and blood products can be administered and will remain in the circulation. The shock seen in burn patients results from multiple small leaks as a sequela from disruption of capillary integrity. This occurs both at the burn site and in unburned tissue. Until capillary integrity is restored, fluids given intravenously will leak out of circulation. The only way to effectively keep "the tank" filled is to continuously pour in fluid at the same rate that fluid is leaking out.

Crystalloids are utilized for this purpose as they most closely resemble the solute concentrations of extracellular fluid lost in burn injury. A bolus of fluid will simply increase the leak rate and then allow the tank to empty: For this reason, fluid boluses are discouraged in burn resuscitation. Instead, it is preferable to increase the rate of continuous fluid infusion until the rate of leakage is matched. Capillary integrity is usually restored between 12 and 24 hours post injury, at which point fluids remain in circulation. Colloid solutions are normally given for burn resuscitation at this point to draw extravasated crystalloid back into circulation.

For several hours after a burn injury, cardiac output is depressed. With appropriate resuscitation, cardiac output normalizes around 24 hours postburn [20, 21]. At this point, cardiac output increases to 2–2.5 times predicted normal levels [20]. The increase in cardiac output is accompanied by a drop in systemic vascular resistance to 40–80% normal values [20, 21]. In addition to changes in cardiac output, burn patients develop a sustained hypermetabolic response, which may be related to centrally mediated release of catecholamines, glucagon, and cortisol [20, 22]. This results in increased heat production, elevation of core temperature, and an upregulation of the central thermoregulatory set point [20]. Leukocyte counts in the 14,000–18,000 range are seen unrelated to the presence of infection [20]. The hypermetabolism, elevated cardiac output, and low systemic vascular resistance will often persist until the burn wound is healed or surgically closed [20, 22], a process that may take months. The pattern of fever, leukocytosis, elevated cardiac output, and low systemic vascular resistance is normal in burn patients, and does not, by itself, indicate a septic state or the need for intravenous antibiotics [20].

Burn patients have poor temperature autoregulation because the loss of skin integrity results in increased heat loss to the environment [20]. Although hypermetabolic, burn patients can easily become *hypothermic* if not kept warm, especially during transport. This includes the use of blankets and other external heating devices such as the Bair Hugger, as well as increasing airframe cabin temperature when possible.

Dermal Burn Classification

In 1953, Jackson defined the three concentric layers of burn injury as the zones of hyperemia, stasis, and coagulation [23]. The zone of hyperemia is superficial injury, which will usually heal by itself. The zone of coagulation is full-thickness injury, which will not heal, and requires excision and surgical closure or grafting. Between these areas is the zone of stasis, consisting of cells that are injured but not lethally injured. These zones are a key to understanding burn resuscitation. Under-resuscitation will make the zone of stasis hypoxic, and over-resuscitation will make the zone of stasis edematous, in either case causing cell death and increasing the burn area that will require excision and grafting. In current practice, burn injuries are classified both by size (TBSA)

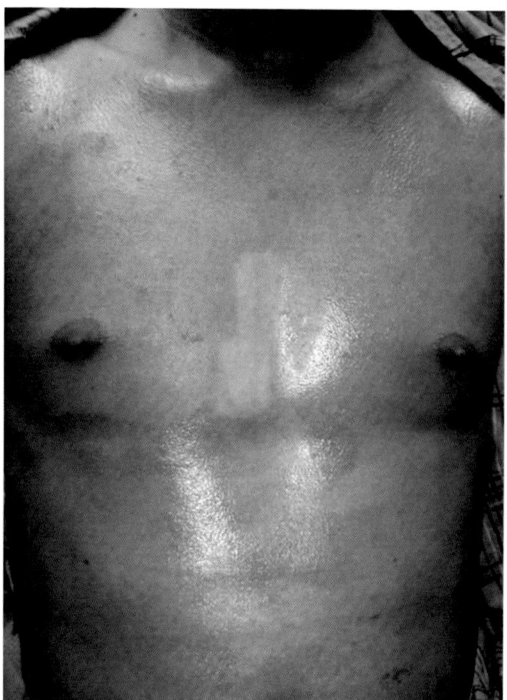

Fig. 17.1 First-degree burn involving the chest

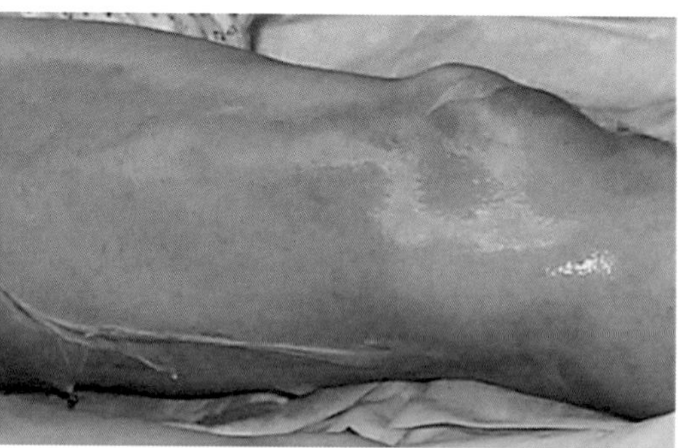

Fig. 17.2 Second-degree burn involving the inner thigh and leg

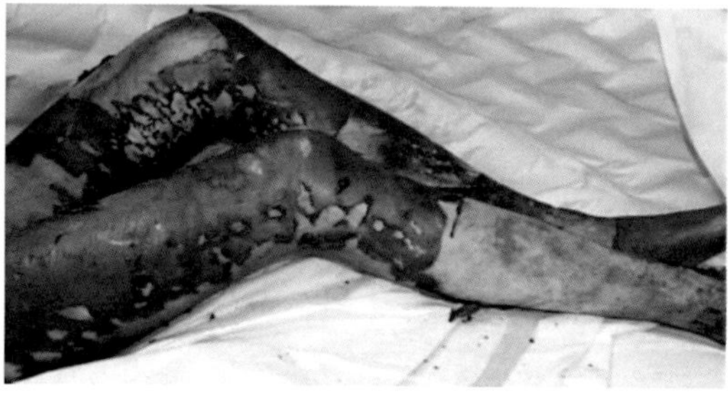

Fig. 17.3 Third-degree burns involving both legs

and by depth. Depth may be classified either by degree or as partial thickness/full thickness.

First- and second-degree burns are termed partial thickness. First-degree burns involve only the epidermis (Fig. 17.1). Since the epidermis continually regenerates, first-degree burns are usually of little clinical significance and are not included in burn size calculation for either fluid resuscitation calculations, ABA criteria for Army Burn Center referral, or for triage purposes.

Second-degree burns involve the dermis to varying depths and are very painful. They typically have blisters or a wet appearance, are pink or erythematous, feel soft and pliable to touch, and blanch with finger pressure. Hot water scalds typically produce a second-degree burn injury. Flash burns can produce either first-degree or superficial second-degree injury (Fig. 17.2). Direct flame contact or clothing ignition usually produces a third-degree burn.

Third-degree, or full-thickness, burns extend fully through both the epidermis and dermis (Fig. 17.3). Because nerve endings have been destroyed, third-degree burns are insensate. The skin may be cold and chalky-white; dark, brown, or black; or even charred. Third-degree burns do not blanch with finger pressure. The texture is hard and leather-like.

Eschar is the term given to leathery full-thickness injury. Circumferential eschar on extremities may restrict circulation, and circumferential eschar on the torso may restrict chest movement and respiration, particularly when capillary leak followed by fluid resuscitation results in edema of the underlying tissue. When this happens, a bedside procedure termed escharotomy is performed to relieve the constriction.

Inhalation Burns

Approximately 10–20% of burn injuries are accompanied by smoke inhalation injury. The presence of smoke inhalation increases the predicted mortality by up to 20% over mortality attributed to age and burn size [25]. Smoke inhalation injury makes the lungs more susceptible to infection, and the combination of inhalation injury and superimposed pneumonia increases mortality by up to 60% [25].

Smoke is a complex substance consisting of more than 400 known toxins [26, 27] and particles of various sizes. The major toxin is carbon monoxide. There are several components to smoke inhalation injury. The first is hypoxia. A fire burning in a closed space rapidly utilizes oxygen and can continue to decrease ambient oxygen levels to 10–15% [26, 27]. Humans in this environment die of asphyxia or become profoundly hypoxic. Temperatures within a burning building can reach 1000–2100 °F (537–1160 °C) [26, 27]. Breathing superheated air causes thermal burns of the oropharynx, which can become progressively edematous. The heat exchange mechanisms of the upper airway are sufficient enough to keep heat from the infraglottic airway. The water-soluble toxins in smoke precipitate in the trachea and the smaller particles end up in lung parenchyma. This results in a chemical tracheitis or pneumonitis. The injury below the epiglottis is not a true thermal injury unless steam is inhaled.

Inhaled carbon monoxide binds to hemoglobin forming carboxyhemoglobin, which hinders oxygen carrying-capacity as the affinity of carbon monoxide for hemoglobin is 210 times greater than for oxygen [28]. Carboxyhemoglobin can be measured by oximetry but is usually not reported on standard arterial blood gas analysis unless requested. Standard I-stat arterial blood gas cartridges do not measure carboxyhemoglobin. Carboxyhemoglobin is read as oxygenated hemoglobin on pulse oximetry resulting in false elevation of saturation. The treatment of carbon monoxide poisoning is administration of 100% oxygen. The half-life of carboxyhemoglobin is 5–6 hours when the patient is breathing room air and 30–90 minutes when breathing 100% oxygen [28]. Carbon monoxide poisoning will often have already been treated by the time the flight transport team first encounters the burn patient.

Diagnosis

The signs and symptoms of smoke inhalation are nonspecific. Facial burns, singed nasal hair, voice hoarseness, and carbonaceous sputum raise suspicion of inhalation injury but lack specificity. The best clinical correlate is a history of an indoor fire combined with loss of consciousness.

Initially, patients are usually asymptomatic and have normal chest radiographs. Progression to airway loss or respiratory failure can be rapid. A patient displaying hoarseness, change of voice, or other respiratory symptoms represents impending airway loss and requires immediate intubation. Respiratory failure from smoke inhalation may result in severe hypoxia precluding safe aeromedical evacuation. This usually occurs in the first few post-burn days.

Aeromedical Evacuation Consideration for Inhalation Burns

Specialized ventilation techniques such as high-frequency percussive ventilation (HFPV) are utilized by the burn flight team to transport patients in respiratory failure from inhalation injury and represent a standard of care at many burn centers [29]. At the Army Burn Center, Cioffi et al. demonstrated that the prophylactic use of HFPV in patients with inhalation substantially lowered the rate of pneumonia and increased survival [30].

A commonly used HFPV ventilator during AE is the Volume Diffusive Respirator (VDR, Percussionaire, Sandpoint, Idaho), which is powered by oxygen and compressed air rather than by electricity. With medical air supplied by either cylinder or air compressor, the oxygen requirements are 15–18 gaseous liters per minute, with an additional 24 l a minute required by the attached nebulizer [31]. When compressed air is unavailable, the airline is connected to the oxygen supply, further increasing oxygen requirements. The first in-flight use of the VDR ventilator was a 125-mile rotary wing transport of a patient with a 92% TBSA burn in 1992, performed using four oxygen cylinders containing a total of 12,000 gaseous liters. Based on the large gas requirements required, in-flight use of the VDR was discontinued until 2012, when the first transatlantic flight using the VDR was accomplished on a C-17 aircraft. The C-17 represents an ideal aeromedical evacuation platform, having two built-in

Dewar flasks providing a total of 150 liquid liters or 120,600 gaseous liters of medical grade oxygen [31]. This allows safe transcontinental transport of war casualties from Landstuhl, Germany, to San Antonio, TX.

In 2011, we published our wartime experience in the transport of 33 burn patients with a total distance of 174,145 air miles using high-frequency percussive ventilation on C-17 aircraft [31]. The mean burn size was 55.2% total body surface area (range 1–95% TBSA). Of the 33 patients, 30 had associated trauma with a mean Injury Severity Score of 33.4 (range of 2–75). This included six patients with abdominal compartment syndrome who had decompressive laparotomy preflight and who were successfully transported with the abdominal cavity covered only with temporary dressings [31]. During the 12-hour flight from Germany to San Antonio, the VDR ventilator normally consumes 30 liquid liters (equals 24,120 gaseous liters) of oxygen per patient at normal ventilator settings assuming that a compressed air source is also used.

Chemical Burn Injuries

Chemical burn injury is uncommon and comprises 2.1% of admissions to the Army Burn Center [32]. Chemical burns are classified by mechanism of injury: acid, alkali, or organic compound. Acid burns cause coagulation necrosis and bind to skin protein, which forms an eschar, producing a less severe injury. Alkali burns result in liquefaction necrosis, disrupting skin proteins and producing a deeper injury. Skin contact with organic chemicals can result in both cutaneous injury and systemic toxicity—typically renal or hepatic failure. The fumes of organic compounds may cause unconsciousness or pulmonary injury [6].

Specific Chemicals

Hydrofluoric Acid

There are two special types of chemical burns that transport teams need to be aware of because of the potential for associated cardiac arrhythmia. These are burns caused by either hydrofluoric acid or white phosphorus. Hydrofluoric acid is a weak inorganic acid that causes minimal skin damage but results in severe pain upon reaching deep tissue. Hydrofluoric acid burns can result in profound hypocalcemia, and death from cardiac arrest can occur with burns as small as 2.5% body surface area [33]. Hydrofluoric acid burns are treated with topical, subcutaneous, and or intra-arterial calcium compounds, which are titrated to pain relief [33].

The cardiac effects of hypocalcemia include QT prolongation, bradycardia, and ventricular fibrillation [33]. If electrocardiographic changes are present, immediate intravenous calcium administration is indicated and should not be deferred while calcium levels are measured [33]. In addition to blood calcium, blood magnesium and phosphate should be replaced as indicated [33]. Several days of calcium administration are often required.

White Phosphorus

White phosphorus burns can also cause life-threatening hypocalcemia or hyperphosphatemia in as little as 1 hour postburn [32]. Sudden death can occur with burns of 10–15% TBSA, and there is no reliable predictor of which patients will develop electrolyte abnormalities [32]. Electrocardiographic monitoring is mandatory, and calcium and phosphate levels should be monitored for at least 48–72 hours [32].

White phosphorus particles embedded in the wound can spontaneously ignite (oxidize) producing a yellow flame with white smoke [32]. This is prevented with serial surgical debridement to remove all embedded particles and by keeping the wound wet with sterile saline [32]. Removed particles should be placed under water to prevent re-ignition [32]. Phosphorus particles glow under ultraviolet light, and a Woods lamp is a useful guide to debridement. Topical copper sulfate solutions were previously utilized to facilitate particle identification but can cause renal failure or fatal massive intravascular hemolysis and are no longer indicated [32].

Sulfur Mustard

Medical planning in advance of Operation Iraqi Freedom assumed that chemical weapons including sulfur mustard would be employed against Coalition Forces [8]. This fortunately was not the case, but several sulfur mustard casualties did occur in the course of the war and were transported back to the United States for treatment. Sulfur mustard exposure to the skin produces chemical burns that usually present as erythema, which then may progress to blisters [34]. Experience in World War I and in the Iraq-Iran War of 1980–1988 shows that sulfur mustard casualties overwhelmingly are produced by vapor rather than liquid exposure and are nearly always first- and second-degree burns rather than deeper injury [34].

Mustard vapor rapidly penetrates skin, where highly reactive metabolites immediately bind to peptides, protein, and DNA [34]. For this reason, after a few minutes, the active chemical is not present in tissue, in biologic fluids, or in the fluid found in blisters, and such fluids pose no special (chemical) risk to caregivers [34]. Clothing contaminated with sulfur mustard may cause continued skin exposure, deepening the skin injury. Off-gassing from contaminated clothing may result in lung injury. Contaminated clothing should be immediately removed and the skin decontaminated as described in the following.

Initial Treatment of Chemical Burns

Chemical burns are small but frequently full-thickness injury requiring grafting [33]. The initial treatment of chemical burn injury is to irrigate the affected area with water until the pain significantly decreases or the skin pH normalizes. This may take 20 minutes or more for acid burns but usually requires several hours for alkali burns. Initial decontamination, irrigation, and burn wound care will normally be performed prior to arrival of the flight team.

The effects of mustard on the skin cannot be halted by decontamination after a few minutes of exposure. However, decontamination does lower the risk of active chemical exposure to medical personnel [35]. Decontamination can be accomplished with soap and water, 0.5% hypochlorite solution, or both [35] and obviously should be performed before putting a patient on the aircraft. There are no specific burn modalities approved by the US Food and Drug Administration (FDA) for the treatment of mustard gas burns, and standard treatments for thermal burns such as silver sulfadiazine or Silverlon® (Argentum Medical LLC, Willowbrook, Illinois) dressings are used for this purpose.

Aeromedical Evacuation Considerations for Chemical Burns

The most important aspect of initial management is to adequately flush the burned area with water until the pain significantly decreases or stops. Normally, this should be completed before flight is attempted. Flushing aboard the aircraft will create contaminated runoff, which will have to be contained. Clothing with chemical contamination should be removed prior to flushing and should not be transported in the aircraft.

While all chemical burns meet American Burn Association criteria for transfer to a burn center, in practice, the average burn size of a chemical burn is usually significantly smaller than the thermal burns admitted to a burn center. This usually means that transport can be delayed if necessary. In particular, if cardiac arrhythmia secondary to hypocalcemia is present (hydrofluoric acid or white phosphorus burns), transfer should be delayed until hypocalcemia, hypomagnesemia, and hyperphosphatemia have been corrected and the electrocardiogram has normalized. White phosphorus particles that remain embedded in skin may re-ignite on contact with hair, and transport of white phosphorus injuries is usually delayed until complete debridement and removal of all particles has been completed.

Electrical Burns

Electrical burns are also uncommon and comprise 4–7% of burn center admissions [33]. In addition to direct tissue injury from electrical contact, associated injuries may include thermal burns from clothing ignition, thoracic or lumbar compression fractures from muscle tetany, or cervical spine injuries from associated falls. Direct current poorly penetrates intact skin and causes approximately one-third of the tissue damage seen with alternating current injuries. Contact with electricity at 1000 V or higher is termed "high-voltage injury"; extremity fasciotomies and amputations are commonly required in this setting.

Alternating current that passes across the chest has a tendency to induce cardiac disturbances. Up to 37% of electric injuries may have an associated arrhythmia, although the most common rhythms encountered are sinus tachycardia (which is normal in burn patients) and nonspecific ST-T changes [33]. Lethal arrhythmias (asystole, ventricular tachycardia, or fibrillation) may be seen but almost always occur either on-scene or within hours of injury [33]. Massive muscle injury elsewhere in the body makes serial monitoring of cardiac enzymes inaccurate in the prediction of myocardial injury.

Different body tissues have different resistance to the passage of electricity, and electricity views a human extremity as several resistors in parallel. Bone has high resistance and thus impedes electrical flow and becomes heated, similar to the heater wire in a toaster. After the current is turned off, the bone continues to radiate heat internally into fascial compartments, causing muscle swelling, necrosis, and compartment syndromes. At the same time, the skin may dissipate heat to the environment and remain unburned. With electrical injury, it is entirely possible to have dead muscle found under intact and unburned skin.

Electrical injury can cause lysis of red blood cells and necrosis of myocytes, resulting in hemoglobinuria or myoglobinuria and characteristic dark-colored urine (Fig. 17.4). Renal failure frequently results, and associated hyperkalemia from myocyte lysis is made worse in the setting of renal failure. It is neither necessary nor practical to measure urine myoglobin or hemoglobin in a deployed setting; diagnosis is assumed whenever the urine is dark following electrical injury.

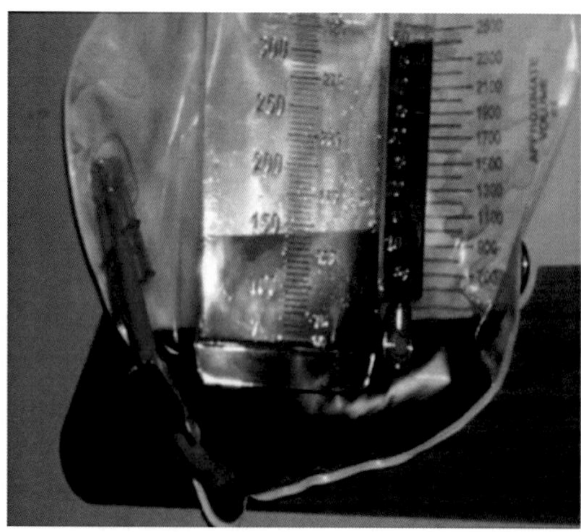

Fig. 17.4 Myoglobinuria in a urine collection bag. (Photograph by Dave Barillo, MD)

If the diagnosis is in question, the detection of red blood cells on urine dipstick testing in the absence of red blood cells seen on light microscopy confirms the presence of myoglobinuria.

Resuscitation After Electrical Burns

Because electrical injuries are three-dimensional, resuscitation formulas are less accurate and provide only a starting point. The endpoints of resuscitation are also confusing and depend upon urine color. Patients with electrical injury and normal-colored urine are resuscitated like any other burn patient with a desired endpoint of 30–50 cc urine output per hour. If the urine is dark, fluids should be increased to force diuresis, with a goal of 75–100 cc of urine per hour. Sodium bicarbonate can be added to the resuscitation fluid to alkalinize the urine: Myoglobin is more likely to precipitate in renal tubules in an acidic environment. Failing these maneuvers, mannitol may be added as an osmotic diuretic if the patient is adequately volume resuscitated, with the understanding that diuretic administration will render urine output useless as an endpoint of resuscitation. At some point, urine color will begin to lighten. When a normal urine color has been restored, fluid administration is decreased with a goal of 30–50 cc of urine per hour.

Aeromedical Evacuation Considerations for Electrical Burns

Flight considerations for patients with electrical injury include assessment and management of hyperkalemia and protection of any associated fractures in transit. Hyperkalemia may become severe, life threatening, and difficult to treat; recurrent or refractory hyperkalemia points to a diagnosis of inadequately managed compartment syndrome or unresected dead muscle. When either is suspected, flight of the patient should be deferred pending completion of surgical exploration and debridement. Neither CCAT nor burn flight teams routinely carry insulin in their drug boxes. If treatment of hyperkalemia in flight is anticipated, adequate calcium, insulin, dextrose, and bicarbonate should be obtained from the sending facility before leaving for the flight line.

Preflight Treatment and Stabilization

Fluid Resuscitation

Fluid resuscitation is required of most serious burn injuries. To estimate fluid resuscitation requirements, the size of the cutaneous burn must be determined. Burn size is estimated with the rule of nines or with a Lund and Browder chart [36]. First-degree burn is not included in burn size estimates: the important figure is the combined size of second- and third-degree burns. The rule of nines is based on the fact that most adult body parts have either 9% or 18% total body surface area. Each arm has 9%, each lower extremity has 18%, and the anterior and posterior torsos are 18% each (Fig. 17.5). It is important to understand that these values refer to the entire anatomic structure; a 9% burn of the upper extremity involves burn covering fingertip to shoulder of both the dorsal and volar surfaces. Smaller burns may be estimated from comparison with the palm of the patient, which is 1% of the body surface area. A different rule of nines diagram is used for children, where the head comprises up to 19% body surface area and the lower extremities comprise 14% (Fig. 17.5). The rule of nines provides a quick estimate and is usually employed prehospital. On arrival to definitive care, burn size is reassessed with a Lund and Browder chart to obtain a more accurate estimate (Fig. 17.6) [14, 36].

Circulation is assessed by examination of the patient and the resuscitation records. During the first 48 hours of acute burn resuscitation, the typical patient will be managed by several different surgical and flight teams. For this reason, hourly completion of the Joint Trauma System burn resuscitation flowsheet is highly encouraged (Fig. 17.7).

Heart rate and urine output are the primary indicators of adequacy of resuscitation. Blood pressure, base deficit, and arterial pH are useful adjuncts, but are not primary resuscitation endpoints. The flight transport team will not normally be required to calculate and start initial burn resuscitation. Nevertheless, it is useful to know the resuscitation formulas to be able to tell if ongoing resuscitation is adequate.

Classic burn resuscitation methods include the Modified Brooke and Parkland formulas. Both were designed for burn injury alone and are less useful in the setting of blast injury/multiple trauma complicated by a large thermal burn. It is crucial to understand that both formulas are merely estimates and, in practical terms, provide only a starting point of resuscitation. The 24-hour fluids needed are calculated by multiplying patient weight in kilograms times the combined size of second- and third-degree burn, times either a factor of 2 (Modified Brooke) or 4 (Parkland). A 100 kg patient with a 25% second-degree burn and a 25% third-degree burn (50% TBSA) would require 100 × 50 × 2 cc or 10,000 cc in the first 24 hours using the Modified Brooke formula or 100 × 50 × 4 cc (20,000 cc) using the Parkland formula. In both cases, first-degree burn is not included in burn size estimate.

Half of the 24-hour calculation is delivered in the first 8 hours postburn, with the remainder given in the next 16 hours. Using this example, the intravenous (IV) rate would be then started as 5000 cc/8 hours (625 cc/h using the Modified

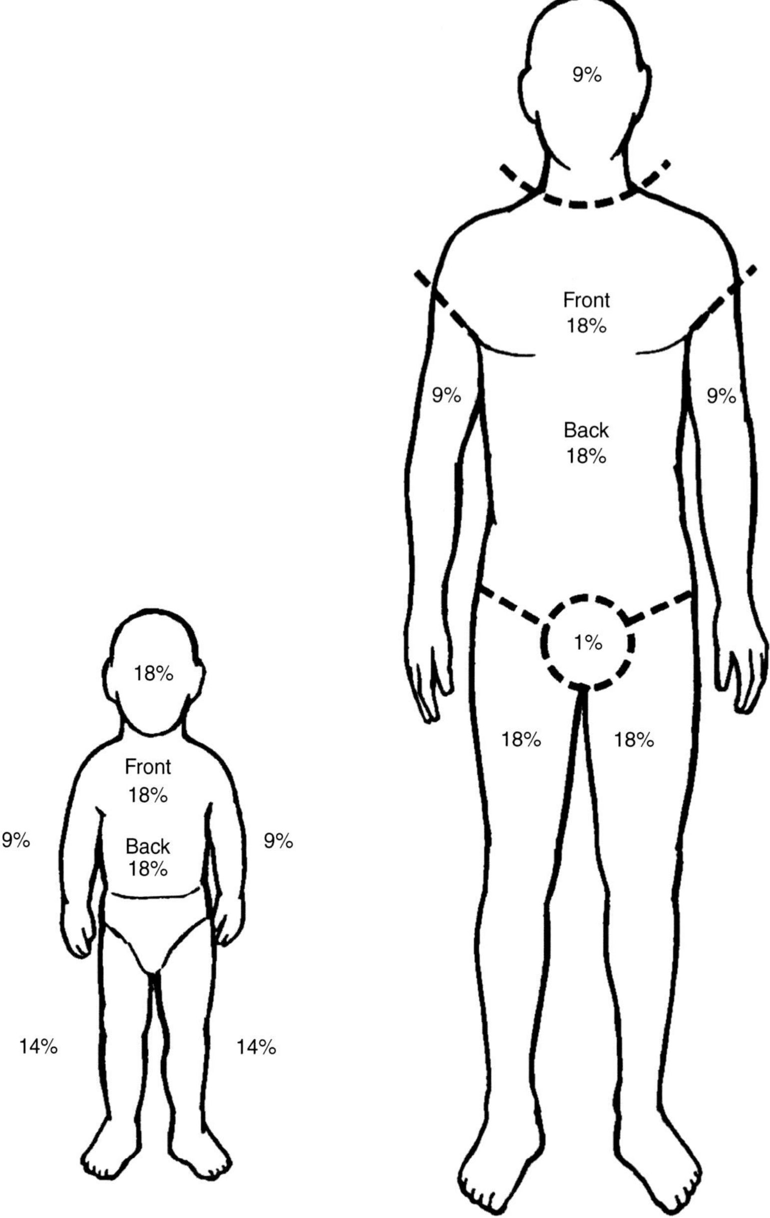

Fig. 17.5 Rule of nines for estimating total body surface area

Brooke Formula, or at 1250 cc/h using the Parkland formula). The first 8 hours starts at the time of the burn injury. If the patient arrives unresuscitated 4 hours postinjury, then the 8-hour fluid volume would be programmed for delivery over the next 4 hours. The resuscitation fluid of choice is Ringer's lactate.

A simpler method of calculating fluid resuscitation, developed during the current conflict, is the rule of ten [37]. For a patient between 40 and 70 kg, the total second- and third-degree burn size is calculated and multiplied by 10. For a patient with a 70% TBSA burn, the initial IV fluid rate would be 700 cc/h. Resuscitation is then adjusted hourly based urine output and heart rate. If the patient weighs more than 80 kg, 100 cc/h of fluid is added for each 10 kg over 80 kg.

Area	Birth to 1 year	1–4 years	5–9 years	10–14 years	15 years	Adult	2nd degree	3rd degree	Total	Donor areas
Head	19	17	13	11	9	7				
Neck	2	2	2	2	2	2				
Anterior trunk	13	13	13	13	13	13				
Posterior trunk	13	13	13	13	13	13				
Right buttock	2½	2 ½	2 ½	2 ½	2 ½	2 ½				
Left buttock	2 ½	2 ½	2 ½	2 ½	2 ½	2 ½				
Genitalia	1	1	1	1	1	1				
Right upper arm	4	4	4	4	4	4				
Left upper arm	4	4	4	4	4	4				
Right lower arm	3	3	3	3	3	3				
Left lower arm	3	3	3	3	3	3				
Right hand	2 ½	2 ½	2 ½	2 ½	2 ½	2 ½				
Left hand	2 ½	2 ½	2 ½	2 ½	2 ½	2 ½				
Right thigh	5 ½	6 ½	8	8 ½	9	9 ½				
Left thigh	5 ½	6 ½	8	8 ½	9	9 ½				
Right leg	5	5	5 ½	6	6 ½	7				
Left leg	5	5	5 ½	6	6 ½	7				
Right foot	3 ½	3 ½	3 ½	3 ½	3 ½	3 ½				
Left foot	3 ½	3 ½	3 ½	3 ½	3 ½	3 ½				
						Total				

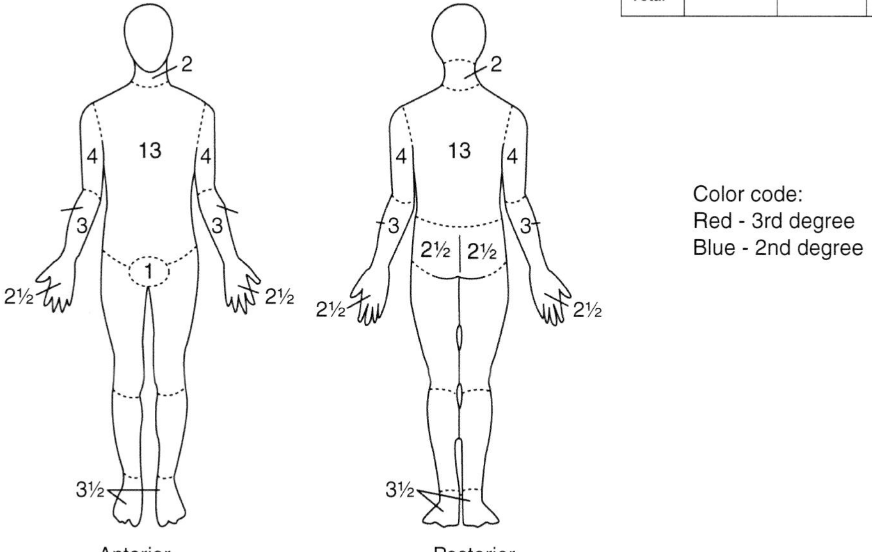

Fig. 17.6 Lund and Browder chart for estimating total body surface area, with burn estimate by age and area. (Adapted from [26] and U.S. Department of Health and Human Services http://www.remm.nlm.gov/burns.htm)

JTS BURN RESUSCITATION FLOW SHEET (1 OF 3)

Date		Initial Treatment Facility			
Name	SSN	Pre-burn estimated weight (kg)	%TBSA (Do not include superficial 1st degree burn)	Calculate Rule of Tens (if >40<80kg, %TBSA × 10 = starting rate for LR	Calculate max 24hr volume (250 ml × kg) Avoid over-resuscitation, use adjuncts if necessary
Date & Time of Injury		BAMC/ISR Burn Team DSN 312-429-2876; Yes No			

Tx Site/ Team	HR from burn	Local Time	Crystalloid* (LR) / Colloid	Total	UOP (Target 30-50ml/hr)	Base Deficit/ Lactate	Heart Rate	MAP (>55) / CVP (6-8 mmHg)	Pressors (Vasopressin 0.04 u/min) Bladder Pressure (Q4)
	1st								
	2nd								
	3rd								
	4th								
	5th								
	6th								
	7th								
	8th								
	9th								
	10th								
	11th								
	12th								
	13th								
	14th								
	15th								
	16th								
	17th								
	18th								
	19th								
	20th								
	21st								
	22nd								
	23rd								
	24th								
Total Fluids:									

Fig. 17.7 Joint Trauma System flow sheet

The rule of ten meets acceptable standards of resuscitation in 92% of cases and is much easier to use than the traditional formulas. The rule of ten can also serve as a resuscitation guide in flight. Knowing that the burn size is 70% allows the flight transport team to estimate that the initial fluid rate was 700 cc/h. If the team picks this patient up with an IV rate of 100 cc/h and a low urine output, the problem will be obvious.

It cannot be overemphasized that burn resuscitation is a continuous and dynamic process and that the burn formulas provide only a starting point. Adequacy of resuscitation must be reassessed at least *hourly* for the first 48 hours. Resuscitation is adequate when the urine output is between 30 and 50 cc/h and the heart rate is in the 100–120 beats per minute range. The target heart range is higher than usual guidelines for trauma patients because of burn hypermetabolism. If conscious, a well-resuscitated burn patient should also have a clear sensorium. Because full-thickness burn is insensate, it is not unusual to have a fully conscious burn patient prior to intubation.

Fluid administration must be assessed and adjusted at least hourly. If the urine output is under 30 cc/h for 2 hours, then the IV rate should be increased by 20–30%. If the urine output is more than 50 cc/h for 2 hours, then the IV rate should be decreased by 20–30%. Bolus administration of fluid simply makes the capillaries leak faster and should be avoided. At 24 hours postburn, the actual fluid volume is calculated by dividing the total fluid intake by initial body weight and burn size. The goal is a resuscitation that calculates out to be between 2 and 4 cc/kg body weight/% burn at that time.

At 24 hours, capillary integrity is mostly restored, and intravenous 5% albumin is started. In difficult resuscitations, "early albumin" can be started early at 8–12 hours. Albumin need is calculated based upon the burn size according to Joint Trauma System Clinical Practice Guidelines (Table 17.2) [14]. Albumin is continued until 48 hours postburn, at which time fluid choice and rate are based upon clinical status and laboratory studies. Both over- and under-resuscitation can be deadly. Over-resuscitation increases tissue edema and may hasten the need for intubation or escharotomy.

Unique to the current conflict is the significant incidence of abdominal compartment syndrome requiring decompressive laparotomy.

A 12-hour resuscitation volume of greater than 237 ml/kg (16 l in a 70 kg male) appears to be a threshold for development of abdominal compartment syndrome [38]. Abdominal compartment syndrome results in decreased renal blood flow, renal failure, intestinal ischemia, and respiratory failure unless promptly recognized and treated by abdominal escharotomy, peritoneal drain placement, or decompressive laparotomy [38]. Decompressive laparotomy for abdominal compartment syndrome is associated with a 60–100% mortality rate [38].

Table 17.2 Infusion rate for 5% albumin during burn patient resuscitation [13]

	Total body surface area		
Weight	30–49%	50–69%	70–100%
<70 kg	30[a]	70	110
70–90 kg	40	80	140
>90 kg	50	90	160

[a] ml/hour

Prior to implementation of current Joint Trauma System resuscitation guidelines, 13% of patients with burns >20% TBSA underwent decompressive laparotomy in theater [39]. Implementation of Joint Theater Trauma System resuscitation guidelines has resulted in a significant ($p = 0.03$) decrease in the composite endpoint of abdominal compartment syndrome and mortality [39]. The development of abdominal compartment syndrome with need for decompressive laparotomy in a patient with a large burn is almost universally fatal: All efforts to avoid over-resuscitation in theater and in flight must be made.

It is useful to assess the adequacy of resuscitation at 12–18 hours (or as early as 8 hours) to see if a difficult resuscitation is occurring. By assuming that present IV rate will be continued to the 24-hour mark and adding this total to fluid already given, the adequacy of resuscitation can be assessed. A large-volume resuscitation is considered to be 6 cc/kg/% TBSA burn or larger. Large-volume resuscitation may be due to associated traumatic injury, associated inhalation injury, electrical injury, very deep or massive burns, or to errors in calculation. When a patient is on track for a large-volume resuscitation, alternative resuscitation strategies [14, 38, 39] are indicated. These include the early institution of 5% albumin at 8–12 hours rather than at 24 hours; every 4-hour measurement of bladder pressures to assess for intra-abdominal hypertension; and measurement of subclavian or internal jugular central venous pressure, with a goal central venous pressure of 6–8 mmHg [14]. When central venous pressure goals are reached, fluid increases in response to low urine output should be deferred, as low output may represent renal insufficiency or failure rather than under-resuscitation at this point. The addition of intravenous vasopressin at 2.4 units per hour (0.04 units/minute) and norepinephrine at 2–20 μg/kg/min should be considered [14, 38].

Examination of the patient for adequate circulation should include assessment of peripheral pulses. Diminished or absent pulses in one extremity might indicate dressings that are too tight or an extremity in need of escharotomy. If all pulses are diminished, the patient should be assessed for under-resuscitation or hypovolemia. Adequate intravenous access is important. Most burn references recommend two large-bore peripheral intravenous lines [19], but in practice, most patients are flown with double- or triple-lumen central venous lines, large-bore percutaneous catheter introducers, or a combination. Arterial and venous lines should be sewn into place, not taped, prior to transfer. Where possible, extremities should be elevated in flight, but pulses should be checked with the extremity not elevated. Due to tissue edema, pulses may not be palpable, and Doppler signals will have to be obtained.

If circulation is adequate and dressings are dry, it is not always necessary to assess the burn wound prior to a short flight. If there is any question, however, the wounds should be carefully examined, as bleeding from an escharotomy or fasciotomy site will be difficult to control in flight. In flight, the burn wounds covered with Silverlon® and gauze dressings will remain covered and only require periodic moistening (but not soaking) with water.

Pain Management

It has been said that "pain is the ultimate narcotic antagonist" [40]. This is not to suggest that pain is desirable but to point out that some patients maintain their vital signs only because of stimulation. In such cases, administration of small IV doses of narcotics will result in profound hypotension. A patient that becomes hypotensive following administration of small doses of IV narcotics is hypovolemic, until proven otherwise, and raises concern for a missed traumatic injury. When this occurs preflight, it is prudent to delay or defer flight until the cause of the hypotension is addressed and until missed associated injuries have been ruled out.

In flight, pain is managed with intravenous narcotics and sedation is managed with either intravenous benzodiazepenes, ketamine, or propofol. Most burn courses stress the need for frequent small doses of intravenous narcotics, and ICU algorithms are moving away from benzodiazapenes and from continuous administration in favor of as-needed dosing. In practice, however, the flight transport team will normally pick up an intensive care unit patient who has already had pain and sedation issues managed and who is already on continuous narcotic and sedative infusions at an effective dose. While most ICU physicians and nurses have a favorite choice of narcotic or sedative, in reality all of the commonly available medications work, and it is counterproductive to demand that functioning IV drips be discontinued and replaced with one's choice of narcotic and sedative prior to flight.

If pain and sedation are already adequately controlled, our practice is to leave the patient on whatever pain and sedation regimen is currently running. Neuromuscular blockade is avoided unless absolutely necessary to obtain synchrony with the ventilator or to lower elevated intracranial or intra-abdominal pressures. Neuromuscular blockade is not started until adequate analgesia and sedation are addressed.

Propofol Infusion Syndrome

Propofol infusion syndrome is a theoretic concern when propofol is administered for prolonged periods (>48 hours) and at high rates (>4 mg/kg/h) [41]. While rare, propofol infusion syndrome is an "all or none" phenomenon with sudden onset and usually fatal outcome. The syndrome results in metabolic acidosis, rhabdomyolysis of skeletal and cardiac muscle, severe and refractory hypotension, myocardial and renal failure, and bradycardia [41]. We have had at least one suspected case of propofol infusion syndrome in flight, which resulted in the death of the patient soon after landing.

When inadequate sedation requires high doses of propofol (>60 μg.kg/min), our practice is to add 100 mg (2 cc) of ketamine to the propofol bottle producing "ketafol." In the emergency medicine literature, ketafol is also mixed in 1:1 or 1:4 ratios [42]. Ketamine has strong analgesic and dissociative anesthetic properties. In meta-analyses, the combination of ketamine and propofol is associated with fewer respiratory complications and fewer cardiac complications of hypotension and bradycardia compared to propofol alone [43].

Escharotomy

Escharotomies are among the most misunderstood procedures in burn care. An escharotomy is a bedside procedure performed on *circumferential full-thickness* burns to relieve actual or impending vascular compromise. The tissue edema caused by capillary leak and fluid resuscitation contributes to the need for escharotomy, and over-resuscitation hastens this need. Paresthesias or diminishing pulses in an extremity are the usual indication. Escharotomy is normally **not required** in second-degree burns or in noncircumferential burns.

Chest escharotomies are performed for circumferential full-thickness burns that are interfering with chest movement and hindering oxygenation or ventilation. An increase in airway pressures on volume-controlled ventilation or a deteriorating respiratory status on pressure-controlled ventilation suggests the need for chest escharotomy. However, in combat practice, serial examinations by the same surgical team are impractical.

Escharotomy Procedure

Escharotomy is a bedside procedure performed with knife or electrocautery (Fig. 17.8). Since full-thickness burn is insensate, general anesthesia is not necessary, but small doses of intravenous narcotics and sedatives are often utilized. An incision is made only to the deep border of the dermis and carried along the entire length of the full-thickness burn. It is neither necessary nor desirable to take the incision through subcutaneous fat or to the level of the fascia.

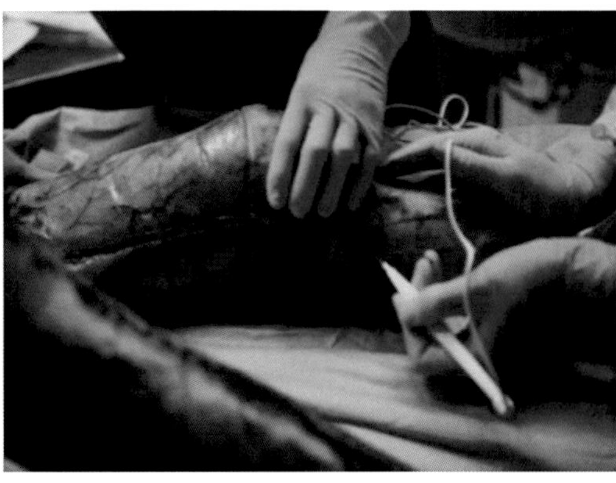

Fig. 17.8 Escharotomy on the inner aspect of the left thigh and leg

Methods differ according to location. For the chest, a shield-shaped incision is made along the anterior or mid-axillary lines and connected to a bilateral subcostal incision and a transverse upper chest incision just inferior to the clavicles (Fig. 17.9). For the upper extremity, the arm is placed in an anatomic position and a mid-radial or mid-ulnar incision is made. On the lower extremities, the incision is in the mid-medial or mid-lateral line. On the extremities, if one incision fails to restore circulation, a second incision is made along the opposite side of the extremity. Bleeding is controlled with electrocautery.

As pressure is relieved, the incision will widen and bleeding will restart. For this reason, it is prudent to leave the incision site undressed for 30 minutes for serial observation and hemostasis as new bleeding occurs. If escharotomy fails to restore circulation, adequacy of resuscitation should be reassessed, particularly if circulation is poor in all extremities. Escharotomy of the fingers is controversial, as there is little contained in the fingers other than bone and tendon, which are not critically oxygen-sensitive. Fingers sufficiently burned to require escharotomy frequently result in amputation. Neck or penile escharotomies are not indicated, although the foreskin sometimes requires surgical division when edema precludes urethral catheterization.

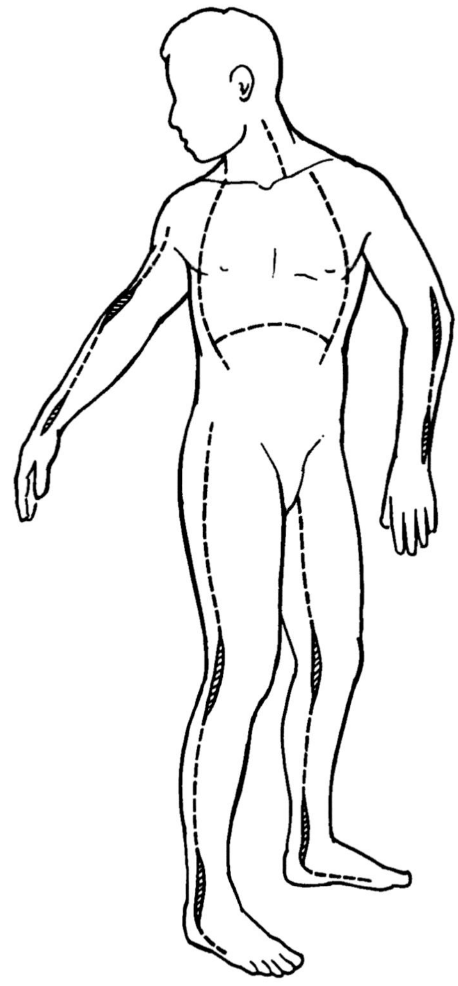

Fig. 17.9 Recommended sites for escharotomy incisions

Patients with electrical burns or with combined burn and traumatic injury (particularly extremity fractures) may require **fasciotomy**, which is a surgical procedure performed in the operating room. Isolated burn injury in the absence of electrical injury, multiple trauma, or fractures **almost never** requires fasciotomy. The prophylactic use of fasciotomy in this setting is strongly discouraged. Unnecessary fasciotomy complicates burn wound management, and fasciotomy sites often bleed in flight. In nonburn patients, fasciotomy may be indicated for increased compartment pressures related to fractures or prolonged or unknown ischemic times.

If possible, the need for fasciotomy should be confirmed with measurements of compartment pressures. An exception is prophylactic fasciotomy following limb revascularization, which is usually done immediately following the revascularization procedure [24, 44]. When lower extremity fasciotomy is required, all four compartments of the leg should be completely opened, with particular attention to the anterior compartment. Fasciotomy of the upper extremity should include the dorsal, volar, and mobile compartments of the forearm. In electrical injuries, release of the median nerve at the carpal tunnel and ulnar nerve in the canal of Guyan is frequently performed at the same time as forearm fasciotomy.

Aeromedical Evacuation Considerations

Prophylactic escharotomies are commonly performed prior to aeromedical transport in circumstances where circumferential full-thickness burns of the extremities or torso are present, the total body surface area is large, and a large-volume resuscitation is anticipated. Elevation of the extremity is also important and should be continued in transit. If escharotomy or fasciotomy has been recently performed, dressings should be removed and the wounds inspected for bleeding preflight if the situation permits.

Infection Prophylaxis

Infection can develop in untreated burn wounds after several days, and topical antimicrobials are utilized to decrease wound colonization. Deep burn wounds are normally avascular, and prophylactic systemic antibiotics are neither effective nor indicated. Whether or not to apply a topical antimicrobial cream for transport will depend on anticipated time and distance.

In civilian practice, use of topical antimicrobial agents is discouraged prior to burn center arrival, as these creams will have to be removed by the burn team to assess the wounds. Instead, covering the burn surface with a clean (nonsterile), dry sheet is advocated.

The Army Burn Center uses an alternating agent approach, applying mafenide acetate (Sulfamylon®) cream during the day and silver sulfadiazine (Silvadene®) cream at night—the combination providing broader antimicrobial coverage than either agent alone. Burned ears are continuously covered with mafenide to prevent development of chondritis [45, 46].

Silver-Nylon Stretch Wrap Burn Dressings

The burn flight team approach to wound coverage has changed during the present conflicts. In the past, the burn flight team would normally apply both creams preflight after assessment of the wounds on the theory that the patients were already receiving burn center care by the team. During OIF and OEF, it was not unusual for the team to simultaneously transport several patients with burns >50% body surface area on the same flight. As each dressing change requires several nurses and several hours, the logistics of performing multiple every-12-hour dressing changes proved daunting. Additionally, many of the wounds were combined burn and trauma, including open fractures and extremity amputations. For this reason, it soon became standard practice to utilize a silver-containing antimicrobial stretch wrap dressing (Silverlon®) as the topical treatment of choice (Fig. 17.10) [45, 46].

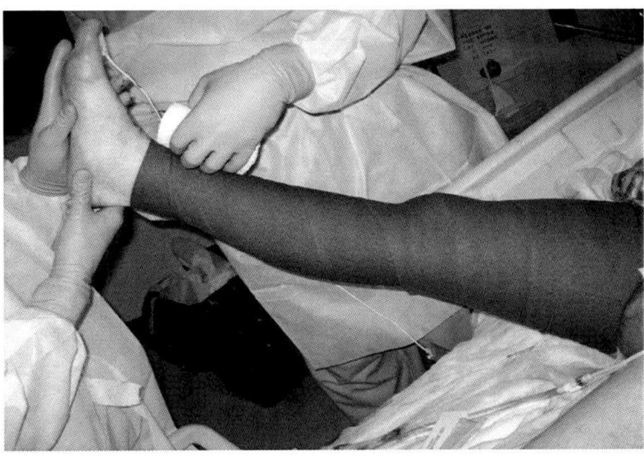

Fig. 17.10 Silverlon dressing placement over a leg burn

These stretch silver-nylon dressings now represent the standard of care for burn aeromedical evacuation. Silver ion is bacteriostatic against Gram-positive and Gram-negative bacteria as well as yeast-like organisms [20, 46]. Silverlon® dressings can be left in place for up to 7 days and simply require periodic moistening with water. A one-time preflight dressing change using Silverlon® at Landstuhl Regional Medical Center precluded the need for BID dressings or changes in flight. Silverlon® dressings were also extensively utilized in-country at US medical facilities in Iraq and Afghanistan, decreasing both the logistic and personnel burdens of providing burn care in austere environments [46].

Ventilation Considerations

Breathing is assessed by auscultation, observation of chest wall motion, and examination of arterial blood gas results and the chest radiograph. Our policy is to place a chest tube if there is any indication of a pneumothorax, including small and asymptomatic pneumothoracies found as incidental findings on computed tomography (CT) scan. If chest wall motion is limited by circumferential full-thickness burns, chest escharotomy should be performed preflight.

Ideally, our team prefers to have an arterial partial pressure of oxygen (PO_2) of 100 torr or greater on a fraction of inspired oxygen (fiO_2) of 0.5 or less on the ground at the referring facility. When this cannot be accomplished, alternative ventilation modes are employed, or rarely, the flight is delayed to give the flight team an additional 24 hours to optimize the patient.

The standard CCATT issue ventilator (Uni-Vent 754®, Impact Instrumentation, Inc., West Caldwell, New Jersey) provides assist-control (A/C), synchronized intermittent mandatory ventilation (SIMV), and continuous positive airway pressure (CPAP) modes. Some teams are also equipped with LTV 1000 ventilators (Pulmonetic Systems, Cardinal Health, Minneapolis, Minnesota), which may be utilized in volume, pressure, or inverse ratio pressure modes. Burn flight teams carry TXP® transport ventilators

(Percussionaire, Sandpoint, Idaho), a pressure-limited ventilation mode that we have utilized as a primary ventilator for burn transport for more than 20 years [47]. A modification of the TXP called the Duotron transport ventilator (Percussionaire, Sandpoint, ID) utilizes two TXP ventilators attached to a common manometer [48]. One TXP provides pressure-limited ventilation, while the second provides a high-frequency component.

With the availability of C-17 aircraft, it is now possible to transport burn patients utilizing high-frequency percussive ventilation (HFPV) in flight. A burn flight team switches to this mode when either volume- or pressure-limited ventilation modes have failed to provide adequate gas exchange. The in-flight use of HFPV requires both large volumes of oxygen and significant expertise on the part of the transport team and should not be attempted by those without experience in the use of this modality in ground-based practice.

A 30-minute trial prior to flight with the patient connected to the transport ventilator is desirable. If ventilation or oxygenation cannot be adequately managed with the standard CCAT ventilator, then the flight transport team should change over to the LTV or VDR ventilator if available. Failing this, the team should consider delaying transport of the patient to allow the ground team more time for patient optimization. Burn flight teams carry TXP, Duotron, VDR-4, and LTV ventilators and in addition can provide airway pressure release ventilation (APRV) in flight using the Drager Oxylog 5000 transport ventilator (Drager Medical) with local flight waiver. The burn team should be notified when a severe inhalation injury patient is first received downrange, so that appropriate ventilator preparation in Germany can be arranged before the patient arrives.

Other Aeromedical Evacuation Considerations

Burn patients with injuries of 20% body surface area or larger should have a functioning nasogastric tube and Foley catheter prior to flight. Prophylaxis against stress ulceration should be provided with either H_2 blockers or proton pump inhibitors. Deep venous thrombosis prophylaxis is provided either with subcutaneous unfractionated or low molecular weight heparin. Long-range aeromedical transfer does not increase the rates of deep venous thrombosis in burn patients who are given proper prophylaxis [49]. Prophylactic intravenous antibiotics are not indicated for burn injury but may be required for associated traumatic injury. Prophylaxis against hospital- (or aircraft-) acquired pneumonia includes elevating the head on a backrest attached to the NATO stretcher where practical.

Aeromedical Evacuation Timing for Burn Patients

Patients with serious burn injuries should be transported to specialized treatment centers as soon as possible, both because the intensive and extensive care required, but also because of the need to rapidly excise and graft burned tissue. Military burn patients who are injured overseas should be transported to the United States as soon as they can be stabilized. The ideal window is in the first 72 hours after injury, before hemodynamic and respiratory complications can worsen.

The decision to send a burn patient to the next level of care is made by the staff surgeon managing the patient and the validating flight surgeon. The flight transport team will usually first encounter the patient several hours preflight and has the responsibilities of ensuring that the patient is stable enough to get to the next stop and that the team is appropriately equipped for the flight. In general, problems encountered on the ground will only get worse in the air, and every effort should be made to optimize the patient's condition before going to the flight line.

Burn size is not a deterrent to flight. Our policy is that no US service member is considered as expectant or nonsalvagable. We have successfully flown several patients with burns in excess of 95% TBSA from Germany to San Antonio. The patient is not going to expire in flight from the burn wound itself: It is the details of airway, breathing, and circulation that will present the greatest challenges.

Final Preflight Evaluation

Where possible, the patient should be evaluated at the referring medical facility rather than on the flight line or in the aircraft. We follow the sequence advocated by the Advanced Trauma Life Support and Advanced Burn Life Support curricula, including primary and secondary surveys. The primary and secondary surveys should also be repeated at appropriate intervals in flight.

Adequacy and patency of the airway should be assessed. If the patient is not already intubated and there is any question about a safe and adequate airway, elective endotracheal intubation should be performed preflight, using a # 8 or larger endotracheal tube [14] to facilitate subsequent fiber-optic bronchoscopy and suctioning of secretions in-flight. Tube changes in the first few postburn days are complicated by resuscitation-related airway edema, and a patent but functioning small-sized tube should not be electively replaced in this timeframe. Tape will not stick to burned skin, and the endotracheal tube should be secured with umbilical ties.

Burn Team Equipment Requirements

Both the US Army burn flight team and USAF CCAT teams are equipped to deal with multiple patients and many different medical conditions. This requires that both teams travel with many bags or cases full of medical equipment. As medical problems develop in flight, a common sight is to have several team members simultaneously searching through multiple equipment bags to find the drug or device necessary to remedy the problem. To avoid this problem, several of our surgeons began to purchase and carry their own emergency medical equipment in a personal rucksack. In response, we developed an emergency bag containing most of what is required to manage the first 10 minutes of adult ICU emergencies [50]. On a typical flight, three identical bags are carried, one each by the surgeon, nurse, and respiratory therapist. When the destination is reached, this allows team members to split up for ground transport to the burn center in different ambulances and still have adequate emergency supplies.

Common In-Flight Problems

Once flight has commenced, the biggest problems encountered with burn patients are agitation, hypotension, and adequacy of resuscitation. Agitation may indicate hypoxia, inadequately controlled pain, inadequate sedation, hypovolemia, or benzodiazepene withdrawal from abrupt discontinuation. Reassessment of resuscitation, medication administration, and arterial blood gasses is indicated. Unfortunately, treatment of agitation by increase in analgesics or sedatives will often precipitate the second problem: hypotension.

Hypotension

Hypotension can be multifactorial. The most common cause is under-resuscitation, but adrenal insufficiency, hypocalcemia, or a poorly functioning arterial line should also be considered. It is useful to confirm arterial catheter pressure measurements with a blood pressure cuff—a maneuver made difficult by the presence of bulky burn dressings. Neither arterial nor cuff blood pressure measurements are absolutely accurate in burn patients, and trends, rather than individual readings, should be followed. Hourly notation of fluid administration, urine output, and blood pressure on the Joint Theater Trauma System burn resuscitation flowsheet may reveal trends pointing to the cause of the hypotension. Joint Theater Trauma System Burn Clinical Practice Guidelines should be followed.

The optimal mean arterial pressure for the burn patient must be individualized, and often patients will maintain adequate organ perfusion at mean arterial pressures (MAPs) lower than 70 mmHg [14, 39]. In the burn intensive care units at Army Burn Center, we maintain a goal of a mean arterial pressure of 60 mmHg or above and sometimes accept a MAP in the 55 mmHg range. This is also a reasonable level in flight if the patient is otherwise stable and continues to make adequate urine. Failing this, vasopressin is added at a dose of 0.04 units per minute (2.4 units per hour) and not titrated. Next, central (jugular or subclavian) venous pressure is measured and optimized (central venous pressure of 6–8 mmHg). If hypotension persists, a norepinephrine drip is started and titrated to a MAP of 60 mmHg. Acidemia (pH < 7.20), hypocalcemia, or adrenal insufficiency may cause catecholamine-resistant shock [32, 33]. The iStat® arterial blood gas analyzer (Abbott Laboratories, Abbott Park, Illinois) can be utilized to assess venous oxygen saturation, arterial pH, and ionized calcium level. We have found that the hemoglobin results produced by the iStat at altitude are unreliable, and should not be depended upon. Adrenal insufficiency is treated with 100 mg of intravenous hydrocortisone. If hypotension responds to hydrocortisone, the dose should be repeated every 8 hours.

High rates of propofol administration can cause hypotension by a variety of mechanisms, including inhibition of catecholamine release [51]. It is sometimes necessary to add a norepinephrine drip at a low dosage so that sufficient pain and analgesia medications can be delivered. Hypovolemia should always be considered in this scenario. Unfortunately, adding a pressor in this circumstance can complicate management, as infusions of norepinephrine, epinephrine, or dopamine can decrease blood propofol levels, at least in animal models [52], thus requiring an increase in propofol infusion rate once the catecholamine drip is started.

Conclusion

Compared to other conflicts, aeromedical transport teams are now tasked with the more rapid movement of less stable patients. The effectiveness of the joint CCAT/burn flight team approach to long-range AE of burn patients has been proven in multiple missions in Operations Enduring Freedom and Iraqi Freedom [16]. Even the largest of burns can be safely flown back to the United States given proper preparation, training, adequate personnel, and correct equipment. A key to successful burn care is compulsive use and reliance on the Joint Trauma System burn resuscitation flow sheet and assiduous avoidance of over-resuscitation. Problems on the ground can be exacerbated during AE, and continuous reassessment of the primary survey is important. Experience with this approach has demonstrated that transcontinental AE of burn patients may be safely performed by using the essential combination of the *Right Team*, the *Right Tools*, and the *Right Techniques*.

References

1. US Department of Defense/US Transportation Command (TRANSCOM) memorandum: utilization of specialized burn patient management during patient movement operations dated December 07, 2004.
2. Emergency War Surgery, Third United States Revision. Washington, DC: Borden Institute, Walter Reed Army Medical Center; 2004. http://www.dtic.mil/dtic/tr/fulltext/u2/a428731.pdf. Accessed 16 July 2018.
3. American Burn Association: Burn Incidence and Treatment in the United States: 2016. http://ameriburn.org/who-we-are/media/burn-incidence-fact-sheet/. Accessed 16 July 2018.
4. American Burn Association: Burn Care Resources Directory in North America; 2014. http://ameriburn.org/.
5. American Burn Association/American College of Surgeons. Guidelines for the operation of burn centers. J Burn Care Res. 2007;28(1):134–41.
6. Barillo DJ, Craigie JE. Burn injury. In: Hurd WW, Jernigan JG, editors. Aeromedical evacuation: management of the acute and stabilized patient. New York: Springer; 2003.
7. Bowen TE, Bellemy RF, editors. Emergency war surgery, second United States revision of the emergency war surgery NATO handbook. Washington, DC: US Government Printing Office; 1988.
8. Cancio LC, Horvath EE, Barillo DJ, Kopchinski BJ, Charter KR, Montalvo AE, et al. Burn support for operation Iraqi freedom and related operations, 2003–2004. J Burn Care Rehabil. 2005;26(2):151–61.
9. Eldad I, Torem M. Burns in the Lebanon War 1982: "The blow and the cure". Mil Med. 1990;155:130–2.
10. Owen-Smith MS. Armoured fighting vehicle casualties. J R Army Med Corps. 1977;123:65–76.
11. Shafir R, Nili E, Kedem R. Burn injury and prevention in the Lebanon War 1982. Isr J Med Sci. 1984;20:311–3.

12. Shirani KZ, Becker WK, Rue LW, Mason AD, Pruitt BA Jr. Burn care during operation desert storm. J US Army Medical Dept. 1992;PB 8-92-1/2:37–9.
13. Cioffi WG, Rue LW, Buescher TM, Pruitt BA Jr. A brief history and the pathophysiology of burns. In: Zajtchuk R, editor. Textbook of military medicine part 1, vol. 5. Washington, DC: US Government Printing Office; 1990.
14. Driscoll IR, Mann-Salinas EA, Boyer NL, Pamplin JC, Serio-Melvin ML, Salinas J, et al. US department of defense, Joint Trauma System. Joint Trauma System Clinical Practice Guideline: Burn Care (CPG ID: 12); May 11, 2016. http://jts.amedd.army.mil/assets/docs/cpgs/JTS_Clinical_Practice_Guidelines_(CPGs)/Burn_Care_11_May_2016_ID12.pdf. Accessed 16 July 2018.
15. Hurd WW, Jernigan JG. Introduction. In: Hurd WW, Jernigan JG, editors. Aeromedical evacuation, management of acute and stabilized patients. New York: Springer; 2003.
16. Renz EM, Cancio LC, Barillo DJ, White CE, Albrecht MC, Thompson CK, et al. Long range transport of war-related burn casualties. J Trauma. 2008;64(2 Suppl):S136–44.
17. Pruitt BA Jr, Goodwin CW, Cioffi WG. Thermal injuries. In: Davis JH, Sheldon GF, editors. Surgery – a problem solving approach. 2nd ed. St. Louis: Mosby Co; 1995.
18. Yowler CJ, Fratianne RB. Current status of burn resuscitation. Clin Plast Surg. 2000;27(1):1–10.
19. Mozingo DW, Barillo DJ, Pruitt BA Jr. Acute resuscitation and transfer management of burned and electrically injured patients. Trauma Q. 1994;11(2):94–113.
20. Barillo DJ, McManus AT. Infection in burn patients. In: Cohen J, Powderly WG, editors. Infectious diseases. 2nd ed. London: Mosby International; 2003.
21. Pruitt BA Jr, Mason AD, Moncrief JA. Hemodynamic changes in the early postburn patient: the influence of fluid administration and of a vasodilator (hydralazine). J Trauma. 1971;11:36–46.
22. Pruitt BA Jr, Goodwin CW, Cioffi WG. Thermal injuries. In: Davis JH, Sheldon GF, editors. Surgery – a problem solving approach. St. Louis: Mosby-Year Book; 1995. p. 643–719.
23. Jackson DM. The diagnosis of the depth of burning. Br J Surg. 1953;40:588–96.
24. Hirshberg A, Mattox KL. Top knife: art and craft in trauma surgery. Castle Hill Barns: TFM Publishing Ltd; 2005.
25. Shirani KZ, Pruitt BA Jr, Mason AD Jr. The influence of inhalation injury and pneumonia on burn mortality. Ann Surg. 1987;205:82–7.
26. Barillo DJ. Diagnosis and treatment of cyanide toxicity. J Burn Care Res. 2009;30(1):148–51.
27. Barillo DJ, Goode R, Esch V. Cyanide poisoning in fire victims – analysis of 364 cases and review of the literature. J Burn Care Rehabil. 1994;15(1):46–57.
28. Jordan BS, Barillo DJ. Pre-hospital care and transport. In: Carrougher G, editor. Burn care and therapy. Chicago: Mosby-Year Book, Inc.; 1998.
29. Paulsen SM, Killyon GW, Barillo DJ. High-frequency percussive ventilation as a salvage modality in adult respiratory distress syndrome: a preliminary study. Am Surg. 2002;68(10):852–6.
30. Cioffi WG, Rue LW, Graves TA, McManus WF, Mason AD Jr, Pruitt BA Jr. Prophylactic use of high-frequency percussive ventilation in patients with inhalation injury. Ann Surg. 1991;213(6):575–82.
31. Barillo DJ, Renz EM, Wright GR, Broger KP, Chung KK, Thompson CK, et al. High-frequency percussive ventilation for intercontinental aeromedical evacuation. Am J Disaster Med. 2011;6(6):369–78.
32. Barillo DJ, Cancio LC, Goodwin CW. Treatment of white phosphorus and other chemical burn injuries at one burn center over a 51 year period. Burns. 2004;30(5):448–52.
33. Winfree J, Barillo DJ. Non thermal injuries. Nurs Clin North Am. 1997;32(2):275–96.
34. Hurst CG, Petrali JP, Barillo DJ, Graham JS, Smith WJ, Urbanetti JS, et al. Vesicants. In: Tuorinsky SD, editor. Medical aspect of chemical warfare. Washington, DC: Borden Institute; 2008. p. 259–309.
35. Braue EH, Boardman CH, Hurst CG. Decontamination of chemical casualties. In: Tuorinsky SD, editor. Medical aspect of chemical warfare. Washington, DC: Borden Institute; 2008. p. 527–57.
36. Lund CC, Browder NC. The estimation of areas of burns. Surg Gynecol Obstet. 1944;79:352–8.
37. Chung KK, Blackbourne LH, Renz EM, et al. The rule of ten: a simplified approach to calculation of the initial fluid rate in adults. J Burn Care Res. 2008;29(2):S120.
38. Chung KK, Blackbourne LH, Wolf SE, White CE, Renz EM, Cancio LC, et al. Evolution of burn resuscitation in operation Iraqi freedom. J Burn Care Res. 2006;27(5):606–11.
39. Ennis JL, Chung KK, Renz EM, Barillo DJ, Albrecht MC, Jones JA, et al. Joint Theater Trauma System implementation of burn resuscitation guidelines improves outcomes in severely burned military casualties. J Trauma. 2008;64:S146–52.
40. Bandersnatch F. Surgical blunders and how to avoid them. Gainesville: Triad Publishing; 1990.
41. Fodale V, LaMonaca E. Propofol infusion syndrome: an overview of a perplexing disease. Drug Saf. 2008;31(4):293–303.
42. Miner JR, Moore JC, Austad EJ, Plummer D, Hubbard L, Grey RO. Randomized double-blinded clinical trial of propofol, 1:1 propofol/ketamine, and 4:1 propofol/ketamine for deep procedural sedation in the emergency department. Ann Emerg Med. 2015;65(5):479.
43. Jalili M, Bahreini M, Doosti-Irani A, Masoomi R, Arbab M, Mirfazaelian H. Ketamine-propofol combination (ketafol) versus propofol for procedural sedation and analgesia: systemic review and meta-analysis. Am J Emerg Med. 2016;34:558–69.
44. Joint Trauma System. Clinical Practice Guideline: Vascular Injury. Defense Health Agency. 12 Aug 2016.

https://jts.amedd.army.mil/assets/docs/cpgs/JTS_Clinical_Practice_Guidelines_(CPGs)/Vascular_Injury_12_Aug_2016_ID46.pdf Last Accessed on 5 April 2019.
45. Aurora A, Beasy A, Rizzo JA, Chung KK. The use of a silver-nylon dressing during evacuation of military burn casualties. J Burn Care Res. 2018;39(4):593–7.
46. Barillo DJ, Pozza M, Brandt MM. A literature review of the military uses of silver-nylon dressings with emphasis on wartime operations. Burns. 2014;40s:s24–9.
47. Barillo DJ, Dickerson EE, Cioffi WG, Mozingo DM, Pruitt BA Jr. Pressure-controlled ventilation for the long-range aeromedical transport of patients with burns. J Burn Care Rehabil. 1997;18(3):200–5.
48. Galvez E, Park MS, Harshbarger TL, et al. Evaluation of the Duotron, a high frequency pressure cycled transport ventilator. J Burn Care Rehabil. 1999;20(1, part 2):S201.
49. Chung KK, Blackbourne LH, Renz EM, Cancio LC, Wang J, Park MS, et al. Global evacuation of burn patients does not increase the incidence of venous thromboembolic complications. J Trauma. 2008;65(1):19–24.
50. Barillo DJ, Renz E, Broger K, Moak B, Wright G, Holcomb JB. An emergency medical bag set for long-range aeromedical transportation. Am J Disaster Med. 2008;3(2):79–86.
51. Han L, Fuqua S, Quanlin L, Zhu L, Hao X, Li A, et al. Propofol-induced inhibition of catecholamine release is reversed by maintaining calcium influx. Anesthesiology. 2016;124:878–84.
52. Myburgh JA, Upton RN, Grant C, Martinez A. Epinepherine, norepinepherine and dopamine infusions decrease propofol concentrations during continuous propofol infusion in an ovine model. Intensive Care Med. 2001;27:276–82.

18 Patients Requiring Mechanical Ventilation

Dario Rodriquez Jr. and Richard D. Branson

Introduction

Aeromedical evacuation (AE) of the critically ill and injured patient requires careful consideration and preparation long before the mission takes place. Key elements are selection of the appropriately skilled staff, good communication, equipment adequate for the needs of the patient, and a healthy respect for the task at hand. Mechanical ventilation adds to this complexity, and clinicians should be cognizant of the impact of the transport environment on patient/platform and methods to mitigate untoward consequences (Fig. 18.1).

This chapter will review the relevant gas laws that explain the impact of altitude on patients, equipment, and caregivers. We will discuss the impact on patient assessment and monitoring created by barometric pressure changes. The AE environment also creates a number of limitations, including low light, high ambient noise, vibration, and limited resources. The principles of ventilation that are universal to patients with respiratory failure will be discussed and the important characteristics of ventilators for transport reviewed.

D. Rodriquez Jr. (✉)
CMS, USAF (ret.), Research Health Science, CSTARS, Cincinnati, OH, USA

Department of Aeromedical Research, En Route Care Research Division, USAF School of Aerospace Medicine, University of Cincinnati, Cincinnati, OH, USA
e-mail: RODRIQDO@ucmail.uc.edu

R. D. Branson
Department of Surgery, Division of Trauma/Critical Care, University of Cincinnati, Cincinnati, OH, USA

School of Aerospace Medicine, Wright Patterson Air Force Base, Dayton, OH, USA

Impact of Altitude on Mechanically Ventilated Patients

Altitude Physiology

Ascent to altitude is accompanied by a fall in barometric pressure according to Boyle's Law. Boyle's Law essentially states that at a constant temperature, the volume of a gas is inversely proportional to its pressure. A fall in pressure at altitude is associated with an increase in gas volume and a reduction in gas density. This "thinning" of the air results in a decrease in the partial pressure of oxygen at altitude despite a constant concentration. Dalton's Law states that the total pressure of a mixture of gases is equal to the sum of the partial pressures of each gas. Together, these laws describe the effect of hypobaric hypoxia. Caregivers should be knowledgeable of the impact of hypobarism on patients, themselves, and equipment. The basic gas laws govern these alterations (Table 18.1).

W. W. Hurd, W. Beninati (eds.), *Aeromedical Evacuation*,
https://doi.org/10.1007/978-3-030-15903-0_18

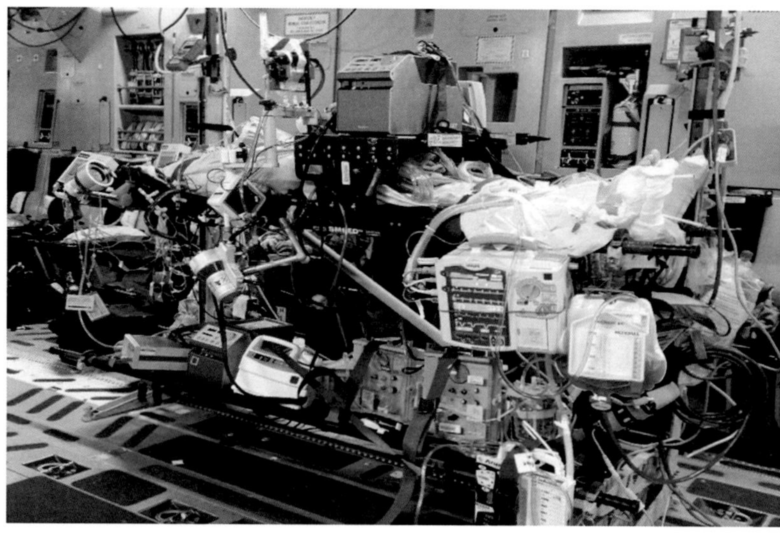

Fig. 18.1 An injured soldier aboard a C-17 requiring mechanical ventilation during aeromedical evacuation. (Photo by Capt John-Michael Fowler)

Table 18.1 Gas laws governing physiologic changes associated with altitude

Law	Formula	Patient impact	Equipment effects
Boyle's	$P_1 \times V_1 = P_2 \times V_2$	Gas in a trapped space increases with ascent. (Pain and discomfort from gastrointestinal, dental, sinus, ocular gas) Expansion of untreated pneumothorax Evaluate intubated patients for ear block when agitation increases Gas volumes increase by 25% at 5000 feet, by 50% at 10,000 feet, and by 100% at 18,000 feet	Cuff pressure in endotracheal or laryngeal tubes increases Air in IV bags or air splints expands with altitude, falls with descent Prefilled syringes lose medication Ventilators deliver inaccurate tidal volumes
Dalton's	$P = P_1 + P_2 + P_3 + P_4 + P_n$	Hypobaric hypoxia with increasing altitude Increased oxygen requirements	
Gay-Lussac's Law	$P_1/T_1 = P_2/T_2$	The human physiologic temperature range is narrow, no patient impact	Pressure in gas cylinders increases with increased temperature and falls with decreasing temperature
Henry's	$P = k_H c$	Decompression illness Pain in joints	Creation of gas bubbles in IV solutions or blood IV pump failure

P pressure, *T* temperature, *V* volume, *p* partial pressure of the solute above the solution, k_H Henry's law constant, *c* the concentration of solute in solution, *IV* intravenous

The partial pressure of oxygen in the atmosphere (PiO_2) is calculated as the sum of barometric pressure (P_B) and the fraction of oxygen (FIO_2):

$$PiO_2 = P_B \times FIO_2.$$

The FIO_2 of air is 0.21, and thus P_B and ambient air PiO_2 decrease as barometric pressure decreases with increasing altitude:

$$\text{At sea level: } PiO_2 = 760\,\text{mm Hg} \times 0.21 = 159\,\text{mm Hg}$$

$$\text{At 8000 feet: } PiO_2 = 564\,\text{mm Hg} \times 0.21 = 118\,\text{mm Hg}$$

The effective FIO at various altitudes is shown in Table 18.2.

Alveolar oxygen (PaO_2) is further diminished by the presence of water vapor and carbon dioxide (CO_2) as described by the alveolar air equation:

$$PaO_2 = FIO_2\left(P_B\text{-}PH_2O\right) - PaCO_2\ /\ \text{Respiratory Exchange Ratio}\left(\text{RER}\right)$$

This results in $PaO_2 = 100$ mm Hg at sea level and $PaO_2 = 59$ mm Hg at 8000 feet. This assumes a constant for PH_2O of 47 mm Hg and a $PaCO_2$ of 40 mm Hg. At this altitude, passengers will have a mean fall in arterial oxygen saturation measured by pulse oximetry (SpO_2) of approximately 4.4%.

These effects have little impact on healthy individuals but can have serious consequences for patients with lung disease. As a result, patients with hypoxemia at sea level will require additional oxygen at AE cruising altitude. Patients with pulmonary hypertension will encounter hypoxia and increases in pulmonary artery pressures.

Henry's Law states that the amount of gas dissolved in solution varies directly with the partial pressure of that gas over the solution. While the simplest observation of Henry's Law is the opening of a carbonated beverage to atmospheric pressure, dissolved gas in tissues can represent a concern. Gas in solution or moving out of solution is the basis for decompression illness. While decompression sickness is unlikely during normal flight, sudden decompression can create symptoms, even at modest altitudes.

Table 18.2 Change in partial pressure and effective oxygen with altitude

Altitude (feet)	Barometric pressure (mm Hg)	Effective oxygen %	Partial pressure of oxygen (PiO_2) mm Hg
0	760	20.9	159
3000	681	18.6	143
6000	609	16.6	127
8000[a]	564	15.4	118
15,000	429	11.8	90
20,000	349	9.4	73

[a]Maximum cabin altitude in commercial and military refueling or cargo aircraft

Air Transportation of Mechanically Ventilated Patients

Military experience with long-distance AE over the last decade has resulted in dramatic advances in our ability to transport mechanically ventilated patients by improving both our techniques and equipment [1–3]. Critical elements for successful AE include communication, coordination, and planning. However, the single most important improvement has been the development and utilization of specialized Critical Care Air Transport Teams (CCATTs) for transport of these extremely high-risk patients. CCAT teams are composed of a critical care physician, a nurse with intensive care unit (ICU) experience, and a respiratory therapist.

Transportation of mechanically ventilated patients is associated with a number of challenges and consequential risks (Table 18.3). Transportation by ground vehicle or rotary wing aircraft requires the coordinated movement of the patient with a large amount of equipment with continuous patient monitoring in an isolated environment that is often noisy and cramped. Transportation by fixed-wing aircraft adds the risks associated with increased altitude.

Table 18.3 Adverse events reported for mechanically ventilated patients during aeromedical evacuation

Accidental extubation	Hypothermia
Air embolus	Hypoxia
Altered mental status	Incorrect patient identification
Arrhythmia	Increased intracranial pressure
Bleeding	Loss of airway
Cardiac arrest	Need for restraints
Equipment failure (ventilator, monitors, IV pump)	Obstructed airway
Hemodynamic instability	Oxygen failure/depletion
Hypertension	Pneumothorax
Hypotension	Spinal destabilization
	Ventilator-associated pneumonia

IV intravenous

Team composition is an integral component of planning for movement of mechanically ventilated patients. It is essential that experienced critical care practitioners make up the members of the transport team. Many patient transfers can be managed by a registered nurse and respiratory therapist, particularly when the transport is a relatively short distance. A physician should be part of the transport team for long-distance AE and for short-distance transports when a patient is unstable, e.g., requiring vasoactive drugs or having an arterial line or pulmonary artery catheter in place. The American College of Critical Care Medicine has defined standards for care of patients during transport [4].

Acute Respiratory Distress Syndrome Patients

Movement of mechanically ventilated patients with acute respiratory distress syndrome (ARDS) requiring mechanical ventilation is associated with a number of additional challenges. US Air Force Lung Teams were created to address the issues of patients requiring more sophisticated levels of ventilator support. To date, AE teams have transported more than 400 patients with ARDS, including 24 with severe ARDS, using sophisticated ventilators or extracorporeal membrane oxygen (ECMO) techniques with few complications [5, 6]. Patients with severe ARDS and an arterial partial pressure of oxygen to inspired oxygen ratio (PaO_2/FIO_2) < 70 were most likely to suffer in-flight hypoxemia. Wilcox et al. demonstrated that under care of a Critical Care Transport Team, many patients with hypoxemic respiratory failure had improved oxygenation upon arrival at the receiving facility after AE [7].

Aeromedical Evacuation Oxygen Delivery Systems

All ventilators require an oxygen supply source. This need can be fulfilled using integral aircraft oxygen systems, liquid oxygen systems, compressed gas cylinders, or oxygen concentrators. When finite oxygen sources are used, a minimum of 150% of the calculated oxygen need should be available for each AE flight because of the potential for unforeseen delays during AE transport.

Integral Aircraft Oxygen Systems

In order to administer oxygen to a large number of patients, C-17 aircraft are equipped for AE so that patients can be connected directly to an existing aircrew oxygen system. The large systems integral to military transport aircraft provide an abundance of oxygen sufficient for most AE flights.

Portable Therapeutic Liquid Oxygen System

When AE is performed in the C-130/KC-135, AE patients cannot be connected directly to an existing aircrew oxygen system. In this situation, patient oxygen is administered using the Next Generation Portable Therapeutic Liquid Oxygen System (NPTLOX, Essex Industries, St. Louis, Missouri) (Fig. 18.2). The NPTLOX is a low-pressure portable 20.0-liter liquid oxygen storage

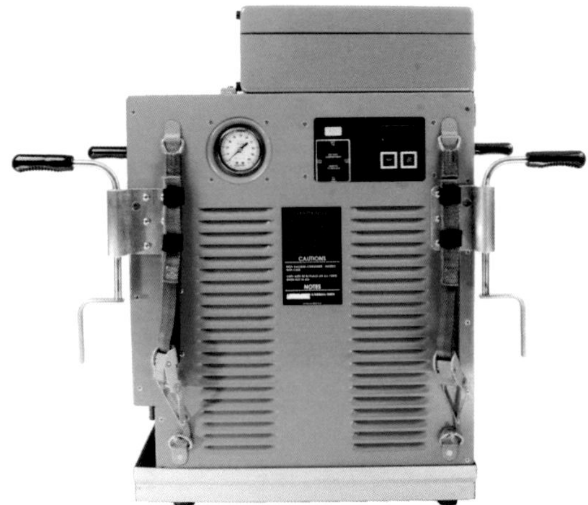

Fig. 18.2 Next Generation Portable Therapeutic Liquid Oxygen System (NPTLOX) used for USAF aeromedical evacuation. (Photo courtesy of Essex Industries, St. Louis, MO)

and gaseous delivery system. It can supply up to 17,200 gaseous liters of oxygen at a maximum flow rate of 66 liters per minute at 50 psig. It has three flow control valves that can deliver oxygen to three patients simultaneously with different flow rates, from 0.5 to 15 liters per minute. The six quick disconnect outlet ports can supply 50 psi of oxygen to mechanical ventilators or other patients.

The NPTLOX system weighs <100 pounds when full and can be carried by two AE personnel to be mounted in the aircraft. It does not require external power and uses two 9-V batteries for the quantity indicator. The system has been tested to military standards.

Oxygen Cylinders

Rotor wing transport usually is accomplished with an E cylinder or a number of E cylinders yoked together. These cylinders provide 660 liters of gas per cylinder. Note that aluminum cylinders and some new cylinders have a greater capacity than previous generations. An H cylinder contains 6900 liters and may be required for longer-distance transports. An H cylinder is 152 cm in height and weighs 68 kg, rendering it portable only on a cart. Oxygen cylinders are often used for short-duration AE flights in the C-21, and cylinder duration must be carefully calculated prior to departure. However, oxygen cylinders are rarely used for AE flights in military refueling or cargo aircraft transporting multiple patients in flights of several hours of duration.

Oxygen Concentrators

Oxygen concentrators concentrate oxygen from ambient air to supply an oxygen-enriched gas stream. Oxygen concentrators are designed for home and ambulatory oxygen delivery to individual patients but can provide low-flow oxygen to a ventilator to provide FIO_2 close to 50%. These portable devices can provide oxygen continuously if electrical power is maintained. A recently introduced ventilation system, VOCSN (Ventec Life Systems Inc.), includes an integral oxygen concentrator capable of pulse dosing oxygen at the beginning of inspiration to maximize FIO_2 delivery [8–10].

Transport Ventilators

Mechanical Ventilation Principles

Mechanical ventilation is instituted to support gas exchange, reduce the work of breathing, and prevent ventilator-induced lung injury [11]. A joint task force of medical societies recently published clinical practice guidelines for the care of mechanically ventilated patients [12]. The following recommendations are based on these guidelines.

Evidence overwhelmingly supports both tidal volume (V_T) and pressure limitation of positive-pressure breaths. This includes the use of a V_T based on predicted body weight, initial V_T of 4–8 ml/kg, and maintenance of plateau pressure (Pplat) <30 cm H_2O. Predicted body weight is based on height measurement, as height is the major determinant of lung volumes, not actual body weight. Predicted body weight for men = 50 + 2.3 (height in inches – 60) and for women = 45.5 + 2.3 (height in inches – 60).

The V_T range allows the adjustment based on patient comfort and acid-base balance. At a low V_T, if the patient exhibits signs of air hunger, V_T can be increased in 1 ml/kg increments to reduce dyspnea. This should be done while watching the Pplat. If acidosis and hypercarbia are encountered, increases in V_T are warranted to maintain pH > 7.25. Continued air hunger and acid-base abnormalities may be treated with sedation and if necessary neuromuscular blockade. It is important to note that the data suggests there is no "safe" V_T, as reduction in Pplat below the 30 cm H_2O threshold is consistently associated with improvements in mortality [12].

Positive end-expiratory pressure (PEEP) maintains end-expiratory lung volume, lung recruitment, and oxygenation. The application of PEEP is often governed by local fetish and tradition. A minimum PEEP of 5 cm H_2O should be used in all ventilated patients with the exception of those undergoing cardiopulmonary resuscitation (CPR). This is often termed "physiologic PEEP"—an unproven concept. However, compared to no PEEP, 5 cm H_2O PEEP improves oxygenation, decreases the work of breathing, limits ventilator-induced lung injury secondary to atelectrauma, maintains expiratory lung volume, and improves compliance.

Setting PEEP can be accomplished by monitoring compliance, oxygenation, respiratory mechanics, or more sophisticated techniques. In ARDS, low levels of PEEP, 5–10 cm H_2O, are generally sufficient for mild forms of the disease ($PaO_2/FIO_2 > 200 < 300$) [13]. In moderate ($PaO_2/FIO_2 > 100 < 200$) to severe ARDS ($PaO_2/FIO_2 < 100$), higher levels of PEEP (10–25 cm H_2O) are associated with shorter ventilator days, reduced mortality, and less frequent use of rescue therapies [14].

The effect of increasing PEEP depends on lung recruitability, which varies widely in ARDS. In patients with low recruitability, increasing PEEP leads to alveolar over-distention and harm. If the lung is recruitable, increasing PEEP improves compliance, reduces ventilator-induced lung injury, and provides a benefit. If an increase in PEEP is associated with a smaller increase in Pplat (PEEP increase of 5 cm H_2O with a Pplat change of 2 cm H_2O), recruitment is presumed, and the benefit of PEEP outweighs potential harm. If an increase in PEEP is associated with a larger increase in Pplat (PEEP increase of 5 cm H_2O with a Pplat change of 8 cm H_2O), overdistension is likely, and the harm exceeds any benefit.

The adjustments of V_T, PEEP, and FIO_2 cannot be made in isolation. The principles of lung protection require that appropriate targets for oxygenation and airway pressures are maintained. This may require a reduction in V_T following an increase in PEEP to maintain both oxygenation and Pplat <30 cm H_2O. Appropriate targets for SpO_2, pH, and $PaCO_2$ should be determined for individual patients. Evidence demonstrates worsened outcomes in severe traumatic brain injury/post cardiac resuscitation associated with hyperoxic events [15, 16]. Hyperoxia occurring with the initiation of mechanical ventilation has been found to have a negative impact on mortality, supporting judicious application of oxygen levels to maintain appropriate SpO_2 [17]. During AE, SpO_2 targets of 94% or greater prior to ascent may help reduce the negative effects of inadvertent in-flight hypoxemia.

Pressure- Versus Volume-Controlled Ventilation

Much has been discussed about the value of pressure- versus volume-controlled ventilation and the mode of ventilation during ventilatory support. However, the use of pressure- versus volume-controlled ventilation has never been shown to impact outcome. Use should be guided by clinician experience and preference.

Volume-controlled ventilation has the advantage of using a square flow waveform allowing assessment of respiratory mechanics and control of overdistension. The fixed flow of volume ventilation, however, can be associated with increases in the work of breathing and asynchrony. Pressure-controlled ventilation limits the applied pressure and provides a variable flow to meet patient demands, perhaps improving patient comfort. However, pressure control can allow large V_Ts with patient effort and violate lung-protective principles. An adaptive pressure breath delivers breaths with a variable pressure to maintain a selected V_T. This type of ventilation control is commonly referred to as pressure-regulated volume control (PRVC) ventilation and has the combined advantages and disadvantages of both volume and pressure control. Importantly, in PRVC, increased patient effort not only allows V_T above lung-protective goals but does so by offloading the work of breathing to the patient.

Ventilation Mode

The mode of ventilation is equally controversial and often based on clinician preference. The most common modes include continuous mandatory ventilation (CMV), intermittent mandatory ventilation (IMV), and pressure support ventilation (PSV). There are at least a dozen different modes that run the gamut from providing full support or partial support of minute ventilation.

Despite intense opinions, no mode of ventilation has ever been demonstrated to improve outcomes compared to another mode. During flight, the use of CMV (also known as assist/control ventilation) using either a volume or pressure control is currently considered to be the safest choice.

Rate Considerations

Under normal conditions, a set respiratory rate of 12–15 breaths per minute and an I/E of 1:1 to 1:2 is a sufficient starting point. In CMV, this allows the patient to select a rate greater than this value if necessary. In patients with chronic obstructive pulmonary disease (COPD) characterized by hyperinflation and airflow limitation, an I/E of 1:3 or greater may be required to prevent air trapping and auto-PEEP.

Device Characteristics of Transport Ventilators

A number of sophisticated transport ventilators have been developed and tested for airworthiness for use during AE (Fig. 18.3). There are a number of important characteristics shared by these transport ventilators:

- *Weight* – A portable ventilator is one that can be carried by a nurse or therapist from the transfer facility to the aircraft. In practice, devices weighing less than 15 pounds are desirable.
- *Durability* – Ventilators should be compact, simple to operate, durable, and unaffected by extremes of heat, cold, or vibration. Proper shielding is required to limit emission of electromagnetic energy.
- *Airworthiness* – The ventilator should not interfere with operation of the communications or aircraft and must be federally approved for use aboard aircraft.
- *Power* – While some devices use pneumatic power from compressed gas, these devices are commonly impacted by hypobarism and have excessive gas consumption. The newest devices use lead acid or lithium ion batteries. Battery life is impacted by the type of delivery system (turbine vs. piston), PEEP, type of breath (pressure control requires greater energy consumption than volume control), FIO_2, and lung mechanics. Battery life is typically listed at nominal settings, and in the sickest patients, the actual battery life may be a third of that nominal value.
- *Gas consumption* – Gas consumption is typically oxygen or compressed gas used by the ventilator to operate, but that is not delivered as part of the patient's minute ventilation. Fluidic and pneumatic devices have the highest gas

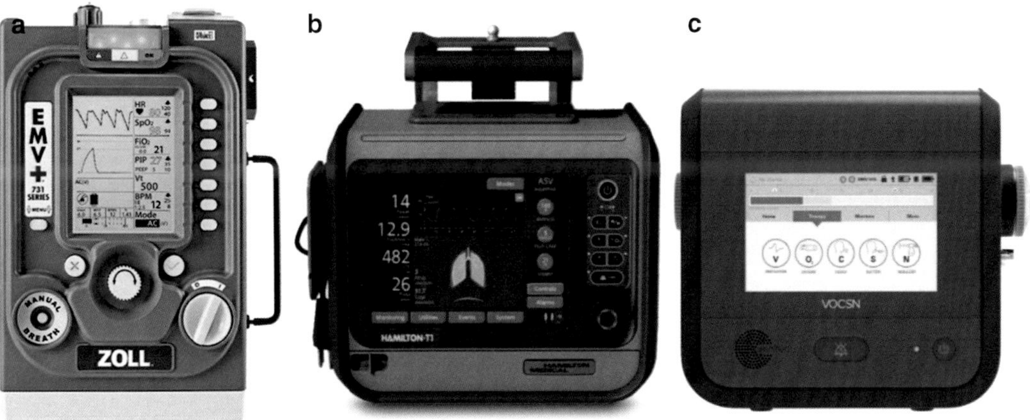

Fig. 18.3 Three new transport ventilators: (**a**) EMV+ 731 (ZOLL Medical, Chelmsford, Massachusetts), (**b**) the Hamilton-T1 (Hamilton Medical, Bonaduz, Switzerland), and (**c**) Ventec VOCSN. (Ventec Life Systems, Bothell, Washington)

consumptions. Ideally, gas consumption should be less than 5 L/min.

- *Controls* – Controls should be easy to access and difficult to inadvertently change. At a minimum the controls for respiratory rate and tidal volume should be independent.
- *Safety* – Appropriate alarms and monitoring should be integral to the ventilator. Monitoring airway pressures and delivered V_T is essential. Alarms should be visual and aural, as the noise inside many aircraft prohibits hearing alarms. An anti-asphyxia valve is required in case of ventilator failure. Monitoring of battery life and gas consumption is ideal. Alarms for low battery life and loss of source gas are required.
- *Assembly and disassembly* – The ventilator circuit and components should be impossible to reassemble improperly. Reconnection of the circuit during flight can be a challenge.

Ventilator Performance

The currently available transport or portable ventilators have performance characteristics comparable to intensive care unit (ICU) devices. Transport ventilators should be able to deliver consistent tidal volume and minute ventilation regardless of patient respiratory mechanics. The work of breathing should be comparable to ICU ventilators and the trigger should be PEEP compensated. Volume and pressure breaths should be available, and CMV and PSV are minimum mode capabilities. A PEEP range of 0–25 cm H_2O should be available. The range of V_T should be 50–800 ml. The long-term holdover of 2.0 L V_Ts on ventilators is unnecessary and potentially dangerous.

Ventilators certified by the US Federal Aviation Administration (FAA) for aeronautical use (i.e., Airworthiness Release certified) must be able to compensate for changes in altitude. Ventilators with a piston-based design deliver a constant tidal volume regardless of the altitude. The volume of the piston is the same; this device is not compensated but simply volume constant due to its archetype. Blower-based devices (turbines, blowers, etc.) are impacted by changes in barometric pressure, typically delivering up to 20% greater V_T at 8000 feet. A device that is "altitude compensated" monitors barometric pressure and changes the output to maintain a constant V_T. Importantly, not only is volume delivery inaccurate in uncompensated devices, but volume monitoring can be inaccurate as well—particularly in ventilators using a variable or fixed orifice pneumotachometer. As an example, the LTV-1200 ventilator is not altitude compensated, while the Impact 754 and 731 as well as the Drager portable ventilators are all altitude compensated. Some ICU ventilators (Medtronic 980) are altitude compensated, while others are not (Drager Evita-4). Because of their inability to compensate for out-of-range changes in gas density, some ventilators alarm and continue to operate, while others cease to operate. The LTV-1000 delivers larger tidal volumes while displaying a volume that is smaller than actually delivered. Figure 18.4 demonstrates a Hamilton-T1 display the ventilator failure passing through 13,000 feet in an altitude chamber. Failure of a ventilator to provide altitude compensation requires some additional thought: Should the ventilator cease to operate and alarm or continue to operate and alarm [18–25]?

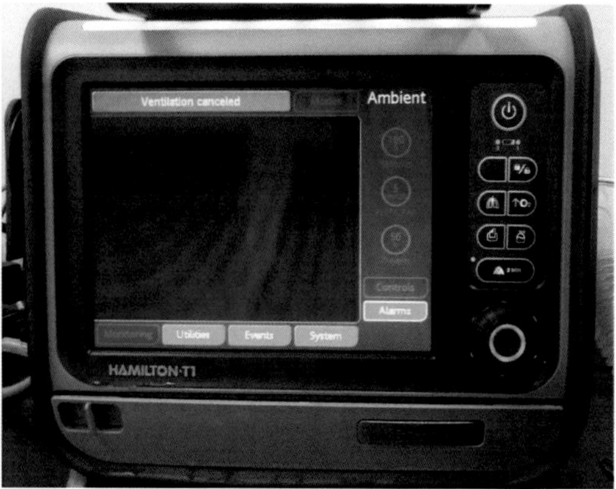

Fig. 18.4 Ventilator failure can suddenly occur when the compensation is unable to maintain tidal volume at higher altitudes, particularly during either explosive or gradual decompression

Ancillary Devices

Humidifiers

A passive humidification device, heat and moisture exchanger or "artificial nose," is ideal for transport. These devices reclaim exhaled heat and moisture and return it to the patient on the following inspiration. Increases in resistance of heat and moisture exchangers can occur in the presence of hemoptysis, pulmonary edema, and excessive secretions. Monitoring airway pressures for signs of partial or complete occlusion is required. When choosing a heat and moisture exchanger, a low dead space (<50 ml) is desirable to allow lung-protective tidal volumes.

Endotracheal Tubes

During invasive ventilation, the endotracheal tube serves as a conduit for ventilation and protects the lower airway from aspiration. An endotracheal tube cuff filled with air is sensitive to changes in barometric pressure, increasing during ascent and potentially causing tracheal injury. On descent, a fall in cuff pressure may allow aspiration of secretions around the cuff into the lower airway—a precursor to ventilator-associated pneumonia. Manual control of the cuff is difficult during the entire flight pattern. Several new devices that allow continuous monitoring and maintenance of cuff pressures have been developed for use during AE [26–28].

Transport Ventilator Versus Manual Ventilation

Manual ventilation is often used during short-distance transports as it is inexpensive and simple and needs only human power. During manual ventilation, however, the volume, frequency, and pressure applied are typically unknown. A number of studies have reported hyperventilation and acute respiratory alkalosis during manual ventilation resulting in cardiovascular complications. For this reason, manual ventilation should be used during long-distance AE only in emergency situations [29].

Adjuncts to Mechanical Ventilation

In the presence of refractory hypoxemia, a number of techniques can be used to improve gas exchange.

Cabin Altitude Restriction

Cabin altitude restriction can reduce the impact of hypobarism and associated hypoxia on critically ill patients. However, cabin altitude restriction often requires cruise altitude restrictions. This results in a reduction in aircraft performance, in terms of decreased air speed, increased fuel consumption, and increased flight duration [30]. For this reason, cabin altitude restriction should be requested only when oxygenation of critical patients cannot be maintained by other means.

The cabin altitude in a C-17 is equivalent to a modern civilian airliner, which can maintain a cabin altitude pressure of 6500–7000 feet above sea level even at the highest cruise altitudes. At most cruising altitudes, the KC-135 can maintain a cabin pressure altitude of commercial aircraft of less than 8000 feet. However, cabin pressures can exceed 8000 feet when flow at pressure altitudes above 43,000 feet [31]. The C-130 can maintain a cabin pressure-altitude of 5000 feet at its standard cruise altitude of 28,000 feet. The C-21, despite its many other limitations, can maintain a cabin pressure-altitude equal to sea level at a cruise altitude of 22,000 feet. At its maximal cruise altitude of 41,000 feet, the C-21 maintains a cabin pressure altitude of 8000 feet.

Recruitment Maneuvers

A recruitment maneuver is accomplished by increasing lung volumes through manipulation of PEEP, V_T, or both. There are several methods, but the safest and most effective appears to be a stair step increase in PEEP while maintaining a constant inspiratory pressure. This maneuver can be accomplished over 2–3 minutes. A successful recruitment maneuver improves compliance and SpO_2 and should typically be followed by an increase in PEEP to maintain recruitment [12].

Inhaled Pulmonary Vasodilators

Inhaled nitric oxide (INO) and aerosolized epoprostenol have been shown to improve oxygenation in the short term by selectively dilating blood vessels next to open alveoli. This improvement in ventilation/perfusion (V/Q) matching is not associated with a mortality benefit. The use of INO during transport has been described and in at least one report is associated with more successful transport of a patient with ARDS referred to an ECMO center [32]. Equipment specific for transport using INO is commercially available.

Prone Position

Prone positioning improves the distribution of ventilation by altering pleural pressure gradients in lung tissue. Unique among many of the adjuncts to mechanical ventilation, prone positioning is associated with a decrease in mortality in severe ARDS. Prone positioning can be accomplished with manpower or with a specialty bed. Prone positioning complicates assessment of the patient, risks loss of the airway, and renders cardiopulmonary resuscitation (CPR) almost impossible. Prone positioning is also associated with increases in skin tissue breakdown. The use of prone positioning has been described during AE but should be done so with an abundance of caution [33, 34].

High-Frequency Ventilation

High-frequency ventilation (HFV) includes a variety of techniques including high-frequency jet ventilation (HFJV), high-frequency oscillation (HFO), and high-frequency percussive ventilation (HFPV). While each HFV technique has been accomplished during transport, size, weight, and gas consumption commonly restrict use. HFJV and HFO are most commonly used in neonatal and pediatric transport. More recently, HFO has been associated with worse outcomes in adults and should not be routinely performed [12].

HFPV can be delivered by the volumetric diffusive respirator and has been championed by a few despite the lack of any meaningful outcome data [35]. Importantly, the pneumatic operation of HFPV is impacted significantly by changes in altitude, increasing delivered volumes and PEEP. This is particularly a concern with the volumetric diffusive respirator, as monitoring of V_T is absent and pressure monitoring is accomplished with an analog manometer.

Noninvasive Ventilation

Noninvasive ventilation refers to ventilation via a tight-fitting face or nasal mask. The use of noninvasive ventilation in COPD is a standard of care and is associated with reduced mortality, morbidity, hospital stay, and costs during an exacerbation [36]. Similarly, the use of the related mask continuous positive airway pressure (CPAP) technique for cardiogenic pulmonary edema is associated with improved outcomes. Avoiding intubation and its unintended consequences is one of the key attributes of noninvasive ventilation and CPAP. The use of noninvasive ventilation and CPAP during AE is evolving and should offer similar benefits. The main caveat is failure of noninvasive ventilation at altitude requires emergent intubation—always a risky proposition during flight. Using noninvasive ventilation or CPAP should be accompanied by preparation for failure, including the appropriate personnel and equipment to perform intubation. High-flow, heated, and humidified nasal oxygen is a promising method of noninvasive support, but the need for a heated humidifier limits the use in AE.

Extracorporeal Membrane Oxygen

The use of extracorporeal membrane oxygenation (ECMO) for cardiac and respiratory failure has grown exponentially over the last few years. ECMO has been used during transport for decades and can be lifesaving in select circumstances. New technology for ECMO is smaller, lighter, and infinitely more portable than previous devices. The use of ECMO during flight remains a challenge and fraught with risk. Additional equipment and surgical intervention is difficult in the face of equipment failure or dislodgment. However, it appears that the use of ECMO for transport will continue to grow. Centers exploring this option should be aware of the costs, training, and experience required for successful program implementation [37, 38].

References

1. Mason PE, Eadie JS, Holder AD. Prospective observational study of United States (US) Air Force Critical Care Air Transport team operations in Iraq. J Emerg Med. 2011;41:8–13.
2. Galvagno SM, Dubose JJ, Grissom TE, Fang R, Smith R, Bebarta VS, Shackelford S, Scalea TM. The epidemiology of Critical Care Air Transport Team operations in contemporary warfare. Mil Med. 2014;179(6):612–8.
3. Ingalls N, Zonies D, Bailey JA, Martin KD, Iddins BO, Carlton PK, Hanseman D, Branson R, Dorlac W, Johannigman J. A review of the first 10 years of critical care aeromedical transport during operation Iraqi freedom and operation enduring freedom: the importance of evacuation timing. JAMA Surg. 2014;149(8):807–13.
4. Warren J, Fromm RE Jr, Orr RA, Rotello LC, Horst HM. Guidelines for the inter- and intrahospital transport of critically ill patients. Crit Care Med. 2004;32:256–62.
5. Fang R, Allan PF, Womble SG, Porter MT, Sierra-Nunez J, Russ RS, Dorlac GR, Benson C, Oh JS, Wanek SM, Osborn EC, Silvey SV, Dorlac WC. Closing the "care in the air" capability gap for severe lung injury: the Landstuhl Acute Lung Rescue Team and extracorporeal lung support. J Trauma. 2011;71(1 Suppl):S91–7.
6. Blecha S, Dodoo-Schittko F, Brandstetter S, Brandl M, Dittmar M, Graf BM, Karagiannidis C, Apfelbacher C, Bein T, DACAPO Study Group. Quality of inter-hospital transportation in 431 transport survivor patients suffering from acute respiratory distress syndrome referred to specialist centers. Ann Intensive Care. 2018;15;8(1):5.
7. Wilcox SR, Saia MS, Waden H, Genthon A, Gates JD, Cocchi MN, McGahn SJ, Frakes M, Wedel SK, Richards JB. Improved oxygenation after transport in patients with hypoxemic respiratory failure. Air Med J. 2015;34(6):369–76.
8. Blakeman TC, Rodriquez D Jr, Britton TJ, Johannigman JA, Petro MC, Branson RD. Evaluation of oxygen concentrators and chemical oxygen generators at altitude and temperature extremes. Mil Med. 2016;181(5 Suppl):160–8.
9. Blakeman TC, Rodriquez D Jr, Gerlach TW, Dorlac WC, Johannigman JA, Branson RD. Oxygen requirement to reverse altitude-induced hypoxemia with continuous flow and pulsed dose oxygen. Aerosp Med Hum Perform. 2015;86(4):351–6.
10. Rodriquez D Jr, Blakeman TC, Dorlac W, Johannigman JA, Branson RD. Maximizing oxygen delivery during mechanical ventilation with a portable oxygen concentrator. J Trauma. 2010;69(Suppl 1):S87–93.
11. Fan E, Needham DM, Stewart TE. Ventilatory management of acute lung injury and acute respiratory distress syndrome. JAMA. 2005;294(22):2889–96.
12. Fan E, Del Sorbo L, Goligher EC, Hodgson CL, Munshi L, Walkey AJ, et al; American Thoracic Society, European Society of Intensive Care Medicine, and Society of Critical Care Medicine. An Official American Thoracic Society/European Society of Intensive Care Medicine/Society of Critical Care Medicine clinical practice guideline: mechanical ventilation in adult patients with acute respiratory distress syndrome. Am J Respir Crit Care Med. 2017;195(9):1253–1263.
13. Bime C, Fiero M, Lu Z, Oren E, Berry CE, Parthasarathy S, Garcia JGN. High positive end-expiratory pressure is associated with improved survival in obese patients with acute respiratory distress syndrome. Am J Med. 2017 Feb;130(2):207–13.
14. Acute Respiratory Distress Syndrome Network, Brower RG, Matthay MA, Morris A, Schoenfeld D, Thompson BT, Wheeler A. Ventilation with lower tidal volumes as compared with traditional tidal volumes for acute lung injury and the acute respiratory distress syndrome. N Engl J Med. 2000;342(18):1301–8.
15. Rincon F, Kang J, Vibbert M, Urtecho J, Athar MK, Jallo J. Significance of arterial hyperoxia and relationship with case fatality in traumatic brain injury: a multicentre cohort study. J Neurol Neurosurg Psychiatry. 2014;85:7.
16. Kilgannon JH, Jones AE, Shapiro NI, Angelos MG, Milcarek B, Hunter K, Parrillo JE, Trzeciak S. Association between arterial hyperoxia following resuscitation from cardiac arrest and in-hospital mortality. JAMA. 2010;303(21):2165–71.
17. Page D, Ablordeppey E, Wessman BT, Mohr NM, Trzeciak S, Kollef MH, Roberts BW, Fuller BM. Emergency department hyperoxia is associated

with increased mortality in mechanically ventilated patients: a cohort study. Crit Care. 2018;22:9.

18. Blakeman T, Britton T, Rodriquez D Jr, Branson R. Performance of portable ventilators at altitude. J Trauma Acute Care Surg. 2014;77(3 Suppl 2):S151–5.
19. Blakeman T, Rodriquez D Jr, Petro M, Branson R. Evaluation of intensive care unit ventilators at altitude. Air Med J. 2017;36(5):258–62.
20. Blakeman TC, Rodriquez D Jr, Britton TJ, Johannigman JA, Petro MC, Branson RD. Performance of portable ventilators following storage at temperature extremes. Mil Med. 2016;181(5 Suppl):156–9.
21. Blakeman TC, Rodriquez D, Dorlac WC, Hanseman DJ, Hattery E, Branson RD. Performance of portable ventilators for mass-casualty care. Prehosp Disaster Med. 2011;26(5):330–4.
22. Blakeman TC, Rodriquez D Jr, Hanseman D, Branson RD. Bench evaluation of 7 home-care ventilators. Respir Care. 2011;56(11):1791–8.
23. Blakeman TC, Rodriquez D, Branson RD. Accuracy of the oxygen cylinder duration calculator of the LTV-1000 portable ventilator. Respir Care. 2009;54(9):1183–6.
24. Rodriquez D Jr, Branson RD, Dorlac W, Dorlac G, Barnes SA, Johannigman JA. Effects of simulated altitude on ventilator performance. J Trauma. 2009;66(4 Suppl):S172–7.
25. Rodriquez D Jr, Branson R, Barnes SA, Johannigman JA. Battery life of the "four-hour" lithium ion battery of the LTV-1000 under varying workloads. Mil Med. 2008;173(8):792–5.
26. Branson R, Rodriquez D Jr. Cuff pressure confusion: solutions are abundant. Air Med J. 2017;36(5):223.
27. Blakeman T, Rodriquez D Jr, Woods J, Cox D, Elterman J, Branson R. Automated control of endotracheal tube cuff pressure during simulated flight. J Trauma Acute Care Surg. 2016;81(5 Suppl 2 Proceedings of the 2015 Military Health System Research Symposium):S116–20.
28. Britton T, Blakeman TC, Eggert J, Rodriquez D, Ortiz H, Branson RD. Managing endotracheal tube cuff pressure at altitude: a comparison of four methods. J Trauma Acute Care Surg. 2014;77(3 Suppl 2):S240–4.
29. Blakeman TC, Branson RD. Inter- and intrahospital transport of the critically ill. Respir Care. 2013;58(6):1008–23.
30. Butler WP, Steinkraus LW, Burlingame EE, Fouts BL, Serres JL. Complication rates in altitude restricted patients following aeromedical evacuation. Aerosp Med Hum Perform. 2016;87(4):352–9.
31. Heimbach RD, Sheffield PJ. Protection in the pressure environment: cabin pressurization and oxygen equipment. In: DeHart RL, editor. Fundamentals of aerospace medicine. Philadelphia: Lea and Febiger; 1985. p. 110–3.
32. Teman NR, Thomas J, Bryner BS, Haas CF, Haft JW, Park PK, Lowell MJ, Napolitano LM. Inhaled nitric oxide to improve oxygenation for safe critical care transport of adults with severe hypoxemia. Am J Crit Care. 2015;24(2):110–7.
33. Guérin C, Reignier J, Richard J-C, et al; PROSEVA Study Group. Prone positioning in severe acute respiratory distress syndrome. N Engl J Med. 2013;368(23):2159–2168.
34. DellaVolpe JD, Lovett J, Martin-Gill C, Guyette FX. Transport of mechanically ventilated patients in the prone position. Prehosp Emerg Care. 2016;20(5):643–7.
35. Barillo DJ, Renz EM, Wright GR, Broger KP, Chung KK, Thompson CK, Cancio LC. High-frequency percussive ventilation for intercontinental aeromedical evacuation. Am J Disaster Med. 2011;6(6):369–78.
36. Nava S, Hill N. Non-invasive ventilation in acute respiratory failure. Lancet. 2009;374(9685):250–9.
37. Fan E, Gattinoni L, Combes A, Schmidt M, Peek G, Brodie D, et al. Venovenous extracorporeal membrane oxygenation for acute respiratory failure: a clinical review from an international group of experts. Intensive Care Med. 2016;42(5):712–24.
38. Bryner B, Cooley E, Copenhaver W, Brierley K, Teman N, Landis D, Rycus P, Hemmila M, Napolitano LM, Haft J, Park PK, Bartlett RH. Two decades' experience with interfacility transport on extracorporeal membrane oxygenation. Ann Thorac Surg. 2014;98(4):1363–70.

Medical Casualties

19

J. Christopher Farmer, Thomas J. McLaughlin, and Robert A. Klocke

Introduction

The transport of critically ill patients from one location to another is inherently perilous. Although this is true even for in-hospital conveyances (e.g., down the hall to accomplish a computed tomography scan), the risk is considerably greater during long-distance aeromedical evacuation (AE) because the only expertise and medical equipment available is that which was enplaned with the patient. For this reason, AE of medical casualties (especially those needing intensive care) requires extensive preplanning and careful preparation for both predictable and unanticipated problems.

During the last two decades, what has most changed is our ability to externally "control" patient hemodynamic and respiratory systems during transport with extracorporeal membrane oxygenation (ECMO). For our very sickest intensive care unit (ICU) patients, we are less constrained by our limited ability to pharmacologically and mechanically manipulate cardiorespiratory host physiology because we can partially to fully support these organ systems with venoarterial and veno-venous ECMO.

Unfortunately, this ability does not mitigate the risk of AE transport. For example, many of these labile patients have ongoing vasodilatory shock requiring vasopressor support during transport. Additionally, the life-threatening and sudden risk of equipment and device malfunction during transport is substantially higher. Finally, more devices means more cubic space and more people are required to accomplish AE transport. This further complicates the transport process.

Ultimately, the ability to prepare for AE is limited by the amount of personnel, equipment, and supplies that will fit on an aircraft (Fig. 19.1). Therefore, successful transport of medical casualties depends on (1) a thorough understanding of the medical conditions that afflict the patient, (2) knowledge of potential or likely physiological complications and how vital en-route monitoring will be accomplished, (3) a clear response plan if AE transport processes aggravate existing medical conditions, and (4) response planning for device malfunction during transport. Simply put, take

J. C. Farmer (✉)
Col, USAF, MC, FS (ret.), Department of Critical Care Medicine, Mayo Clinic Hospital, Phoenix, AZ, USA
e-mail: Farmer.j@mayo.edu

T. J. McLaughlin
Colonel, USAF, MC, SFS (ret.), Department of Emergency Medicine, Texas A&M University College of Medicine, Bryan, TX, USA

Department of Emergency Medicine, CHRISTUS Health/Texas A&M Spahn Emergency Medicine Residency, Corpus Christi, TX, USA

R. A. Klocke
Department of Medicine, Jacobs School of Medicine and Biomedical Education, State University of New York at Buffalo, Buffalo, NY, USA

W. W. Hurd, W. Beninati (eds.), *Aeromedical Evacuation*,
https://doi.org/10.1007/978-3-030-15903-0_19

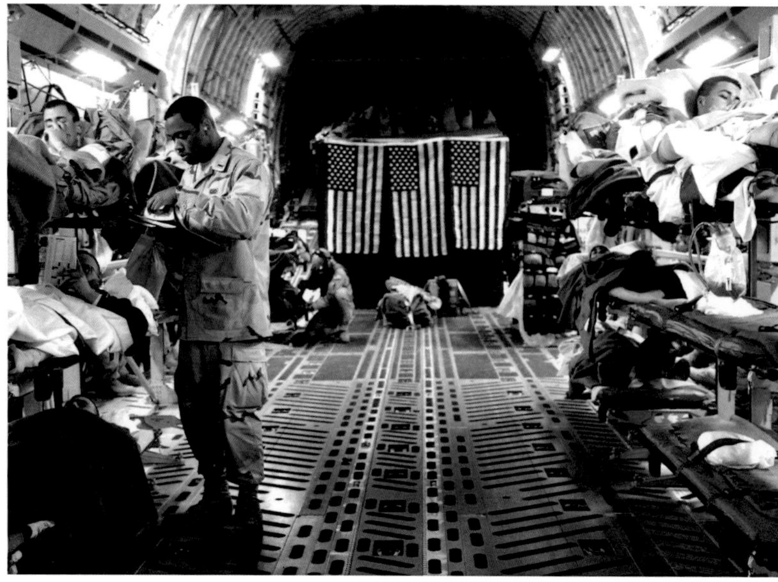

Fig. 19.1 Aeromedical crew members treat injured Haitians during aeromedical evacuation on a C-130 from Port-au-Prince, Haiti, to Dobbins Air Reserve Base, Georgia, after a devastating earthquake. (New York National Guard photo by Staff Sgt. Peter Dean)

only what is necessary, but ensure what you have is what you actually need and that you can successfully recognize and adapt if anything "breaks!"

Definition of Terms

Medical Evacuation Versus Aeromedical Evacuation

The first important distinction to be made is between medical evacuation (MEDEVAC) and aeromedical evacuation (AE)—two clearly different processes that are often confused because they have much in common. MEDEVAC is defined as transportation of casualties from the site of injury to a medical facility or between relatively nearby medical facilities [1]. This includes both ground transportation and air transportation, most commonly by rotary-wing aircraft. In the civilian sphere, MEDEVAC is the majority of air transportation, and the most common scenario is transportation of trauma patients from the site of a motor vehicle accident to an emergency department. In the military, the MEDEVAC system is designed to transport combat and noncombat casualties to the closest field medical facility or between medical facilities within the theater.

In contrast, AE is defined as the long-distance (usually >300 miles) air transportation of casualties between medical facilities. In the civilian sphere, this is likely to be a shorter distance between an emergency department and an ICU to a higher level of care at another facility. It is usually performed using rotary-wing aircraft. However, it has also been clearly demonstrated that transportation of patients over distances greater than 800 miles is safe [2]. For military AE, the distance of transport is often measured in thousands of miles and fixed-wing aircraft are almost exclusively used. The similarities between AE and MEDEVAC are obvious, especially when transporting critically ill patients by air.

Elective Versus Urgent Aeromedical Evacuation

Elective Aeromedical Evacuation

Elective AE is characterized by relatively unlimited time for planning prior to transportation. In most cases, elective AE takes place after definitive therapy, when the rigors of air travel are unlikely to result in medical decompensation. Although these patients are stable and convalescing, some may be critically ill and require high levels of in-flight medical care and support requirements. In addition, even the most stable patients may experience complications and become unstable when exposed to the sometimes-rigorous AE environment.

For the critically ill patient, the goal of elective AE is seamless critical care from the point of transfer through arrival at the accepting facility. The most significant determination of the quality of transport care is the training and expertise of the medical attendants. To this end, medical attendants should be knowledgeable in the environment of flight as well as the provision of critical care.

Elective AE of a medical casualty is most commonly performed to transport a patient to a facility capable of a higher level of care. It is also used to transport a patient from a foreign environment where the culture, language, and medical capabilities are significantly different. In every case, the decision to transfer a patient should be made with consideration of (1) the risks to the patient of *not* being transferred, (2) the risks inherent to AE, and (3) the expected benefits of the transfer. Regardless of the reason, elective AE patients should be stable with a secure airway and have demonstrated an appropriate response to therapy, including stable vital signs prior to transport.

Urgent Aeromedical Evacuation

Medical casualties may sometimes have to be transported by AE after having received only enough therapy to "stabilize" their disease process. Common reasons for urgent AE include:

1. Transportation to a facility capable of a higher level of care when appropriate care is not available locally.
2. Removal from a military theater of operations.
3. Removal from a disaster area where local medical facilities are saturated.

Table 19.1 provides examples and a partial list of conditions that commonly require urgent AE to a higher level of care. These seemingly disparate conditions are similar in that they all possess an increased risk for en route deterioration. A significant proportion of these transport risks relate to acute airway compromise and inability to oxygenate/ventilate. In some patients, rapid airway deterioration requires immediate recognition and definitive intervention to avoid loss of life. Next, refractory shock not responsive to infusion therapies constitutes another broad category of significant transport risks. Finally, device malfunction is the last aggregate category of major transport risk. For all of these risk categories, continuous and comprehensive physiological monitoring is essential in order to promptly recognize impending disasters and permit preemptive intervention.

A surprisingly large number of previously healthy patients develop life-threatening cardiac syndromes (e.g., infarction, pump failure, or uncontrolled hypertension) in relatively austere locations, necessitating transfer to higher levels of care. Because of lack of appropriate medical facilities locally, these patients often require transfer during the most unstable phases of their diseases [3]. Complete evaluation and definitive treatment are often unfeasible prior to AE. This results in reliance on state-of-the-art

Table 19.1 Medical conditions that may require urgent aeromedical evacuation (AE) to a higher level of care

Primary respiratory conditions
Acute, severe hypoxemic respiratory failure requiring advanced mechanical ventilation and/or nonconventional respiratory support (e.g., ECMO)
Acute, severe right heart failure
Submassive and massive pulmonary embolism
Other causes of acute pulmonary hypertension
Primary cardiovascular conditions
Myocardial infarction and unstable angina requiring intervention
Cardiogenic shock
Life-threatening arrhythmias
Hemodynamic instability and collapse
Undifferentiated refractory shock
Accelerating severe sepsis
Acute multiple organ failure
Acute kidney injury (AKI) requiring intervention
Fulminant hepatic failure
Gastrointestinal hemorrhage requiring nonsurgical intervention
Intensive care unit (ICU) conundrums
Refractory status epilepticus
Hematological emergencies

ECMO extracorporeal membrane oxygenation

monitoring throughout AE for timely detection of complications that may develop during the natural progression of the disease.

Description of Patients' Conditions

It is vitally important that we use precise, consistent, commonly understood, and quantifiable terms to describe a patient's medical condition. A patient who is described as "critically ill" by one provider may be depicted as "stable" by another. For example, a patient with primary respiratory failure on a mechanical ventilator requiring adjustment once or twice daily is critically ill but is also stable. This contrasts with patients with respiratory failure secondary to evolving acute respiratory distress syndrome (ARDS), who are both critically ill and unstable. The relative risk involved in moving these two patients on ventilators is drastically different and is influenced by the patient's medical condition, the equipment available, and the experience level of the providers caring for the patient.

Safe AE is dependent on reliable communication between all involved physicians to ensure that the right personnel and equipment are available. Using the same terminology to express the difference in acuity of illness is one of the most fundamental requirements of critical-care-related casualty transport. While this is vital for critically ill patients, it is also true for medical casualties of lesser acuity.

Stable Versus Stabilized Versus Unstable Patients

Patients who require AE can be divided into three basic groups: (1) stable, (2) stabilized, and (3) unstable. *Stable* patients are those patients who are extremely unlikely to medically decompensate during a prolonged flight either because their medical condition is not life-threatening, their physiology has not been in flux, or they are in the convalescent stage of their illness or injury. For the purposes of this book, stable patients are transported by elective AE and are classified as "routine" using the standard AE patient nomenclature (see Chap. 7).

The second group is *stabilized* patients: those who have received sufficient medical care to allow them to be transported by AE but are at significant risk of becoming unstable during the flight. These include patients transported by urgent AE (when a patient's serious condition cannot be adequately treated locally) and are termed "special" by standard AE patient classification because they require special equipment or expertise for AE.

The final AE group is made up of *unstable* patients. These patients require active and aggressive intensive care throughout AE for survival. These patients are also classified as both urgent and special and may be more common during military operations and natural disasters. In response to US military doctrinal changes, AE of both stabilized and unstable patients is now common. For this reason, the AE system developed the Critical Care Air Transport Teams (CCATT) made up of intensive care providers trained to use sophisticated air-transportable intensive care equipment (see Chap. 9).

Variables Influencing Long-Distance Aeromedical Evacuation

Stressors of Flight

Successful AE of medical casualties requires a clear understanding and insight of the stressors of flight on a patient. These stressors can be considered in three broad categories: (1) physical, (2) mechanical, and (3) environmental.

The most important *physical* stressors are the consequence of altitude-induced changes in cabin pressure on the patient and the adjunctive medical devices used en route. The physiological implications of these effects will be discussed later in the respiratory and cardiovascular sections.

Mechanical stressors include aircraft-specific factors, such as vibration, noise saturation, and poor lighting. Noise and vibration render auditory diagnostic assessment difficult or impossible. For this reason, medical equipment must provide ample visual cues, especially for alarms

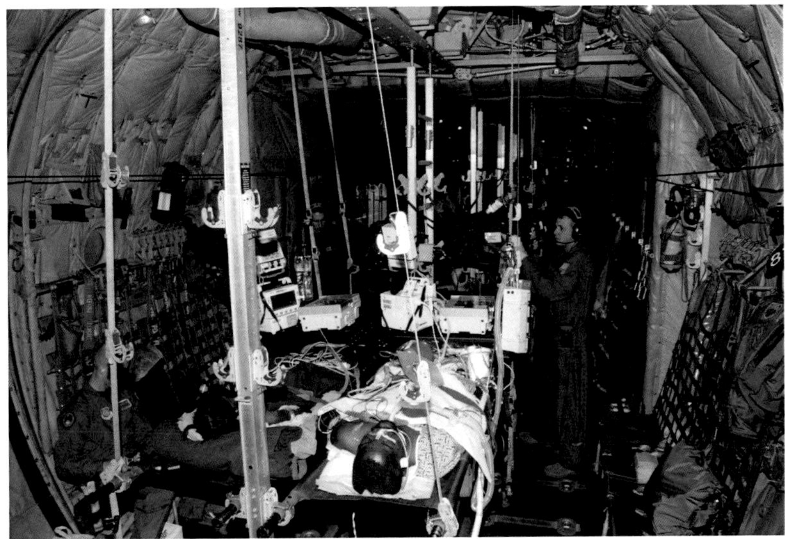

Fig. 19.2 An aeromedical evacuation mission from Balad Air Base, Iraq, to Ramstein Air Base, Germany. The C-17 Globemaster can be configured to transport up to 36-littered patients and 48 ambulatory patients using a three-tier litter system. (USAF US Air Force Photo by Master Sgt. Scott Reed)

on devices such as mechanical ventilators and cardiac monitors. This problem may be compounded when AE of multiple patients results in a high patient-to-provider ratio (Fig. 19.2). In this potentially low-light environment, visual alarms must reliably attract the caregivers' attention (e.g., by blinking incessantly).

Finally, the most important *environmental* stressors include those related to extremes of temperature and low humidity. Failure to account for these variables can significantly complicate patient management.

Decreased Pressure

At the altitude flown during routine fixed-wing AE, the cabin pressure in a pressurized aircraft is equivalent to an altitude of approximately 8000 ft. above sea level. This lower pressure significantly decreases the amount and rate of oxygen that diffuses across alveolar-capillary membrane surfaces. For this reason, the flight altitude must be restricted for patients with severe lung disease and unresolvable hypoxemia at the normal cabin altitude. Even with a partial altitude restriction (i.e., 3000–7500 ft) during fixed-wing AE, the partial pressure of oxygen (PaO_2) in a majority of casualties may be compromised to <60 mm Hg [4].

Altitude restriction for AE aircraft creates a significant cost in terms of speed and fuel efficiency; thus, it should only be used when essential. The obvious result is increased duration of the flight, related to both decreased air speed and increased refueling stops. This, in turn, increases the overall risk to the patient transport and must be carefully accounted for during the AE planning phase.

Oxygen Therapy

All AE patients should receive an amount of oxygen equivalent to that received prior to transport in order to minimize risk of hypoxemia. This requires maintenance of the same inspired oxygen partial pressure (P_IO_2) [5]. Even though the inspired fraction of oxygen is constant at all altitudes, the reduction of barometric pressure with ascent to altitude decreases the ambient P_IO_2 according to the following formula:

$$P_IO_2 = [PB - PH_2O] \times F_IO_2$$

where PB is ambient barometric pressure and PH_2O is the partial pressure of water vapor that is dependent on the patient's temperature. At 37 ° C, body temperature, PH_2O is 47 mm Hg.

Although PH_2O will vary with patient temperature, for practical purposes it can be assumed

Table 19.2 Barometric pressure at indicated altitude and standard temperature

Altitude (feet)	Barometric pressure (mm Hg)	Barometric pressure – 47 (mm Hg)	Temperature (° C)
0	760	713	15.0
1000	733	686	13.0
2000	706	659	11.0
3000	681	634	9.1
4000	656	609	7.1
5000	632	585	5.1
6000	609	562	3.1
8000	564	517	−0.8
9000	542	495	−2.8
10,000	523	476	−4.8
11,000	503	456	−6.8
12,000	483	436	−8.8
14,000	446	399	−12.7
16,000	412	365	−16.7
18,000	379	332	−20.7
20,000	349	302	−24.6
22,000	321	274	−28.6
24,000	294	247	−32.5
26,000	270	223	−36.5

to be constant over the range of temperatures present in patients. Thus, the required F_IO_2 to maintain P_IO_2 constant during exposure to a lower barometric pressure can be calculated as follows:

$$\text{Required } F_IO_2 = F_IO_2 \times [PB_1 - 47]/[PB_2 - 47]$$

where F_IO_2 is the current F_IO_2, PB_1 the current barometric pressure, and PB_2 the barometric pressure at the new altitude (Table 19.2).

For example, if a patient is in a location 1000 feet above sea level and is receiving an FiO_2 of 0.50 but will be transported at a cabin altitude of 8000 feet to a hospital located 4000 feet above sea level, the following calculations illustrate the required F_IO_2 during transport and after arrival:

$$\text{In-flight required } F_IO_2 = 0.50(686)/517 = 0.66$$

$$\text{Destination required } F_IO_2 = 0.50(686)/609 = 0.56$$

Pneumothorax

An unrecognized pneumothorax can have a devastating effect on respiratory system function during AE. Even a small pneumothorax on the ground may become a life-threatening tension pneumothorax at altitude because gas trapped in this closed space expands as the aircraft ascends. For this reason, special efforts should be made to diagnose a simple pneumothorax prior to flight in high-risk patients, such as trauma or mechanically ventilated patients. In general, a thoracostomy tube or pigtail catheter should be inserted in all patients with a pneumothorax prior to AE, even in the absence of symptoms. Once inserted, the chest tube should never be clamped during transport but must instead be vented using a one-way (e.g., Heimlich) valve, a water seal, or a continuous suction device.

Effects on Equipment

The risk of altitude-related gas expansion is also a concern for air-containing medical devices, such as a Foley catheter or endotracheal tube. On the ground, air in an endotracheal tube cuff is extremely unlikely to expand to the point of causing tracheal injury. However, during ascent, the cuff can expand to a sufficient diameter to rupture the trachea and/or obstruct the endotracheal tube, especially in the event of cabin decompression. For this reason, the US Air Force (USAF) AE system insists that all patients with endotracheal and tracheostomy tubes have the cuffs filled with sterile saline rather than air prior to takeoff. If air is left in the cuff, pressures must be measured and documented frequently during AE.

Low Humidity

The fresh air supply of the aircraft, obtained from the surrounding atmosphere, becomes progressively drier as altitude increases. As a flight progresses, moist air is continuously replaced by drier air, resulting in a decreasing humidity within the aircraft. The cabin humidity may drop as low as 5% after 2 hours and as low as 1% after 4 hours of flight. This low humidity may result in symptoms of dry mouth, chapped lips, hoarseness, or sore throat among crew members and patients.

Long flights with such low humidity may complicate patients' underlying medical conditions. Respiratory secretions become more viscous and can result in impaired gas exchange, thus contributing to hypoxia and even major airway and segmental bronchial obstruction. Humidified oxygen should be used for all patients requiring oxygen therapy. Warmed, humidified air should be supplied to tracheostomy patients, even if supplemental oxygen is not given.

Low ambient humidity also increases insensible fluid losses in all patients but especially those who are flown >4 hours, have large surface area open wounds, or require mechanical ventilation. For patients with large open wounds, insensible fluid losses can be limited by covering the wound or affected extremity with a non-permeable plastic sheet. In high-risk patients, this increased insensible fluid loss may increase the risk of hypovolemia, and thus sufficient large-bore intravenous (IV) catheters should be placed prior to takeoff. In the event of cardiovascular deterioration, fluid resuscitation needs to be increased accordingly.

Temperature Changes

As altitude increases, the temperature outside the aircraft decreases an average of 2 ° C (3.6 ° F) for every 1000 feet. These temperature changes may not be adequately ameliorated by the aircraft climate control system, potentially exposing a patient to a significant variation in temperature. In addition, during long-distance AE, significant temperature variation commonly develops in different locations of the aircraft cabin.

Exposure to temperature extremes for an extended period may result in motion sickness, headache, disorientation, fatigue, discomfort, and irritability. It will also increase metabolic rates, resulting in increased oxygen consumption. For patients with tenuous pulmonary reserve capacity, significant physiological compromise can result.

Technology Required for Transportation

Medical equipment commonly used for critical care in fixed medical facilities may not function properly in an aircraft, primarily because of the changes in cabin pressure. For this reason, a number of devices have been modified and, after extensive testing, approved for military AE by Air Force Research Laboratories for medical devices. All AE aircraft must be capable of providing electrical power for medical equipment, and this is often accomplished by using an inverter. The inverter transforms aircraft power to 110 V/60 Hz—the wall source power almost exclusively used in US hospitals. In a dedicated ambulance aircraft, this is never an issue; however, AE is routinely accomplished in one of a number of possible aircraft, depending on availability. In every case, the aeromedical crew must make sure that the appropriate power source is available for any necessary medical equipment.

Monitoring Devices

The most commonly used devices during AE are electronic monitoring devices. These include a cardiac monitor, external blood pressure monitor, arterial line monitor, pulse oximetry, end-tidal CO_2 monitor, in-line O_2 analyzer, Wright spirometer, and cuffolator (endotracheal tube cuff pressure measurement device) (Table 19.3) [6].

Aeromedical Evacuation Implications of Specific Medical Conditions

Pulmonary Conditions

Respiratory considerations are paramount for successful AE. The effects of altitude, while

Table 19.3 Medical equipment approved for use during aeromedical transport

Monitoring devices
Pulse oximetry (SpO_2)
External blood pressure measuring device
Cardiac monitor
Arterial line monitor
End-tidal CO_2 monitor
In-line O_2 analyzer
Wright spirometer
Cuffolator (endotracheal tube cuff pressure measurement device)
Defibrillators
Paddle model
"Hands-off" model
Ventilators
Adult/child
Infant
Portable laboratory instruments
Arterial blood gases
Hemoglobin and hematocrit
Electrolytes
Miscellaneous
Codman ventriculostomy package
Suction pumps and tubing
Advanced cardiac life support (ACLS) resuscitation bag
Warming blankets
Infusion pumps
Battery-powered portable bronchoscope with internal light source
Portable point of care ultrasound device

inconsequential to a healthy individual, may be devastating to the compromised patient. Therefore, a crucial AE concern is identification of patients susceptible to hypoxia so that the effects of altitude can be prevented or recognized before deleterious impact.

Pneumothorax

An untreated pneumothorax is a contraindication to AE (Table 19.4). A pneumothorax of any size must be treated prior to flight because expansion of intrapleural air with aircraft ascent can compress functioning lung tissue and compromise oxygenation. Tension pneumothorax can develop as continued expansion of trapped air shifts the mediastinal contents toward the opposite hemithorax. The resultant compression of the vena cava decreases venous return, resulting in decreased cardiac output and potential cardiopulmonary collapse.

Table 19.4 Contraindications to aeromedical evacuation (AE) of medical patients

Absolute[a]
Untreated pneumothorax
Chest tube without one-way valve, water seal, or suction
Uncorrected or refractory severe arterial oxygen desaturation
Refractory life-threatening shock
Uncontrolled life-threatening cardiac arrhythmias
Pneumoencephaly without venting or drainage
Moribund or agonal state
Relative[b]
Myocardial infarction within 1 week
Unstable angina
Cardiogenic shock
Severe anemia (hemoglobin <7 mg/dL)
Severe substance withdrawal or violent psychosis

[a]Contraindication only to elective AE
[b]Contraindication to elective or urgent AE

Tension pneumothoraces must be treated immediately with a needle thoracostomy followed by the insertion of a chest tube. The chest tube should be connected to a Heimlich valve or other one-way valve system to prevent further expansion of the pneumothorax. Lack of a one-way valve on a chest tube is another contraindication to AE.

Acute Respiratory Failure

The AE transportation of patients with acute respiratory failure requires meticulous planning, special equipment (i.e., respirator, pulse oximeter, etc.), and, in almost every case, accompaniment by a respiratory therapist or critical-care physician.

The patient's precarious medical condition may be made worse by altitude-associated hypoxia requiring careful adjustment of the respirator. In addition, equipment and incompatibility of supplies such as connectors are often a problem, especially at interface points where the responsibility for care of a patient is transferred from one group of clinicians to another. Patients may quickly deteriorate while clinicians try to fix these problems. For this reason, the respiratory therapist is an irreplaceable resource for troubleshooting and improvising. A well-prepared respiratory therapist will bring a supply of the most common fittings and the necessary tools to connect them.

The most difficult types of respiratory failure patients to transport by AE are those with ARDS. As the aircraft ascends, the altitude-related hypoxia will often result in decreased oxygenation for "borderline" ARDS patients. Unfortunately, increasing the inspired oxygen concentration alone may not improve oxygenation because these patients have a marked degree of pulmonary shunting. The most effective way to improve oxygenation is to re-expand collapsed alveoli, thereby increasing functional residual lung capacity (FRC). This is accomplished with a combination of positive pressure ventilation and positive end-expiratory pressure (PEEP). Recent work has demonstrated the value of PEEP in correcting altitude-associated hypoxia in an animal model of ARDS [7]. Changes in cabin pressure make adjustment of respirator settings extremely difficult. This, plus the nature of ARDS, puts the patient at increased risk of pulmonary barotrauma during AE.

Today, the relative availability of veno-venous ECMO has added an additional useful tool to the management of patients with refractory, severe, acute hypoxemic respiratory failure. Table 19.5 outlines current indications for considering ECMO to facilitate successful AE transport. These are adapted from the Extracorporeal Life Support Organization (ELSO) 2015 document, "Guidelines for ECMO Transport" [8]. Typically, ECMO therapies are either initiated by the sending ICU team prior to transport, or the transport team accomplishes the vascular cannulation themselves prior to AE transport. Dependence upon inhaled nitric oxide ($_{I}$NO) to treat hypoxemic respiratory failure is no longer an absolute contraindication to AE, since $_{I}$NO can be safely administered during transport.

The intent of veno-venous ECMO is to achieve adequate oxygenation and ventilation without exposing the patient's lungs to the damaging effects of aggressive positive pressure invasive mechanical ventilation. However, the successful utilization of ECMO requires sophisticated procedural skills, highly advanced knowledge of the specific physiology of ECMO circuits and their impact on native circulation and gas exchange, the ability to accurately interpret and act on ECMO-specific laboratory and hemodynamic parameters, and active education and quality programs that ensure all involved providers are up to date with these skills and knowledge.

Table 19.5 Indications for the use of extracorporeal membrane oxygenation (ECMO) prior to aeromedical evacuation (AE) in patients with failure of mechanical ventilator support and refractory hypoxemia/hypercapnia

Determination by the managing physician that there is an unacceptable risk of deterioration during transport
Presence of air leak syndrome that is likely to worsen during transport
Inability to achieve acceptable patient oxygenation without high-frequency oscillatory ventilation (HFOV), which is currently not available for AE patient.
Refractory septic/cardiogenic shock despite aggressive inotropic/pressor support ECMO indication primarily in neonatal and pediatric patients Degree of pre-transport hypoperfusion/hypotension/acidosis predicts further deterioration during transport
Other clinical scenarios which may necessitate ECMO transport: Worsening acute respiratory distress syndrome (ARDS) or other etiology of acute refractory respiratory failure at a center not capable of providing ECMO ECMO support initiated at referring center for primary cardiac failure and patient needs transport to transplant center for evaluation for possible orthotopic heart transplantation (OHT) or other cardiac intervention Patient who is a possible candidate for lung transplantation requires ECMO for safe transfer to transplant center Patient placed emergently and unexpectedly on ECMO support at center without resources to maintain patient on long-term ECMO support

Adapted from Dirnberger et al. [8]

Chronic Obstructive Pulmonary Disease

Chronic obstructive pulmonary disease (COPD) refers to the triad of asthma, emphysema, and chronic bronchitis. Each of these diseases involves airway obstruction in some manner and predisposes a patient to complications associated with the flight environment.

Both acute and subacute aggravating factors can predispose these patients to complications both at sea level and during flight [9]. Acute factors that can result in immediate respiratory deterioration include pneumothorax, pulmonary embolism, and lobar atelectasis. Subacute factors that can result in a slower deterioration include acute bronchitis, pneumonia, small pulmonary emboli, segmental atelectasis, minor trauma such as rib fractures or small pulmonary contusions, and metabolic factors. In addition, gastric distention secondary to decreased cabin pressure may limit diaphragmatic excursion and reduce vital capacity.

During AE, the COPD patient should be observed for early signs and symptoms of hypoxia, including tachycardia, tachypnea, dyspnea, hypertension, confusion, restlessness, and headache. Pulse oximetry should be used during AE to continuously monitor the oxygenation of COPD patients.

Arterial oxygen saturation is ≥95% in normal healthy patients at sea level. Patients with COPD frequently have lower readings (88–90%), which appear to be tolerated chronically and do not require oxygen supplementation. However, any drop in a patient's oxygen saturation requires immediate evaluation of ventilation and initiation of oxygen therapy to restore oxygenation to an acceptable value (≥ 90%).

The use of high levels of supplemental oxygen therapy in patients with COPD can be relatively dangerous since increased oxygen may decrease the patient's hypoxic drive to breathe, resulting in acute respiratory acidosis. This usually occurs in unstable patients with an acute exacerbation rather than in patients with compensated respiratory acidosis. Although a patient's arterial PCO_2 may rise somewhat with judicious use of supplemental oxygen, in most cases marked respiratory acidosis is avoided. However, an unstable patient with an acute exacerbation of COPD cannot be transported without significant risk unless personnel and facilities are available for in-flight endotracheal intubation and mechanical ventilation. Obviously, such patients are not candidates for elective AE.

In patients requiring mechanical ventilation, several factors need to be considered. Ventilators should be plugged into an external power source if possible to conserve battery power, and sufficient battery reserve should be present to operate the ventilator for 1.5 times the expected flight duration. Expected oxygen utilization should be carefully calculated using the patient's minute ventilation. At least 1.5 times the expected oxygen utilization should be available on board the aircraft.

As gases expand with ascent to altitude in accordance with Boyle's law, air in an endotracheal tube cuff will expand as well—although usually not enough to cause injury to the trachea. Rapid decompression, however, could result in tracheal rupture or obstruction of the distal outlet of the endotracheal tube. Endotracheal cuff pressures may be monitored with the use of a cuffolator pressure monitor. Alternatively, the endotracheal tube cuff can be filled with saline, which will not expand with ascent to altitude. The expansion of gas at altitude also requires that the tidal volume of ventilators be recalibrated at altitude to avoid barotrauma. Patients should be closely monitored with cross-reference to the patient, cardiac monitor, and ventilator. In cases where the patient's respiratory status is unclear, an arterial blood gas may be able to provide guidance. Finally, a high index of suspicion should be maintained for development of a pneumothorax in patients who demonstrate respiratory distress or cardiopulmonary decomposition.

Cardiovascular Conditions

Myocardial Infarction and Unstable Angina

A diseased and recently injured heart has a limited ability to compensate for the additional cardiovascular stresses imposed by AE. One of the greatest threats to a diseased heart is hypoxia. Patients with ischemic heart disease demonstrate decreased oxygen saturation during AE, with a reported oxygen saturation of <90% in approximately 20% of patients [10]. This drop in oxygen saturation increases both myocardial workload and oxygen demand and can result in clinical deterioration of patients with little cardiac reserve.

There are other cardiovascular stresses imposed by AE related to the physiology of flight. These include acceleration during takeoff, which can decrease cardiac output by decreasing venous return, especially if litter patients are transported with their head positioned forward. The low humidity associated with flight may cause mild dehydration, thus increasing cardiac workload. Finally, the stress of flight can result in the increased release of catecholamines and autonomically induced dysrhythmias [11].

Because of the increased risk of complications immediately after a myocardial infarction (MI), historically elective AE is relatively contraindicated until at least 1 week after the acute event.

A study of 196 patients who traveled on commercial aircraft after an MI found that while complications occurred in <5% of patients, the majority of these occurred in patients transported <14 days following the event [12]. Additional time for recovery before elective AE may be indicated based on factors that could predispose the patient to complications in flight. These factors include extensive coronary disease, a difficult postinfarction course, limited cardiovascular reserve, and a substantial need for medications.

In contrast to commercial transport of post-myocardial infarction patients, AE utilizing dedicated air ambulances and experienced medical personnel may be achieved earlier. Essebag and colleagues [13] retrospectively reviewed transport of 109 patients with serious cardiovascular disease by commercial and dedicated air ambulance flights as long as 10 hours duration. Of these patients, 51 who were transported by air ambulance had suffered myocardial infarctions, and one-half of these were complicated (Killip class II, III, or IV). In 16 patients transported >7 days postinfarction, there were no in-flight complications. Five of 35 patients transferred 0–7 days postinfarction suffered complications during AE. Four patients had chest pain and one exhibited arterial desaturation. All patients responded to conventional measures and had no sequelae. These data underscore the importance of experienced teams in successful urgent AE. Although data in the literature is sparse, it is clear that the closer in time to the myocardial infarction, the more likely serious events will occur. AE of patients with MI during the initial phases of their illnesses should be carried out only after careful planning and in the presence of experienced critical-care personnel.

AE of patients with unstable angina should be attempted only when absolutely necessary because of their tenuous medical condition. Castillo and Lyons [14] reported outcome data on 59 patients with unstable angina who underwent transoceanic AE. Unfortunately, in-flight data were only available on 31 of the patients. Of these, six patients had in-flight events (three with chest pain, one each with arterial desaturation, headache, and hypertension). None suffered a myocardial infarction during AE. Of the 31 patients with available in-flight data, there were no reported arrhythmias. It is not clear if this data are applicable to all cases of unstable angina considering the relatively benign outcomes in most of the 59 patients (five with congestive heart failure, two with eventual myocardial infarction, and one death). Patient selection for AE may have been responsible for the generally favorable outcomes reported. Unfortunately, there are no prospective controlled studies published in the literature regarding AE of patients with severe cardiovascular problems.

Several basic principles should be applied when AE is required for patients with severe coronary disease or recent MI. Pulse oximetry should be used to make certain that the patient's oxygen saturation is adequate and stable. Appropriate cardiac drugs must be available, including antiarrhythmic and vasoactive drugs, sedatives, and analgesics. IV access is important for fluid therapy and the administration of cardiac drugs. Cardiac monitoring should be used in any patient at risk of dysrhythmia. Central venous and/or arterial monitoring may be necessary in unstable patients. A cardioversion unit should be readily available. In all cases, the patient should be accompanied by critical-care specialists trained in the treatment of acute complications of coronary artery disease.

Congestive Heart Failure and Cardiogenic Shock

The stresses of flight may significantly worsen the cardiovascular state of a patient with congestive heart failure and thus are historically a relative contraindication to elective AE, especially in class 3 and 4 congestive heart failure. The hypoxia associated with ascent to altitude may worsen the patient's condition by predisposing to tachyarrhythmias and acute myocardial ischemia. Hypoxia also increases right ventricular afterload by an increase in pulmonary arterial pressure. Unfortunately, even a small increase in afterload can result in cardiovascular decompensation and cardiogenic shock in those patients with significant right ventricular failure. Oxygen supplementation to prevent hypoxia and monitoring arterial saturation by pulse oximetry are indicated.

Decreases in preload may also result in cardiac decompensation in these patients. During flight, decreased cabin pressure may predispose to loss of intravascular volume into the interstitial space (i.e., third spacing). Some patients might have inadequate cardiac reserve to compensate for the increased myocardial workload resulting from the compensatory increased heart rate and contractility. The resulting interstitial edema often will manifest clinically as a dry cough, while progression to alveolar edema will appear as pink, frothy sputum.

If urgent AE is required, critical-care specialists prepared to detect and treat deterioration in the patient's condition must be available. A patient with congestive heart failure should be positioned with the head oriented toward the front of the aircraft so that the acceleration during takeoff will not transiently exacerbate the congestive failure. ECMO (venoarterial) may be required prior to AE transport in order to better stabilize a patient's hemodynamic profile during extreme and refractory situations.

Pacemakers

The vibration of flight, in particular in rotary-wing aircraft, may actuate pacemakers with activity-sensing functions and increase the pacemaker rate [15]. This may have significant implications for patients with severe cardiovascular disease as they may be unable to tolerate a prolonged tachycardic rate. The increased rate is easily correctable by placing a magnet over the pacemaker and converting it to a non-inhibited unsynchronized paced rhythm.

Dysrhythmias

The early recognition and treatment of dysrhythmias is essential in the safe aeromedical transport of patients. Dysrhythmias should be treated the same as would be treated at ground level. When at altitude, however, special attention should be given to ensuring the patient is receiving adequate oxygenation and ventilation. Defibrillation and cardioversion can be performed during flight, provided that standard safety precautions are observed to ensure the safety of medical attendants, crew members, and other patients. Although defibrillation has demonstrated no adverse effect upon an aircraft's instruments, navigation, or electrical supply, aircrew members should be notified prior to use of this intervention.

Other Medical Conditions

Anemia

Anemia seriously reduces tolerance to a hypoxic environment. At 100% oxygen saturation, the maximum O_2 concentration for a patient with hemoglobin reduced to 7 g/dL will be only 9.8 ml/dL. To compensate for this decreased oxygen-carrying capacity, cardiac output must increase. If a patient's compensatory mechanisms are compromised, slight reductions in arterial oxygenation may produce hypoxic symptoms. Alternatively, increased cardiac stress in a patient with borderline cardiac reserve may result in angina, MI, or heart failure. Accordingly, severe anemia (<7 mg/dL) is a relative contraindication to AE. At this level, even healthy individuals are at risk.

Patients should be transfused with whole blood or packed red blood cells in order to optimize cellular oxygen delivery. In patients with active coronary artery disease, the transfusion threshold may be higher (HgB >8.5 g/dL). If transfusion is unavailable, either altitude restriction should be imposed to maintain a cabin pressure equal to sea level or sufficient supplemental oxygen should be administered to ensure maximum possible oxygen saturation.

Mild anemia is usually well tolerated by healthy individuals during AE; however, supplemental oxygen may be administered. This is especially important during pregnancy, when most patients have physiological anemia and the stresses imposed by pregnancy make them more likely to become symptomatic (see Chap. 21).

Patients who have or are at risk of cardiac disease are at special risk of hypoxia-related complications with any degree of anemia. If transfusion is not practicable, pulse oximetry and supplemental oxygen to maintain a saturation of >90% are the mainstay of treatment. Patients must be closely monitored for decompensation. Symptoms that do not respond to increased oxygen may require altitude restriction or diversion to the nearest appropriate medical facility.

Gastrointestinal Diseases

The gastrointestinal (GI) tract normally contains some gas that expands during ascent. In healthy individuals, gas expansion is rarely problematic at cabin pressures at or below 8000 ft. equivalent because of the resilience of the intestinal walls and the ability to relieve the increased pressure through belching or flatulence. On occasion, intraluminal gas expansion during flight may cause abdominal discomfort because of tight clothing or restraining devices. Also, gas expansion in the splenic flexure of the colon can cause upper-left quadrant fullness and a pressure radiating to the left side of the chest that can be confused with the pain of cardiac ischemia.

In contrast, patients with GI disorders (e.g., bowel obstruction, ileus, or motility problems) may have significant difficulties during flight. Excessive gas production and the inability for gas to be normally transported through the intestines place patients at risk of significant problems related to gas expansion during flight. In addition to abdominal discomfort and pain, the patient may suffer from nausea, vomiting, shortness of breath, and, in extreme cases, vagal symptoms.

All patients known to have GI disorders should have a nasogastric tube placement prior to flight. During flight, the tube should normally be attached to a low-flow suction device. If suction is not available, an open nasogastric tube may be of some use, whereas a clamped tube will not.

Patients with colostomies may have an increased amount of bowel elimination during flight due to the increased peristaltic motion stimulated by intraluminal gas expansion. All such patients should have their colostomy bag replaced immediately prior to AE, and extra bags should be available. Excess flatus and gas expansion in the bag may require careful release in some cases.

Airsickness

Airsickness occurs in some people as a result of abnormal labyrinthine stimulation from unaccustomed pitching, rolling, yawing, accelerating, and decelerating forces experienced during flight. The result is a predictable sequence of symptoms that progress from lethargy, apathy, and stomach awareness to nausea, pallor, and cold eccrine perspiration and finally to retching and vomiting and total prostration.

Motion sickness can complicate the care of patients and their attendants and on occasion incapacitate an AE crew member. Interventions should be initiated promptly following the onset of early signs and symptoms and include the administration of oxygen, placing the patient in a supine position with restricted head motion and a cross-cabin orientation if possible, cooling of the environment, and the administration of antiemetic medications.

Neurological Disorders

The care of the nontraumatic neurological patient entails the prevention of complications associated with their underlying medical condition. In the case of paralyzed patients, special attention should be paid to ensuring pressure-sensitive areas of the body are protected from injury. Those patients on Stryker frames should be turned on a prescribed basis, usually 2 hours in the supine position and 1 hour in the prone position.

Some patients may have increased intracranial pressure as a result of trauma, cranial surgery, or infection such as bacterial meningitis. For these patients, steps should be taken to prevent factors that are known to increase intracranial pressure further, such as vomiting, hypoxia, and seizure activity.

Patients with a seizure disorder may be at increased risk during AE because hypoxia lowers seizure threshold. For this reason, a therapeutic level of an anticonvulsant medication should be documented prior to flight, and supplemental oxygenation should be provided. The treatment of seizures during flight begins by ensuring that the patient's oxygenation and ventilation are adequate, followed by administration of anticonvulsive medication.

General treatment of the obtunded or comatose patient includes an in-dwelling urinary catheter and IV fluid administration. These patients must be observed closely throughout flight because they are at increased risk of airway compromise and aspiration of gastric contents [16].

Acute Kidney Injury and Renal Failure

Patients with acute kidney injury requiring renal replacement therapies should undergo dialysis immediately prior to all long-distance AE flights. For patients requiring continuous renal replacement therapies (CRRT), this should be continued during AE transport, unless the patient can be safely transitioned to intermittent hemodialysis (IHD) prior to transport. The ability to perform IHD is limited by the presence or absence of hemodynamic stability. During overseas AE the aeromedical crew should be aware of when the next dialysis treatment is required so that arrangements can be made en route if required. Serum electrolytes should be routinely reassessed for patients with acute kidney injury, even if they are not yet dialysis dependent.

Alcoholism

The importance of considering the special need of the alcoholic patient is made clear by the special AE categories used to designate these patients (see Chap. 7, Table 7.2). Alcoholism may be the primary reason for AE or an undiagnosed disease process in a patient being transported for another condition. The major risk in either case is acute alcohol withdrawal, which can be fatal if unrecognized or untreated.

Alcohol withdrawal symptoms develop within 8–24 hours after the reduction of ethanol intake and peaks between 24 and 36 hours. These symptoms range from mild withdrawal characterized by insomnia and irritability to major withdrawal typified by autonomic hyperactivity resulting in tachycardia, fever, diaphoresis, and disorientation.

To minimize the risk of alcohol withdrawal during AE, patients known to be alcoholic should be sufficiently observed prior to flight. Alcohol withdrawal symptoms that present unexpectedly in-flight require the prompt recognition and treatment of symptoms. A high index of suspicion is required in patients who are not known to be alcoholic.

Mild alcohol withdrawal symptoms may be effectively treated with supportive care alone, such as reassurance, personal attention, and general nursing care (Table 19.6). If the symptoms progress, moderate to severe withdrawal should be treated with pharmacological doses of benzodiazepines. Withdrawal symptoms unresponsive to benzodiazepines may benefit from haloperidol. A low-dose dexmedetomidine infusion may also help with symptom management during AE transport. If IV hydration is given with glucose-

Table 19.6 Patient care plan: alcohol withdrawal syndrome

1. Administer medications as appropriate—sedatives to counteract the depressant withdrawal syndrome
2. Thiamine to prevent Wernicke's encephalopathy
3. Vitamin replacement for malnourishment
4. Antacids to reduce potential gastritis symptoms
5. Monitor vital signs
6. Follow patient safety protocols because major brain functions may be impaired
7. Keep environmental stimuli at a low level as excessive stimulation leads to hallucinations and agitation
8. Provide adequate hydration and caloric intake
9. Observe for signs of increasing tremors or confusion indicating impending delirium tremens

containing fluids, these patients should first receive magnesium and thiamine to prevent the precipitation of Wernicke's encephalopathy.

Severe Sepsis

Sepsis is a dysregulated host response to infection that can include severe hemodynamic instability with relentless shock. It may present in a spectrum of signs and symptoms that range from extremely subtle in the early phases of the disease to complete cardiovascular collapse. The constellation of signs and symptoms of sepsis include fever, chills, tachycardia, tachypnea with respiratory alkalosis, and findings of end-organ hypoperfusion. Although fever is common in sepsis, patients may present with hypothermia, especially neonates or elderly patients. With decreased perfusion of tissues in septic shock, severe metabolic acidosis is a common additional complication.

The goal of the treatment of sepsis should be the infection source control prior to the onset of the cascade of cellular, microvascular, and cardiovascular events that lead to severe sepsis with shock. Therefore, treatment is often initiated prior to the specific identification of a causative organism/infection source. Empirical treatment is recommended using broad-spectrum antibiotics chosen to cover the organisms most likely to be responsible for the sepsis. The patient's history of illness or trauma is especially helpful in determining the choice of antibiotics.

Supportive therapy is essential in maintaining adequate oxygenation and hydration. Adequate ventilation with supplemental oxygen will correct hypoxia and its associated symptoms. IV fluid therapy will enhance tissue perfusion and oxygen delivery. In those cases where septic shock does not respond to fluid therapy, treatment with vasoactive pharmacological agents such as dopamine may result in increased cardiac output and improved tissue perfusion.

Monitoring for signs and symptoms attributable to early sepsis is essential in patients who have conditions that are predisposed to this development and subsequent progression to septic shock. Initial evaluation of the patient's oxygenation and tissue perfusion is a priority because the aeromedical environment may predispose a patient to hypoxia and dehydration, compounding the effects of sepsis upon the respiratory and cardiovascular systems. Early intubation and mechanical ventilation may be required in these patients. IV fluid administration is important in maintaining appropriate blood pressure and tissue perfusion. Anemia may be extremely detrimental in patients with sepsis. Although healthy individuals in the aeromedical environment may tolerate mild anemia, septic patients who are anemic are at increased risk and may require transfusion to maintain oxygenation of tissues.

Biologic and Chemical Casualties

Patients contaminated with chemical or biologic agents as a result of occupational exposure or terrorist event may sometimes need AE transportation. External decontamination is the first important consideration and must be performed prior to AE for all patients exposed to chemical or biologic agents. Once patients are decontaminated, the degree of further precautions needed during AE will be determined by the actual or suspected agent involved and the patient's medical condition. To protect medical personnel and other patients, precautions should be used when transporting any patient exposed to chemical or biologic agents, as outlined in Chap. 20 and the excellent review of Withers and Christopher [17].

Both the incubation period prior to symptomatic disease and the time of greatest infectivity vary greatly for different biologic agents. Diseases that are transmissible during the incubation period present the greatest challenge. Because the infected individual cannot be identified on the bases of clinical findings, the chance of secondary infection of other personnel is increased, and preventive measures cannot be applied selectively.

Patients confirmed or suspected to have a highly infectious or contagious disease can be isolated during AE using the Vickers aircraft transport isolator (VATI) (see Chap. 20, Fig. 20.2)—an air transport isolator. A stretcher isolator is a lightweight unit for initial patient retrieval, where the patient is then transferred to the air transport isolator in or near the aircraft. This allows for full nursing capability provided by an isolation team from the US Army Medical Research Institute of Infectious Diseases to care for patients in transit. All air passing in and out of the unit travels through a high-efficiency particulate air filter. If the unit is accidentally punctured, negative pressure within the unit prevents potentially contaminated air from contaminating the cabin air. Gloved sleeves within the unit facilitate care of the patient. A few diseases are considered by the World Health Organization (WHO) to be internationally quarantinable and are thus a contraindication to elective AE. Authorization by both command (if military) and diplomatic authorities must be obtained prior to AE across international borders.

In both the civilian and military spheres, the possibility exists of chemical contamination as a result of either occupational exposure or terrorist activities. Onset of symptoms is usually rapid after exposure to most chemical agents, although symptoms may be delayed for several hours after exposure to some agents. Patients exposed to chemical agents must be thoroughly decontaminated prior to AE. Treatment may be required throughout the AE flight. Medical attendants must be familiar with appropriate therapies for various chemical agent exposures.

References

1. Department of the Army. Medical evacuation in a theater of operations: tactics, techniques, and procedures. Washington, DC: US Government Printing Office; 1991. FM 8-10-6
2. Valenzuela TD, Criss EA, Copass MK, Luna GK, Rice CL. Critical care air transportation of the severely injured: does long distance transport adversely affect survival? Ann Emerg Med. 1990;19:169–72.
3. Fromm RE, Haiden E, Schlieter P, Cronin LA. Utilization of special services by air transported cardiac patients: an indication of appropriate use. Aviat Space Environ Med. 1992;63:52–5.
4. Henry JN, Krenis LJ, Cutting RT. Hypoxemia during aeromedical evacuation. Surg Gynecol Obstet. 1973;136:49–53.
5. Saltzman AR, Grant BJB, Aquilina AT, Ackerman NB Jr, Land P, Coulter V, Klocke RA. Ventilatory criteria for aeromedical evacuation. Aviat Space Environ Med. 1987;58:958–63.
6. [no authors listed] Transporting critically ill patients. American College of Critical Care Medicine, Society of Critical Care Medicine, and American Association of Critical-Care Nurses. Health Devices. 1993;22:590–1.
7. Lawless N, Tobias S, Mayorga MA. FiO_2 and positive end-expiratory pressure as a compensation for altitude-induced hypoxemia in an acute respiratory distress syndrome model: implications for air transportation of critically ill patients. Crit Care Med. 2001;29:2149–55.
8. Dirnberger D, Fiser R, Harvey C, Lunz D, Bacchetta M, Frenckner B, et al. Extracorporeal Life Support Organization (ELSO) Guidelines for ECMO Transport. May 2015. https://www.elso.org/Portals/0/Files/ELSO%20GUIDELINES%20FOR%20ECMO%20TRANSPORT_May2015.pdf. Accessed 18 July 2018.
9. Ekström M. Clinical usefulness of long-term oxygen therapy in adults. N Engl J Med. 2016;375:1683–4.
10. Bendrick GA, Nicolas DK, Krause BA, Castillo CY. Inflight oxygenation saturation decrements in aeromedical evacuation patients. Aviat Space Environ Med. 1995;66:40–4.
11. Tyson AA Jr, Sundberg DK, Sayers DG, Ober KP, Snow RE. Plasma catecholamine levels in patients transported by helicopter for acute myocardial infarction and unstable angina pectoris. Am J Emerg Med. 1988;6:435–8.
12. Cox GR, Peterson J, Bouchel L, Delmass JJ. Safety of commercial air travel following myocardial infarction. Aviat Space Environ Med. 1996;67:976–82.
13. Essebag V, Lutchmedial S, Churchill-Smith M. Safety of long distance aeromedical transport of the cardiac patient: a retrospective study. Aviat Space Environ Med. 2001;72:182–7.
14. Castillo CY, Lyons TJ. The transoceanic air evacuation of unstable angina patients. Aviat Space Environ Med. 1999;70:103–6.
15. Gordon RS, O' Dell KB, Low RB, Blumen IJ. Activity-sensing permanent internal pacemaker dysfunction during helicopter aeromedical transport. Ann Emerg Med. 1990;19:1260–3.
16. Kalisch BJ. Intrahospital transport of neuro ICU patients. J Neurosci Nurs. 1995;27:69–77.
17. Withers MR, Christopher GW. Aeromedical evacuation of biological warfare casualties: a treatise on infectious diseases on aircraft. Military Med. 2000;165(suppl 3):1–21.

20 Aeromedical Evacuation of Patients with Contagious Infections

Brian T. Garibaldi, Nicholas G. Conger, Mark R. Withers, Steven J. Hatfill, Jose J. Gutierrez-Nunez, and George W. Christopher

Introduction

The operational decision to evacuate patients with communicable diseases or those who are biologic warfare casualties is complicated by many factors, including the etiologic agent involved. Unlike nuclear or chemical casualties, patients with contagious infections may transmit disease after external decontamination. Further, theater medical facilities might be overwhelmed by a mass-casualty disaster after an epidemic or biologic warfare attack, necessitating rapid evacuation.

A comprehensive review of the aeromedical evacuation (AE) of patients with contagious infections would have to contain elements from several diverse disciplines. These would include disaster medicine, air transport medicine, critical care medicine, the ergonomics and aerobiology of aircraft interiors, infection control, international aviation law and diplomacy, and the operational requirements and constraints of the US Air Force (USAF) and other military and civilian services. We have limited the discussion in this chapter to the ecology of aircraft interiors, disease transmis-

B. T. Garibaldi (✉)
Department of Medicine and Physiology, Division of Pulmonary and Critical Care Medicine, Johns Hopkins Biocontainment Unit, Johns Hopkins University School of Medicine, Baltimore, MD, USA
e-mail: bgariba1@jhmi.edu

N. G. Conger
Col, USAF, MC, Wright Patterson Air Force Base, Dayton, OH, USA

Division of Infectious Disease, Department of Internal Medicine, Wright State University School of Medicine, Dayton, OH, USA

M. R. Withers
COL, MC, USA (ret.), Office of Medical Support & Oversight, U.S. Army Research Institute of Environmental Medicine, Natick, MA, USA

S. J. Hatfill
Department of Clinical Research and Leadership, Department of Microbiology, Immunology, and Tropical Medicine, George Washington University Medical School, Washington, DC, USA

J. J. Gutierrez-Nunez
Col, USAF, MC (ret.), University of Puerto Rico School of Medicine, Department of Medicine, San Juan Veterans Administration Medical Center, San Juan, PR, USA

G. W. Christopher
Col, USAF, MC (ret.), Medical Countermeasure Systems, Joint Program Executive Office for Chemical and Biological Defense, Fort Belvoir, VA, USA

W. W. Hurd, W. Beninati (eds.), *Aeromedical Evacuation*,
https://doi.org/10.1007/978-3-030-15903-0_20

sion onboard aircraft, and highlights of the elements of military and civilian AE capabilities for patients with contagious infections or biologic warfare exposures. Unresolved issues will be identified with the goal of stimulating discussion and future research.

Airframe as a Microbial Environment

The engineering parameters of aircraft ventilation and pressurization are well known and tested extensively by aircraft manufacturers. While most studies of aircraft cabin air quality have focused on tobacco by-products and other chemical contaminants, few have addressed the ecology of airborne microbes. The few available studies of the aerobiology of aircraft interiors suggest that the modern aircraft interior is a less likely venue for disease transmission than most public places [1].

The risk of transmitting infections in modern aircraft under normal conditions is probably equal to, or lower than, the risks in other crowded enclosures. This is related to the excellent ventilation systems built into modem aircraft. However, when the ventilation system is not functioning (as is often the case prior to takeoff), the aircraft cabin environment increases the risk for transmission of airborne viruses such as measles and influenza.

Ecology of Aircraft Cabin Air

Air vented into most aircraft cabins is sterilized during pressurization. To maintain an internal cabin atmosphere equivalent to less than 8000 ft. above mean sea level while at altitude, pressurized air is extracted from the main jet engine compressor, where it has been subjected to both high temperature (more than 250 °C) and pressure (450 psi). The air is then cooled by a series of heat exchangers and vented into the cabin [2].

Microbial survival times are also altered by variations in relative humidity [3]. Because air at altitude has low relative humidity (10–15%), the resultant compressed cabin air does also. Low humidity inhibits bacterial growth and stability but increases the survival and infectivity of certain airborne viruses [4]. The influenza virus was found to survive longer in dry air (relative humidity <50%), while poliovirus survived longer in humid air (relative humidity >50%) [5].

Ventilation: Air Distribution Systems and Airflow

The three most important factors that determine the incidence of infections spread by airborne particles in an enclosed space are the susceptibility of those exposed, the duration of exposure, and the concentration of infectious droplets or droplet nuclei. The concentrations of droplets and droplet nuclei increase when the generation rate is high, when the static volume of enclosed air is small, and when fresh air ventilation is low. Ventilation of any enclosed space decreases the concentration of airborne organisms logarithmically, removing approximately two-thirds of the airborne droplets per air exchange [6].

The mechanism by which air is circulated through most large aircraft cabins depends on several factors. When on the ground, fans recirculate cooled or conditioned air throughout the cabin. When the engines are off, ventilation is provided in one of two ways: Either an auxiliary power unit runs the cabin ventilation system or preconditioned air is supplied by connecting a ground air-conditioning unit to an air manifold. In some aircraft, no fresh air is taken in until pressurization is begun at altitude. However, older military transport aircraft (such as the C-130 Hercules) use pressurized air from the engines for ventilation whether on the ground or aloft. At altitude, compressed air enters continually while air is vented overboard via an outflow valve. First-generation jet airliners (e.g., Boeing 707s, Boeing 727s, DC-9s) and most military transports use 100% ambient (fresh) air for cabin supply [7].

The airflow design for most large aircraft is either circumperipheral or longitudinal. For both designs, conditioned air typically enters the cabin at standing head level. With the circumperipheral design, air circulates from aircraft skin to mid-cabin and then down and back to the vents near the skin at floor level on the same side. With the longitudinal design, air circulates from the aircraft skin in the midsection to outflow valves either fore or aft. The outflow valves are sometimes along the hull (two on the Boeing 707: one at the forward edge of the wings and the other near the tail) or elsewhere along the fuselage (below the right cockpit floor in the C-130).

The type and direction of airflow during an AE flight have important implications for airborne spread of infection. In general, the circumperipheral mode is preferable to the longitudinal because it minimizes aircrew exposure to contaminated air. With the longitudinal design, the direction of airflow should be adjusted so that it is aftward by closing the forward outflow valves. In the C-9A Nightingale, cabin airflow is "top to bottom, front to back," and therefore, contagious patients are placed as far aft and as low as possible.

The airflow for the C-141 takes on special importance because of its history as the main strategic AE airframe for the US military. This aircraft also had a longitudinal airflow design, where the air enters both on the flight deck and the aft cargo compartment. Air then flows toward two outflow valves located above the aft pressure bulkhead [8]. Therefore, potentially infectious patients were placed as far aft and as high as possible. The ventilation patterns of the C-17 transport, which may assume some of the strategic AE missions in the future, remain to be characterized [9].

The risk of airborne infection to the flight crew is related to the flight deck airflow design. In many commercial airliners, such as the B-707, the flight crew is somewhat protected by the independent flight deck ventilation system. As noted previously, the C-141 flight crew is protected by the longitudinal system, where the air enters on the flight deck and flows aftward through the cabin. This is in contrast to the C-130, where the flight deck personnel may be at increased risk because all cabin air is drawn to the cockpit, where it is vented out [10].

Commercial airline cabin airflow has two important design features that may reduce respiratory droplet or airborne transmission. First, most cabins feature a flow design that is both circumperipheral and laminar, with air entering overhead, flowing down the sides, and exiting through vents above the floor. Second, they have relatively high air exchange rates, typically ranging from 15 to 20 exchanges per hour. This exceeds both the 12 air exchanges per hour that maintain air quality in modern office buildings and the 12 exchanges per hour recommended by the US Centers for Disease Control and Prevention (CDC) for the hospital isolation rooms of patients with active tuberculosis [11]. Unfortunately, the purging of air within the cabin may not always be uniform because of the laminar flow design. There may be decreased air circulation in fore and aft areas, resulting in stagnant zones; animal studies demonstrate that increased ventilation decreases airborne transmission in confined spaces [12, 13]. It is important to remember that ventilation alone is not sufficient to prevent all transmission of airborne pathogens [14].

High-Efficiency Particulate Air (HEPA) Filtration

Jet engine efficiency is decreased by the extraction of compressor air for delivery to the cabin because this air is not available for additional thrust. To economize, commercial airliners use systems that partially recycle cabin air, rather than continuing to supply 100% fresh air from the engines. The fraction of recirculated air ranges from 24% to 66% [15]. The use of recirculated air may reduce air quality due to the recirculation of aerosolized contaminants. To counter this, most airlines have installed high-efficiency particulate air (HEPA) filters in their recirculation systems. These are 99.7% effective for removing particles of 0.3 μ(mu)m diameter or larger.

Although HEPA filters were originally installed for passenger comfort (e.g., for removing tobacco smoke), they also appear to reduce the risk of transmission of airborne pathogens [16, 17]. The droplet nuclei carrying measles, varicella, and tuberculosis are typically 5 μ(mu)m or less in diameter. A study commissioned by the US Department of Transportation to evaluate the levels of bacteria, fungi, carbon dioxide, ozone, and tobacco products in recirculated airliner cabin air found that microorganism concentrations did not reach levels considered hazardous to health [18].

Microbial Aerosols in Aircraft

In response to concerns generated by lethal viral hemorrhagic fevers, and a possible need to transport patients with these diseases by air, the ventilation and air-conditioning systems on pressurized, long-range transport aircraft were studied to evaluate the aerodynamics of aerosolized microorganisms [19]. The two aircraft evaluated were the Lockheed Martin C-130E Hercules (the aircraft used for most tactical AE) and the Boeing 707–347C. At the time, the aviation engineering knowledge of ventilation and air pressure changes on these aircraft was extensive. The movement of smoke particles was observed, and the dispersion of aerosolized spores of a nonpathogenic organism (*Bacillus subtilis* var. *globigii*) was assayed at multiple cabin sites under various pressure and ventilation conditions. Results of both smoke and spore studies suggested that the optimal location for placing a highly infections patient in the 707 would be the left rear of the cabin. When the aircraft was pressurized and the forward outflow valve was closed, contamination was largely restricted to the rear area, placing the flight crew at minimal risk if they stayed forward.

In view of its airflow design, it was no surprise that there was substantial drift of smoke from the cargo hold of the C-130 into the flight deck [19]. Approximately 3% of the spores released in the aft cabin reached the flight deck, probably enough to transmit infection over a prolonged flight if the organism had been infectious. The relative locations of the bleed valves and outflow valve would make plastic diaphragms impractical. One conclusion of the study was that high-containment isolators would be required to evacuate patients with potentially lethal contagious diseases in a C-130. These isolators would protect the flight crew and medical workers and allow refueling stops without alarming foreign governments, which might otherwise refuse international landing clearances (Fig. 20.1). These types of isolators are still used by non-US military forces for AE transport [20]. The US military and civilian transportation services have adopted a slightly different approach as will be discussed later.

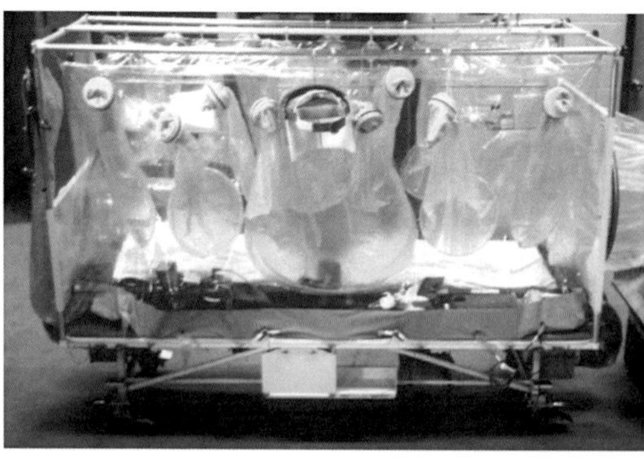

Fig. 20.1 The Vickers aircraft transport isolator (ATI) is designed for prolonged patient transportation and in-flight care. (Reprinted with permission from [59])

A second conclusion of the study was that such patients should only be transported in long-range jet aircraft with the air distribution characteristics similar to those of a Boeing 707. However, significant air contamination occurs within the cabin while these aircraft taxi for takeoff with the recirculation fans functioning. To avoid this, the starboard engines should be operated with the forward outflow valve closed, thus ensuring rapid air exchanges within the cabin. Potentially infectious patients should be boarded through the rear passenger hatch and then placed in the left rear of the cabin facing aft. To protect the flight crew, patients and medical workers should venture no further forward than mid-cabin and flight crew no further aft than that same point.

These concepts were applied, without empiric validation, in 1974, when the aft area in a 707 was used to transport a patient with Lassa fever [21]. A 707 was selected because it was capable of a nonstop flight to Germany, obviating potential difficulties obtaining permission to refuel in a third country. This dedicated AE utilized extensive and unprecedented precautions to transport the patient (a German physician) from Lagos, Nigeria, to Hamburg. The patient was isolated in the rear of the cabin, and a "neutral zone" was created using two polyvinyl chloride partitions. The outflow valves were configured to create a longitudinal pressure gradient in the cabin so that airflow was from the forward to the aft section. Finally, to avoid microbial dissemination via recirculated air, the starboard engines were started to allow pressurization prior to boarding the patient through the aft door. After transporting the patient, the aircraft interior was fumigated with vaporized formalin for 6 hours, and there were no secondary cases.

Between 1987 and 1994, the air was sampled for microorganisms on 36 domestic and international flights, including small and large jet airliners and turboprop commuter aircraft [22]. It was assumed that all microbial contamination originated from passengers and crew because the air taken in from the engines was presumably sterile. It was also assumed that lower levels of microbial air contamination would correlate with a lower risk of disease transmission, although this has not been validated clinically. Control samples were taken at urban locations such as buses, malls, streets, and airports. Microorganisms were quantified by counting colony-forming units (CFUs) after 72 hours incubation, but no attempt was made to identify the organisms.

This study found no significant differences between air at sea level and higher sites nor between coach, business, first-class, or galley sections [22]. The highest counts came from samples taken near outflow vents, about 1 foot above floor level. Interestingly, the microbial air contamination found during flight was significantly lower than that found in cities, buses, and public buildings. Decreased passenger movement (e.g., during sleep) correlated with lower numbers of CFU. The authors concluded that "the small number of microorganisms found in US airliner cabin environments does not contribute to the risk of disease transmission among passengers." [22]

Disinfection of Aircraft

Disinfection of the aircraft is an important element to consider in the AE of infectious disease patients. The World Health Organization (WHO) specifies basic advice on hygiene and sanitation [23] but does not provide details on standard operating procedures (SOPs) or disinfectants to use. In 2014, the Lufthansa group implemented and shared SOPs for the safe decontamination of commercial aircraft, taking into consideration passenger and crew safety, aircraft operability, aircraft instillations, and aircraft certifications. Lufthansa Technik Central Laboratories studied the effects of several alcohol-based, formaldehyde-based, and oxygen-releasing disinfectants on aircraft materials including glass, metal, electric conduits, synthetics, and seat covers to determine the safe application and techniques to be used on their airline fleet [24].

Survey of Infectious Disease Transmission in Aircraft

The risk of transmitting infections in aircraft has probably been exaggerated [25]. Most reports of disease transmission onboard aircraft describe foodborne outbreaks on commercial airliners [26], a discrete area of relevance to AE. The following is a brief summary of the transmission of several common pathogens.

Tuberculosis

Tuberculosis is an obvious concern aboard AE aircraft because it is a common and serious disease usually spread via airborne transmission, especially in confined spaces [27]. Three conclusions about the risk of tuberculosis spread can be drawn from the limited number of published retrospective cohort studies of tuberculosis exposures aboard aircraft. First, the risk of tuberculosis transmission aboard an aircraft is apparently no greater than in other confined spaces, with reported conversion rates of 2–4% [28, 29]. Second, the duration of exposure appears to be important, with several studies reporting no tuberculosis transmission after exposure to an infectious patient after flights less than 9 hours in duration [30, 31]. Finally, the risk of conversion appears much greater for those seated within two rows of an infectious passenger on airlines with a laminar air flow system [32]. Based on this information, the CDC recommended that "those known to be infectious travel by private transportation rather than by commercial aircraft" [28].

The CDC has also suggested three criteria to determine which passengers and flight crew members should be notified of the possibility of tuberculosis exposure [28]. First, the person with tuberculosis was infectious at the time of the flight. Infectiousness can be assumed if the person was symptomatic with acid-fast bacilli (AFB) smear-positive, cavitary pulmonary, or laryngeal tuberculosis or has transmitted the disease to household or other close contacts. Second, the exposure was prolonged (i.e., duration of flight exceeded 8 hours). Finally, passengers and flight crew who were at greatest risk for exposure based on proximity to the infectious passenger should be given priority for notification. Routine tuberculosis screening for airline crew members has not been recommended as an occupational health measure.

Influenza

Air travel has significantly altered the epidemiology of influenza. Since the 1950s, it has become clear that influenza pandemics have followed major air transportation routes. Influenza has also been transmitted during flight. Because of confinement in a closed space associated with flight, these cases most likely constitute common-source, single-exposure outbreaks rather than the usual linear "person-to-person-to-person" epidemics.

Based on published reports, several conclusions can be drawn. First, prolonged ground delays may increase the risk, especially if the air ventilation system is not functioning. In one such report, 72% of the passengers became ill and there was a strong association of the rate of illness with the duration of exposure to the ill passenger [33]. Thus, a second conclusion is that the length of exposure is important. But, in contrast to tuberculosis, even patients exposed for less than 1 hour appear to be at significant risk. Third, the attack rate of influenza aboard a well-ventilated airliner appears to be higher than the general community attack rate during epidemics (10–20%) but less than the rate for boarding schools or nursing homes (>50%) [34].

A major problem with influenza is that individuals do not show signs of infection until several days after they have become infected. During this time, the influenza virus multiplies in the cells lining the upper respiratory tract and sheds into the environment around the infected individual. The infected person may feel slightly unwell but nowhere ill enough to miss work or travel, and they can transmit the virus to others around them. Individuals infected with influenza A virus are usually infectious for at least 1–2 days before the onset of symptoms. After several days of infection, individuals develop fever and the other classical symptoms of influenza, and they remain infectious up to 5–7 days after becoming ill [35]. Infants and immunocompromised individuals can shed influenza virus particles for up to 21 days.

Respiratory protection alone is not fully protective against influenza virus exposure, infection, and severe disease because the human eye is a target for entry of some influenza A virus strains into the human respiratory tract. Both the cornea and the conjunctival epithelial cells contain the sialic acid molecules that serve as the receptors for the H protein of the influenza virus [36]. When the human eye contacts a suspended small-particle influenza virus-laden aerosol from an infected patient's cough or sneeze, surface tension can draw the viral particles to the epithelial cells onto the ocular surface where they adhere. Once adherent, the nasolacrimal drainage system can drain attached viruses from the eye surface through the tear ducts into the nasopharynx within 30 minutes.

Measles

Measles is one of the most contagious infectious diseases, with an attack rate of about 80% among susceptible, casual contacts. Spread by droplet nuclei, virions can survive in the air for several hours. During the early 1980s, more than 500 measles cases per year were either imported to the United States or acquired from imported cases. Most of the imported cases were associated with air travel, and several secondary cases were acquired during flight [37].

An important aspect of measles transmission is that it may occur before the patient becomes symptomatic, a day or two before the end of the incubation period. In one report, eight passengers became infected on a single flight even though no ill or coughing passengers were observed during the flight [38].

Smallpox

During the Intensified Smallpox Eradication Program (1967–1980), concern was extremely high that smallpox would be reintroduced to Europe or the United States from endemic areas by air travel. Consequently, smallpox vaccinations and boosters were recommended for national and international flying personnel [39]. From 1959 to 1973, 27 of the 29 known cases of smallpox imported to Europe were associated with air travel. None were acquired during flight, as all case patients traveled during the incubation period [40]. There is one case of potential infection during air travel, but it is unclear whether transmission occurred in the air or in a terminal [41].

Viral Hemorrhagic Fevers

Viral hemorrhagic fevers (VHFs) are caused by a taxonomically diverse group of RNA viruses and feature a febrile syndrome with severe vascular abnormalities. In general, they are associated with high rates of morbidity and mortality. With the exception of Lassa fever, little is known about their transmissibility during air transport.

Prior to the Ebola outbreak of 2014–2015, much of the attention paid to AE for viral hemorrhagic fevers focused on Lassa fever. The mortality and communicability of Lassa fever had engendered a cautious approach to these patients in the West from both the medical and aeromedical communities. As reported above, an infected patient transported from Lagos to Germany was the sole patient on a C-141, and the patient together with the aeromedical crew were quarantined from the flight crew [22]. Perhaps the most unusual AE in history occurred when a CDC worker with Lassa fever and his wife were transported from Sierra Leone to the United States on a C-141 [42]. For lack of an isolation chamber, they were both sealed for the duration of the flight in an Apollo space capsule that had been flown from a US military warehouse in Germany.

Fortunately, the risk of transmission of Lassa fever, both on the ground and during commercial flight, appears to be low. There have been two reports of inadvertent exposure of large numbers of susceptible individuals to patients with Lassa fever in Western hospitals without evidence of secondary transmission [43, 44]. On at least four occasions, passengers with Lassa fever have traveled on commercial overseas flights without a single secondary case occurring [42–45]. This suggests that the apparently high transmission rate of Lassa fever in West African hospitals may be due to local infection control practices [43, 45].

Based on these reassuring reports, it was suggested that Lassa fever patients could be safely transported by AE using simple barrier infection control techniques [43, 46]. However, the WHO strongly discourages the transport of Lassa fever patients from endemic to non-endemic areas, stating that this should be undertaken only in exceptional circumstances and should be accomplished using special precautions including high-containment isolators [47].

The Ebola outbreak of 2014–2015 provided the largest experience for the AE of patients with viral hemorrhagic fevers. A number of healthcare workers who acquired the infection while caring for patients in West Africa were transported to healthcare facilities in developed countries for treatment. While several of these patients were transported by military services [20], the majority of patients were transported using civilian aircraft that were contracted to provide AE services by government agencies [48]. Phoenix Air, a commercial transport service based in the United States, transported 21 confirmed Ebola patients and 19 high-risk exposures [49]. In all cases, AE providers used special precautions and some form of high-containment isolation system during transport. There were no reported cases of Ebola transmission to the healthcare workers or personnel of these AE flights.

Severe Acute Respiratory Syndrome (SARS)

The international spread of respiratory disease due to the severe acute respiratory syndrome (SARS) coronavirus was accelerated by long-distance travel of symptomatic and incubating patients from Hong Kong to Vietnam, Canada, the United States, and Europe [50]. The risk of transmission during air travel was underscored by a cluster of 22 cases acquired during a flight from Hong Kong to Beijing, traced to a 73-year-old superspreader. However, another flight carrying four symptomatic patients led to only one secondary case, and a flight carrying a patient during incubation resulted in no additional cases [51]. Surveillance of passengers in seven flights carrying symptomatic SARS patients to the United States identified no transmission events [52]. An analysis of SARS transmission during commercial flights carrying symptomatic SARS patients to Singapore disclosed transmission in only one of three flights, for an attack rate of less than 1%. The authors concluded that SARS was less communicable than influenza during air travel [53].

In-Flight Preventive Measures

The most effective method to minimize disease transmission is to defer AE of infectious patients until after the period of communicability. Unfortunately, there are many situations in which infectious patients must be evacuated, and AE planners must be ready to respond.

Early diagnosis of communicable diseases is the key to prevent transmission. Only then can disease-specific, transmission-based precautions be promptly implemented. Attempts are currently underway to develop portable, rapid diagnostic tests, such as enzyme-linked immunosorbent assays and genetic typing, which can be used in the field. In the presence of a biologic warfare threat, patients will be screened for incubating infections (e.g., smallpox) prior to being transported for other indications to minimize the risks of evacuation-related epidemics.

When a casualty is determined to be infectious, the most obvious preventive measure would be to defer AE until after the communicable period. However, such casualties might need evacuation sooner for tactical or other reasons. The use of restricted flights for transportation of cohorts with specific communicable diseases would obviate the risk of patient-to-patient transmission but offer little protection to either the aeromedical or flight crews.

When transporting any infectious patient, standard infection control practices are essential. Additional transmission-based precautions are necessary for certain infections. CDC guidelines mandate the use of surgical masks for diseases transmitted by droplets (e.g., influenza) and fit-tested HEPA-filtered masks for diseases transmitted by droplet nuclei (e.g., tuberculosis) in hospitals. These guidelines have been adapted for use in aircraft [54]. The USAF is currently developing a comprehensive regulation on infection control on aircraft.

Judicious patient placement should be used to minimize the transmission of disease by respiratory droplet or droplet nuclei based on the ventilation characteristics of the specific aircraft. For example, infectious patients are placed as far aft and as *low* as possible in the C-9A but as far aft and as *high* as possible in a C-141 [8]. The ventilation pattern of the C-17 transport remains to be characterized [9].

The C-130 is potentially the most problematic from an infectious disease perspective because cabin air is vented out through the cockpit [10]. In high-risk situations, the flow of cabin air can be reversed aftward by opening the safety valve located in the cargo door [55]. Unfortunately, the aircraft cannot be pressurized in this configuration, necessitating an altitude restriction. As an additional protective measure, the recirculation fan in the cargo compartment can be turned off to prevent recirculation of droplet nuclei.

In a commercial airliner, HEPA filtration confers some level of protection. This may become an important factor in a large conflict, where Boeing 767 passenger aircraft might be used to transport a large number of potentially infectious ambulatory patients. However, this is unlikely to be a major benefit to AE, since the Civil Reserve Air Fleet (CRAF) program, wherein Boeing 767s could be converted into air ambulances, no longer exists (see Chap. 8).

Another possible approach is airflow compartmentalization, where plastic partitions, neutral zones, contaminated zones, and pressure gradients are used in an attempt to minimize cross-contamination [22]. Although this approach might be considered in exceptional cases, no protocols for these measures currently exist for use in US AE aircraft, primarily because they have yet to be proven effective in practice.

High-Containment Isolation Systems

High-containment isolation systems can be used for transporting a limited number of patients with highly contagious, potentially lethal diseases. Unfortunately, these isolators are limited in both number and capability and require specially trained teams of medical personnel. These isolators are necessary for the implementation of the extremely strict CDC infection control guidelines for the care and AE of patients with infections such as arenavirus, filovirus, and bunyavirus hemorrhagic fevers [37, 56–59]. They have been deployed for evacuating patients with suspected or proven VHF and active pulmonary tuberculosis [20, 48, 60, 61]. Although valuable for evacuating limited numbers of patients, they would not be suitable for evacuating mass casualties. A number of isolators are currently available. Table 20.1 compares and contrasts the capabilities of current high-containment isolation systems.

Air Transportable Isolator (ATI)

The air transportable isolator (ATI) is the oldest isolator that is currently in use (Fig. 20.1) [59]. Phillip Trexler developed the first model in 1975 to provide care for patients with severe immunodeficiency based on technology that was used for gnotobiotic animal research [62]. Two years later he developed a negative pressure version of the ATI to isolate patients with high consequence pathogens [63].

The ATI is a transparent polyvinyl chloride envelope suspended on a portable frame (221 cm × 69 cm × 86 cm; weight 112 kg). The envelope incorporates gloved sleeves, "half-suits," and transfer and docking ports for patient ingress and egress and for introducing supplies. Negative air pressure is maintained by an electrical air handling system powered by either the aircraft electrical system or rechargeable portable batteries. HEPA filters are utilized on both the air intakes and exhaust.

Challenge studies demonstrated that the system contained aerosolized bacteriophage during isobaric and hypobaric conditions and could withstand rapid decompression. The isolator can be equipped with portable oxygen tanks, cardiac monitors, pulse oximeters, intravenous fluids and tubing, medications, sphygmomanometers, and defibrillators. To minimize the risk of puncturing the isolator, phlebotomy is minimized, and a needleless intravenous (IV) system can be used. Sharp instruments are avoided.

Communication between patients and caregivers is limited by poor sound transmission through the envelope, noise generated by the air exchange

Table 20.1 Comparison of current high-containment isolation systems

	ATI	ABCS	CBCS	TIS
Max no. of patients	1	1	4	8
Direct patient care	Limited	Yes	Yes	Yes
Aircraft	C-17	Gulfstream G-III	Modified Boeing 767	C-17, C-130

ATI air transportable isolator, *ABCS* aeromedical biological containment system, *CBCS* containerized biocontainment system, *TIS* transportation isolation system

system, and background aircraft noise but can be improved with handheld two-way radios. Physical examinations are difficult to conduct through the gloved sleeves. Suction capabilities are limited, and mechanical ventilation is not feasible.

Contraindications to transport in the Vickers ATI included acute respiratory failure or the presence of gas trapped within closed body cavities that may pressurize at high altitudes (e.g., pneumothorax, ileus, or bowel obstruction) [64, 65].

The US Army Medical Research Institute of Infectious Diseases (USAMRIID) used the ATI as part of its Aeromedical Isolation Team until 2007 [66]. The ATI was used in the AE of two Ebola patients to the United Kingdom by the Royal Air Force (RAF) during the 2014–2015 Ebola outbreak. Prior to the Ebola outbreak, the RAF had maintained three ATIs and had used them on only four occasions. During the outbreak, the RAF increased their capacity to 28 isolators.

Aeromedical Biological Containment System (ABCS)

In 2005, Phoenix Air was asked by the CDC to help develop a transport system for patients with SARS. Manufactured by Production Products in St. Louis, the result was the Aeromedical Biological Containment System (ABCS) (Fig. 20.2). While the ABCS was never used to transport SARS patients, the US Department of State enlisted Phoenix Air to use the ABCS for AE of two US medical personnel who contracted Ebola in West Africa in 2014.

Providers are required to wear personal protective equipment in order to enter the ACBS containment area and provide care. This is in contrast to the ATI, which contains the patient and allows providers external access. The ABCS uses a metal exoskeleton to support an internal plastic liner that creates an airtight isolation chamber. The patient is placed in the chamber, and an anteroom

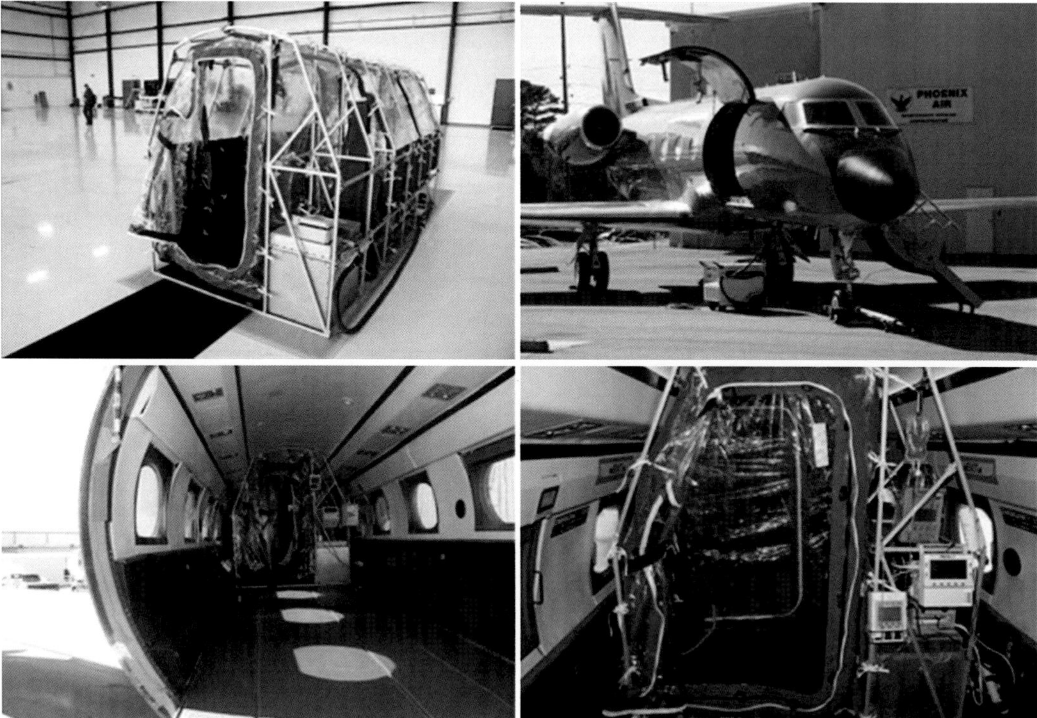

Fig. 20.2 The Aeromedical Biological Containment System (ABCS) was used by Phoenix Air to transport Ebola patients to the United States and Europe during the 2014–2015 outbreak on a modified Gulfstream G-III. (Photos courtesy of Michael Fleuckiger from Phoenix Air)

allows healthcare personnel to don personal protective equipment (PPE) before entering. The chamber is maintained at negative pressure using an air pump, and both the air intake and exhaust are HEPA filtered. Exhaust air is pumped through a valve in the aircraft fuselage. The entire chamber is placed inside a modified Gulfstream G-III aircraft, in which the direction of cabin air has been reversed to flow fore to aft. The ABCS was used for 38 transports during the Ebola outbreak of 2014–2015 [49, 67].

Containerized Biocontainment System (CBCS)

Recognizing that the ABCS is only able to transport one patient at a time, Phoenix Air worked with the Paul G. Allen Foundation, the US Department of State, and MRIGlobal to create the Containerized Biocontainment System (CBCS) (Fig. 20.3). The CBCS is a 44-foot cargo container that can hold up to four patients who all have the same highly infectious disease. The container has a medical staff room, an anteroom, and a patient treatment area. The entire container is maintained under negative pressure, and air intake and exhaust are HEPA filtered. Two containers can fit in a modified Boeing 747 or a military cargo transport [49, 68]. While the CBCS has not been used to transport a confirmed patient, it has been used in three large-scale drills, including the international transport of 11 standardized patients from Sierra Leone to the United States as part of Operation Tranquil Shift in 2017 [69].

Transportation Isolation System (TIS)

In response to the Ebola outbreak, the USAF worked with Production Products to develop

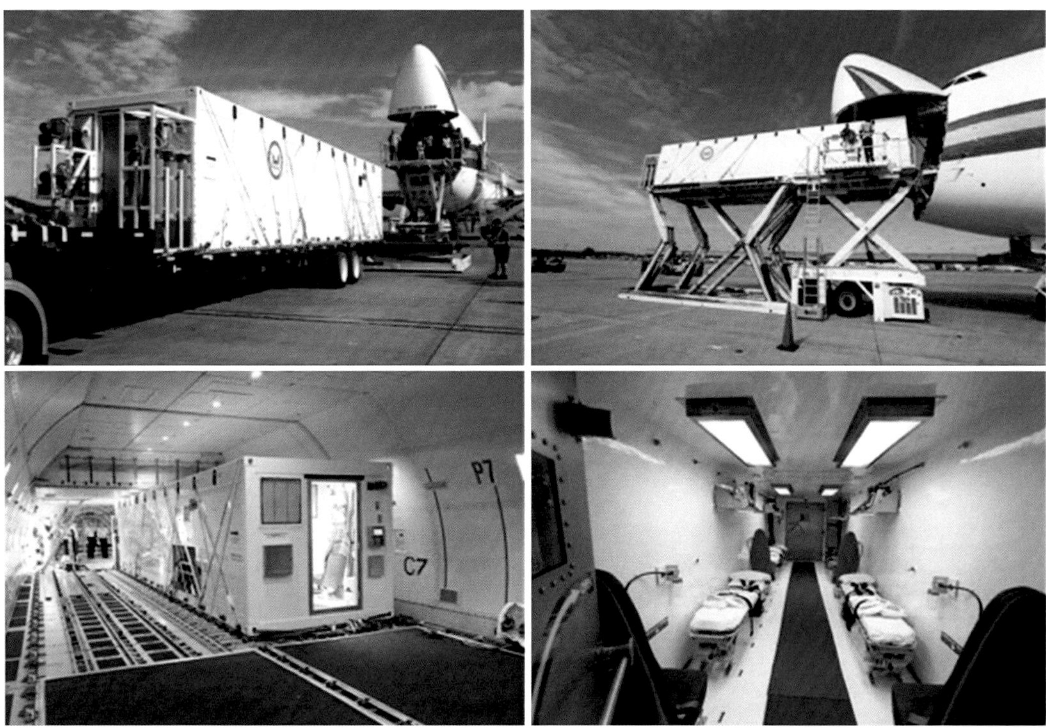

Fig. 20.3 The Containerized Biocontainment System (CBCS) was developed to transport up to four patients with highly infectious diseases on a modified 747 or military cargo plane. (Photos courtesy of Michael Fleuckiger from Phoenix Air)

the Transportation Isolation System (TIS). The TIS is similar in design to the ABCS in that it has an exoskeleton that is draped with plastic sheeting. The TIS is modular and can combine two patient care pods, each with the capacity to hold four patients. The entire unit is under negative pressure and has an anteroom for providers to don PPE. All intake and exhaust air is HEPA filtered. The TIS can be loaded onto a C-17 or C-130 Super Hercules. In total, the Air Force commissioned 25 TIS units during the Ebola outbreak [70]. While it has never been used for confirmed case transport, the TIS has been successfully deployed in several military exercises (Fig. 20.4).

Aircrew Chemical/Biological Protective Systems

Aircrew Eye/Respiratory Protection (AERP) System

The USAF has anticipated the possible future challenge of operating in a chemically contaminated environment by introducing the Aircrew Eye/Respiratory Protection (AERP) system, which is in essence a gasmask for aviators (Fig. 20.5) [71]. Transport aircraft have been equipped with the AERP system, and these could be used to protect aeromedical crew members from infection. The system consists of a mask-

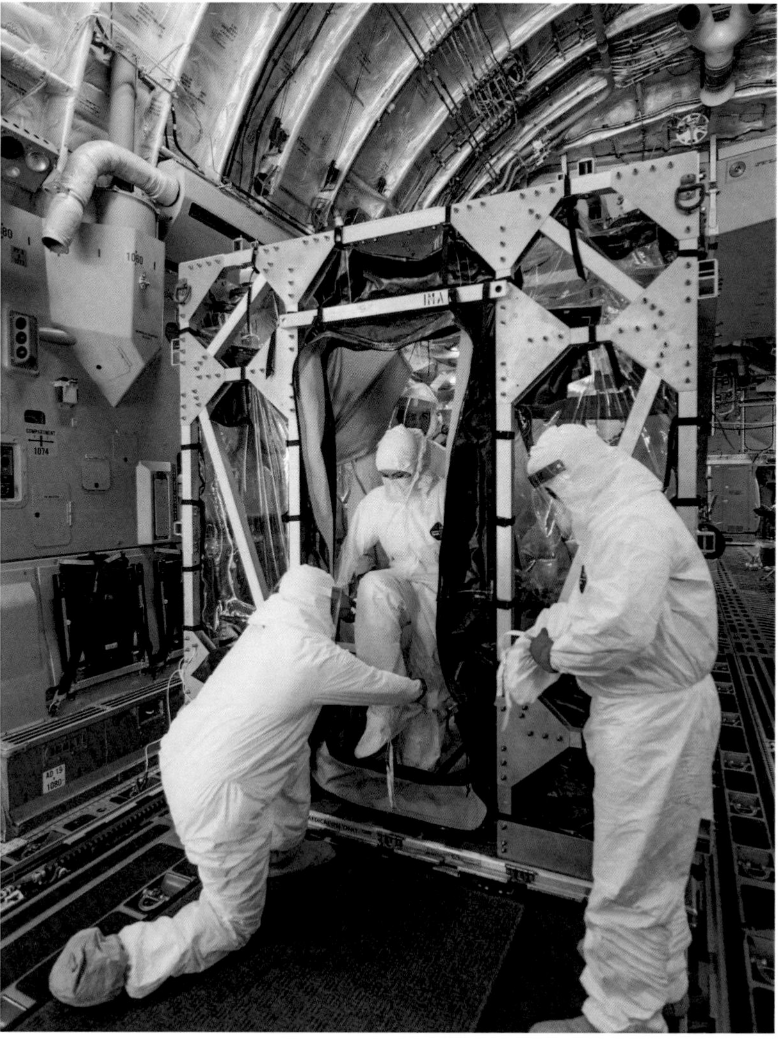

Fig. 20.4 The USAF Transportation Isolation System (TIS) is a modular system that can transport up to eight patients with highly infectious diseases. AE crew members wearing personal protective equipment are exiting the TIS during Exercise Mobility Solace at Joint Base Andrews, Maryland (US Air Force Photo/Airman Megan Munoz)

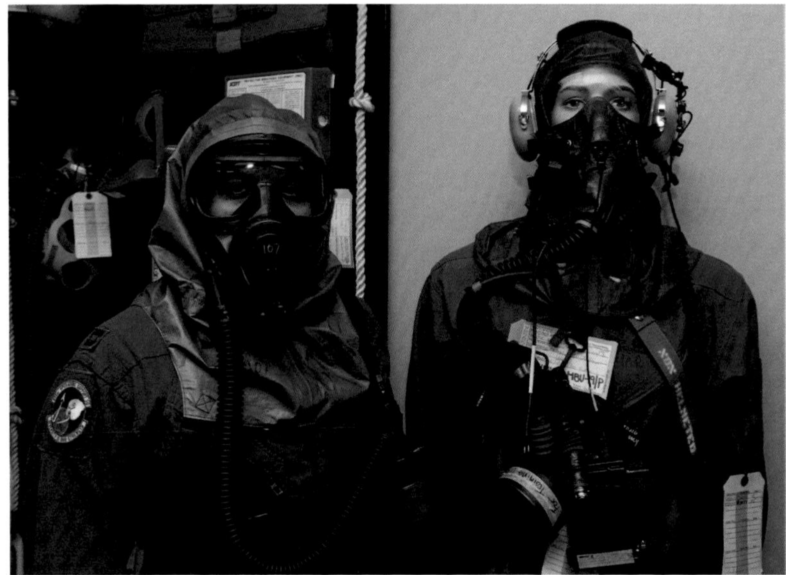

Fig. 20.5 An aircrew member wears the XM69 Aircrew Chemical, Biological, Radiological, and Nuclear (CBRN) Defense system while standing next to a mannequin wearing the legacy US Air Force Aircrew Eye/Respiratory Protection (AERP). (US Air Force photo/Senior Airman Zachary Cacicia)

hood assembly, a blower, and an intercommunication unit. The C-9A, which is no longer in service with the USAF, could be configured to carry eight AERP stations located throughout the aircraft. There are fewer such stations on the C-17, C-130, and C-141 aircraft.

During flight, regulated aircraft oxygen is passed through the filter/manifold subassembly to the mask for breathing, while filtered ambient air is used to provide visor defogging. On the ground, filtered ambient air is used. The AERP blower is powered by the aircraft electrical system or by batteries. The AERP system is available in most aircraft used for military AE, and all aeromedical crew members routinely train for its use during emergencies [72].

Aircrew Chemical, Biological, Radiological, and Nuclear (CBRN) Defense System

The newest USAF chemical biological protective system, the XM69 Aircrew Chemical, Biological, Radiological, and Nuclear (CBRN) Defense system, was developed in conjunction with the Department of Defense [73]. This system is to be utilized by aviators from all four US military branches.

The system is designed to be more comfortable and with decreased acquisition and sustainment costs. It is currently undergoing testing and evaluation to establish reliability and determine maintainability. The goal is to replace all AERPs with the XM69 system for all aircrew members, regardless of the airframe they fly.

US Military Policies for Evacuating Contagious Patients and Biologic Warfare Casualties

Historical Review

Aeromedical evacuation of US service members with contagious diseases has been routinely undertaken since the establishment of a military AE service in 1942. During World War II, C-46 Commandos, C-47 Skytrains, and C-54 Skymasters were reconfigured to carry litters after unloading military cargo, becoming air ambulances on their return flights to the United States [74].

Air transportation was soon determined to be the most desirable method of evacuation for all but the sickest of active tuberculosis patients [75]. Those with large tension cavities or therapeutic pneumothoraces could not be moved by air because intrapleural gas volume would double as these unpressurized aircraft ascended from sea level to 18,000 ft. In most cases, patients were held at hospitals of embarkation until a sufficient number accumulated to fill a dedicated flight of tuberculosis patients. A trained nurse was usually present, and strict "sanitary precautions" and "proper isolation" were practiced. However, the aeromedical personnel were not screened with tuberculosis skin tests [75]. Consequently, the number of new tuberculosis infections occurring during these early air evacuations is unknown.

In 1954, the first aircraft specifically designed and dedicated to routine air medical transport, the C-131A Samaritan, entered service. It could carry specialized medical equipment and was capable of cabin pressurization. In 1961, the Boeing 707 jet was modified by the military to become the C-135 Stratolifter and soon became the mainstay of the first permanent intercontinental airlift system. Meanwhile, the C-130 Hercules began to see use for tactical AE. In 1965, the C-141 Starlifter began to replace the C-135 for strategic (i.e., overseas) AE. This jet aircraft represented a quantum increase in patient load, range, speed, and control of cabin environment.

During the Vietnam War, helicopters moved wounded from the battlefield to medical treatment facilities in rear areas. From there, C-130 Hercules, C-123 Providers, and C-7 Caribous moved them to rear airfields, where C-141 Starlifters embarked on intercontinental routes. AE became so efficient that evacuees were sometimes received in a continental US medical facility within 24 hours of wounding. Large-scale actions in Vietnam in 1968 demonstrated the ability of the AE system to successfully respond to periodic surges of patients.

In 1968, the USAF received its first C-9A Nightingale, a military version of the McDonnell Douglas DC-9 specifically designed and dedicated for AE. New features included a special area for patient isolation and intensive care, a hydraulic ramp to facilitate enplaning of litter patients, integrated electrical and suction outlets, and medical supply and storage equipment cabinets. The C-9A fleet was decommissioned in 2005. The USAF currently conducts aeromedical evacuation by adapting a variety of aircraft including the C-130 and C-17.

The cornerstone of the current infection control program is adherence to the CDC guidelines for infection control. Any infections thought to have been acquired during AE are to be reported to the Air Mobility Command Surgeon's Office, Scott Air Force Base (AFB), Illinois. To date, no cases have been reported.

Biologic Warfare Casualties

Military doctrine regarding all aspects of the medical management of biologic warfare casualties, including AE, is currently under development. Much of the existing joint and USAF doctrine relevant for the AE of nuclear, biologic, and chemical casualties does not clearly differentiate between these three groups. Clearly, there are significant differences among the diseases produced by these three weapons of mass destruction.

The USAF Surgeon General has developed interim guidelines for the AE of biologic warfare casualties. These guidelines are based on rational infection control procedures recommended for the infectious diseases caused by potential agents. Before these interim guidelines can be implemented locally, they must be approved by the appropriate theater commander-in-chief (a nonmedical general officer) and theater surgeon.

A key element of any successful approach to the treatment and transportation of biologic warfare casualties is early and rapid identification of exposure, clinical diagnosis, and laboratory confirmation using field diagnostic tests [76]. To meet this need, the USAF is preparing to deploy multiple specialized teams and has developed a portable device that can quickly identify organisms by genetic typing. It is now projected that these teams will interface with the AE system as integral components of aeromedical staging facilities.

International Legal and Regulatory Aspects

In the 1970s, widely publicized outbreaks of Lassa and Ebola fevers in Africa spurred considerable interest among airline officials and public health authorities. In retrospect, inappropriate and unnecessary measures were instituted at airports in many countries to minimize the risk of disease importation. In commenting upon what he considered a deplorable state of affairs, Michel Perin of Air France's Central Medical Service wrote:

> Most airline companies refuse to admit aboard passengers known, or believed, to have contagious diseases. Such stringency can scarcely be justified by reference to laws or regulations, whether national or international. It introduces the risk of arbitrary, mistaken, or prejudiced conduct. It does not seem logical because airlines learn about only a small fraction of the contagious persons who travel, and public health is much more greatly endangered by unknown infectious persons. Normal hygienic conditions aboard planes usually suppress the risk of contagion of most diseases. The possibility of refusing admission should be given to airlines in certain cases, according to their doctor's appreciation. [77]

Perin suggested that exclusionary rules should be applied "only against someone who refuses to comply, or seems incapable of complying, with the conditions intended to make him harmless, or against someone who has such an infectious disease that it would be impossible to make him harmless to others" [77].

Insight into how the international community reacts to even rumors of highly contagious diseases among airline passengers can be gleaned from events of August and September 1994. An epidemic of plague in the Indian city of Surat resulted in panic and chaos. Many of the inhabitants, including most physicians, evacuated themselves from the city. Panic spread rapidly to commercial air carriers, with all but two international airlines canceling flights to India. Indians deplaning at airports around the world were evaluated for signs of plague, and, in Canada, airport workers donned gloves and masks [78]. Eleven febrile Indian passengers were promptly quarantined when they deplaned in New York City. None had plague, but four were found to have malaria, one had dengue fever, and one had typhoid fever [79].

The most recent experience with Ebola in 2014–2015 further highlighted the potential for panic in response to a highly infectious disease. After the start of the outbreak, several US lawmakers called for a complete travel ban on individuals from Liberia, Sierra Leone, and Guinea, despite the fact that such a ban would be extremely difficult to enforce and would have had a negative economic impact on those countries in the midst of a crisis [80]. In a somewhat ironic display of paranoia, the Louisiana Department of Health and Hospitals, in conjunction with the Governor's Office for Homeland Security and Emergency Preparedness, banned individuals who had traveled to those West African countries from attending the American Society of Tropical Medicine and Hygiene conference in New Orleans [81].

Ultimately, several countries, including the United States, implemented extensive travel screening protocols at airports to detect patients at risk for Ebola and to monitor them for development of disease once they entered the country [82]. The US restricted entry from Ebola-affected countries to five designated airports [83]. Two individuals developed active Ebola infection after arriving by international flight [83, 84]. A third patient, a nurse who contracted the disease while caring for the first Ebola patient in the United States, traveled by domestic airline before she became symptomatic [85]. There were no reported cases of Ebola transmission on any international or domestic flights. It has been postulated that enhanced travel and border health measures helped to curtail the spread of the outbreak [82]. However, an extensive review by the

Department of Homeland Security Inspector General found several serious deficiencies in the US Ebola screening effort [86].

The WHO International Health Regulations (IHR) (2005) [87] stipulate that the pilot in command of an aircraft is required to inform authorities at destination airports of any health concerns stipulated by "Article 38 Health Part of the Aircraft General Declaration" (unless not required by the destination "State Party") before or at the time of landing. The Declaration requires reporting of passengers or crew who may have a communicable disease, described as a fever (temperature 38 °C/100 °F or greater) associated with one or more of the following signs or symptoms: appearing obviously unwell; persistent coughing; impaired breathing; persistent diarrhea; persistent vomiting; skin rash; bruising or bleeding without previous injury; or confusion of recent onset, as well as cases of illness disembarked during a previous stop, and information on treatments received during the flight.

The IHR also stipulates that:

> The Aircraft shall not be prevented for public health reasons from calling at any point of entry. However, if the point of entry is not equipped for applying health measures, the aircraft may be ordered to proceed at its own risk to the nearest suitable port of entry, unless the aircraft has an operational problem which would jeopardize safety. The aircraft may be restricted to a particular area of the airport with no embarking and disembarking. However, the aircraft shall be permitted to take on, under supervision of the competent authority, fuel, water, food and supplies. [87]

If disembarking is allowed, public health authorities may implement options that range from quarantine, isolation, and treatment, placing suspect persons under health surveillance, to no specific health measures.

US Military Regulations

The US military services have regulations that govern the transport of infected passengers. One of the most relevant of these regulations for the AE of potentially contagious patients is USAF Regulation 161–4, which requires aircraft commanders to request an inspection by a quarantine official when an ill passenger has any of the following symptoms and signs: (1) a temperature of 100 °F (38 °C) or greater accompanied by a rash, lymphadenopathy, or jaundice, or that has persisted for over 48 hours; (2) diarrhea defined as three or more loose stools or a greater than normal amount of loose stool for that person in a 24-hour period; and (3) death due to illness other than physical injuries [88]. The implications of this relatively imprecise and abstruse statement could be considerable. Medical planners must be aware of these regulations because failure to implement their provisions may have international repercussions.

Unanswered Questions

Certain aspects of our current understanding of the AE of contagious patients remain unresolved. We offer the following questions about issues that may warrant future research:

1. Will additional smoke and simulant dispersal studies be done in various current AE aircraft to determine optimal aircraft type and patient configurations for AE of patients with contagious diseases?
2. Would the use of HEPA-filtered recirculated air reduce the risk of disease transmission in USAF aircraft that could potentially be used for tactical or strategic AE?
3. What is the utility of ultraviolet (UV) light in reducing transmission of airborne infections in aircraft?
4. What is the role of methods such as vaporized hydrogen peroxide in decontaminating aircraft after transport of patients with highly infectious diseases?
5. Should the United States pursue international agreements regarding the entry of military aircraft carrying contagious disease patients into other countries under certain conditions?

Acknowledgments The opinions and assertions herein are those of the authors and do not purport to reflect official positions of the Department of the Army, Department of the Air Force, or Department of Defense. The authors would like to thank Michael Flueckiger from Phoenix Air for providing information about biological containment systems.

References

1. Martin TE. Al Jubail–an aeromedical staging facility during the gulf conflict: discussion paper. J R Soc Med. 1992;85(1):32–6.
2. Clayton AJ, O'Connell DC, Gaunt RA, Clarke RE. Study of the microbiological environment within long- and medium-range Canadian Forces aircraft. Aviat Space Environ Med. 1992;47:12.
3. Harper G. The influence of environment on the survival of airborne virus particles in the laboratory. Des archiv fur die virusforschung. 1963;13:64–71.
4. Buckland FE, Tyrrell DAJ. Loss of infectivity on drying various viruses. Nature. 1962;195:2.
5. Hemmes JH, Winkler KC, Kool SM. Virus survival as a seasonal factor in influenza and poliomyelitis. Nature. 1960;188:430–1.
6. Nardell EA. Dodging droplet nuclei: reducing the probability of nosocomial tuberculosis transmission in the aids era. Am Rev Respir Dis. 1990;142(3):501–3.
7. Harding RM. Aviation medicine. 3rd ed. London: BMJ Publishing Group; 1993. p. 120–2.
8. Anonymous. Flight manual, USAF series c-141b aircraft (to tc-141b-t). Washington, DC: US Government Printing Office; 1998.
9. Ewing J. C-17 globemaster iii: Amc's air-lifter of the future. Aerospace Medical Association's 69th Annual Scientific Meeting. Seattle; 1998.
10. Anonymous. Flight manual, USAF series c-130-b, c-130e, and c-130h aircraft (to 1c-130-b-1). Washington, DC: US Government Printing Office; 1996.
11. Jensen PA, Lambert LA, Iademarco MF, Ridzon R. Guidelines for preventing the transmission of mycobacterium tuberculosis in health-care settings, 2005. MMWR. 2005;54(RR-17):1–140.
12. Schulman JL, Kilbourne ED. Airborne transmission of influenza virus infection in mice. Nature. 1962;195(4846):1129–30. https://doi.org/10.1038/1951129a0.
13. Andrews CH, Glover RE. Spread of infection from the respiratory tract of the ferret. I. Transmission of influenza a virus. Br J Exp Pathol. 1941;22:7.
14. Nardell EA, Keegan J, Cheney SA, Etkind SC. Airborne infection: theoretical limits of protection achievable by building ventilation. Am Rev Respir Dis. 1991;144(2):302–6.
15. Harding R. Cabin air quality in aircraft. BMJ. 1994;308(6926):427–8.
16. Driver CR, Valway SE, Morgan W, Onorato IM, Castro KG. Transmission of mycobacterium tuberculosis associated with air travel. JAMA. 1994;272(13):1031–5.
17. Hendley J. Risk of acquiring respiratory tract infections during air travel. JAMA. 1987;258:1.
18. Nagda NGT. Airliner cabin environment: contaminant measurements, health risks, and mitigation options. Washington, DC: US Department of Transportation; 1989.
19. Clayton A. Lassa fever – to air evacuate or not. AGARD-CP. 1975;169:1.
20. Ewington I, Nicol E, Adam M, Cox AT, Green AD. Transferring patients with Ebola by land and air: the british military experience. J R Army Med Corps. 2016;162(3):217.
21. Renemann HH. Transportation by air of a lassa fever patient in 1974. Aeromedical implications of recent experience with communicable disease, agard conference proceedings no 169. Neuilly sur Seine: Advisory Group for Aerospace Research and Development; 1975.
22. Wick RL, Irvine LA. The microbiological composition of airliner cabin air. Aviat Space Environ Med. 1995;66:5.
23. Anonymous. Guide to hygiene and sanitation in aviation. Geneva: World Health Organization; 2009.
24. Klaus J, Gnirs P, Hölterhoff S, Wirtz A, Jeglitza M, Gaber W, et al. Disinfection of aircraft: appropriate disinfectants and standard operating procedures for highly infectious diseases. Bundesgesundheitsblatt Gesundheitsforschung Gesundheitsschutz. 2016;59(12):1544–8.
25. Ritzinger F. Aeromedical review 4-65 disease transmission by aircraft. Brooks AFB, TX: USAF School of Aerospace Medicine; 1965.
26. Tauxe RV, Tormey MP, Mascola L, Hargrett-Bean NT, Blake PA. Salmonellosis outbreak on transatlantic flights; foodborne illness on aircraft: 1947–1984. Am J Epidemiol. 1987;125(1):150–7.
27. Houk VN, Baker JH, Sorensen K, Kent DC. The epidemiology of tuberculosis infection in a closed environment. Arch Environ Health. 1968;16:10.
28. CDC. Exposure of passengers and flight crew to mycobacterium tuberculosis on commercial aircraft, 1992–1995. MMWR. 1995;44:4.
29. Miller MA, Valway S, Onorato IM. Tuberculosis risk after exposure on airplanes. Tuber Lung Dis. 1996;77(5):414–9.
30. McFarland J, Hickman C, Osterholm M, MacDonald K. Exposure to mycobacterium tuberculosis during air travel. Lancet. 1993;342(8863):112–3.
31. Baxter T. Low infectivity of tuberculosis. Lancet. 1993;342(8867):371.
32. Kenyon TA, Valway SE, Ihle WW, Onorato IM, Castro KG. Transmission of multidrug-resistant mycobacte-

rium tuberculosis during a long airplane flight. N Engl J Med. 1996;334(15):933–8.
33. Moser MR, Bender TR, Margolis HS, Noble GR, Kendal AP, Ritter DG. An outbreak of influenza aboard a commercial airliner. Am J Epidemiol. 1979;110(1):1–6.
34. Association APH. In: Chin J, editor. Control of communicable diseases manual. Baltimore: United Book Press; 2000.
35. Carrat F, Vergu E, Ferguson NM, Lemaitre M, Nightmare S, Leach S, Valleron AJ. Time lines of infection and disease in human influenza: a review of volunteer challenge studies. Am J Epidemiol. 2008;167(7):775–85.
36. Belser JA, Lash RR, Garg S, Tumpey TM, Maines TR. The eyes have it: influenza virus infection beyond the respiratory tract. Lancet Infect Dis. 2018;18(7):e220–7.
37. CDC. Management of patients with suspected viral hemorrhagic fever. MMWR. 1988;37:16.
38. Slater P. An outbreak of measles associated with a New York/Tel Aviv flight. Travel Med Int. 1995;13:4.
39. Halgelsten JO, Jessen K. Air-transport, a main cause of smallpox epidemics today. Aerosp Med. 1973;44(7):3.
40. Fenner F, Henderson DA, Arita I, Jezek Z, Ladnyi ID. Smallpox and its eradication. Geneva: World Health Organization; 1988.
41. CDC. Smallpox—stockholm. MMWR. 1963;12:3.
42. Garrett L. The coming plague: newly emerging diseases in a world out of balance. New York: Farrar, Straus and Giroux; 1994.
43. Fisher-Hoch SP, Craven RB, Forthall DN, Scott SM, Price ME, Price FM, et al. Safe intensive-care management of a severe case of Lassa fever with simple barrier nursing techniques. Lancet. 1985;326(8466):1227–9.
44. Cooper CB, Gransden WR, Webster M, King M, O'Mahony M, Young S, et al. A case of Lassa fever: experience at St Thomas's Hospital. BMJ (Clin Res Ed). 1982;285(6347):1003–5.
45. Schlaeffer F, Bar-Lavie Y, Sikuler E, Alkan M, Keynan A. Evidence against high contagiousness of Lassa fever. Trans R Soc Trop Med Hyg. 1988;82(2):311.
46. Hotton JM, Bousquet M, Barry B, Lamour O. Aeromedical evacuation of patients with Lassa fever. Aviat Space Environ Med. 1991;62:909–10.
47. WHO. Viral hemorrhagic fevers: report of the WHO expert committee. WHO Tech Rep Ser. 1985;721:5–126.
48. Esler D. The Ebola business. Business and Commerical Aviation. January 2016. https://aviationweek.com/bca/how-phoenixair-entered-ebola-business.
49. McWhirter C, McKay B. Special Planes Are Lifeline for Ebola Patients. The Wall Street Journal. 2015.
50. Lim MK, Koh D. Sars and occupational health in the air. Occup Environ Med. 2003;60(8):539–40.
51. Olsen SJ, Chang H-L, Cheung TY-Y, Tang AF-Y, Fisk TL, Ooi SP-L, et al. Transmission of the severe acute respiratory syndrome on aircraft. N Engl J Med. 2003;349(25):2416–22.
52. Vogt TM, Guerra MA, Flagg EW, Ksiazek TG, Lowther SA, Arguin PM. Risk of severe acute respiratory syndrome–associated coronavirus transmission aboard commercial aircraft. J Travel Med. 2006;13(5):268–72.
53. Wilder-Smith A, Paton NI, Goh KT. Short communication: low risk of transmission of severe acute respiratory syndrome on airplanes: the Singapore experience. Tropical Med Int Health. 2003;8(11):1035–7.
54. Control CfD. Preventing spread of disease on commercial aircraft: guidance for cabin crew 2017 [cited November 5, 2018]. Available from: https://www.cdc.gov/quarantine/air/managing-sick-travelers/commercial-aircraft/infection-control-cabin-crew.html.
55. Anonymous. Flight manual, USAF series c-130h aircraft (to 1c-130h-1). Washington, DC: US Government Printing Office; 1996.
56. CDC. Update: management of patients with suspected viral hemorrhagic fever-United States. MMWR. 1995;44:5.
57. Hill EE, Mckee KT. Isolation and biocontainment of patients with highly hazardous infectious diseases. J US Army Med Dept. 1991;PB 8-91-1/2:10–4.
58. Wilson KE, Driscoll DM. Mobile high-containment isolation: a unique patient care modality. Am J Infect Control. 1987;15(3):120–4.
59. Christopher GW, Eitzen EM. Air evacuation under high-level biosafety containment: the aeromedical isolation team. Emerg Infect Dis. 1999;5(2):241–6.
60. Clausen LB, Bothwell TH, Isaäcson M, Koornhof HJ, Gear JH, McMurdo J, Payn EM, Miller GB, Sher R. Isolation and handling of patients with dangerous infectious disease. S Afr Med J. 1978;53:6.
61. Clayton A. Containment aircraft transit isolator. Aviat Space Environ Med. 1979;50:6.
62. Trexler PC, Spiers AS, Gaya H. Plastic isolators for treatment of acute leukaemia patients under "germ-free" conditions. BMJ. 1975;4(5996):549–52.
63. Trexler PC, Emond RT, Evans B. Negative-pressure plastic isolator for patients with dangerous infections. BMJ. 1977;2(6086):559–61.
64. Withers MR. Aeromedical evacuation of biological warfare casualties: a treatise on infectious diseases on aircraft. Mil Med. 2000;165(11):21.
65. Hutchinson JG, Gray J, Flewett TH, Emond RT, Evans B, Trexler PC. The safety of the Trexler isolator as judged by some physical and biological criteria: a report of experimental work at two centres. J Hyg. 1978;81(2):311–9.
66. Kortepeter MG, Kwon EH, Hewlett AL, Smith PW, Cieslak TJ. Containment care units for managing patients with highly hazardous infectious diseases: a concept whose time has come. J Infect Dis. 2016;214(suppl 3):S137–41.

67. Esler D. Protection from contagion. Business and Commerical Aviation. January 2016. https://aviationweek.com/bca/protectioncontagion-phoenix-airs-aeromedical-biological-containment-system-gulfstream-iii.
68. Glatter R. The new weapon in the fight against Ebola and other deadly pathogens. Forbes. 2015;13:2015.
69. Morton J. UNMC looks to expand cooperation with pentagon on highly infectious diseases. April 13, 2017.
70. Anonymous. Mobile isolation unit for highly contagious fits air force cargo planes. Stars and Stripes; 2016.; Available from: https://www.stripes.com/news/mobile-isolation-unit-for-highly-contagious-fits-air-force-cargo-planes-1.399701.
71. Anonymous. Human systems center (brooks afb, tex), products and progress. Available from: http://www.brooks.af.mil/hsc/ya/yac/aerp.htm.
72. Anonymous. Flight manual, USAF series c-9a aircraft (to 1c9-a-1). Washington, DC: US Government Printing Office; 1997.
73. Zachary Cacicia. New aircrew masks tested at dover 2016: Available from: http://www.amc.af.mil/News/Article-Display/Article/785873/new-aircrew-masks-tested-at-dover/.
74. Merwin CA. U.S. Air Force patient airlift: from balloons to high-speed jets. J Air Med Transp. 1990;9(1):18–22.
75. Coates J. Internal medicine in world war ii. Vol ii. Infectious diseases. Washington, DC: Office of the Surgeon General, Department of the Army; 1963.
76. Reed K. Draft of united states air force concept of operations (conops) for management of biological warfare casualties (unpublished 2nd draft); 1997.
77. Perin M. Transportation in commercial aircraft of passengers having contagious diseases. Aviat Space Environ Med. 1976;47:5.
78. Wills C. Yellow fever, black goddess: the co-evolution of people and plagues. Reading: Helix Books, Addison-Wesley Publishing Co; 1996.
79. CDC. Detection of notifiable diseases through surveillance for imported plague—New York, September–October 1994. MMWR. 1994;43:3.
80. Dastin J. U.S. Airlines point to additional problems of any Ebola travel ban. Reuters; 2014. Available from: http://www.reuters.com/article/us-health-ebola-usa-airlines/u-s-airlines-point-to-additional-problems-of-any-ebola-travel-ban-idUSKBN0IH2CT20141028.
81. Asgary R, Pavlin JA, Ripp JA, Reithinger R, Polyak CS. Ebola policies that hinder epidemic response by limiting scientific discourse. Am J Trop Med Hyg. 2015;92(2):240–1.
82. Cohen N. Travel and border health measures to prevent the international spread of Ebola. MMWR Suppl. 2016;65(3):11.
83. CDC. Enhanced Ebola screening to start at five U.S. airports and new tracking program for all people entering U.S. from Ebola-affected countries; 2014.
84. Botelho GW, Wilson J. Thomas Eric Duncan: first Ebola death in the U.S.: CNN; 2014. Available from: http://www.cnn.com/2014/10/08/health/thomas-eric-duncan-ebola/index.html.
85. News A. Nurse who contracted Ebola called CDC before flight, official says; 2014.
86. Department of Homeland Security, Office of Inspector General, Report No. OIG-16-18. Ebola response needs better coordination, training and execution; January 6, 2016 [cited November 14, 2018]. Available from: https://www.oig.dhs.gov/assets/Mgmt/2016/OIG-16-18-Jan16.pdf.
87. Anonymous. In: WHO, editor. International health regulations. 3rd ed. Geneva, Switzerland: World Health Organization Press; 2005.
88. USAF. Quarantine regulations of the armed forces. Departments of the navy, army, and the air force. Washington, DC: US Government Printing Office; 1992.

Aeromedical Evacuation of Obstetric and Gynecological Patients

21

William W. Hurd, Jeffrey M. Rothenberg, and Robert E. Rogers

Introduction

Obstetric and gynecological diagnoses remain the most common reasons for hospital admissions in the United States [1]. This is related in part to the fact that childbirth occurs almost exclusively in a hospital setting. In addition, problems related to the female reproductive tract are relatively common in women of all ages, but especially in women of reproductive age. Together, childbirth and hysterectomy account for more than 30% of all inpatient surgical procedures performed annually in the United States [1]. The implications for long-distance civilian aeromedical evacuation (AE) are obvious.

W. W. Hurd (✉)
Col, USAF, MC, SFS (ret.), Chief Medical Officer, American Society for Reproductive Medicine, Professor Emeritus Department of Obstetrics and Gynecology, Duke University Medical Center, Durham, NC, USA

Formerly, CCATT physician and Commander, 445th ASTS, Wright-Patterson Air Force Base, Dayton, OH, USA
e-mail: whurd@asrm.org

J. M. Rothenberg
Obstetrics-Gynecology, St. Vincent Hospitals, Indianapolis, IN, USA

R. E. Rogers (Deceased)
COL, MC, USA (ret.), Department of Obstetrics and Gynecology, Indiana University School of Medicine, Indianapolis, IN, USA

Obstetrics and gynecology has taken on increased importance in military medicine as well. The active-duty military population is now made up of more than 15% women, who are almost exclusively of reproductive age [2]. In addition, the majority of active-duty and retired men have wives who often utilize the military medical care system. This is especially true overseas, where civilian medical care might not be available or adequate. With more than 450,000 active-duty troops and their dependents stationed overseas, large portions of the personnel who utilize overseas the military medical system are female [3]. The AE implications related to the significant number of obstetric and gynecological patients treated in military medical facilities should not be underestimated, and contingency plans should be immediately available.

Even during armed conflict, gynecological considerations remain surprisingly important. Although active-duty dependents are no longer a major consideration, many of the medical problems experienced by women living under field conditions are gynecological in nature. A recent example is the Persian Gulf War. Prior to and during the offensive actions in Kuwait and Iraq, more than 600,000 US military personnel were billeted under field conditions, many for more than 6 months. Women made up 7% of the active-duty personnel in the theater. However, more than 17% of the sick call visits were by women, and more than 25% of these visits were for gynecological problems [4].

W. W. Hurd, W. Beninati (eds.), *Aeromedical Evacuation*,
https://doi.org/10.1007/978-3-030-15903-0_21

One unanticipated result of billeting a large number of men and women together under field conditions for an extended period was inadvertent pregnancy. Because pregnancy is an administrative indication for reassignment outside of the theater of operations, pregnancy became the single most common reason for AE of women during Operations Desert Shield and Desert Storm [5].

This chapter will explore both the obstetric and gynecological implications for AE. Uncomplicated and complicated pregnancies will be examined at all stages, including the first, second, and third trimesters and the postpartum period. Information on emergency delivery is also included. Chronic and acute gynecological conditions and considerations for AE of the postoperative gynecological patient will be discussed.

Obstetric and Gynecological Emergency Equipment

An important consideration for AE of the obstetric and gynecological patient is the availability of equipment specific to these problems. Because many specialized instruments are not routinely available without preplanning, an ob/gyn emergency kit should be made available. This is composed of instruments that are commonly used for both obstetric and gynecological problems. In addition, the kit should include instruments specific to emergency vaginal delivery (Table 21.1).

The kit should include instruments for evaluation and be prepared for vaginal lacerations or vaginal bleeding including speculums, suturing instruments and materials, and scissors. Instruments and equipment specific for delivery of infants include cord clamps, suction bulbs, and towels. A relatively important piece of equipment for an emergency vaginal delivery in a confined area is a bedpan. This is used to elevate the buttocks during emergency delivery, as described later. Various types of gauze and padding are also essential. This includes gauze for packing a vaginal laceration or the vagina in the event of uterine hemorrhage. Obstetric menstrual pads are included for both gynecological vaginal bleeding and normal postpartum bleeding. In addition, specific medication might be required when transporting high-risk pregnant patients (see specific diagnoses later).

Table 21.1 Emergency obstetric and gynecological (ob/gyn) kit

Sterile preassembled ob/gyn kit
Instruments: Vaginal speculum (Graves and Pederson) Needle holder Suture scissors Thumb forceps Large (Russian) Small (Allis) Ring forceps (2) Single-tooth tenaculum Vascular clamps Large (Kelly) hemostat (2) Small (Crile) hemostat (2) Bandage scissors
Cord clamp
Suction bulb
Towels
Gauze, 4 × 42″ (40)
Gauze 2″ tape, 10 ft (for packing)
Sterile gloves
Thermal absorbent blanket and head cover (for newborn infant)
Bedpan (to elevate buttocks)

Obstetric Patients

Uncomplicated Pregnancy

Flight imposes little risk to the healthy pregnant woman or her fetus. Pregnant women have flown millions of hours in commercial aircraft at all stages of gestation without a documented increase in the risk of any pathologic or physiological events associated with pregnancy. The few studies that have been published have not demonstrated an increased risk associated with flying during pregnancy for spontaneous abortion, venous thromboembolism during pregnancy, or premature labor during flight [6, 7]. However, one recent questionnaire study found that excessive flying during pregnancy (an average of seven flight, each >7 h in duration) was associated with preterm delivery at an average of 36 weeks' gestation versus 39 weeks' gestation for controls [6].

This is not to say that there are no medical implications related to flying during pregnancy. Sudden, potentially catastrophic events might occur at any time in pregnancy and are more common near term. The space constraints and the relative isolation from immediate medical care that often occurs during flight must be taken into account both by potential pregnant passengers and the flight crew.

Effects of Altitude

During routine commercial flights, the maximum cabin pressure is equal to an altitude of approximately 8000 ft. This results in a 25% decrease in PO_2 in a healthy pregnant adult breathing ambient air from 80 to 60 mmHg [8]. Fortunately, this drop has no appreciable effect on a healthy pregnant woman or her fetus. However, in pathologic conditions where the fetus might suffer from decreased oxygenation, supplemental oxygen should be given as a matter of course.

Immobilization

Prolonged immobilization is probably the most significant medical consideration for the pregnant patient during a long flight. Pregnant women have increased coagulability for hormonal reasons, leading to an increased risk of venous thrombosis [9]. In late pregnancy, increased intra-abdominal pressure from the pregnancy decreases venous return from the lower extremities, thus increasing the risk of venous thrombosis further. The risk of lower-extremity venous stasis might be increased even further in a sitting position with the knees flexed. However, no study to date has demonstrated an increased risk of venous thromboembolism during long-distance flight for pregnant women [6].

Regardless, it is recommended that women flying late in pregnancy in a seated position should ambulate at frequent intervals throughout the flight in an effort to minimize their risk of venous thromboembolism [10]. However, this is often not always practical in the space-limited environment of military AE aircraft. A semi-recumbent position afforded by reclining the seat back might also help with venous return. Pregnant women at high risk for venous thromboembolism can be treated with low-dose heparin therapy [9].

Effects of Gravitational Forces

Pregnant women might be more susceptible to the effects of increased gravitational force (g-force). During take-off and landing, both commercial and military passengers experience a slight increase in g-forces. For most people, the effects of this slight increase are negligible. However, there is an increased susceptibility to orthostatic hypotension during the second half of pregnancy as a result of increased venous pooling in the lower extremities. This might also explain an apparent increased sensitivity to g-forces in late pregnancy. In one report, pregnant women transported by military AE after 34 weeks experienced "dizziness and shadowing of vision" during descent that responded to supplemental oxygen [10].

Onset of Labor During Flight

A potential concern in late pregnancy is the onset of labor or any one of the normal or pathologic processes associated with labor during a prolonged flight. Each year, the sudden onset of labor, rupture of the amniotic membranes, or bleeding in pregnancy during flight requires emergency diversion of commercial airlines [10]. Because of the significant implications of this, the International Air Transport Association has recommended that pregnant women should not fly on commercial aircraft after the 36th week of pregnancy (the 35th week for overseas flights) to minimize the risk of such an event occurring during flight [11]. US Air Force (USAF) regulations recommend against elective air transfer of pregnant women beyond the 34th week of gestation for the same reason [12].

Fortunately, there is usually a matter of hours between the onset of labor and delivery of the infant in most women. At term, labor lasts an average of 8–12 h [9]. However, some women deliver less than 2 h after the onset of painful contractions. For this reason, the onset of obvious labor during a commercial flight is best treated by diversion to the nearest large airport and evaluation of the laboring patient in a hospital setting.

If AE is required during the last month of an uncomplicated pregnancy, the availability of obstetric emergency supplies and an attendant who is trained in emergency vaginal delivery is a reasonable precaution.

A related concern is that the risk of spontaneous ruptured membranes might be increased by the changes in pressure associated with flight. It has long been suspected that subtle changes in atmospheric pressure might increase the risk of spontaneous rupture of membranes [13]. Anecdotal evidence suggests that the rapid increase in pressure associated with landing of commercially pressurized aircraft might increase the risk of membrane rupture near term [11].

Problems During the First Half of Pregnancy

First-Trimester Bleeding: Miscarriages

Bleeding is extremely common during the first trimester of pregnancy, defined as the first 13 weeks after the last menstrual period. During this time, it has been estimated that more than one-third of pregnant women experience some bleeding in early pregnancy. At least 20% of all clinical pregnancies will end in spontaneous abortion, commonly referred to as a "miscarriage."

When a woman has bleeding in the first trimester, consideration should always be given to the possibility that the patient actually has an ectopic pregnancy, discussed in more detail later. The importance of making this diagnosis lies in the fact that minimal external vaginal bleeding can be associated with life-threatening intra-abdominal hemorrhage from an ectopic pregnancy. For this reason, ultrasound should be used to verify that the pregnancy is intrauterine in any patient with first-trimester bleeding [14].

Once an ectopic pregnancy has been excluded, the spontaneous abortion can be further classified according to stage of progression. A "threatened" abortion describes a pregnancy in which any spotting or bleeding is occurring. Fortunately, the first sign of a spontaneous abortion, relatively light bleeding, almost always occurs days to weeks before progression to the heavy bleeding and cramping [14]. Heavy bleeding can occur during the later stages of a spontaneous abortion, which is termed an "inevitable" spontaneous abortion if the cervix is open but no tissue has been passed, or "incomplete abortion" if some, but not all, tissue has been passed vaginally. In some cases, the bleeding can be heavy enough to constitute a medical emergency. The final stage of most spontaneous abortions, termed "complete" abortion, is when all tissue has been passed and is usually associated with minimal residual bleeding. The stage of a spontaneous abortion should be verified by ultrasound prior to AE.

A less common condition, termed a "septic" abortion, is when an intrauterine infection complicates a spontaneous or induced abortion. In the past, septic abortions were the common sequelae of illegal abortions. The implications of a septic abortion for AE are similar to a uterine infection related to other causes and are discussed later. Another uncommon condition is a "missed" abortion, defined as a pregnancy in which the fetus is no longer viable but no bleeding or cramping has occurred. This condition can be treated the same as a threatened abortion for the purposes of AE.

Implications for Aeromedical Evacuation

Significant bleeding in the first trimester of pregnancy is a contraindication to elective AE (Table 21.2). Emergency transportation to the

Table 21.2 Contraindications for aeromedical evacuation (AE) of obstetric and gynecological patients

Obstetric patients
First trimester:
Uterine bleeding (especially with cramping)
Suspected ruptured ectopic pregnancy
Second and third trimesters:
Active labor
Uterine bleeding
Cervix >4 cm dilated
Incompetent cervix, untreated
Severe preeclampsia
Postpartum
Heavy vaginal bleeding
Gynecological patients
Pelvic inflammatory disease with peritonitis
Ruptured tubo-ovarian abscess
Heavy vaginal bleeding

Table 21.3 Criteria for aeromedical evacuation (AE): first-trimester bleeding

Elective AE
No bleeding for 48 h with ultrasound evidence of a viable fetus
After fetal nonviability is verified by ultrasound, perform D&C prior to transport
Convalescent period: 24 h after D&C
Urgent AE
Bleeding < normal menstruation
Minimal or no uterine cramping
No signs of intra-abdominal bleeding (e.g., ectopic pregnancy)
Convalescent period: 12 h after D&C

D&C dilation and curettage

nearest appropriate medical facility is required. Patients with minimal spotting might be moved short distances relatively safely if there is no significant cramping and the cervix is closed (e.g., an early threatened abortion) (Table 21.3). Fortunately, few patients will experience heavy bleeding within the first week after the onset of spotting [14].

During contingency operations (e.g., natural disaster or armed conflict), it might be necessary to move pregnant patients who are experiencing more than minimal spotting by AE. Before AE is considered, several conditions should be met to minimize the chance that a threatened abortion will progress to heavy bleeding. The most valuable tool is ultrasound. In a patient with bleeding, the presence of cardiac activity indicates that the chance of miscarriage is less than 5% and thus heavy bleeding is unlikely. If fetal heart tones are observed by ultrasound and no bleeding has occurred for >48 h, AE is relatively safe. In contrast, the absence of cardiac activity with an intrauterine sac >10 mm in diameter 7 or more weeks from the last menstrual period is associated with an increased risk of miscarriage and heavy bleeding [14].

Regardless of the ultrasound findings, the most important clinical consideration is the amount of bleeding and uterine cramping. If the bleeding is less than a menstrual period and there is minimal or no uterine cramping, then urgent AE is reasonable in a contingency situation. However, if the patient is bleeding more than a normal menstrual period or having significant cramping, she should not undergo AE (Table 21.3). In these emergency situations, medical evacuation (MEDEVAC) to the nearest medical facility for cervical dilation and curettage (D&C) might be lifesaving.

Preparation for Aeromedical Evacuation

If AE is required for a patient with a threatened abortion, certain steps should be taken to minimize the risk to the patient during flight. First, it should be verified that the patient's hemoglobin is >12 g/dL so that she will have an adequate reserve should heavy bleeding occur. If the patient is found to be anemic, transfusion prior to transportation might be needed to increase the margin for safety.

In any pregnant patient who is bleeding, an intravenous (IV) catheter should be placed prior to flight because placing it during flight might be difficult. The amount of bleeding will determine whether the patient will require ongoing IV hydration or only a heparin lock. However, in all cases, the ability to quickly start IV fluids is imperative. In addition, the patient needs an adequate supply of obstetric pads to last throughout the flight or longer, should a delay occur.

Potential In-Flight Emergencies

The vaginal bleeding that can be associated with a spontaneous abortion can be massive, resulting in hypovolemic shock. The first step of in-flight treatment of heavy bleeding is a pelvic examination using the equipment in an ob/gyn emergency kit (Table 21.1). With the patient in a supine "frog leg" position (with heels together), a vaginal speculum and concentrated light source are used to inspect the cervix. If tissue is seen protruding through the cervical os, the tissue should be removed by gentle traction with ring forceps. This might result in completion of the spontaneous abortion process and decrease bleeding. However, if significant bleeding continues, emergency treatment consists of tightly packing the vagina with gauze and diversion of the flight to an airfield near a medical facility.

Another, less common, complication of spontaneous abortion is intrauterine infection, termed septic abortion. If a patient with a diagnosis of spontaneous abortion develops a fever, with or without chills, emergency therapy consists of IV hydration and broad-spectrum antibiotics. In most cases, definitive surgical treatment (D&C) can be delayed for several hours with little risk to the patient.

Ectopic Pregnancy

An ectopic pregnancy, usually located in the fallopian tube rather than the uterus, occurs in approximately 1–2% of all pregnancies. In patients at increased risk of tubal pregnancies because of previous pelvic infection or tubal surgery, the ectopic rate can be as high as 15–25% of pregnancies.

A patient with an ectopic pregnancy most commonly presents with vaginal bleeding and unilateral pain 6–8 weeks after her last menstrual period. However, this presentation is neither specific nor sensitive for ectopic pregnancy. A threatened spontaneous abortion can often present with these symptoms. Alternatively, some patients present with atypical symptoms that can range from painless bleeding to severe abdominal pain with hemorrhagic shock.

With modern ultrasound and serum beta-human chorionic gonadotropin (hCG) determination, the diagnosis of ectopic pregnancy is often made well before tubal rupture and intrauterine hemorrhage. The result is that many ectopic pregnancies might be diagnosed days or weeks prior to the need for definitive surgery. In some patients, the tubal pregnancy resolves spontaneously or can be treated medically and surgery avoided [15].

Implications for Aeromedical Evacuation

A diagnosis of ectopic pregnancy is a contraindication for elective AE. Although the chance of sudden tubal rupture and intra-abdominal hemorrhage is small, the inability to treat this emergency by means other than immediate surgery makes AE relatively risky. Once the ectopic pregnancy has been surgically removed, AE is delayed until the patient has recovered from surgery, as discussed later for the postoperative gynecology patient.

A nonsurgical approach for the treatment of ectopic pregnancies has become more popular in the last few years. This involves the use of methotrexate, a chemotherapeutic agent that destroys placental tissue and results in resorption of the ectopic pregnancy [15]. Although this approach is safe in selected patients, there is an approximately 5% risk of tubal rupture requiring emergency surgery. For this reason, patients being treated nonsurgically for ectopic pregnancy should not be transported by elective AE until their serum beta-hCG levels are undetectable.

In contingency operations, or when definitive treatment is not available locally, it might be necessary to transport patients with an ectopic pregnancy. If required, patients with a diagnosis of an unruptured ectopic pregnancy should be transported at the earliest opportunity.

Preparation for Aeromedical Evacuation

When AE is required, certain criteria should be met prior to transportation. First, the patient should be hemodynamically stable. Second, there should be no evidence of intra-abdominal bleeding such as peritoneal signs or free intraperitoneal fluid on ultrasound. Finally, the patient should have a sufficient hematologic reserve (Hgb > 12 g/dL) in case of rupture during transport. An important point to remember is that a vigorous pelvic exam should be avoided in patients suspected of having an ectopic pregnancy to avoid iatrogenic tubal rupture.

Because sudden rupture is always a possibility, IV access should be established prior to flight. This can be either a functioning IV line or a heparin lock. Transportation as a litter patient is imperative.

In-Flight Emergencies

Sudden rupture of an ectopic pregnancy is uncommon prior to 6 weeks' gestation as determined by the last menstrual period. However, the patient might have already been pregnant at the time of the apparent "last menses," making the gestational age 2–4 weeks greater than calculated using this "menses." For this reason, the onset of severe unilateral pain in a patient with a tentative diagnosis of ectopic pregnancy constitutes a medical emergency, with or without signs of peritoneal irritation and hemodynamic instability.

Emergency in-flight treatments include IV hydration and Trendelenburg position. Transfusion with type-specific packed red cells or whole blood is indicated for signs of hypovolemic shock. Because the only definitive treatment for a ruptured ectopic pregnancy is surgical, any sudden changes in the patient's condition is an indication for emergency flight diversion to an airfield with a nearby medical facility.

Lesser degrees of unilateral pelvic pain are common with an ectopic pregnancy. However, it is difficult to differentiate pain related to tubal distension from catastrophic tubal rupture. For this reason, any change in the nature or degree of pelvic pain in a patient with an ectopic pregnancy should be treated as a likely "ruptured ectopic" and considered life-threatening.

Vaginal bleeding is a common occurrence in patients with ectopic pregnancies. For this reason, several days' supply of menstrual pads should be sent with the patient. Heavy vaginal bleeding with a diagnosis of ectopic pregnancy suggests that the patient might actually be having a spontaneous abortion (see above).

Hyperemesis of Pregnancy

Another common problem encountered in the first trimester is hyperemesis. This excessive nausea and vomiting can lead to dehydration and electrolyte imbalances. Treatment consists of supportive measures including IV hydration with electrolyte replacement and antiemetic therapy. No other special considerations are needed for AE.

Problems During the Second Half of Pregnancy

The incidence of problems is somewhat lower in the second trimester of pregnancy but continues to increase thereafter until term. Because of this, all pregnant women should be thoroughly evaluated prior to any long-distance flight, including AE (Table 21.4). This should include at the very least verification of fetal viability by auscultation of fetal heart activity (by fetoscope, Doppler, or ultrasound) and a pelvic examination to verify that the cervix is closed and accurately estimate the gestational age.

Table 21.4 Criteria for aeromedical evacuation (AE): second and third trimesters

Elective AE
≤34 weeks pregnant
No labor for 48 h
Cervical dilation <4 cm
Amniotic membranes intact
No vaginal bleeding for 7 days
Urgent AE
Premature labor effectively stopped for 24 h
Cervical dilation <4 cm
No vaginal bleeding for 24 h

Incompetent Cervix

Approximately 5% of pregnancies are complicated by painless dilation of the cervix, almost exclusively in the middle third of pregnancy. The treatment for an incompetent cervix is strict bed rest until a suture (cerclage) can be placed around the cervix. These patients are at risk for premature rupture of membranes and premature labor and delivery.

Fetal Demise

Intrauterine fetal demise might occur at any time. During the second or third trimester, the earliest sign of this is usually a cessation of fetal movement noticed by the patient. The diagnosis can be suspected by absence of fetal heart tones by auscultation but is verified by ultrasound. After fetal demise, the patient will usually remain asymptomatic for days to weeks. Some patients will experience bleeding, resulting in a second-trimester spontaneous abortion. Later in pregnancy, premature labor might occur. In extreme cases, the patient can experience a disseminated intravascular coagulation. However, this complication is rare in a patient in whom the fetus has been dead for less than 4 weeks [11].

Premature Labor

The single most common complication of the third trimester is premature labor, which occurs in up to 20% of all pregnancies [9]. Premature labor is defined as painful, regular contractions associated with progressive dilatation before 37 weeks' gestation. In some cases, underlying causes can be determined, such as abruptio placentae (see later) or intrauterine infection. However, the vast majority of cases are idiopathic.

The initial treatment for premature labor is bed rest, IV hydration, and medications to decrease uterine contractility, referred to as tocolytics. Intramuscular steroids are commonly given to accelerate fetal lung maturity. In many cases, prolonged treatment with subcutaneous or oral tocolytics is required to decrease the chance of premature delivery.

Premature Rupture of Membranes

Premature rupture of membranes is another relatively common condition. In general, the fetal membranes rupture during labor as a part of the normal delivery process. However, in approximately 5% of patients, ruptured membranes occur prior to the onset of labor and often prior to term. The latency period is defined as the time interval between the rupture of membranes and the initiation of labor. The length of this period is inversely proportional to the gestational age at the time of rupture. In over half of these patients at term, spontaneous labor begins within 12–48 h. If membranes rupture prior to labor, these patients are at increasing risk of intrauterine infections as the interval between membrane rupture and delivery increases. Care should be taken to avoid unnecessary digital examination of the cervix after rupture of membranes.

Third-Trimester Uterine Bleeding

Bleeding from the uterus in the third trimester is a potentially life-threatening problem for both the fetus and mother. These patients can be divided into two major categories: abruptio placentae and placenta previa.

Abruptio Placenta

The most common serious cause of bleeding in the third trimester is abruptio placentae, which occurs in 1–2% of all deliveries. In this situation, the placenta partially or completely detaches prematurely. The result is vaginal bleeding associated with premature labor. This can also result in massive hemorrhage, which can be fatal to the unborn child and potentially to the mother as well. In extreme cases, this can also be associated with disseminated intravascular coagulopathy. Most often in these cases, there will not be enough time to transport the patient before delivery except by short-distance MEDEVAC to the nearest medical facility.

Placenta Previa

The painless bleeding associated with placenta previa occurs in approximately 1% of all pregnancies [9]. In this condition, the placenta is implanted abnormally low in the uterus, such that it partially or completely covers the cervical opening. As uterine contractile actively becomes more common near term, the risk of bleeding increases. Digital cervical examination is contraindicated because this might incite bleeding. This condition can result in massive hemorrhage that can be fatal for both the mother and fetus.

Pregnancy-Induced Hypertension

Another relatively common complication in the third trimester is pregnancy-induced hypertension, or preeclampsia, which occurs in approximately 5% of all pregnancies [9]. The hypertension of preeclampsia is usually accompanied by proteinuria and edema of the hands and face. This condition puts the fetus at risk for abruptio placentae and intrauterine demise and the mother at risk for grand mal seizures, referred to as eclampsia.

The ultimate treatment is delivery of the fetus. However, if the woman is remote from delivery, the treatment often consists of bed rest for mild cases. More serious cases are treated with IV magnesium sulfate to prevent seizures, antihypertensive medications, and induction of labor, regardless of gestational age.

Implications for Aeromedical Evacuation

Women with the aforementioned complications in the second and third trimesters of pregnancy constitute a group of extremely high-risk patients for AE. Contraindications to AE include untreated incompetent cervix, labor (premature or term) that cannot be stopped with tocolytics, any degree of uterine bleeding, and severe preeclampsia (Table 21.2). If facilities are not available locally to treat these conditions, the patient should be transported to the nearest appropriate medical facility by MEDEVAC.

Patients with intrauterine fetal demise can undergo AE as long as their clotting factors (as reflected by prothrombin time, partial thromboplastin time, fibrinogen, and platelets) are within the normal range. Because intravascular coagulation is uncommon and usually occurs after the fetus has been dead for more than 4 weeks, transportation as soon as possible is advisable [9].

Patients with the remainder of these complications can be transported by AE if their condition can be stabilized. A patient with a history of premature labor can be transported if she has been without uterine contractions for >48 h. The fetal position should be verified to be vertex (head down) because unexpected delivery from a breech position can be dangerous for the infant. Tocolytic therapy should be continued throughout the flight to minimize the risk of recurrent labor. Finally, an individual trained to perform a vaginal delivery and the necessary equipment should accompany the patient.

Patients with premature rupture of membranes are at significant risk for premature labor. If labor has not started within 12 h of rupture, AE might be considered. However, tocolytic therapy should be available in case labor starts during the flight. As with premature labor patients, the fetus should be vertex and both trained personnel and equipment for delivery should be available.

Patients with a diagnosis of placenta previa or chronic abruptio placentae should be free of bleeding for at least 24 h prior to AE and should remain at bed rest throughout transport. Patients with the other conditions listed can be moved by AE but should be accompanied by a physician trained in the management of spontaneous vaginal delivery and obstetric complications that might occur. In most cases, urgent AE should be carried out as soon as practical after the diagnosis and the need for transportation is determined and the patient's medical condition is determined to be stable.

Patients with mild preeclampsia can be transported by AE but should be treated in-flight with anti-seizure medicine as a precautionary measure. The most common of these is magnesium sulfate given as a continuous IV infusion (Table 21.3).

Preparation for Aeromedical Evacuation

Prior to AE, the patient should be ascertained to have (1) cervical dilation <4 cm (by visual inspection only in patients with placenta previa), (2) no bleeding or premature labor for 24 h prior to transportation, and (3) adequate hematologic reserve (Hgb >12 g/dL). All patients should be transported by litter in the left lateral decubitus position and must have a functioning IV line in place. Supplemental oxygen (4 L/min by nasal prongs) should also be routinely administered. Continuous fetal monitoring is not required because all conservative treatments for fetal distress (position, hydration, and oxygen) are already in place and definitive treatment (operative delivery) is not possible in-flight. Patients with mild preeclampsia should be treated with anti-seizure medicine as well.

Potential In-Flight Emergencies

In the third trimester, most in-flight emergencies can be treated only with supportive measures in-flight, whereas definitive treatment will require emergency flight diversion to an airfield near a medical facility with obstetric capabilities. Because emergency delivery is a significant risk for many of these patients, they should be accompanied by medical personnel trained in emergency vaginal delivery and an ob/gyn equipment kit (Table 21.1).

Hemorrhage

Treatment of obstetric hemorrhage during flight is limited to supportive measures, including IV fluids, transfusion of whole blood or packed red blood cells, Trendelenburg and left lateral decubitus position, and supplemental oxygen (4 L/min by nasal prongs). Emergency flight diversion with immediate transfer to a medical facility equipped with an operating room might be lifesaving for the mother and child.

After emergency delivery, postpartum hemorrhage can be a problem in as many as 5% of cases. The treatment of this is discussed later in the section on emergency delivery.

Seizure

Eclampsia is the most common cause of seizure during pregnancy and is usually associated with hypertension and proteinuria, as described previously. Emergency treatment consists of maintaining the maternal airway, controlling convulsions, and lowering the blood pressure if the diastolic blood pressure is >100 mmHg [9].

Seizures are most commonly treated with parenteral magnesium sulfate ($MgSO_4$). An initial bolus of 4 g $MgSO_4$ is given intravenously as a 20% solution at a rate of 1 g/min. Maintenance $MgSO_4$ should be given until delivery, usually at a dose of 2 g/h. The patient must be observed closely for respiratory depression related to $MgSO_4$ toxicity. The treatment is calcium gluconate (Ig intravenously administered slowly), which should always be readily available when $MgSO_4$ is used.

If the patient was diagnosed as having preeclampsia prior to AE, she might be already receiving $MgSO_4$. If she is having a seizure despite $MgSO_4$ therapy, the emergency treatment is IV diazepam (10 mg). Although this is an expedient way to treat seizures, there is a risk of respiratory depression that might require respiratory support. In addition, the infant will show signs of respiratory depression if born within 1 h of this treatment.

Fever

When transporting a patient with premature labor or premature rupture of membranes, the development of an elevated temperature is most likely a sign of intrauterine infection (chorioamnionitis). Another common source of infection is pyelonephritis. The fetal heart rate will almost always be elevated with maternal fever. In all cases of maternal fever, treatment consists of IV antibiotics and acetaminophen as an antipyretic. Aspirin and nonsteroidal anti-inflammatory drugs (NSAIDs) should be avoided in late pregnancy. If the patient is not already on oxygen supplementation, this also should be started (4 L/min by nasal cannula). Transfer to a medical facility within 1–2 h is important.

Labor

Regular, painful contractions can occur in any pregnant patient during flight but is most likely to occur in patients previously diagnosed with premature labor or premature rupture of the membranes. The initial treatment is bed rest in a left lateral recumbent position and IV hydration (lactated Ringer's solution at 175 cc/h). If the patient is being given a tocolytic agent, the dose can be increased. Careful monitoring must be done for signs and symptoms of toxicity. Flight diversion and transfer to an obstetric unit will be required if the labor cannot be stopped. In the absence of placenta previa, cervical examination by someone with obstetric experience can give the crew an estimation of how imminent delivery might be. Should the patient experience the urge to push, preparation for vaginal delivery should be made.

Emergency Vaginal Delivery

In-flight vaginal delivery is fortunately an uncommon event. This might be because women in late pregnancy avoid prolonged flights. In addition, there is normally a matter of hours between the onset of labor and the actual delivery in most patients. However, AE flight crews, especially on long overseas flights, should be familiar with the signs of labor and know how to best assist a woman during delivery should this become necessary.

Signs of Labor

In general, labor is a relatively prolonged course of events that begins with regular painful contractions and/or a spontaneous rupture of membranes and ends with vaginal delivery. Labor is usually a long process, averaging 12 h for the first child and 8 h for subsequent deliveries [9]. However, labor can be unexpectedly quick in some cases, especially with premature labor and women who have had several previous children. Once the patient has an urge to push, delivery usually occurs in less than 2 h and sometimes in a matter of minutes, especially in multiparous women. Because of this, an emergency ob/gyn kit and personnel trained to assist with a vaginal delivery should be available any time a pregnant patient is transported in the late second or third trimester of pregnancy.

Stages of Labor

Labor progresses in a predictable manner divided into three stages. The first stage is the regular painful contractions that result in gradual dilation of the cervix. After an average of 8–10 h, the complete dilation of the cervix is coupled with an often irresistible urge to push. The second stage of labor is the descent of the presenting part through the open cervix and ends with delivery of the infant. This usually takes 1–2 h of active pushing, although it can take less than 10 min in some cases. The third stage of labor is the delivery of the placenta, which can be the most dangerous stage for the mother if hemorrhage occurs.

Vaginal Delivery with a Vertex Presentation

In approximately 96% of all deliveries, the fetus descends through the birth canal with the top of the head proceeding first [9]. This vertex presentation is the simplest and safest mode of delivery. Several steps are involved in assisting a vertex vaginal delivery (Fig. 21.1).

When the perineum begins to bulge, or the presenting part becomes visible, the patient should be placed in an appropriate position for delivery. This is usually in a semi-recumbent position, with the back elevated approximately 45° from horizontal. Adequate lateral room should be made to allow the patient to abduct her thighs such that the angle between her thighs is at or near 90°. In this position, the patient's buttocks must be elevated at the time of delivery to allow for the delivery of the anterior shoulder of the infant (see later). A padded, inverted bedpan under the buttocks works well for this propose.

The delivery process itself involves assisting the patient and minimizing the risk of vaginal and peritoneal trauma. Having the patient grasp her knees or behind her knees and pull backward often assists in delivery. As the vertex is seen bulging from the vaginal opening, general pressure is placed on the head so as to avoid explosive delivery. A gentle, slow delivery will minimize the risk of trauma to the perineum, whereas explosive delivery often results in significant vulvar and vaginal lacerations. The hemorrhage associated with severe vulvar and vaginal lacerations can be life-threatening.

Once the infant's face is within view, the head should be gently turned either facing to the right or left thigh and both mouth and nose suctioned with bulb suction. During this time, the mother can be instructed to try to avoid pushing, although this is often not possible for her to do.

The next step is delivery of the infant's shoulders. As the mother pushes, *gentle* downward traction on the infant's head will aid in delivery of the anterior shoulder. Significant traction should be avoided because this can injure the brachial nerves that extend from the infant's neck vertebrae to the upper arm. The inability to deliver the shoulders (shoulder dystocia) is discussed later. Once the anterior shoulder is delivered, general upward traction will assist in the delivery of the posterior shoulder. The remainder of the infant's delivery proceeds relatively quickly because the largest part is the head and the shoulders.

The umbilical cord is clamped twice and cut between the clamps. The infant is then rubbed briskly and dried to stimulate breathing and minimize loss of core temperature. The infant should be wrapped in a warm blanket. A full-term infant might be left in the mother's arms or on her bare chest, then covered during the remainder of the delivery as long as the infant is breathing without difficulty. If the infant is making inadequate respiratory efforts, neonatal resuscitation might be required.

Delivery of the Placenta

The third stage of labor is delivery of the placenta. After delivery of the infant, the cord protrudes

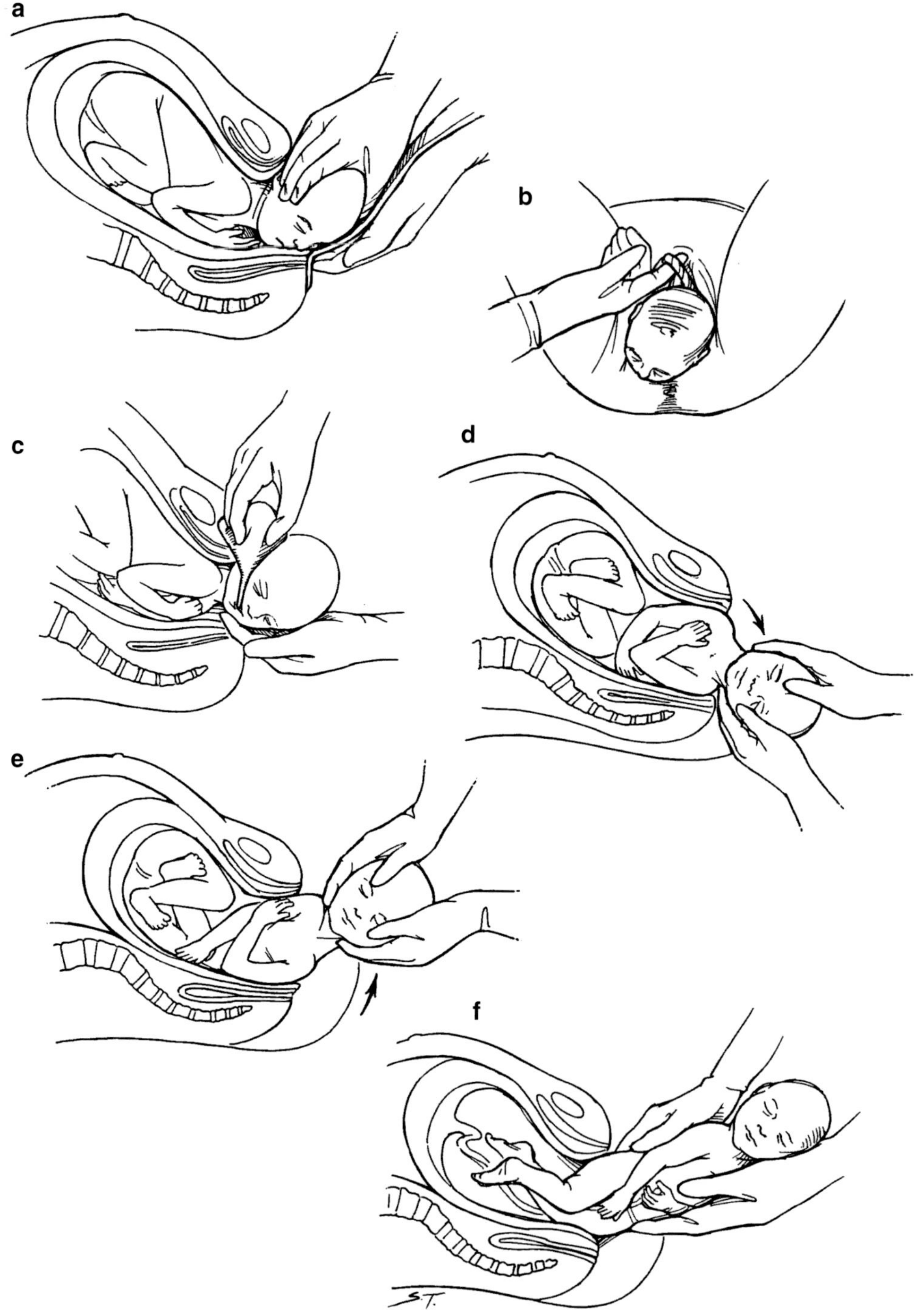

Fig. 21.1 Emergency vaginal delivery, vertex presentation. (**a**) The perineum is supported as the head emerges. (**b**) A nuchal cord is reduced (if present) by lifting it from the posterior neck over the head. (**c**) The mouth and nose are suctioned. (**d**) The anterior shoulder is delivered by maternal pushing and gentle downward traction on the head. (**e**) The posterior shoulder is delivered by continued maternal pushing and gentle upward traction on the head. (**f**) The infant's body is delivered by gentle outward traction

from the vagina. If there is minimal bleeding, the vagina and perineum can be evaluated for lacerations while waiting for the placenta to separate. Usually, placentas will deliver spontaneously within 30 min. If significant vaginal bleeding occurs prior to the placental delivery, gentle downward traction on the umbilical cord and uterine massage might expedite this. Every effort must be made to avoid excessive traction on the umbilical cord, which can result in inversion of the uterus.

Once the placenta is delivered, the uterus should be massaged and the patient administered oxytocin 20 IU/L intravenously at a rate of 200 mL/h until the uterus remains contracted and vaginal bleeding slows. Maternal breastfeeding might also help expedite delivery of the placenta or decrease postpartum bleeding.

Once uterine contracture and hemostasis are assured, any resulting vaginal or perineal lacerations should be repaired with suture under local anesthesia. If no other individual trained in this procedure is available, then closure of lacerations that are not actively bleeding can be delayed until transportation to a medical facility. However, if hemorrhage from the lacerations is a significant problem, temporary hemostatic control can usually be achieved by direct pressure. In extreme cases, tight vaginal packing might be required. The risk of hemorrhage from vaginal and cervical lacerations should not be underestimated because they can potentially lead to hemorrhagic shock in untreated cases. The perineum should be routinely examined in the immediate postpartum period to evaluate for excessive blood loss.

Delivery Complications

Breech Presentation

Approximately 4% of infants are delivered from a breech presentation. Ideally, the presentation of the infant should be determined by ultrasound prior to AE. However, in many cases, ultrasound is not available or the infant changes position between the ultrasound and the flight. For this reason, patients at high risk for delivery should be accompanied by a medical attendant who is experienced in assisting in delivery regardless of the presentation. The steps for assisting a vaginal breech delivery are shown in Fig. 21.2.

Other Abnormal Presentations

Rather than a presentation of a head or breech, an arm or a shoulder might present. This situation is often associated with rupture of membranes and is more common prior to term. In a medical facility, this complication is an indication for cesarean delivery. In any other situation, immediate transportation to a medical facility with an obstetrician and surgical capabilities is the only acceptable approach.

Shoulder Dystocia

Difficulty in delivering the shoulders after the head has been delivered occurs in <1% of all vaginal deliveries. If the shoulders do not deliver with the expulsive efforts of the mother coupled with *gentle* downward traction on the head, several simple techniques might assist in this delivery (Fig. 21.3). An extremely effective procedure is McRobert's maneuver. Two assistants help the mother press her thighs back against her abdomen, while continuing to push (Fig. 21.3a). This changes the angle of the pelvis and often results in delivery of the anterior shoulder with gentle downward traction on the infant.

Another effective approach is suprapubic pressure (Fig. 21.3b). An assistant pushes firmly downward with the heel of their hand immediately above the symphysis pubis. This will often push the anterior shoulder beneath the symphysis pubis and allow delivery to proceed.

If a medical attendant experienced in obstetrics is available, cutting a large episiotomy will also aid in delivery of the shoulders. However, because of the risk of hemorrhage and injury to the infant or mother in inexperienced hands, an episiotomy should only be performed by someone with obstetric expertise.

A final procedure, which takes a significant amount of obstetric skill, is delivery of the posterior arm of the infant (Fig. 21.3c, d). This involves reaching into the vagina, finding the posterior arm, which is pinned against the infant's body, and delivering the entire arm. Once the posterior arm and shoulder are delivered, a hand is placed

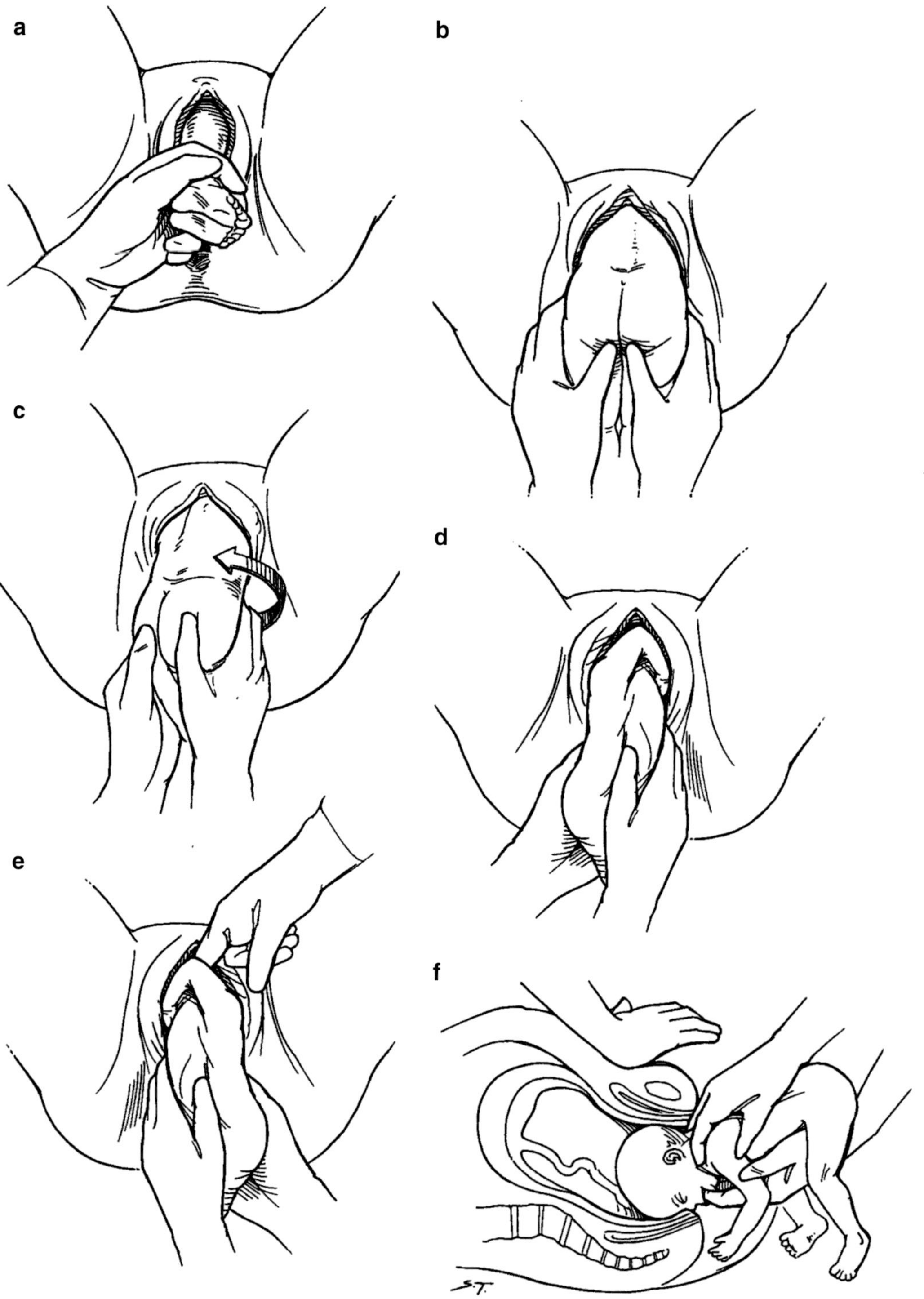

Fig. 21.2 Emergency vaginal delivery, breech presentation. (**a**) The feet are guided out during maternal pushing. (**b**) The infant is delivered to the level of the umbilicus by maternal pushing alone and rotated such that the back is upward. (**c**) The infant is rotated 90° to visualize the left arm (or alternatively the right arm). (**d**) The anterior arm is delivered with a single finger. (**e**) The infant is rotated 180°, and the opposite arm is delivered with a single finger. (**f**) The infant's head is delivered using maternal expulsion and suprapubic pressure. A finger should be placed over the maxillary process and the body kept parallel to the floor

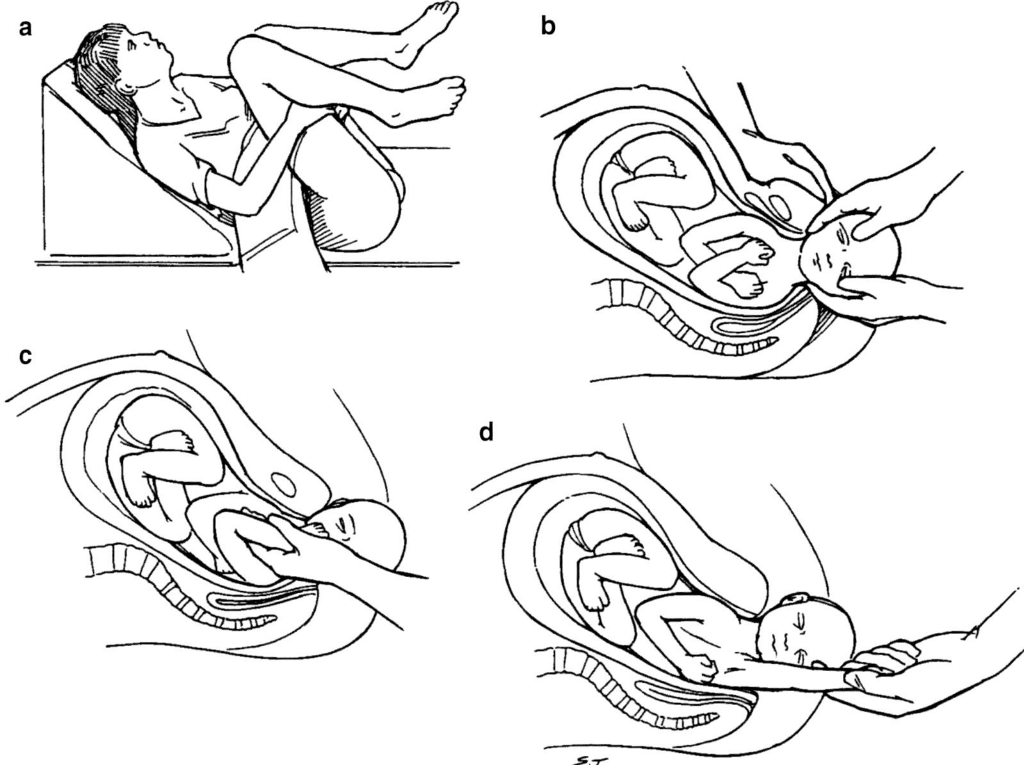

Fig. 21.3 Procedures to deliver the shoulders in a difficult vaginal delivery. (**a**) McRobert's maneuver involves flexing the hips such that the thighs are almost touching the abdomen. (**b**) Suprapubic pressure applied by an assistant may also be helpful. In the most difficult cases (**c**, **d**), the infant is rotated so that the shoulders are near vertical and a hand is reached in posterior to the head. The posterior arm is delivered by sweeping it across the chest and grasping the hand. The infant is then rotated 180° and the process repeated for the opposite arm

on the infant's back and on the abdomen, and the infant is then rotated such that the previously anterior shoulder is now posterior and this arm is likewise delivered. This difficult maneuver might result in significant vaginal lacerations and might fracture the arm of the infant. However, if all other methods for delivering the shoulders have failed, this maneuver can be lifesaving for the infant.

Cord Prolapse

In some patients, spontaneous rupture of the membranes results in prolapse of the cord prior to the delivery of the infant. This is much more common in infants who are not presenting in the vertex (head-down) position. If cord prolapse occurs during the late first stage or early second stage, voluntary maternal pushing by someone who has had children before can result in the delivery of the baby quickly enough to avoid problems. However, if the cervix is not completely open, or if this is the patient's first child, pushing usually takes 1 h or more. The situation can be temporarily mediated by placing a hand in the vagina to keep the presenting part from compressing the cord and cutting off the circulation to the infant. However, unless an emergency cesarean section is carried out in a matter of minutes, prolapse of the cord is usually fatal to the infant.

Postpartum Hemorrhage

Life-threatening hemorrhage immediately after delivery of the infant occurs in approximately 5% of all vaginal deliveries [9]. For this reason, those involved in caring for women who deliver outside of a hospital setting must be familiar with the treatment of postpartum hemorrhage.

Once the infant is delivered, there is usually a period of time when little bleeding occurs prior to delivery of the placenta (see above). As the placenta begins to separate, a significant amount of bleeding often occurs, usually in the range of several hundred milliliters of blood. At this point, the placenta must be delivered so that the uterus can fully contract, because the only way the uterus can achieve hemostasis after delivery is by significant uterine contraction. For this reason, the next step after delivery of the placenta is vigorous transabdominal uterine massage. An experienced operator will often place a hand in the vagina below the uterus to assist in the massage.

The patient should be given intramuscular (IM) or IV oxytocin at this time to expedite uterine contractions. The natural way to release oxytocin is by breast stimulation associated with breastfeeding. A combination of natural or exogenous oxytocin and uterine massage will result in adequate hemostasis in most cases. However, it should be kept in mind that the average blood loss for a vaginal delivery is approximately 500 mL and thus what might appear to a nonobstetrician to be excessive hemorrhage during and immediately after delivery of the placenta is to be expected.

Uterine Inversion

An uncommon but important complication of a normal vaginal delivery is uterine inversion. This is usually a result of too aggressive traction on the umbilical cord. If the placenta is implanted in the top of the uterus (fundus), excess traction on the cord can result in the uterus turning inside out. In this configuration, the uterus can no longer achieve hemostasis by contraction. In this situation, the fundus of the uterus must be pushed back up to return the uterus to its natural configuration. This should be done with the placenta still in place. The final step is vigorous bimanual massage and oxytocin therapy. If replacement of the uterine fundus is not possible, then the patient should be aggressively hydrated as she is transported as quickly as possible to a medical facility.

The Postpartum Patient

The immediate postpartum period is a time of dramatic change in the physiology for both the mother and newborn infant. This is more obvious for the newborn child than for the mother, but these changes have significant implications for AE for both. After either vaginal delivery or cesarean delivery, the patient has to deal with significant physiological changes. After cesarean delivery, the patient must also deal with the expected sequela of major abdominal surgery.

Implications for Aeromedical Evacuation

Elective AE of the postpartum patient and her newborn infant should be delayed for at least 1 week after vaginal delivery. This assures adequate uterine involution, such that postpartum hemorrhage is unlikely to occur. This 1-week recovery time also allows for the complete physiological readjustment and the almost complete healing of any laceration or episiotomy associated with delivery. In addition, most normal newborn infants will also be ready for transportation 1 week after delivery. If either the mother or infant is not ready for transportation, AE should be delayed so that they can be transported together. An exception to this would be if the infant were extremely premature or will require prolonged hospitalization related to another medical condition.

After cesarean delivery, elective AE should be delayed for at least 2 weeks. This is usually more than enough time for the mother to become medically stable from a postpartum perspective, as described previously. However, she needs to recover from major abdominal surgery as well. Prior to elective AE, she should be tolerating a regular diet and be fully ambulatory so that she can travel in a seat rather than a litter. By this time, most women will be able to perform all activities other than heavy lifting.

In a contingency situation, the earliest time the patient should be transported by AE is 24 h after delivery. The mother and child need this period of physiological adjustment immediately after delivery. In addition, postpartum hemorrhage is most likely to occur in the first day after delivery. During this time, many patients will receive IV hydration and a dilute solution of oxytocin until uterine contraction and adequate hemostasis is assured.

Likewise, the newborn infant is carefully observed during the first 24 h for early signs of circulatory or breathing problems. If the infant develops signs of decompensation during AE, this might be difficult to recognize in the flight environment. In addition, expert pediatric care is unlikely to be available.

The mother and newborn infant should be transported together, with rare exception. Thus, if one is taking more time to stabilize after birth, transportation of the other should be delayed. One possible exception would be when the infant has serious medical problems or is extremely premature. If the infant will need to remain hospitalized for weeks to months, the mother might need to be transported separately. If expedient AE of the premature infant is absolutely required, a Critical Care Air Transport Team will need to be involved.

Prerequisites for Aeromedical Evacuation

After either vaginal delivery or cesarean section, the most important requirement for AE is that the patient's postpartum bleeding (lochia) has slowed sufficiently. The bleeding should be <1 obstetric pad per hour with no episodes of "flooding," and the uterus should remain firmly contracted. Continued heavy postpartum bleeding might be due to inadequate uterine contracture, retained intrauterine placenta, or infection, and is a contraindication to AE. Because of the risk of sudden bleeding after delivery, the patient should have adequate hematologic reserve with a Hgb >10 g/mL.

Appropriate wound healing should be assured prior to AE. After a vaginal delivery, any vaginal lacerations or episiotomy should also be healing appropriately. After cesarean delivery, the abdominal incision should be healing normally.

Preparation for Aeromedical Evacuation

The length of time since delivery and any complications the patient had with her pregnancy will dictate preflight preparation. If AE is required in the immediate postpartum period, appropriate pain and nausea medicines should be available. In all cases, the patient should be given a several days' supply of obstetric pads for vaginal bleeding. If the patient developed a uterine infection (endometritis) during or after delivery, continuation of IV antibiotics is usually required until the patient has been afebrile for 4 h. If the patient remains hypertensive after delivery, antihypertensive medication might be required.

All patients, both vaginal delivery and cesarean section, who are transported within 1 week of delivery should be transported in the supine position as litter patients because prolonged sitting might increase the risk of deep-vein thrombosis (DVT). Women who have had cesarean sections will sometimes require continued IV hydration for up to 3 days after delivery until bowel function has returned. Women within 72 h of vaginal delivery should be transported with a heparin lock in place in the event that unexpected hemorrhage should occur.

AE transportation of a newborn infant will take special arrangements. Because a litter is too narrow to accommodate both mother and infant, a separate temperature-controlled incubator will be required (see Chap. 22). The infant will need frequent feedings, and many mothers will be breastfeeding. In general, the most appropriate position for infant feeding by the mother will be in a sitting position. For this reason, the mother will need to be in a stretcher low enough to the deck that she will be able to get up to attend to the infant. She will also need a seat in which to feed or nurse the baby. If the mother is unable to feed and care for the infant, a separate attendant will be required.

Potential In-Flight Complications

Hemorrhage

Postpartum hemorrhage is most likely to occur within 24–72 h after delivery. However, the risk of heavy bleeding decreases with time after delivery but can occur any time within the first month postpartum.

Immediate postpartum bleeding is related to failure of the uterus to adequately contract (i.e., "atony") or less commonly a vaginal laceration.

Should moderate vaginal bleeding continue in the immediate postpartum period, evaluation of the perineum and vagina is important to determine the source. This type of bleeding will usually stop with direct pressure over the bleeding site. If the laceration is higher in the vagina, temporary vaginal packing with laparotomy pads might be effective until definitive treatment can be obtained.

Postpartum bleeding that begins days after delivery may be due to subinvolution of the uterus, which is often associated with subclinical infection and will often respond to antibiotic therapy. Another cause of postpartum hemorrhage is the undiagnosed presence of retained placenta, which usually requires uterine curettage for resolution.

The treatment of postpartum hemorrhage during flight is primarily supportive with IV hydration. If the patient is within 72 h of delivery, lack of uterine contracture might be the cause. In these cases, treatment consists of uterine massage and IV oxytocin (10 U over 2 min) or increasing circulating endogenous oxytocin by breastfeeding. If an obstetrician is available, uterine packing might be attempted. Emergency flight diversion to a facility with obstetric care is required for definitive treatment of postpartum hemorrhage.

Abdominal Pain

Patients might experience severe abdominal pain within the first week after delivery as a result of nonmechanical (paralytic ileus) or mechanical bowel obstruction. Paralytic ileus is usually caused by bowel irritation related to the intra-abdominal blood or infection associated with cesarean delivery. The risk is greatest within the first 48 h of surgery and is uncommon after vaginal delivery. Decreased pressure associated with altitude can result in expansion of trapped gas in the gastrointestinal tract and exacerbate postoperative pain, nausea, and vomiting.

Mild symptoms might be treated with parenteral pain medication and antiemetics. More serious nausea or vomiting is an indication to pass a nasogastric tube. In extreme cases of pain, a decrease in altitude might be helpful.

Postpartum Seizure

Patients who had preeclampsia during pregnancy are at a small risk for a grand mal seizure for the first week after delivery. The risk is highest for the first 24 h after delivery and decreases after this time. For this reason, most patients with a diagnosis of moderate to severe preeclampsia are treated with IV magnesium sulfate for 24 h after delivery. A full 25% of eclamptic seizures occur in the postpartum period, and therefore any woman with a seizure after delivery should be treated as an eclamptic.

The treatment for seizures is IV or IM antiseizure medication. This can be diazepam (10 mg) given every 30 min for a total of 30 mg until the seizures have stopped. Following the cessation of seizure, the treatment is supportive and includes IV hydration, a lateral position to avoid aspiration, oxygen supplementation (4 L/min by nasal prongs), and close observation for signs of respiratory suppression. Should this patient have problems with respiration, temporary bag-mask ventilatory assistance might be required.

Infection

Infection is a relatively common postpartum complication. In most cases, this will follow an infection during pregnancy. However, even in some patients without intrapartum infection, endometritis will manifest within the first 4 weeks after delivery. The primary symptom of endometritis is uterine tenderness with increased vaginal bleeding. A more advanced infection usually presents with fevers, chills, and purulent vaginal discharge.

The primary treatment is IV hydration and oral antipyretics. If antibiotics are available, a broad-spectrum antibiotic can be started intravenously or orally as a first line of therapy until a medical facility can be reached. Flight diversion will rarely be necessary unless the patient appears to be getting septic.

Breast Engorgement

Although engorgement is not truly a medical emergency, this common postpartum problem can be distressing to the patient. Breast engorgement commonly occurs 2 or 3 days after delivery and is usually less dramatic in women who are breastfeeding. However, it can occur both in those patients who choose breastfeeding and those who do not.

The treatment for breastfeeding patients is to increase the frequency of nursing the infant. The treatment for non-breastfeeding patient is exactly the opposite. Breast stimulation should be minimized. Breast binding, by wrapping the upper thorax with an elastic bandage, will decrease engorgement and the discomfort. Engorgement can sometimes be associated with significant temperature elevation. Antipyretics and analgesics will help with both the discomfort and the fever associated with engorgement.

The Gynecological Patient

Chronic Gynecological Conditions

Patients with chronic gynecological conditions might require AE (Table 21.5). These conditions include such diverse conditions such as endometriosis, gynecological malignancies, and intractable menstrual abnormalities. The symptoms vary with the diagnosis. However, the three most common gynecological symptoms these patients might have are vaginal bleeding, nausea, and lower abdominal pain.

Table 21.5 Criteria for aeromedical evacuation (AE): high-risk gynecological conditions

Elective AE
Pelvic infections:
Afebrile for 48 h after cessation of parenteral antibiotics
Abnormal uterine bleeding:
Bleeding etiology has been diagnosed and treated
Bleeding < normal menstrual flow
Postoperative:
1 week after minor surgery or laparoscopy
4 weeks after major surgery
Urgent AE
Pelvic infections:
No evidence of abscess rupture
Abnormal uterine bleeding:
No heavy vaginal bleeding for 12 h
Hgb > 12 g/dL
Postoperative:
12 h after minor surgery or laparoscopy
24 h after major surgery

Implications for Aeromedical Evacuation

The risk of in-flight problems for patients with chronic gynecological conditions is low. Asymptomatic patients might be transported at any time. The risk of symptoms with gynecological malignancies increases over time, so these patients should be transported as soon as possible after the diagnosis is made.

Patients with advanced gynecological malignancies are at risk for vaginal bleeding, anemia, and gastrointestinal symptoms. A supply of gynecological pads should always be available. If the patient has experienced any abnormal vaginal bleeding, preparations should be made for the possibility of vaginal hemorrhage during flight. Significant hemorrhage is treated with IV fluid expansion and flight diversion. In extreme cases, tight packing of the vagina might be required to slow the bleeding until transfer to a medical facility can be arranged.

Patients with significant gastrointestinal symptoms—including nausea, vomiting, and abdominal pain—should be transported with an IV line in place for hydration. Significant vomiting and abdominal distension might require a nasogastric tube.

Finally, abdominal pain might require treatment with parenteral pain medications or antiemetics. The onset of severe colicky abdominal pain at altitude suggests expanding trapped intestinal gas. If the pain does not respond to standard doses of pain medication or gastric intubation, decreasing altitude might help.

Genital Trauma, Including Sexual Assault

Trauma to the external female genitalia can be significant enough to impair functionality for days or weeks. These injuries are most commonly straddle-type injuries where the patient has fallen forcefully on an object such as a beam or crossbar of a bicycle. These types of blunt traumas to the external genitalia might result in nothing more than bruising. However, significant vulvar and vulvovaginal hematomas are possible.

When a patient is found to have significant genital trauma, the possibility of rape should be considered. In these cases, psychological considerations are important because many rape victims might suffer from significant posttraumatic distress. Even with minimal physical trauma, rape victims might have to be evacuated from the theater if they are unable to carry out their military function.

Medical treatment of blunt genital trauma most commonly involves observation with decreased activity until the signs and symptoms resolve. Symptomatic pain relief includes ice packs acutely, followed by heat and oral pain medication.

Lacerations, even those that are relatively superficial, might bleed significantly because this is a relatively vascular area. Direct pressure is usually all that is required to stop the bleeding. In severe cases, vaginal packing might be required. Surgical repair might be required to stop arterial bleeding or to close clean, deep lacerations. Prophylactic antibiotic coverage is recommended because vulvar and vaginal lacerations are prone to infection.

Penetrating peritoneal injuries might involve not only the vagina and external genitalia but also the rectum and bladder. In extreme cases, surgical exploration might be required to rule out injury to the intra-abdominal organs.

Implications for Aeromedical Evacuation

Patients with serious genital injuries should be allowed to recover for 7 days after definitive surgical treatment before elective AE. This will decrease the risk of bleeding or infection developing during the flight and dramatically reduce the amount of pain the patient will experience. In contingency situations, urgent AE might be carried out as soon as 12 h after vulvovaginal surgery if the patient is otherwise medically stable.

As with any condition with a possibility of significant blood loss, the patient should have an adequate hematologic reserve (Hgb >12 g/mL). Patients with significant vulvar edema should be transported by litter with a bladder catheter. In addition to any required antibiotics, the patient should have an adequate supply of menstrual pads.

Psychological support prior to and during AE is especially important in the case of sexual assault. The relatively prolonged periods of isolation and removal from normal psychosocial support inherent in long-distance AE will increase the stress on the patient. Agitated patients might benefit from the short-term use of a sedative or hypnotic during the flight (e.g., zolpidem 10 mg PO).

The mode of AE will depend on the severity of the injury and the length of recovery before AE. If the injury makes prolonged sitting uncomfortable, the patient should be transported by litter. Patients transported in a seated position might require analgesics during flight.

Potential in-flight complications include increased vaginal bleeding and infection. These problems are discussed later under postoperative gynecological care. The sexual assault victim might suffer from a panic attack as part of a posttraumatic stress syndrome. This will usually respond to the acute administration of an anxiolytic (e.g., diazepam 5–10 mg PO, IM, or IV).

Gynecological Pelvic Infections

Pelvic infections, most commonly in the form of pelvic inflammatory disease (PID), are relatively frequent in the reproductive-aged population. The most common presenting symptoms are the triad of pelvic pain, vaginal discharge, and fever. However, PID can have an indolent onset and might be confused with gastroenteritis or appendicitis. Gynecological examination usually reveals a purulent cervical discharge and tenderness of the cervix, uterine fundus, and adnexa. Leukocytosis is common. The differential diagnosis includes appendicitis, ectopic pregnancy, ruptured ovarian cyst, and ovarian torsion.

When a diagnosis of PID is made early in the course of the disease, the patient can be treated as an outpatient with a combination of IM and oral antibiotics (e.g., ceftriaxone 150 mg IM plus doxycycline 100 mg PO bid × 10 days). For more serious cases of PID—indicated by fever, leukocytosis, significant nausea, peritoneal signs, or a pelvic mass—the patient should be treated as an inpatient.

The most serious sequelae of PID are pelvic abscesses, which occur in 5–10% of patients. Pelvic abscesses are suggested by palpable adnexal masses. Once PID has advanced to this stage, effective treatment consists of prolonged bed rest and high-dose antibiotics. Surgical drainage is frequently required. Rupture of a pelvic abscess is a medical emergency that has a presentation similar to a ruptured appendix. Immediate laparotomy is indicated and might be lifesaving.

Implications for Aeromedical Evacuation

A ruptured tubo-ovarian abscess is a contraindication to AE. For this reason, patients with PID and signs of peritoneal irritation—such as rebound tenderness, decreased bowel sounds, shoulder pain, or nausea and vomiting—should not be transported by AE. Although these signs could be the result of PID alone, they might also be the result of a ruptured or leaking pelvic abscess. A ruptured tubo-ovarian abscess has a significant mortality rate, even with immediate surgical treatment [16].

Patients with mild PID (no leukocytosis, fever, or abscess) might be transported by AE at any time. Elective AE of patients with more serious cases of PID should be delayed until the convalescent phase of their illness. These patients should be treated as inpatients with parenteral and oral antibiotics. AE should be delayed until the patient has been afebrile for at least 24 h and is able to tolerate oral hydration and feeding. She should be ambulatory with minimal or no pelvic pain.

Urgent AE might be required in a contingency situation for a patient with a pelvic abscess. Surgically drained prior to AE is ideal, particularly when the patient continues to have significant pain and fever. Vaginal drainage can be performed when the abscess is bulging into the posterior cul-de-sac. If not, abscess drainage can be performed using an ultrasound-guided needle transvaginally or a laparoscopic approach. If drainage is not possible, AE should be delayed if possible until the patient has remained afebrile for 48 h and has no sign of peritoneal irritation. Forceful pelvic exams should be avoided because this might increase the risk of abscess rupture. These patients should be transported on a litter with continuous IV hydration and parenteral antibiotics.

Preparation for Aeromedical Evacuation

For elective AE, the patient should be recovered to the point that she is fully ambulatory, tolerating a regular diet, and taking only oral antibiotics. Most can be transported in a sitting position. If she is known to have a resolving tubo-ovarian abscess, establishment of a heparin lock is a reasonable precaution in case of in-flight abscess rupture.

When urgent AE is required during the acute phase of more serious PID, the patient will require continuous IV hydration and IV antibiotics. These patients might not yet be tolerating a regular diet and should be transported by litter. Many patients will require pain and antinausea medication during flight.

Potential In-Flight Complications

The most serious complication of PID is the sudden rupture of a tubo-ovarian abscess. The movement required for AE might increase this risk. It is unlikely that changes in cabin pressure during AE increase this risk.

The primary symptom of a ruptured tubo-ovarian abscess is an acute increase in abdominal pain with signs of peritonitis. This might be accompanied by signs of sepsis and progress to shock if untreated. In-flight treatment is supportive and consists of IV hydration and supplemental oxygen. If the patient is no longer taking IV antibiotics, coverage with a broad-spectrum antibiotic (e.g., a second- or third-generation cephalosporin) is appropriate. Any rapid deterioration of a patient's condition with a known tubo-ovarian abscess is an indication to divert to the nearest airfield with a nearby medical facility.

A less serious complication is the recurrence of fever and/or pelvic pain in a patient recovering from PID. If the patient has no history of a pelvic abscess, and otherwise appears stable, treatment should consist of recumbence, oral pain medication, antipyretics, and antibiotics. If possible, the patient should be given IV fluids and antibiotics. Flight diversion might be required if the patient becomes unstable.

Abnormal Uterine Bleeding

Excessively heavy or frequent bleeding is a common occurrence among reproductive-aged women. The differential diagnosis includes pregnancy (see previous sections on spontaneous abortion and ectopic pregnancy), anovulatory bleeding, infection, and malignancies. In postmenopausal-aged women (usually >50 years of age), any uterine bleeding is abnormal and uterine cancer is more common. Clinical evaluation includes a pregnancy test (in pre-menopausal women), complete blood count, Pap smear, and physical examination. Endometrial biopsy is commonly performed in women >40 years of age with abnormal bleeding.

The treatment for gynecological bleeding depends on the diagnosis. Anovulatory bleeding is usually treated with hormones, whereas infection is treated with antibiotics. D&C might be required for definitive diagnosis and treatment.

In cases of cervical or endometrial malignancy, hemorrhage is usually related to neovascularity of the tumor itself. Lesser degrees of bleeding might be treated with vaginal packing until definitive treatment with surgery or radiation can be carried out. Extreme cases of bleeding might require emergency hysterectomy. If the necessary expertise is available, radiographic selective cauterization and embolization of the bleeding vessel might be used.

Implications for Aeromedical Evacuation

Uncontrolled, heavy vaginal bleeding from any cause is a contraindication to AE. Definitive diagnosis and treatment (i.e., hysteroscopy and D&C) is required prior to AE.

Patients with limited bleeding resulting from anovulation or endometritis might be safely transported by elective AE. Likewise, those with light bleeding after definitive treatment with D&C can safely undergo AE. If abnormal bleeding is treated nonsurgically with hormones or antibiotics, elective AE should be delayed until 1 week after the last episode of heavy bleeding to minimize the risk of recurrent hemorrhage during flight.

A patient with significant vaginal bleeding resulting from endometrial or cervical cancer should be definitively treated prior to elective AE. After radiation therapy or selective embolization, the patient should be observed for at least 1 week to minimize the risk of recurrent hemorrhage. If the definitive treatment includes hysterectomy, AE should be delayed as discussed below for postoperative gynecological patients.

In a contingency situation, urgent AE might be required for patients with continuous or recent episodes of heavy vaginal bleeding. The only appropriate approach is transportation of these unstable patients to the nearest appropriate medical facility (i.e., MEDEVAC). The patient will require a functioning large-bore IV line and readily available blood products.

Preparation for Aeromedical Evacuation

Evaluation prior to AE includes a pregnancy test (for women of reproductive age), complete blood cell count, and physical examination. The patient's Hgb should be >12 g/dL so she will have an adequate reserve should she begin hemorrhaging during AE. An adequate supply of menstrual pads to last several days should be available. An ob/gyn emergency kit should be available (Table 21.1).

After definitive treatment, patients need no special preparation and might be transported as ambulatory. If a patient is at high risk for recurrent heavy bleeding during flight, she should have a functioning IV line in place, type-specific blood products available, and must be a litter patient.

Potential In-Flight Complications

The obvious risk is recurrent heavy vaginal bleeding. This risk is not increased by cabin pressure changes but might be increased by patient movement, in particular in cases of gynecological malignancy. Vaginal bleeding of any etiology might be massive enough to result in hypovolemic shock.

The in-flight treatment of vaginal bleeding includes IV hydration and supplemental oxygen. Vaginal inspection with a speculum, followed by tight vaginal packing with gauze, might temporarily slow the bleeding. Diversion of the flight to the nearest airfield and emergency transportation to the nearest medical facility will usually be required.

Postoperative Gynecological Patients

Many gynecological conditions require surgery for definitive therapy. Because gynecological procedures are some of the most common major operations performed, an understanding of these patients is important for AE.

Gynecological procedures are often divided into three general categories: major, minor, and laparoscopic. The majority of laparoscopic procedures are minor in nature. However, because the peritoneal cavity is entered, and because there is a <1% incidence of major complications, post-laparoscopy patients should be considered separately from those undergoing other minor surgery [17].

Other common minor gynecological procedures are uterine D&C and hysteroscopy. Minor cervical procedures include cervical loop electrosurgical excision procedure (LEEP) or cone biopsy, where the center portion of the cervix is removed using an electrocautery, scalpel, or laser. Mini-laparotomy (incision <6 cm) for tubal ligation or removal of an ovarian cyst is also considered minor surgery. Vulvar and vaginal biopsies also fit into this category.

The most common major gynecological procedure is hysterectomy. This is most commonly performed laparoscopically, with or without robotic assistance, or through a vaginal incision. Difficult hysterectomies are sometimes performed through an abdominal incision. Hysterectomy can be performed with or without the removal of the ovaries. Other major gynecological procedures include vaginal surgical repairs, bladder suspensions, and laparotomy for removal of pelvic masses.

Laparoscopic complications are most often related to introduction of sharp instruments through small incisions and include injury to the intestines, bladder, and blood vessels [17]. These most often are discovered at the time of surgery, but the diagnosis might be delayed for several days after surgery. Later complications of laparoscopy include infection, delayed bleeding, and occult injury of the bowel or urinary tract.

Implications for Aeromedical Evacuation

Prior to elective AE, the postoperative gynecological patient should be allowed to recover to the point that she is ambulatory, tolerating regular diets, and her pain has decreased to the point that she is able to tolerate the rigors of long-distance flight in a sitting position. After minor or laparoscopic gynecological surgery, the patient will usually be ready for AE after a 1-week recovery time. After uncomplicated major surgery, elective AE should be delayed for 3 or 4 weeks, depending on the patient's rate of recovery.

If urgent AE is required during a contingency situation, the risk to the patient increases. The sooner a patient undergoes transportation after surgery, the greater the risk of in-flight complications. For this reason, AE should be delayed for a minimum of 24 h after major gynecological surgery or 12 h after minor gynecological surgery. This will allow the healing process to begin and reduction of the surgical hemorrhage risk. In addition, it will allow the patient to recover from the effects of anesthesia. Finally, the measured Hgb level will more accurately reflect the patient's hemodynamic state because equilibration takes several hours after the acute blood loss associated with surgery.

Preparation for Aeromedical Evacuation

Patients who are almost completely recovered from gynecological surgery need little preparation. They should ready for transportation in a sitting position but might still require oral pain medication. Some patients might still be experiencing vaginal bleeding and thus will need menstrual pads.

If the patient is transported within 1 week of major surgery, probably the most important consideration is the Hgb level. Postoperative patients should have an Hgb $\geq$ 12 mg/dL prior to AE. Most patients will need to be transported by litter. Adequate medication for pain and nausea should be available.

If AE is required within 24 h of major gynecological surgery, the patient should have a functioning IV line. Patients without return of normal bowel function should be actively hydrated. These patients should be transported by litter and have parenteral pain and antinausea medications available. Patients should be routinely fitted with elastic stockings for leg compression to decrease the risk of deep-vein thrombosis.

Potential In-Flight Complications

The risk of postoperative complications decreases with time after surgery. For this reason, complications will be relatively uncommon during elective AE in the convalescent period. If AE is required prior to recovery, complications that rarely occur outside the hospital setting might occur during flight.

Intra-abdominal Hemorrhage

The most common early postoperative complication is intra-abdominal hemorrhage. This complication almost always occurs within the first 24 h of surgery and thus will be unlikely to occur in patients transported after this initial recovery period. However, the movement to which the patient is subjected during AE might result in hemorrhage in the days immediately following surgery.

The signs of intra-abdominal hemorrhage include increased abdominal discomfort and hemodynamic instability. Late signs are abdominal distention and hypovolemic shock. If intra-abdominal hemorrhage is suspected in flight, supportive measures include intravascular volume expansion and supplemental oxygen. Emergency diversion of the flight to an airfield near a medical facility might be lifesaving.

Pulmonary Embolism

A potential early complication of major gynecological surgery is pulmonary embolism, which accounts for almost half of all deaths after gynecological surgery [18]. It is also the second most common cause of death after nonmedical abortion and the most frequent cause of postoperative death in patients with uterine or cervical cancer. The risk is increased in patients who are over 40 years of age or obese or have a history of DVT [18].

The clinical presentation of pulmonary embolism is sudden onset of shortness of breath, chest pain, tachypnea, and tachycardia. The patient might have symptoms of DVT of the leg, such as unilateral leg edema, pain, or erythema.

As with many postoperative complications, the primary approach is preventive. After major gynecological surgery, most patients are treated with leg compression devices (elastic stockings or intermittent pneumatic compression devices) until fully ambulatory. Because of decreased cabin pressure at altitude, the pneumatic devices cannot be used during AE but elastic stockings should be continued.

Patients at high risk for DVT are also treated with prophylactic heparin in the perioperative period. A standard approach is subcutaneous unfractionated heparin or low-molecular-weight heparin until the patient is ambulatory. For patients being transported by AE with 72 h of surgery, the use of either elastic stockings or heparin is a reasonable precaution [19].

Emergency in-flight management of pulmonary embolism is limited to supportive therapy, including IV hydration and oxygen. If the symptoms warrant, flight diversion and transportation to the closest medical facility might be required. Modern management of pulmonary embolism consists of full anticoagulation. In severe cases, clot lysis with streptokinase or urokinase might be required. Surgery might be required for recurrent emboli and massive emboli resulting in cardiovascular collapse.

Abdominal Pain

Some postoperative patients might experience increased abdominal pain during AE. If the pain is acute, intra-abdominal hemorrhage should be considered, as discussed previously. However, a more common cause of postoperative abdominal pain is related to gas trapped in the bowel. It is not uncommon for postoperative patients to have a temporary obstruction related to bowel irritation, referred to as paralytic ileus. It usually spontaneously resolves within 1 week of surgery. Bowel obstruction that does not resolve is more likely to be mechanical in nature, related to intra-abdominal adhesions, or an errant suture.

Even in the hospital, bowel obstruction condition can lead to abdominal distension and colicky pain usually associated with nausea and vomiting. The pain might be worsened by expansion of bowel gas associated with decreased cabin pressure in-flight. Treatment is gastric decompression with a nasogastric or orogastric tube, IV hydration, and supportive therapy with pain and antinausea medicine. It is unlikely for this complication to require emergency flight diversion. However, complete medical reevaluation of the patient at the next scheduled stopover is mandatory.

Postoperative Infection

One of the most common postoperative complications in the first week after surgery is infection. Even with the use of prophylactic antibiotics, clinically significant infection occurs in 5% of hysterectomies [20]. One of the most common sites of postoperative infection is the abdominal incision. The clinical presentation is redness and induration around the incision, with or without purulent discharge. Other sources of infection in a postoperative patient with a fever or signs of sepsis might be more difficult to determine. Infection at the vaginal cuff after hysterectomy or infections of the urinary or pulmonary tract are difficult to diagnose during flight.

If a postoperative patient develops fever or signs of sepsis in-flight, the primary treatment consists of IV hydration and oral antipyretics. If available, broad-spectrum antibiotics can be instituted. Flight diversion is necessary if the patient exhibits signs of advanced sepsis, such as tachycardia or hypotension.

Incisional Bleeding

A relatively common postoperative complication is bleeding from the operative site. Although hemostasis in the subcutaneous tissue is achieved prior to enclosure, patient movement and the normal healing process can sometimes result in significant bleeding. In general, this will occur in the first 48 h after surgery. Later bleeding from the wound might represent infection. After most gynecological procedures, the bleeding will come from an abdominal incision. After hysterectomy and vaginal procedures, the bleeding might come from the vaginal incision.

Treatment for in-flight bleeding from an abdominal incision consists of direct pressure over the bleeding site and placement of an overdressing over the original dressing. When possible, the dressing should be removed to evaluate the wound. In most cases, the wound will remain intact and a pressure dressing will minimize further bleeding. Uncontrollable bleeding will require further evaluation at a medical facility.

Heavy vaginal bleeding in the postoperative patient is a more difficult problem. If a physician with gynecological experience is available, the vaginal cuff can be evaluated using a speculum and focused light source. A discrete bleeding site might be selectively clamped and ligated. Vaginal packing might be most helpful in controlling postoperative bleeding.

Dehiscence

A serious, but fortunately uncommon, wound complication is dehiscence. This is defined as disruption of all layers of the abdominal or vaginal incision, including skin, subcutaneous, fascia, muscle, and peritoneum. The most serious variant of wound dehiscence is evisceration, where peritoneal cavity contents spill out. Dehiscence is usually related to sudden increases in abdominal pressure from coughing or patient movement. Obesity, wound infections, diabetes, and malignancies increase the risk of wound dehiscence.

The treatment for wound dehiscence in-flight is support of the wound with a pressure dressing and an abdominal binder. A binder can be made by wrapping an elastic bandage around the abdomen over a thick dressing. If evisceration occurs, the bowel should be covered with a moist, sterile towel or dressing. If available, this dressing should be covered with a layer of plastic (e.g., trash bag) to limit loss of body heat and moisture. Every effort should be made to avoid compromising the blood supply to the bowel because bowel hypoxia might cause necrosis and necessitate bowel resection. Emergency flight diversion for emergency medical care is mandatory.

References

1. Hall MJ, DeFrances CJ, Williams SN, Golosinskiy A, Schwartzman A. National hospital discharge survey: 2007 summary. Natl Health Stat Rep. 2010;29:1–20.
2. Department of Defense. 2015 demographics profile of the military community. Available at: http://download.militaryonesource.mil/12038/MOS/Reports/2015-Demographics-Report.pdf. Accessed 18 July 2018.
3. Brown D, Skye Gould S. The US has 1.3 million troops stationed around the world — here are the major hotspots. Business Insider. Aug 31, 2017. Available at: http://www.businessinsider.com/us-military-deployments-may-2017-5/#us-troops-are-deployed-in-hotspots-around-the-world-including-places-like-iraq-syria-and-afghanistan-1. Accessed 18 July 2018.
4. Hines JF. A comparison of clinical diagnoses among male and female soldiers deployed during the Persian Gulf war. Milit Med. 1993;158:99–101.
5. Hanna JH. An analysis of gynecological problems presenting to an evacuation hospital during operation desert storm. Milit Med. 1992;157:222–4.
6. Chibber R, Al-Sibai MH, Qahtani N. Adverse outcome of pregnancy following air travel: a myth or a concern? Aust N Z J Obstet Gynaecol. 2006;46(1):24–8.
7. Lauria L, Ballard TJ, Caldora M, Mazzanti C, Verdecchia A. Reproductive disorders and pregnancy outcomes among female flight attendants. Aviat Space Environ Med. 2006;77(5):533–9.
8. Huch R, Baumann H, Fallenstein F, Schneider KTM, Holdener F, Huch A. Physiologic changes in pregnant women and their fetuses during jet air travel. Am J Obstet Gynecol. 1986;154:996–1000.
9. Cunningham FG, Leveno KJ, Bloom SL, Spong CY, Dashe JS, Hoffman BL, Casey BM, Sheffield JS. Williams obstetrics. 24th ed. Columbus: McGraw-Hill Education; 2014.
10. Barry M, Bia F. Pregnancy and travel. JAMA. 1989;26:728–31.
11. Breen JL, Gregori CA, Neilson RN. Travel by airplane during pregnancy. NJ Med. 1986;82:2979.
12. Connor SB, Lyons TJ. US air force aeromedical evacuation of obstetric patients in Europe. Aviat Space Environ Med. 1995;66:1090–3.
13. Polansky GH, Varner MW, O'Gorman T. Premature rupture of the membranes and barometric pressure changes. J Reprod Med. 1985;30:189–91.
14. Hurd WW, Whitfield RR, Randolph JF, Kercher M. Expectant management vs elective curettage for the treatment of spontaneous abortion. Fertil Steril. 1997;68:601–6.
15. Stovall TG, Ling FW. Single-dose methotrexate: an expanded clinical trial. Am J Obstet Gynecol. 1993;168:1759–62.
16. Rosen M, Breitkopf D, Waud K. Tubo-ovarian abscess management options for women who desire fertility. Obstet Gynecol Surv. 2009;64(10):681–9.
17. Hurd WW, Pearl ML, DeLancey JOL, Quint EH, Garnett B, Bude RO. Laparoscopic injury of abdominal wall blood vessels: a report of three cases. Obstet Gynecol. 1993;82:673–6.
18. Thompson JD, Rock JA, Jones HW III. TeLinde's operative gynecology. 10th ed. Philadelphia: Lippincott Williams & Wilkins; 2011.
19. Clagett GP, Anderson FA Jr, Heit J, Levine MN, Wheeler HB. Prevention of venous thromboembolism. Chest. 1995;108:312S–34S.
20. Berek JS. Berek and Novak's gynecology. 15th ed. Philadelphia: Lippincott Williams & Wilkins; 2011.

22 Overview of Pediatric and Neonatal Transport

T. Jacob Lee, Angela M. Fagiana, Robert J. Wells, Howard S. Heiman, William W. Hurd, and Matthew A. Borgman

Introduction

The specialty of pediatrics was one of the earliest to recognize the benefit of moving patients between medical treatment facilities. The impetus for this was to both maximize patient outcomes and conserve medical resources. By 1900, the Chicago Lying-In Hospital had developed specific equipment for transporting newborn infants. By 1950, the New York City Department of Health had set up a newborn transportation system to serve a network of hospitals, complete with specific transportation equipment and teams and a central dispatcher. During 1950–1952, this system moved more than 1200 patients between hospitals [1].

Many areas of the United States developed regional neonatal intensive care units (ICUs) during the 1960s and 1970s as a result of both the

T. J. Lee (✉)
Maj, USAF, MC, Pediatric Critical Care, Critical Care Air Transport, Department of Pediatrics, Brooke Army Medical Center, Joint Base San Antonio-Fort Sam Houston, San Antonio, TX, USA
e-mail: thomas.j.lee80.mil@mail.mil

A. M. Fagiana
Maj, USAF, MC, Neonatal Transport, Department of Neonatology, Brooke Army Medical Center, Fort Sam Houston, TX, USA

Department of Pediatrics, F. Edward Hebert School of Medicine – Uniformed Services University, Bethesda, MD, USA

R. J. Wells
Col, USAF, MC, CFS (ret.), Formerly, Department of Pediatrics, University Of Texas MD Anderson Cancer Center, Houston, TX, USA

Formerly Commander, 445th ASTS, Wright-Patterson AFB, Dayton, OH, USA

H. S. Heiman
COL, MC, USA (ret.), Neonatal Transport, Department of Pediatrics, Neonatal-Perinatal Division, Cohen Children's Medical Center of Greater New York, Northwell Health, New Hyde Park, NY, USA

W. W. Hurd
Col, USAF, MC, SFS (ret.), Chief Medical Officer, American Society for Reproductive Medicine, Professor Emeritus Department of Obstetrics and Gynecology, Duke University Medical Center, Durham, NC, USA

Formerly, CCATT physician and Commander, 445th ASTS, Wright-Patterson Air Force Base, Dayton, OH, USA

M. A. Borgman
LTC, MC, USA, Pediatric Critical Care Services, Brook Army Medical Center Simulation Center, Joint Base San Antonio - Fort Sam Houston, San Antonio, TX, USA

Department of Pediatrics, F. Edward Hebert School of Medicine - Uniformed Services University, Bethesda, MD, USA

W. W. Hurd, W. Beninati (eds.), *Aeromedical Evacuation*,
https://doi.org/10.1007/978-3-030-15903-0_22

significant medical progress in this area and the increasing difficulty of supporting such units. This regionalization further increased the number of infants being transported.

As the size of the regions increased, the potential benefits of aeromedical evacuation (AE) compared to traditional ground transport became obvious. Early reports of this mode of transport were encouraging and included 53 infants transported by large fixed-wing military aircraft (Operation Baby Lift, 1969–1970) and 101 infants moved by both rotary-wing and small fixed-wing aircraft by St. Anthony's Air Transport Service (Denver) from 1972 to 1973 [2, 3].

The advantages of transporting neonates to regional ICUs quickly became apparent to other pediatric subspecialists. The subsequent development of regional pediatric ICUs and regional centers for trauma, dialysis, and transplantation further increased the need for interhospital transport of pediatric patients. In response, the American Academy of Pediatrics published guidelines for both air and ground transport in 1986, with subsequent revisions in 1993, 2000, 2006, and 2016 [4]. In addition, many pediatric subspecialty textbooks in neonatology, pediatric intensive care, and pediatric emergency medicine routinely contain chapters on transport consideration for neonatal and pediatric patients.

Understanding the difference between neonatal and pediatric patients is fundamental to the transport team's utilization of appropriate treatment guidelines and equipment. Earlier US Air Force (USAF) doctrine for Critical Care Air Transport Teams (CCATTs) delineated the age range for neonatal care as birth to 3 months, and 3 months to 14 years for pediatric care, although this has been removed from the most recent updates [5–7]. National standards for delineating neonatal versus pediatric critical care transport teams do not exist and are, therefore, determined by local/regional medical and transport entities and standards of care. Generally speaking, while there is a small amount of overlap, neonatal transport applies for preterm and term infants, any infant under 5 kg, and when Neonatal Resuscitation Program (NRP) algorithms would be appropriate for patient resuscitation (i.e., less than 30 days of life and all premature infants), and pediatric transport applies when Pediatric Advanced Life Support (PALS) algorithms would be appropriate for patient resuscitation (i.e., greater than 3 days of life, assuming full term at birth, to 25 years) [8].

This chapter will first cover pediatric transport goals and the composition, training, and equipment of pediatric transport teams. Next, several common general pediatric conditions moved via AE and the AE implications will be described. Finally, common neonatal conditions requiring AE will be discussed.

Pediatric Transportation

Transportation Goals

The ultimate goal of pediatric AE is to rapidly bring the patient to a higher level of care. To do this successfully, three tasks must be accomplished. First, the transport team must assess the patient's needs with the assistance of the referring medical care providers. A key determination at this point is which personnel are necessary for the transport team. The second task is to determine if the patient is stable enough to transport. This determination is a joint responsibility of the referring medical care providers and the transport team after they have arrived on scene. The final task is to maintain stability of the patient throughout the course of movement between medical treatment facilities, mitigating the stresses associated with AE as well as potential progression of the underlying medical problem.

Transport Team Composition

The composition of the transport team is determined by the transporting facility and will usually depend on patient age and needs, potential complications, financial support, and other local system considerations. A transport team is most commonly composed of some combination of the following personnel: pediatric critical care, emergency, or neonatal nurse; respiratory therapist; emergency medical technician; subspecialty trained physician (e.g., pediatric intensivist, neonatologist, emergency medicine physician); physicians in training (e.g., resident or fellow); transport physician; or advanced practitioner (e.g., nurse practitioner or physician assistant). Not all teams require physicians, especially when the patient population and conditions are fairly heterogeneous. Typically, physicians, if available, might participate in selected transports only for extremely ill patients. There is a physician, however, always designated as the "medical control" to help guide and advise the transport team when she/he is not attending. According to the American Academy of Pediatrics, the most common team composition is RN-RT, with many dedicated teams providing neonatal and pediatric transport, and physicians participating in 9.4–20% of transports [4].

Ideally, all pediatric and neonatal transport service directors should be physicians with expertise in the evaluation and treatment of pediatric or neonatal disease and injury. These expert pediatricians include board-certified specialists in neonatalogy, pediatric emergency medicine, or pediatric intensive care. Although personally participating in only a minimal portion of patient movements, they are responsible for administrative, technical, and medical decision making, as well as education and training of transport teams. Actual transport team members must have pediatric and/or neonatal skills that support the anticipated needs of the patient transported. In reality, it is sometimes difficult for regional planners to construct expert pediatric emergency teams. When expert pediatricians are unavailable, various levels of technicians, nurses, and physicians in training can be utilized to maximize the pediatric skills of the team [9].

Basing a transport system at a pediatric center of excellence, although not required, allows for the accomplishment of two important objectives. First, the primary team members located at these centers can establish and maintain their clinical skills. Second, other pediatric specialists available at these centers serve as a large pool to draw from in the event their skills are required for a specific pediatric transport. When a team is augmented by a specialist with little background in pediatric transport, good communication between the expert and the transport team is essential to assure that patient care is not compromised.

Team Training

Both the Commission on Accreditation of Medical Transport Systems and the American Academy of Pediatrics provide the extensive, specific training content and currency requirements for aeromedical transport teams [4, 8]. This training must include flight preparations, physiology, and safety. Members of neonatal and pediatric transport teams, whether separate or combined, require specialized training in neonatal and/or pediatric resuscitation, stabilization of infants and children for transport, and the frequently encountered diseases in each respective age group. Well-organized educational programs on these topics are offered by the American Heart Association, the American Academy of Pediatrics, and the American College of Emergency Physicians. Additionally, advanced training and experience – most often in neonatal, pediatric, or pediatric cardiac ICUs – for team members is usually required, depending on team composition and required transport missions. The S.T.A.B.L.E. course is specifically designed for the stabilization of critically ill neonates and should be taken by providers transporting these patients.

Continuing education for all team members is crucial to the maintenance of knowledge and skills. Those efforts should include not only operational and medical aspects of transport but also strategies for enhancing team communication skills and stress management.

Transport Team Supplies and Equipment

Supplies

Neonatal and pediatric transport supplies should be maintained independent from each other and from adult supplies. Although this will result in some duplication of materials, it is necessary to avoid the potential danger that can result from confusion of medication doses and concentrations, and will help ensure adequate level of supplies.

Table 22.1 Neonatal and pediatric transport equipment

Neonatal equipment	Pediatric equipment
Transport incubator with thermoregulation capabilities	Transport litter
Monitors with appropriately sized devices:	Securement harness
3-lead ECG	Blankets
Respiratory rate	Monitors with appropriately sized devices:
Pulse oximetry	3-lead ECG
Temperature (skin, core +/– air)	Respiratory rate
Blood pressure (noninvasive)	Pulse oximetry
Ventilator with appropriate tidal volume capability and appropriately sized accoutrements:	Temperature (skin, core +/– air)
Circuit	Blood pressure (noninvasive)
Humidification device	Ventilator with appropriate tidal volume capability and appropriately sized accoutrements:
$EtCO_2$	Circuit
In-line suction	Humidification device
Airway management devices:	$EtCO_2$
Laryngoscope and blades – Sizes 00, 0, and 1	In-line suction
Endotracheal tubes, cuffless – 2.0–4.0 Fr	Airway management devices:
OPA/NPA	Laryngoscope and blades – Sizes 1–3
Portable compressed gas (oxygen and air) at 50 psi	Endotracheal tubes, cuffed – 3.0–7.5 Fr
Oxygen blender with flow meter up to 15 LPM	OPA/NPA
Nitric oxide delivery system (when required)	Emergency cricothyroidotomy kit
Portable suction unit	Portable compressed gas with oxygen +/– air at 50 psi
Point of care blood gas analyzer	Oxygen blender with flow meter up to 15 LPM
Vascular access devices, with insertion kit:	Nitric oxide delivery system (when required)
Peripheral IV – 24/25 ga	Portable suction unit
Arterial line – 2.5 Fr	Point of care blood gas analyzer
Umbilical venous and arterial catheters	Vascular access devices, with insertion kit:
Intraosseous line kit	Peripheral IV – 21–25 ga.
Infusion pumps, syringe pumps	Central venous line – 4.0–7.0 Fr.
Point of care glucose analyzer	Arterial line – 2.5 or 3.0 Fr.
Appropriate IV fluids – D5W, D10W, D5, or 10NS	Intraosseous line kit.
Gastric decompression catheters – OG/NG	Infusion pumps, syringe pumps
Foley catheters	Appropriate IV fluids – D10W, D25W, D5NS, NS
Defibrillator-cardioverter with pediatric pads	Gastric decompression catheters – OG, NG
Prostaglandin infusion availability	Foley catheters
	Defibrillator-cardioverter with pediatric and adult pads
	Intracranial pressure monitor

ECG electrocardiography; *OPA* oropharyngeal airway; *NPA* nasopharyngeal airway; *LPM* liters per minute; *IV* intravenous; *OG* orogastric; *NG* nasogastric

Equipment

Pediatric and neonatal transport equipment must be lightweight, compact, durable, and easily secured to function well in the AE environment. An example list of pediatric and neonatal equipment is shown in Table 22.1. Some basic equipment for pediatric transportation, such as cervical collar and backboard, are part of the standard emergency medical service inventory and may not need to be duplicated by the pediatric transport team, but this should be verified prior to departure to receive the patient.

There are special considerations that need to be taken into account when choosing or establishing transport equipment. Any electrical equipment must have extended battery capability due to the potential for lack of power outlets for extended periods of time en route. Other equally important considerations are the effects of flight on equipment performance and the effects of the equipment on the aircraft. Performance of pediatric

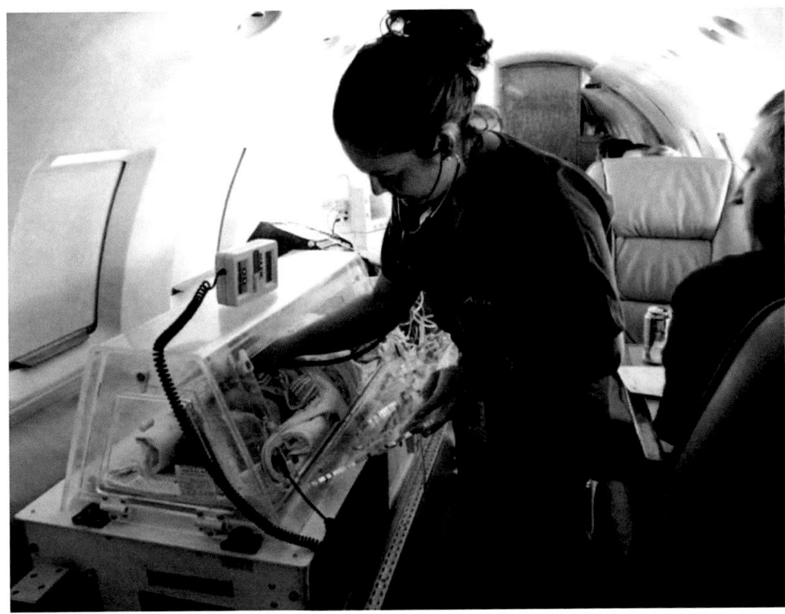

Fig. 22.1 An incubator aboard a Beech King Air 200 aircraft flown by Intermountain Health Care Life (Salt Lake City). (Photo courtesy of AirMed International, Birmingham, AL)

transport equipment should be thoroughly tested for the stresses of flight, including altitude-related changes in pressure, temperature, and humidity, acceleration–deceleration forces, vibration, and the electromagnetic environment of the airframe. In addition to adversely affecting the performance characteristics, these stresses may significantly shorten the useful life of the equipment [6]. Because of these environmental stresses, an effective biomedical maintenance program is critical.

In addition, the effects of pediatric transport equipment on the aircraft must be thoroughly tested to verify that the electromagnetic emissions of the equipment do not interfere with the performance of aircraft avionics, including communications and navigational devices [6]. Extensive safety and performance evaluation of equipment for AE has been carried out by both the U.S. Air Force Research Laboratory and the U.S. Army Aeromedical Research Laboratory [10, 11]. Unfortunately, the majority of the transportation equipment that has been tested and approved for use on aircraft (e.g., infusion pumps and ventilators) was designed for treatment of adult patients. In many cases, it may not be appropriate for use in pediatric patients if it lacks accuracy at the small volumes that must be delivered for pediatric and especially neonatal patients.

Incubators

The incubator, or transport isolette, is the focal point of the neonatal transport system because it provides for two of the most critical aspects of transport: thermal support and integrated patient monitoring. It is also the largest and heaviest piece of equipment used in neonatal transport (Fig. 22.1). Thus, it has a significant impact on the final configuration and composition of the entire transport system. Prior to using an incubator for the first time in a particular aircraft, it must be verified that the incubator fits through the aircraft door and can be fixed firmly in place. In rotary-wing and smaller fixed-wing aircraft, the chief pilot must carefully review any impact on weight and balance calculations because an incubator and cart can weigh as much as 285 lb., though newer devices are typically 75–150 lbs.

Ventilators

Although multiple factors affect the choice of ventilator for air medical transport, such as power source requirement and gas consumption, the most important factors are patient age, patient size, and required tidal volumes. Few ventilators available capably deliver <50 ml of tidal volume and until recently have been primarily pneumatic devices. Pneumatic devices offer a wide range of pressure and volume delivery capabilities, but limited choice in ventilator mode. The ventilator most commonly used by the USAF AE system is the Impact Uni-Vent Eagle Model 731 Positive Pressure Ventilator (ZOLL Medical Corporation), which is described in Chap. 18. For neonates, the MVP-10 has been a common choice. Some newer options include the Crossvent 2i+ (for neonates), the Crossvent 3+ (pediatrics/adults), Hamilton T-1 (neonate/pediatrics/adult), and the LTV 1200 Series.

Extracorporeal Membrane Oxygenation

Extracorporeal membrane oxygenation (ECMO; also known as extracorporeal life support) is the use of mechanical devices for days or weeks to support heart and/or lung function to permit treatment and recovery during severe cardiac or pulmonary failure in neonates, children, and adults [12]. The ECMO circuit consists of a pump, membrane oxygenator, conduit tubing, heater, oxygen source, and monitors. In general, ECMO is considered when mortality from the disease state is greater than 50% and indicated when mortality from the disease state is greater than 80%. Contraindications are somewhat relative and include conditions incompatible with life if recovery occurs, conditions that are irreversible even with implementation of ECMO, preexisting conditions affecting quality of life, patient age and size, and futility of therapy [12]. A dedicated team of physicians with ECMO knowledge and experience should guide institutional decisions regarding use of ECMO for patients.

The most common neonatal indications for ECMO are meconium aspiration syndrome, congenital diaphragmatic hernia, and persistent pulmonary hypertension, with 78% of cases overall having a respiratory indication [13]. The current overall survival rates for neonatal ECMO are 73% for pulmonary indications, 42% for cardiac, and 41% for extracorporeal cardiopulmonary resuscitation (ECPR) [14].

Pediatric ECMO encompasses patients aged greater than 30 days to less than 18 years of life. Pulmonary cases represent 38% of total ECMO cases, cardiac 45%, and ECPR 17%. Survival rates are 58%, 52%, and 42%, respectively [14, 15]. The causes of acute respiratory failure in the pediatric patient are too varied to list but

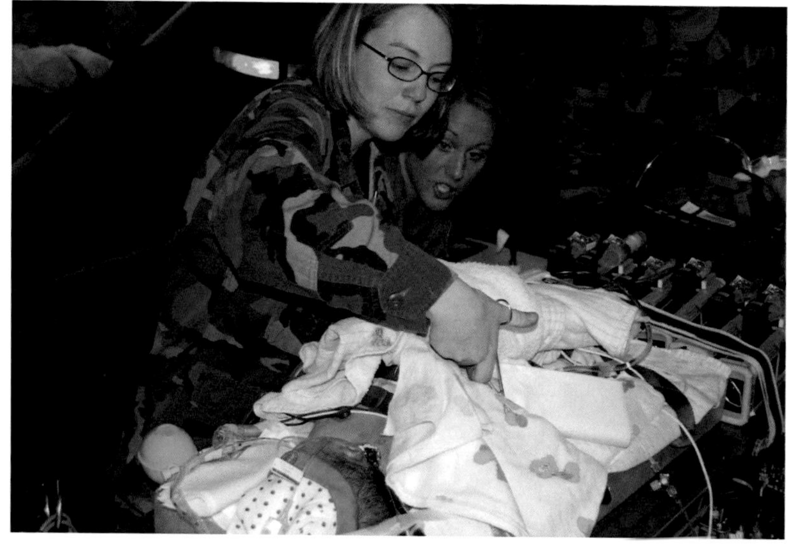

Fig. 22.2 Ground and flight medical crews work together during aeromedical evacuation of a 3-day-old infant requiring extracorporeal membrane oxygen (ECMO) from Puerto Rico to Wilford Hall Medical Center in San Antonio, Texas. (U.S. Air Force photo by Capt. Bruce Hill, Jr.)

most commonly have an infectious etiology – viral or bacterial. ECMO is also utilized for patients with chronic respiratory failure, often as a bridge to lung transplant. ECMO is utilized quite commonly for patients postsurgery for congenital cardiac disease and for acute cardiac failure due to shock, sepsis, and viral cardiomyopathy [16].

With the incorporation of centrifugal pumps, which in some cases are integrated with the oxygenator, ECMO circuits now have a much smaller footprint, and transport routinely occurs in both rotary-wing and fixed-wing aircraft. Patients on ECMO can be transported on almost any size airframe, but team size and supplemental equipment (e.g., medications, blood products, spare parts) make larger aircraft – such as the C-130, C-17, or similar civilian platform – preferable depending on travel distance. Due to the complexity of the equipment and treatment, specialized ECMO transport teams are required (Fig. 22.2).

Transportation Risks

Transportation of neonatal and pediatric patients, either by ground or air, represents a real risk for many reasons. In one study, interfacility transport of premature neonates was associated with a slightly increased risk of advanced intraventricular hemorrhage [17]. In all cases, the risks versus the benefits of transporting an often critically ill patient must be carefully considered. Simultaneously, the added risk of air transport must be measured in light of the availability, duration, and utility of ground transport.

Psychological

When patients are moved between medical treatment facilities, families are usually separated, even if one or more family members accompany the patient. Separation of a child from loved ones or parents from their normal support network may adversely affect the psychological health of both the child and family.

The Aeromedical Environment

The aeromedical environment poses inherent risks to the patients, as well as the team. The simple act of patient movement can put the patient at increased risk of displacing airways or intravascular lines. Movement, plus the vibration associated with flight, can further loosen dressings and disrupt healing wounds. Vibrational stress can increase fatigue, cause shortness of breath, motion sickness, and chest and abdominal pain [4]. The noise in most AE environments exceeds the recommended levels for children and completely precludes the use of auscultation by medical personnel [18]. Noise protection must be provided to the patient. Cooler, less humid cabin air when at flight altitude causes increased insensible fluid losses, increasing the risk of dehydration. Lastly, the variation in lighting often diminishes visual assessment skills.

Thermal Stress

One of the most important aspects of neonatal AE is the maintenance of an optimal thermal environment. However, thermal stress affects both neonatal and pediatric transport patients alike. Cold or heat stress significantly increases both the caloric and oxygen demands of pediatric and neonatal patients. Unlike the older pediatric and adult patient, the neonate is severely limited in his or her capabilities to compensate. Radiative and evaporative heat losses are increased because of the neonate's large body surface area, and this thermal stress can result in profound vital sign disturbances for the neonatal and young pediatric patient. Temperature must be monitored closely. Thermal control measures – such as the incubator and warming mattress for neonates and blankets for pediatric patients – must be utilized.

The purpose of an incubator is to maintain a stable environment in terms of temperature and humidity (Fig. 22.3). Continuous core temperature monitoring of the neonate and the environment is crucial. The transport team

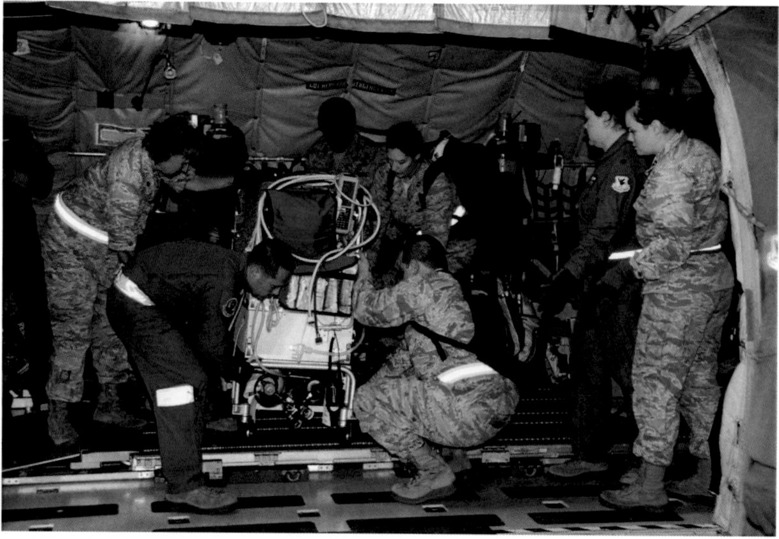

Fig. 22.3 Ground and flight medical crews unload a 2-day-old baby in an incubator from a KC-135 Stratotanker after an aeromedical evacuation flight from Osan Air Base, Republic of Korea, to Tripler Army Medical Center, Hawaii. (U.S. Air Force photo by Staff Sgt. Lauren Padden)

must recognize that monitoring infant axillary temperature alone does not assure that the thermal environment is appropriate, and each time the incubator is opened, the advantage of the regulated environment is temporarily lost until the system re-equilibrates. A table of age and weight should be used to determine the proper neutral thermal air temperature, which ranges from 32 ° C to 36 ° C. While less of a concern, travel in hot environments or significant patient fevers may dictate the provision of cooling measures so that patients do not also overheat.

Effects of Altitude

In contrast to rotary-wing aircraft, which fly at relatively low altitudes, pressurized fixed-wing aircraft usually fly with a cabin altitude equivalent to approximately 8000 ft. Higher altitudes have lower barometric pressure resulting in three primary associated physiologic stressors: gas expansion, decreased oxygen partial pressure, and decreased air humidity. Neonatal and pediatric patients less than 12 months of age have an increased risk of hypoxemia due to anatomic and physiological differences [4]. The effects of these problems are discussed in depth in Chap. 9.

Isolation from Comprehensive Medical Care

The time the patient spends between medical treatment facilities during AE can range from several hours to 10 or more hours. This duration is impacted by multiple factors that should be taken into consideration as best as possible: flying time, ground transport time from the referring hospital to the aircraft and from the aircraft to the receiving hospital, and less predictable events, such as weather and mechanical difficulties of a transport vehicle.

Time during transport away from comprehensive medical care presents multiple problems, especially if the patient's condition deteriorates. Compared to the tertiary care center, limited supplies and equipment are available, and most diagnostic imaging and laboratory tests are unavailable. Equipment failure either due to malfunction or exhaustion of battery power may further complicate required care, and contingency plans should be developed for such emergencies.

Conditions Requiring Transport for Tertiary Care

There is a paucity of published data regarding common neonatal transport conditions. We can assume that the most common admission and transport diagnoses are similar, and those are prematurity, respiratory distress, gastrointestinal conditions, congenital cardiac conditions, and infections. According to unpublished data collected from July 1, 1999, through June 30, 2000, at the University of Cincinnati Children's Hospital and Medical Center, the most common indications for neonatal transport were respiratory insufficiency, related primarily to respiratory distress of the newborn and meconium aspiration syndrome. Gastrointestinal (GI) conditions (e.g., esophageal atresia) were the second most common, followed by congenital cardiac anomalies and infections, such as sepsis [19].

Conditions requiring pediatric transport are more varied. Pediatric patients represent approximately 10% of all transports. Respiratory pathology, injury, and neurologic pathology represent the three most common conditions requiring interfacility transport. Other less common conditions were endocrine, GI, cardiac, and infections, while trauma led to approximately 14% of all pediatric transports [20, 21].

Asthma

Asthma (i.e., reactive airway disease) affects more than 26 million Americans, including 6.1 million children under the age of 18, and of these, nearly 137,000 are hospitalized each year [22]. Between 1999 and 2016, there were 33,307 deaths related to asthma in adults age 15–64 [23]. Deaths related to asthma in children less than 18 years of age represent a small fraction of the total, e.g., 209 deaths in 2016, representing 5.9% of total deaths [22]. From these statistics, the implications for the AE system are obvious.

Implications for Aeromedical Evacuation

Children with severe asthma are at risk during AE for acute exacerbations, probably because of the dry cabin air and the other stresses related to flight. An acute asthma attack is characterized clinically by increased wheezing, respiratory rate, prolonged expiratory phase, and the increased use of accessory muscles [24]. In severe exacerbations, pulse oximetry may be <90% on room air, and the patient will have dyspnea interfering with conversation, being unable to speak with life-threatening exacerbation. Spirometry can be the most objective and accurate measure of severity of exacerbation, but is often unobtainable in young children and in the AE environment.

Treatment of Acute Asthma

All asthma exacerbations should be treated with supplemental oxygen to maintain oxygen saturation ≥90%, inhaled short-acting beta agonist albuterol, and oral systemic corticosteroid (prednisone, prednisolone). For younger children, albuterol should be given 2.5 mg nebulized every 20 minutes for three doses, alternatively 0.5 mg/kg continuous nebulization over 1 hour or four to eight puffs with spacer of albuterol MDI 90 mcg/puff. For older children or adults, 5 mg may be given by nebulizer every 20 minutes for up to 4 hours or 10–20 mg/hr. continuous nebulization. Predinose or prednisolone should be dosed 1–2 mg/kg divided into one to two daily doses, with a maximum of 60 mg/day [24].

Ipratropium bromide inhaled 0.25–0.5 mg every 20 minutes for three doses can be added as an adjunctive treatment with the initial three albuterol doses. Albuterol should be administered via continuous nebulization if symptoms have not improved. If symptoms are still severe despite administered therapies, adjunctive treatments such as subcutaneous epinephrine, subcutaneous terbutaline, or intravenous (IV) magnesium sulfate should be considered [24]. Subcutaneous epinephrine (1:1000 or 1 mg/mL) is dosed 0.01 mg/kg, with a maximum dose of 0.3–0.5 mg, repeated every 20 minutes for a maximum of three doses, and subcutaneous terbutaline is dosed 0.01 mg/kg every 20 minutes for up to three doses. Magnesium sulfate 25–40 mg/kg, maximum dose 2 grams, is infused IV over 20–30 minutes [23]. Long-term therapy will be determined by the receiving physician, but may include a maintenance course of corticosteroids for several weeks.

Upper Airway Obstruction

Upper airway obstruction can occur due to several acute infectious etiologies, including croup, retropharyngeal abscess (RPA), and acute epiglottitis. Croup and retropharyngeal abscess, while causing acute respiratory distress, rarely progress to complete airway obstruction. Croup is typically treated with a single dose of dexamethasone 0.6 mg/kg IV or intramuscular (IM) and can be managed during transport with nebulized racemic epinephrine every 15–20 minutes, as needed. Retropharyngeal abscess rarely causes significant airway compromise and is treated with IV antibiotics and/or surgical drainage. Often, patients with RPA will hold their head and neck turned to one side and present with fever and odynophagia. Any airway obstruction due to RPA will require surgical drainage and further evaluation to determine the extent of any associated deep tissue space infection. During transport, patients should be kept comfortable with IV or PO analgesia – usually acetaminophen 10–15 mg/kg every 6 hours is sufficient – and administration of antibiotics should continue.

Acute epiglottitis is a potentially fatal cause of airway obstruction in both young children and adults and is considered a true emergency. In recent years, there has been a marked decline in the number of pediatric cases of epiglottitis, due to the introduction of efficacious vaccines against *Haemophilus influenzae* type b [25, 26]. However, other bacterial causes are on the rise, there is a growing parental anti-vaccination trend in the United States, and developing countries may not have as robust of vaccination practices as the United States.

Clinical Presentation

The most common symptoms for children are difficulty breathing, stridor, fever, and sore throat, and the child may maintain the leaning forward tripod position. Classically, epiglottitis is most common in children 2–8 years of age, and the four "Ds" have been attributed to the presentation of epiglottitis: drooling, dyspnea, dysphagia, and dysphonia [25, 26].

Implications for Aeromedical Evacuation

Epiglottitis can progress rapidly, within several hours, to complete airway occlusion. If epiglottitis is suspected prior to transport, the patient should be transferred immediately to a pediatric intensive care unit or, ideally, an operating room under the care of a physician experienced in difficult airway management [25, 26]. No further examination of the airway should occur, and all measures to keep the patient calm should be utilized by the AE crew. An intravenous third-generation cephalosporin (ceftriaxone, cefotaxime) is the empiric antibiotic of choice, but should likely be withheld until the airway is secure due to the noxious stimuli of IV placement or IM administration.

An artificial airway will be required in almost 70% of children and more than 20% of adults with acute epiglottitis [27]. It would be most prudent for an artificial airway to be established prior to AE for any patient who has suspected epiglottitis, due to the rapid deterioration that can occur. The decision to intubate if specialists are not available is difficult and may depend on multiple factors. This should be discussed with the accepting facility. Ideally, patients should go to the operating room (OR) for a definitive airway placed in controlled circumstances with ENT and anesthesia. Those who present with severe respiratory distress or actual airway obstruction will require oropharyngeal intubation or surgical intervention (e.g., cricothyrotomy) as part of the initial treatment. A partially open airway can be converted to complete airway obstruction with injudicious maneuvers (e.g., foreign bodies, stable epiglottitis).

If a patient meeting these criteria does not have an artificial airway established prior to AE, they must be closely observed during flight and monitored by pulse oximetry. Administration of humidified oxygen (2 L/minute by nasal prongs) is advisable. If acute respiratory obstruction occurs during flight, facemask ventilation might be attempted prior to intubation. However, high ventilation pressures will likely be required to overcome the resistance of the severely narrowed airway, necessitating a two-handed facemask seal and high oxygen flow rates. Adequate ventilation should be determined by adequate chest wall movement and O_2 saturation of >90% by pulse oximetry. Placement of an endotracheal tube is often extremely difficult. If intubation is not possible and equipment for surgical cricothyrotomy is not available, a needle cricothyroidotomy may be lifesaving.

Seizure Disorders

The most recent Neurocritical Care Society guideline for status epilepticus defines status epilepticus as "5 minutes or more of (i) continuous clinical and/or electrographic seizure activity or (ii) recurrent seizure activity without recovery (return to baseline) between seizures." [28] Seizure etiologies are many and include febrile convulsions (a cause rarely found in adults), metabolic derangements (electrolyte disturbances, hypoglycemia), sepsis, central nervous system (CNS) infection, CNS injury, CNS tumor, drug toxicity or withdrawal, and preexisting epilepsy. However, many seizures are idiopathic, with only 15–20% of children presenting with status epilepticus having an acute symptomatic cause [29]. It is worth noting that both nonconvulsive status epilepticus and refractory status epilepticus have significantly worse mortality rates [28].

Treatment of Seizures

In the convulsing patient, initial supportive, therapeutic, and diagnostic measures need to be conducted simultaneously. The goal of anticonvulsant treatment is the rapid termination of clinical and electrical seizure activity by the prompt administration of appropriate drugs in adequate doses. Attention must be given to the possibility of complicating apnea, hypoventilation, and other metabolic abnormalities. The initial treatment of status epilepticus must involve management of the airway, breathing, and circulation while administering seizure abortive medications, assessing for the underlying cause, and immediately treating any life-threatening causes [28].

Oxygenation

Hypoxemia can be both the cause and consequence of a seizure. In severe episodes, hypoxemia can lead to bradycardia and hypotension. Airway management should occur immediately, and initial treatment is airway maintenance by proper positioning of the head and neck and administration of oxygen, if needed [28]. Oral airways are typically avoided in the setting of seizures as the mouth is clenched shut, so nasopharyngeal airways are utilized. Oxygen should be administered by mask or cannula or ventilation with a bag-valve-mask. In prolonged seizures or when higher doses of antiepileptic drugs causing respiratory depression are necessary, endotracheal intubation should be considered. Intubation may be difficult with an actively seizing patient, and administration of long-acting neuromuscular blocking agents to facilitate intubation is not recommended unless rapid electroencephalogram (EEG) placement can occur to monitor seizure activity. Therefore, priority should be given to administration of antiepileptic drugs, as intubation will be easier to accomplish once seizure activity has stopped.

Maintain Normal Blood Pressure

Hypotension can exacerbate any already existing malfunction of cerebral physiology and function. Hypotension can result from diminished cardiac output, poor vascular tone, or as a result of antiepileptic drug administration that are negative inotropes. Additionally, the underlying pathology causing seizures may contribute to hypotension. Systolic blood pressure and mean arterial pressure should be maintained with fluid resuscitation and vasopressor support to avoid hypotension [28].

Maintain Normal Glucose

Hypoglycemia is a common cause of seizures in children. If hypoglycemia (blood glucose <40 mg/dL) is documented or if it is impossible to obtain the measurement, standard pediatric hypoglycemia treatment should be employed (dextrose 0.5 gm/kg IV; e.g., D25W 2 ml/kg IV). In adult patients when thiamine deficiency is possible due to chronic alcohol use, thiamine should be administered prior to glucose administration. Lastly, pyridoxine (100 mg IV) should be considered for all young pediatric patients presenting with status epilepticus [28, 29].

Administer Antiseizure Medications

The overall goal is to obtain definitive control of status epilepticus as soon as possible [28]. Benzodiazepines are the emergent agent of choice, with IV lorazepam being the preferred. Lorazepam should be administered 0.1 mg/kg IV and may be repeated every 5 minutes up to 4 mg total dose. If there is no IV access, consider midazolam IM, buccal, or intranasal or diazepam rectally. Levetiracetam is increasingly used early due to little cardiopulmonary effects and is dosed 20–60 mg/kg IV push, maximum 3 gm. Second-line agents include fosphenytoin 20 mg PE/kg IV or phenobarbital 20 mg/kg IV, the latter preferred for infants under 6 months. For refractory seizures, consider inducing a medical coma with high-dose pentobarbital or midazolam infusion.

Diabetes Mellitus

Diabetes mellitus is one of the most common chronic diseases among pediatric populations. The two most significant problems associated with diabetes are hypoglycemia due to insulin administration and diabetic ketoacidosis, both of which are potentially severe problems during AE.

Hypoglycemia

All possible measures should be taken to avert severe hypoglycemia in diabetic children. These may include regular monitoring of blood glucose, decreasing insulin dosages, altering insulin regimens for patients with prior severe hypoglycemia, or administering slowly released carbohydrate (e.g., uncooked cornstarch) [30].

Mild-to-moderate hypoglycemia (blood glucose <100 mg/dL) is treated with oral glucose-containing solutions followed by complex carbohydrate. Self-treatment is usually in the form of 4 oz. of juice or soft drink followed by a cookie or candy. Blood glucose testing should be repeated within 30 minutes to ensure resolution of hypoglycemia.

Severe hypoglycemia cannot be identified by a fixed blood glucose value but rather by noticing the physiological symptoms of hypoglycemia, including diaphoresis, tremors, fatigue, dizziness, nausea, vomiting, headache, confusion, or loss of consciousness [31]. When the child is unable to take oral glucose-containing solutions, treatment consists of IV glucose 0.5 g/kg (2 ml/kg of 25% glucose solution) or glucagon administration. Both of these medications should be available when moving insulin-dependent diabetics in the AE system.

The Glucagon Emergency Kit (Eli Lilly and Co, Indianapolis, IN) contains a vial of powdered glucagon (1 mg) together with a syringe prefilled with 1 mL of diluting solution. After reconstitution, children <20 kg are given 0.5 mL by subcutaneous (SC), IM, or IV injection. Larger children and adults are given 1 mL. The time of onset of action varies from 1 to 10 minutes, and the duration of effect ranges from 9 to 32 minutes, depending on the dose and route of administration. The dose may be repeated in 15 minutes, and IV glucose should be administered as soon as available.

Diabetic Ketoacidosis

Diabetic ketoacidosis (DKA) is the most common cause of hospitalization of children with diabetes and has a fatality rate of 0.15–0.3% [32]. DKA is preceded by hyperglycemia secondary to insulin deficiency, either relative or absolute. The resulting decrease in glucose uptake induces hyperketonemia. Both the hyperglycemia and hyperketonemia cause an osmotic diuresis that manifests clinically as dehydration and increased thirst. The dehydration is often worsened by hyperventilation and vomiting that can be either a part of the primary precipitating illness or resulting from the acidosis due to ketosis. Eventually, the hyperosmolality associated with untreated DKA can progress to coma and even death as a result of intracerebral crisis or cardiovascular collapse.

Diabetic children should be evaluated for ketonuria if they have either persistent hyperglycemia (blood glucose >180 mg/dL) or a serious intercurrent illness. Diagnostic criteria for DKA are blood glucose >200 mg/dL, venous pH <7.3 or bicarbonate <15 mmol/L, ketonemia, and ketonuria. The primary goals of therapy are correct dehydration, correct acidosis and reverse ketosis, slowly correct hyperosmolality, restore blood glucose to near normal, monitor for complications of DKA and its treatment, and identify and treat any precipitating event [32].

Initial fluid therapy is aimed at restoring intravascular status and hemodynamic stability due to resulting dehydration. Level of dehydration is difficult to assess but can be assumed to be 5–7% in moderate DKA and 7–10% in severe DKA. Dehydration ≥10% is suggested by weak pulses, oliguria, and hypotension [32]. Volume expansion with 0.9% NaCl should begin immediately with 10–20 mL/kg over 1–2 hours. If peripheral perfusion or blood pressure is not restored with the initial bolus, further bolus doses should be given until this result is achieved. If the patient with DKA presents in shock, 0.9% saline 20 ml/kg should be administered rapidly by large-bore IV [32]. After initial fluid resuscitation, an isotonic fluid, either 0.9% saline, Ringer's lactate, or PlasmaLyte, should be administered at 1.5–2 times calculated maintenance fluid rate for 4–6 hours. Maintenance fluid rate can be calculated by body surface area (1500 ml/m^2/day) or the Holliday-Segar calculation based on body weight (1000 mL for the first 10 kg + 500 mL for the next 10 kg + 20 mL/kg for over 20 kg). In the hospital environment, after the initial 4–6 hours, fluids are changed to hypotonic saline (0.45% saline) with added potassium chloride, potassium phosphate, or potassium acetate, based on patient serum electrolytes. However, given that AE transport rarely exceeds 6–8 hours, continuation of fluid management with isotonic fluid without additives should be sufficient. Bicarbonate therapy is not recommended – potentially causing paradoxical CNS acidosis – but may be necessary if the patient has life-threatening hyperkalemia [32].

Insulin therapy is often initiated 1–2 hours after starting fluid therapy. Blood glucose should be measured after fluid resuscitation prior to starting the insulin infusion. Insulin is administered at 0.05 or 0.1 U/kg per hour by continuous-infusion pump, with studies showing no difference in outcome between the two doses [32]. Lower doses can be utilized if the patient shows a higher degree of insulin sensitivity; i.e., glucose decreases >90 mg/dl per hour. Considering the typical short duration of AE movement and the extensive patient monitoring required, insulin administration is typically withheld during transport until the patient arrives at a tertiary care center, as long as fluid administration is ongoing.

During initial fluid expansion, elevated blood glucose levels can be expected to drop rapidly, potentially 10–15 mmol/L (180–250 mg/dL), even without insulin infusion. In general, rapid changes in serum osmolarity (sodium and glucose) are to be avoided, as this is associated with increased risk of worsening cerebral edema. Once insulin therapy is initiated, the goal is to decrease serum glucose level no more than 5 mmol/L/hr. (90 mg/dL/hr) [32]. If the blood glucose level decreases more than 5 mmol/L/hr. or below the absolute threshold of 17 mmol/L (300 mg/dL), 5% or 10% dextrose should be added to the IV fluids. If serum glucose thresholds are still exceeded despite the addition of 10% dextrose to the IV fluids, further options include adding up to 12.5 dextrose to peripheral IV fluids, increasing fluid administration rates (not to exceed 2.5 times maintenance), or decreasing insulin infusion rate. Ideally, insulin infusion rates will not be decreased below 0.05 units/hr. to prevent recurrence of DKA, but this may be necessary to avert hypoglycemia or precipitous glucose fall. Placement of a central venous line is generally not necessary and intravascular access other than peripheral IV should be avoided due to the higher risk of thrombosis associated with DKA [32].

Cerebral edema represents the most life-threatening complication of DKA, with patients being at risk for cerebral herniation. GCS and other signs of neurological status (e.g., pupillary size and response) should be monitored very closely and frequently. Any deteriorations in neurological status should be considered an emergency. Recommendations against bicarbonate use and insulin bolus administration have reduced rates of cerebral complications and herniation, likely due to diminished shifts in serum osmolarity. If CNS deterioration occurs, the patient with DKA should be treated with emergent protocols for elevated intracranial pressure (ICP), including rapid hypertonic saline administration and hyperventilation. Endotracheal intubation should be avoided due to the risk of increased ICP due to hypoventilation during the intubation and should only be considered after hyperosmotic therapy. If intubation is necessary, careful attention should be made to match their previous minute ventilation to compensate for the metabolic acidosis [32].

Patient monitoring in a hospital setting is extensive and includes monitoring of electrolytes, including sodium, potassium, chloride, and glucose, CNS status, indicators of kidney function, and assessing hydration status. Given the limitations of AE, monitoring during flight should be recorded at 30-minute intervals and include vital signs, GCS score (see Chap. 12), blood glucose, and urine ketones. In addition, fluid intake and output, and insulin administration should be carefully recorded.

Other Pediatric Conditions with Aeromedical Evacuation Implications

Otitis Media and Ear Block

The failure to equilibrate tympanic cavity and atmospheric pressures, usually during descent of an aircraft, can result in aerotitis media (i.e., "aviation otitis"). This acute and potentially chronic inflammation of the middle ear is the result of Eustachian tube obstruction and is especially prone to occur in the presence of an upper respiratory tract infection or otitis media. Preschool-aged children appear to be in particular susceptible to ear pain during both ascent and descent phases of air travel [33].

Certainly, avoiding air travel with acute upper respiratory tract infection or otitis media is ideal. However, air travel may sometimes be required, and these conditions are so common that flying with an undiagnosed otitis media may be unavoidable. Common strategies to prevent or alleviate this condition include chewing, yawning, and swallowing during ascent and especially during descent. Some physicians advocate the administration of oral or nasal decongestants and/or antihistamines prior to take-off because this approach has been found to be effective in adults [34]. For children, administration of oral pseudoephedrine hydrochloride (1 mg/kg, using a 6-mg/mL syrup) 30–60 minutes prior to departure may have some benefit in decreasing the incidence of aerotitis media.

Sickle Cell Disease

Sickle cell disease is an inherited blood disorder that affects about 100,000 Americans, mostly African-Americans [35]. It leaves patients vulnerable to repeated crises that can cause severe pain, multisystem organ damage, and early death. A large study sponsored by the National Institutes of Health published in 1994 showed that almost 15% of children die before the age of 20, most often from infections; but newer studies after the introduction of efficacious vaccinations show reductions in mortality of 68% for children aged 0–3 years, 39% for children aged 4–9 years, and 24% for children aged 10–14 years [35, 36]. The median age of death for patients with sickle cell disease is 42 years for females and 39 years for males, and newer studies have not shown any change in adult mortality [36, 37].

Sickle Cell Pain Crises

Sickle cell pain crises (vaso-occlusive crisis) are acute painful episodes that typically last for 5–7 days but may last for only minutes or persist for weeks. These crises are usually triggered by a physiological stress, such as acute infection, dehydration, extremely hot or cold temperatures, or hypoxia. The result is deoxygenated HbS, which forms rod-like polymers that change the normally round and pliable red blood cells into stiff, sickle-shaped cells. These deformed cells cause vaso-occlusion, which results in a cycle of localized tissue hypoxia leading to further sickling and additional vaso-occlusion. The end result may be tissue infarction and necrosis.

The pain of a sickle cell crisis can be localized or diffuse, constant or intermittent. About half of all patients will also have fever, swelling in the joints of the hands or feet, longbone pain, tachypnea, hypertension, nausea, and vomiting. In the severest forms, organ infarction will manifest. Spleen infarction, usually resulting in severe abdominal pain, has been reported in patients with previously asymptomatic sickle cell trait during unpressurized flight [38]. Rib and/or lung infarction results in an acute chest syndrome consisting of chest pain, dyspnea, fever, and leukocytosis. Other severe manifestations include stroke, pulmonary fat embolism, and seizures [36].

Implications for Aeromedical Evacuation

Many of the stresses associated with AE (e.g., dehydration, extremely hot or cold temperatures, and hypoxia) are known to be triggers for sickle cell crises. For this reason, special efforts should be made to maintain a comfortable cabin temperature with the liberal use of blankets when needed. In addition, all patients with sickle cell disease should be well hydrated, either by frequent drinking or IV fluids.

The need for oxygen during flight remains controversial. Hypoxia associated with increased altitude is known to increase the incidence of sickle cell crises [38]. Nevertheless, sickle cell crises during air travel in pressurized aircraft are extremely uncommon [39]. In general, patients with sickle cell disease can fly on commercial airline flights without supplemental oxygen. However, if a patient is being transported by AE because of a complication associated with their sickle cell disease (i.e., pain crisis, stroke, etc.), it seems prudent to give supplemental oxygen during flight because of the certain health risks associated with crises and is generally indicated to maintain oxygen saturation >95% [40].

Treatment of Sickle Cell Pain Crises

If a patient is transported during a sickle cell pain crisis or a crisis occurs in-flight, the treatment is primarily supportive. The patient should be placed on supplemental oxygen to maintain oxygen saturation >95%. IV hydration with an isotonic solution will help reverse any degree of dehydration, especially in patients experiencing vomiting or known to have kidney impairment.

Pain control is an important aspect of early treatment. Severe pain should be treated with nonsteroidal anti-inflammatory drugs and IV morphine or hydromorphone. Meperidine is no longer recommended due to its side effect profile. Pain medications should be titrated aggressively every 30 minutes, with consideration of increasing doses by 25% until pain is well controlled, and utilization of patient-controlled analgesia (PCA) should be considered [40]. Other additional nonpharmacologic methods, such as heat therapy, may be effective. Once the acute crisis subsides, oral narcotics (e.g., oxycodone or hydrocodone) may be used. It is usually a matter of days until patients are switched to non-narcotic oral analgesics.

The patient must be monitored carefully for signs of oversedation, and naloxone should be readily available in the event of respiratory depression. Other common narcotic side effects include constipation, urinary retention, pruritus, nausea, and vomiting. Diphenhydramine can be given orally for itching and ondansetron may be required to reduce nausea. Additionally, incentive spirometry should be encouraged to prevent acute chest syndrome, and the patient should be screened for other severe complications of sickle cell disease, which may occur simultaneously, such as fever, acute chest syndrome, and acute splenic sequestration.

Pediatric Trauma

Unintentional injuries remain the leading cause of death for all pediatric age groups, with dramatic increases for under 1 year of age and 15–24 years of age [41]. The more common causes of pediatric trauma are motor vehicle accidents, drowning, house fires, homicides, falls, and nonaccidental trauma. Among these, traumatic brain injury is a leading cause of pediatric morbidity and mortality [42]. Differences in development and anatomy cause prepubescent children to be at greater risk for specific injuries and complications.

Due to comparatively larger head size, flexible spinal ligaments, and other vertebral boney developmental differences, younger children and infants are at risk of cervical spinal cord injuries. Cervical spine precautions must be strictly followed. Any injury to the sympathetic nervous system in the upper cervical spine can cause an inadequate patient response to hypoxemia and hemodynamic compromise, causing rapid patient decompensation if not managed appropriately. If upper spinal cord injury is suspected, hypoxemia should be quickly managed and vasoactive infusions may be necessary to stabilize the patient.

Pneumothorax and Pulmonary Contusion

The chest wall of pediatric patients is more compliant, placing the pediatric patient at greater risk of pulmonary contusion and pulmonary barotrauma resulting in pneumothorax [43]. Transport teams should maintain a high suspicion of pneumothorax with any acute respiratory, and potentially hemodynamic, deterioration in the pediatric trauma patient. Pneumothorax can be immediately life-threatening and should be managed similar to adult patients with needle/finger decompression and chest tube placement. No differences exist in the procedure of needle decompression between adults and children, other than considering a smaller angiocath (e.g., 18 ga instead of 14 ga) for the procedure. If the AE team has the appropriate skills and equipment, chest tube placement can occur. A pneumothorax will expand at higher altitudes with lower barometric pressure, and a chest tube should be placed prior to air transport, or the patient may require repeated needle decompression during flight, which is not optimal. Chest tubes should be on suction or have a Heimlich valve attached. Difficulties with respiratory function due to pulmonary contusion typically manifest less acutely, but usually require increased positive end-expiratory pressure (PEEP), either by intubation and mechanical ventilation or continuous positive airway pressure/bilevel positive airway pressure (CPAP/BiPAP), which place the pediatric patient at further risk of pneumothorax.

Intra-Abdominal Injury

Pediatric patients have an increased risk of intra-abdominal injury with trauma, which can cause significant hemodynamic compromise. The abdominal wall muscles are less developed and thinner and therefore offer less protection to abdominal organs and greater transference of energy. The spleen and liver are relatively bigger and often sit below the lowest ribs, making these organs further susceptible to injury. Injury to the highly vascular liver and spleen may cause hemodynamic compromise and should be appropriately managed with fluid and blood component resuscitation following Advanced Trauma Life Support (ATLS) guidelines. The bladder is positioned incompletely in the pelvis and rides up into the abdominal compartment. Injury to the bladder or hollow viscous organs may cause peritoneal signs and should be managed with appropriate fluid resuscitation and immediate surgical evaluation at the receiving medical facility. There are no specific procedures utilized by AE teams to address intra-abdominal injuries, and all require immediate evaluation by a surgical team.

Hypotension

In the pediatric patient, hemodynamic compromise can be difficult to determine and should be treated aggressively. Hypotension is a late and ominous finding. Pediatric patients will typically manifest tachycardia as the initial finding, and transport teams must have an understanding of the variation of normal heart rate and blood pressure by age group and should carry a reference for pediatric vital signs. Above the age of 12 years, adult vital signs are considered normal for the pediatric patient. Below the age of

10 years, systolic hypotension is defined by the formula:

$$70 + 2 \times \text{age}(\text{years})$$

Hypotension should be avoided and aggressively treated; two peripheral IVs (PIVs) should be placed to facilitate fluid and blood component administration. Appropriate IV size will vary by age.

If PIVs cannot be placed, 1–2 pediatric intraosseous lines (IOs) should be inserted. Common pediatric IO sites include the proximal tibial plateau, distal medial tibia, distal femur, and proximal humerus. IO placement should be avoided in extremity fracture proximal to the site of insertion and with underlying bone diseases (e.g., osteogenesis imperfecta), while overlying skin infection is a relative contraindication [44].

Crystalloids should generally be avoided in the setting of hemorrhagic shock. Blood products are typically administered in aliquots of 10–20 ml/kg depending on patient severity and ongoing bleeding. Massive transfusion protocols should be utilized for patients requiring 40 ml/kg of blood products and should approach a 1:1:1 RBC:plasma:platelet ratio as much as is possible [43]. Estimated circulating blood volume is approximately 85–100 ml/kg for neonates, 75–90 ml/kg for infants <6 months, 70–80 ml/kg for 6 months to 12 years, and 65–75 ml/kg for children >12 years [45]. Since infusions and medications are volume based for pediatrics, knowing the patient weight is key, but often unavailable to the AE team. The Broselow tape is commonly used to estimate patient weight, and that, or similar method, should be carried by the transport team in case weight cannot be accurately ascertained.

Traumatic Brain Injury

Pediatric traumatic brain injury (TBI) is one particular subset of trauma patients that may have improved outcomes with shorter injury-to-hospital duration, presumably due to availability of neurosurgical intervention and advanced therapies at the Level 1 trauma center [46]. The transport team may be providing care of a patient both before and after advanced interventions. In general, prevention of secondary injury is the primary goal. It has been clearly shown that hypoxemia and hypotension are associated with worse outcomes. Additionally, serum glucose alterations are detrimental, and increased intracranial pressure (ICP) is associated with worse outcomes [47]. The Brain Trauma Foundation published an update to extensive pediatric TBI guidelines most recently in 2012, but protocol-based application of these guidelines may vary by hospital system and locale [47].

Signs and symptoms of intracranial hypertension are variable, and elevated ICP cannot be accurately determined without direct measurement. A recent study showed that nearly 75% of children with severe traumatic brain injury (GCS ≤ 8) had elevated ICP by direct measurement upon admission to a trauma center [48]. In general, any child with GCS ≤ 8 should be presumed to have increased ICP and be treated accordingly [47]. When a monitoring device has been placed, ICP should be maintained ≤20 mm Hg, although some studies suggest a lower threshold of 15 mm Hg is more appropriate for children <2 years. Cerebral perfusion pressure (CPP), which is calculated as mean arterial pressure (MAP) minus ICP (CPP = MAP − ICP), should be maintained in the range of 40–50 mm Hg for neonates and 50–60 mm Hg for pediatrics, versus 60 mm Hg for adults. Ideally, an arterial monitoring catheter will be placed prior to transport. If there is no monitor placed for ICP measurement, every effort should be made to avoid hypotension.

Early intubation is recommended for severe TBI, and SpO_2 should be maintained >90% for all patients with TBI. Endotracheal intubation should be attempted by an experienced provider utilizing rapid sequence intubation to minimize periods of hypoventilation (which can dramatically increase ICP) and improve success rates [49]. Therefore, transport team composition should be adjusted accordingly. Intubation can be accomplished with etomidate (0.3 mg/kg IV) or ketamine (1–2 mg/kg) and succinylcholine (1 mg/kg IV). Cuffed endotracheal tubes (ETTs) are typically utilized for all pediatric patients, and appropriate ETT size can be estimated by the formula:

$$3.5 + \text{age}(\text{years})/4$$

ETT depth is estimated by the formula:

$$3 \times \text{ETT size}$$

However, appropriate placement in the trachea should be confirmed by standard methods, including equal chest rise and breath sounds, which could be difficult to auscultate during transport. Endotracheal intubation should be completed, when needed, prior to patient transport. Ideally end-tidal CO_2 monitoring should be provided in all head-trauma patients, in addition to routine SpO_2 monitoring; otherwise, repeated blood gas analysis, at least every 1 hour, will be required to track arterial CO_2.

The pediatric brain-injured patient should be kept well sedated and provided adequate analgesia during transport to prevent increased ICP, ideally with agents that are both short-acting, to facilitate repeated neuroexamination and have minimal effects on hemodynamics, and to prevent hypotension and maintain adequate CPP. Fentanyl (starting dose 1 mcg/kg/hr) and versed (starting dose 0.1 mg/kg/hr) are often utilized, although there are no uniform recommendations. Ketamine is no longer thought to increase ICP and can be a useful adjunct or primary agent instead of fentanyl and versed, considering its minimal hemodynamic effects. Propofol can be utilized for short periods, but should be avoided in children <12 years of age for use over 24 hours due to the US Food and Drug Administration (FDA) warning relating to propofol infusion syndrome. Propofol may also contribute to hypotension, which should be monitored. Neuromuscular blocking agents may be utilized to diminish coughing and shivering, and to facilitate intubation, but are typically avoided due to impairment of neurological exam; they should have a short half-life if utilized (e.g., succinylcholine or rocuronium). If ICP elevation is suspected or confirmed, hypertonic saline (3%) should be administered by IV bolus over 15–20 minutes, with the recommend dose of 5–10 ml/kg, and may be repeated every 1–2 hours [47]. Mannitol can be utilized at a dose of 0.5–1 g/kg, but with extreme caution because of its diuretic properties and potential to contribute to hypotension.

Both hyperthermia and hypothermia can be harmful to TBI patients, so in general, the goal during transport is normothermia. Additionally, hypothermia can cause shivering, which may elevate ICP. IV acetaminophen 15 mg/kg can help control pyrexia and additionally provides analgesia.

If an external ventricular drain (EVD) has been placed, the transport team should request cerebrospinal fluid (CSF) drainage goals and hourly limits, as well as drain height set point. The benefits of ICP drainage have not been clearly delineated in the pediatric population, but ICP drainage during periods of acute ICP elevation may be helpful and should be attempted. The transport team will need to adequately secure the EVD and zero the monitor upon loading on the transport vehicle. If there is any evidence of pneumocephaly on initial imaging, surgical removal or craniectomy with decompression will be required prior to air transport and a cabin-altitude restriction of 3000–4000 ft. should be utilized, due to the risk of herniation due to air expansion at higher altitudes.

Therapeutic hyperventilation to reduce ICP should only be utilized for extremely increased ICP and threatening herniation. Prolonged hyperventilation can lead to cerebral vasoconstriction and ischemia. In general, arterial pCO_2 should be maintained 35–40 mm Hg, avoiding hyperventilation to <30 mm Hg during the first 48 hours and elevations of arterial CO_2 at all times, when the concern for increased ICP exists [47].

Hypoglycemia, hyperglycemia, and hyponatremia can be detrimental to the head-injured patient. During transport, normal saline should be run at maintenance rates IV, as detailed previously per the Holliday-Seagar calculation, so as to avoid hyponatremia. If alterations in sodium and water regulation occur (e.g., cerebral salt wasting or syndrome of inappropriate antidiuretic hormone), hypertonic 3% saline can be utilized. Typically, goal serum sodium is >140 mEq/L or 150–160 for elevated ICP. Glucose-containing fluids should be initially avoided, and routine glucose and electrolyte analysis should occur. Even in infants, the stress response to trauma typically prevents hypoglycemia, but dextrose-containing maintenance fluids may be necessary.

The incidence of post-traumatic seizure is approximately 10%, although higher in nonaccidental trauma [42, 47]. Post-traumatic seizure prophylaxis is often recommended with fosphenytoin 20 mEq/kg IV or levetiracetam 20 mg/kg IV [47]. Seizures should be treated aggressively, per the guidelines presented previously in the section "Status Epilepticus."

Other measures that should be utilized are maintaining the head-of-bed elevation at 30 degrees and minimizing airway suctioning and irritation to prevent coughing.

Neonatal Transport

The transition from fetus to neonate involves a miraculous combination of physiological processes. One of the most challenging is establishing independence from the respiratory, circulatory, and homeostatic functions performed by the placenta. As a result, many perturbations can occur in the transition to extrauterine life.

The skills and knowledge required for neonatal AE are very unique. The following section will discuss the timing and special preparations necessary for successful neonatal AE. This will be followed with a discussion of the more common neonatal problems that require transportation and their implications for AE.

Timing for Aeromedical Evacuation

The timing of AE transport of a neonate is dependent on the clinical status of the neonate, as well as the comfort of the referring physician and/or capabilities of the referral facility in providing adequate care for the neonate. Many neonatal transports are carried out on an urgent/emergent basis. If the referral facility has the capabilities, the preference would be to transport a stable patient, but that is often not the case. There needs to be discussion between the physicians at the referring and receiving facilities to determine the most appropriate timing for transport. Parents must consent to transfer with a clear understanding of the risks of transport and their child's prognosis.

Preparation for Aeromedical Evacuation

Careful preparation is necessary prior to neonatal AE to minimize the risk of this often hazardous undertaking. A suggested checklist of this complex process is included in Table 22.2.

Data Collection Prior to Aeromedical Evacuation

The collection of pediatric data is similar to adult data with a few exceptions. For neonatal transport, the mother's history of pregnancy, labor, and delivery becomes important. The neonate's weight, Apgar scores, and gestational age are additional items, as well as confirmation of vitamin K, erythromycin, and hepatitis B vaccine administration. The use of a standardized data collection form for pediatric and neonatology patients is recommended.

Vascular Access

Vascular access with an umbilical venous catheter and umbilical arterial catheter is desirable. The umbilical arterial catheter or a peripheral arterial catheter can be used to continuously monitor blood pressure and provide ease in drawing blood samples. A peripheral intravenous catheter can allow more therapeutic flexibility for administration of fluids and medications that are not compatible. Because heat, vibration, and acceleration–deceleration forces of flight can dislodge adhesives, the team must be ready to reinforce or replace the adhesive on all tubes and lines if they appear unstable.

Table 22.2 Premature neonate aeromedical evacuation checklist

Baseline vital signs and all monitors applied
Vascular access
Umbilical artery and vein
Peripheral intravascular access (as indicated)
Adhesive reinforcement
Skin protection
Thermal management
Incubator prewarmed
Ambient air
Plastic wrap or bowel bag (as indicated)
Thermal mattress (as indicated)
Incubator cover
Preflight imaging
Endotracheal tube placement confirmed
Central line placement confirmed
Chest X-ray
Chest tube care
Heimlich valve
Suction available
Preflight laboratory
Arterial blood gas
Complete blood count
Anemia therapy when indicated
Antibiotic therapy when indicated
Blood glucose normal, dextrose infusion started
Full monitoring applied with gel electrocardiogram leads
Orogastric/nasogastric tube
Sedation adequate
Urethral catheter considered
Patient securing straps applied
Check lines, cables, hoses, and tubing for security and connections
Hearing protection
Parental considerations
Time given for bonding
Consent signed for transport and procedures
Crew alert
Prewarmed cabin
Altitude limitations
Nonmedical attendant
Bring copies of all images and infant's chart

Thermal Management

Closely controlled thermal management will minimize the potentially severe problems associated with hypothermia. The ambient air should be kept 24 ° C or greater in both the ground ambulances and aircraft. The incubator servo-temperature should be set at 36 ° C. A chemical thermal mattress and a cover over the incubator may help maintain temperature in transport, especially in large aircraft cabins. Plastic wrap or bowel bags will minimize evaporative heat loss.

Risk of hyperthermia must also be taken into consideration, particularly during hot summer months. The inside of the transport Isolette can get very hot when there are delays on flight lines or on the ground in aircraft/ambulances with minimal temperature regulation and can lead to hyperthermia and heat stress.

Respiratory Management

One of the most common reasons requiring neonatal transport is respiratory distress. Respiratory distress can be due to respiratory, cardiac, or metabolic conditions or any combination of the three. A decision must be made as to the required respiratory support that will be needed for transport. Due to the limitations of auscultation, visibility, and space en route, intubation can be extremely difficult. If there is any doubt as to their respiratory reserve, the neonate should be intubated and placed on a ventilator prior to transport. Other conditions such as prematurity, seizures, and use of Prostin can also be associated with apnea, so there may need to be a decision to electively intubate prior to transport of these infants with the plan to wean from ventilator support at the receiving institution.

In most cases, respiratory function should be stable prior to AE. In the rare situation where stability cannot be achieved, it must be clear that the benefits of advanced diagnostics and therapeutics at the receiving hospital outweigh the risks of continued resuscitation during flight. If surfactant has been given, the neonate should be observed carefully for signs of improving lung function (e.g., improved chest expansion, improved oxygen saturation) and consideration given to appropriately adjusting ventilator settings prior to movement. Narcotic and sedative therapy (e.g., morphine and midazolam) should be used at doses low enough to avoid respiratory suppression in an effort to promote comfort, control pain, and minimize swings in blood pressure.

As altitude increases, the effective percentage of oxygen in the atmosphere decreases, so neonates very often become more hypoxic at altitude. If the neonate is ventilator dependent and/or requiring a high FiO_2, an altitude restriction may be required to maintain a cabin altitude <2000 ft. in order to mitigate worsening hypoxia. The neonate should be stabilized on the ventilator that is going to be used for transport as far ahead of transport as possible, and ideally, a baseline blood gas should be obtained prior to transport. The ventilator should be connected to hospital medical gases so that the ventilator tank gas can be preserved for transport. A heat moisture exchanger (HME) or some other humidification device should be placed in line to maximize airway humidification and help prevent thick secretions. Even a minor pneumothorax should be treated with a chest tube connected to a Heimlich valve prior to AE because trapped pleural air expands at altitude.

A set of arterial blood gases and serum chemistries should be reevaluated as close to the time of transport as feasible, both to help make ventilator adjustments and guide fluid therapy. Ideally, arterial blood gases on the current ventilator settings should reveal pH >7.25, $PaCO_2$ 40–50 mm Hg, and PaO_2 60–90 mm Hg (exception: pulmonary hypertension; see below). The base deficit should be 5 or better.

Psychosocial Considerations

Every effort should be made to establish a warm and empathetic relationship with the family. The parents are often expecting the birth of a healthy baby, and a deviation from the expected can create significant distress for the parents. They will likely be anxious about the transport of their baby and the potential separation of mother and baby. Every effort should be made to allow the mother to see the baby prior to transport. Ideally, one or both parents should be transported as nonmedical attendants and, if possible, the family unit transported back to the referring hospital as soon as the need for special care has been eliminated.

Final Preparation for Aeromedical Evacuation

Immediately prior to AE, several details must be accomplished. Upon examining the neonate for the last time in the referring facility, a transport flow sheet should be started. Full electronic monitoring should be instituted (temperature, blood pressure, heart rate, respiratory rate, and oxygen saturation) using gel leads to maintain skin integrity. An orogastric (OG) tube should be placed and secured to minimize the effect of swallowed intestinal air on diaphragmatic movement. The OG tube should remain open to allow for gas expansion at altitude. A chest X-ray should confirm all of the following: an OG tube tip in the stomach, ET tube placement in middle third of the trachea, eight to nine rib lung inflation, absence of air-leaks, a normal cardiac silhouette, and appropriate locations of any central lines (e.g., umbilical arterial, umbilical venous, or peripherally inserted central catheters).

Earplugs or muffs should be placed on the neonate (and any nonmedical and medical attendants) to protect hearing. To limit motion during transport, the neonate must be secured adequately with straps with the ET tube clearly visible.

Specific Neonatal Conditions

Prematurity

Extreme prematurity (less than 28 weeks) and the associated extremely low birthweight (<1000 g) create a few of the greatest challenges found in AE, as these neonates often have multiple conditions that make their care extremely complex (Table 22.3). Less extreme degrees of prematurity usually have fewer and less severe forms of these related conditions.

One problem unique to the extremely premature infant is fragile skin. Above all, the skin must be handled gently. To minimize denuded skin and the associated infectious risks, DuoDERM should be applied to the skin prior to use of adherent tape (i.e., when securing the ETT or applying the O_2 sat probe).

Table 22.3 Conditions and complications commonly encountered in extremely premature and extremely low birthweight neonates

Difficult vascular access
Hypothermia
Respiratory distress syndrome
Air leak syndrome
Apnea
Intraventricular hemorrhage
Hypoxia
Hypercarbia
Respiratory and metabolic acidosis
Patent ductus arteriosus
Shock (distributive or cardiogenic)
Disseminated intravascular coagulation
Bacterial or viral infection
Hypoglycemia
Hyponatremia
Hypocalcemia
Hyperkalemia
Immature renal and gastrointestinal function
Limited skin integrity
Increased insensible fluid losses
Absence of parental bonding

Intravenous Fluid Management

Neonatal fluid management can be very challenging, especially in the extremely low birthweight (ELBW) infant. Maintenance fluids within the first 24 hours of life are typically D10W at 80–100 mL/kg per day and are adjusted to maintain hydration and euglycemia. Indicators of potential inadequate fluid replacement are tachycardia (heart rate >160 bpm), hypotension (mean blood pressure that is less than the neonate's gestational age), low urine output (<1 mL/kg per hour), poor capillary refill (>3 sec), a base deficit, or hypernatremia. If attempt at adequate fluid replacement has been met and hypotension or perfusion is still an issue, pressor therapy may be initiated, e.g., dopamine drip at 4–15 μ(mu)g/kg per minute or dobutamine drip at 5–15 μ(mu)g/kg per minute. A urethral catheter is rarely necessary because post-transport diaper weights are sufficient to measure urine output.

Metabolic acidosis is common in premature infants. Judicious use of normal saline boluses (10 mL/kg, repeated up to two to three times) may correct mild acidosis or flush acid out of the tissues in severe acidotic states. A 5% plasmanate or albumin bolus can be substituted in the presence of hypoalbuminemia. If the pH is below 7.20 due to a metabolic acidosis, sodium bicarbonate may be considered (although not routinely given) and carefully given by slow IV bolus (4.2%, 2–4 mL/kg). However, attempts must be made to identify the etiology of the metabolic acidosis and treat the underlying cause.

Intraventricular hemorrhage may be caused by large fluctuations in arterial blood pressure. For this reason, infusing any fluid boluses or flushing any lines at more than 1 mL/minute must be avoided. Therapeutic interventions (e.g., line placement and tracheal suctioning) may initiate or exacerbate intraventricular hemorrhage by temporarily increasing blood pressure, and thus, preprocedure sedation should be considered.

Disseminated Intravascular Coagulation

Disseminated intravascular coagulation (DIC) is suggested in a premature neonate by a platelet count <150,000/mm^3, a decreasing trend in platelet count, or persistent bleeding/oozing from any skin laceration or venous puncture site. If the diagnosis of DIC is made, the neonate should be treated with fresh frozen plasma and/or platelet transfusion prior to transport, especially with an accelerated drop or an absolute platelet count <50,000/mm^3 (consider lower threshold in the extremely preterm infant).

Infection

Bacterial infection is a common cause of prematurity. Ampicillin and gentamicin treatment is often initiated after blood cultures are taken. Cerebrospinal fluid culture is considered when the patient is physiologically stable. Acyclovir treatment for herpes simplex virus can be started based on history or suspicious physical exam.

Hypoglycemia

Hypoglycemia is one of the most common metabolic problems in premature infants. When low blood glucose levels are prolonged or recurrent, they may result in acute systemic effects and neurological sequelae. For this reason, the management of low blood glucose in the first postnatal days is essential [50].

At birth, the sudden discontinuation of the nutrient supply from the mother requires the neonate to mobilize glucose and fatty acids from glycogen and triglyceride depots to meet the energy demands. Unfortunately, infants born prematurely or exposed to certain intrauterine conditions (e.g., malnutrition, maternal diabetes, endogenous fetal hyperinsulinism) may be unable to mount an appropriate and adequate counterregulatory metabolic and endocrine response and thus develop abnormally low plasma glucose concentrations.

Clinical manifestations of hypoglycemia include tremor, sweating, lethargy, floppiness, coma, and seizures. In some cases, hypoglycemia is asymptomatic. However, it remains uncertain as to whether asymptomatic hypoglycemia actually causes brain damage.

Routine measurements of blood glucose concentration should be continued during AE for any infant known to be at risk for hypoglycemia. Glucose monitoring can be initiated as soon as possible after birth, within 2–3 hours after birth and before feeding, or at any time when there are abnormal signs. If the plasma glucose concentration remains <45 mg/dL (2.5 mmol/L) or if abnormal clinical signs develop, IV glucose infusion is administered to raise the plasma glucose.

Respiratory Distress

Increased work of breathing and elevated oxygen requirements can result from a number of conditions to include prematurity and meconium aspiration syndrome. Premature infants have a relative surfactant deficiency that often results in diffuse atelectasis and respiratory insufficiency termed “respiratory distress syndrome.” The frequency and severity of this disorder have been decreased by the use of antenatal steroids and postnatal surfactant administration.

Aspiration of meconium prior to and at the time of birth, termed “meconium aspiration syndrome,” continues to be a common event in both full-term and post-term infants. This syndrome is associated with focal areas of atelectasis, air trapping, and persistent pulmonary hypertension of the newborn with right-to-left shunting through the foramen ovale or ductus arteriosus (DA). Symptoms of respiratory distress can also occur as a result of congenital sepsis, pneumonia, or pulmonary hemorrhage.

Implications for Aeromedical Evacuation

Neonates with respiratory compromise are especially susceptible to the effects of altitude-related hypoxia. In all cases, an altitude restriction should be considered to maximum cabin altitudes <2000 ft. Prior to transport, a ventilator-dependent infant should be assessed for anemia and transfused, if necessary, with packed red blood cells to maintain the hematocrit above 35%.

A pulse oximeter to measure oxygen saturation and/or a portable laboratory device to measure blood gases should be used to assure that the patient is well oxygenated and adequately ventilated. Endotracheal tube suction should be done as needed during transport to clear increased secretions. It is especially important to maximize humidity in the airway through the use of an HME or other humidification device in line with the endotracheal tube.

The transport team must be prepared to identify and manage in-flight hypoxemia or pneumothorax. If a pneumothorax is suspected, it should be treated with needle decompression and chest tube placement (Betadine, 23-gauge butterfly needle, 3-way stopcock, 20-mL syringe, sterile gloves, scalpel, hemostat, and a chest tube).

Diaphragmatic Hernia

This congenital defect occurs in approximately 1 in 3000 live births. A diaphragmatic hernia results in abdominal organs entering the thorax, thus severely affecting lung growth and development. The defect is most commonly on the left side but can be on the right side or, rarely, bilateral. The key physical exam findings include a scaphoid abdomen, severe respiratory distress, shift of the heart sounds, and diminished or absent breath sounds on the affected side. Bowel sounds may be heard in the chest, but all too often are not present in the immediate postnatal period. The result is often a lethal combination of pulmonary hypoplasia and persistent pulmonary hypertension. These infants are at high risk of developing pneumothoraces following resuscitative efforts.

If the diagnosis is known prenatally, the infant should be intubated immediately after delivery. Positive pressure ventilation that is given via bag-valve-mask can cause insufflation of the bowel and result in further compressing already compromised lungs. It is also important that an orogastric tube be placed quickly and placed to continuous suction to keep the bowel decompressed.

Implications for Aeromedical Evacuation

An altitude restriction is recommended to maximum cabin altitudes <2000 ft. It is essential that the gastrointestinal tract remains decompressed and any pneumothorax is treated prior to AE. The impact of altitude-related expansion of gas in the thorax and intestine can be mitigated by placement of a chest tube connected to suction or a Heimlich valve and placement of an orogastric tube to continuous suction, respectively.

The pulmonary hypoplasia and pulmonary hypertension require strategic ventilatory management. Surfactant administration may help mitigate atelectasis in already stiff, hypoplastic lungs. Treatment for pulmonary hypertension is discussed below.

Neonates with larger diaphragmatic defects often present with more severe respiratory distress that requires urgent AE to a tertiary care center where advanced pediatric surgical capabilities, inhaled nitric oxide therapy, and ECMO are available. Fortunately, many neonates afflicted with diaphragmatic hernia are being identified by prenatal ultrasound. In such cases, the pregnant mother often plans to deliver at, or is transported prior to delivery, to a tertiary care center.

Intestinal Obstruction

Intestinal obstruction can present soon after birth. Some obstructions can lead to severe morbidity or death, while others can be stabilized and transported electively. Proximal intestinal obstructions often present antenatally with polyhydramnios. In such cases, the mother will often be transferred to a tertiary care center to allow advanced care of her newborn immediately following birth.

Intestinal obstruction from a volvulus or congenital obstruction may present in the neonatal period with bilious vomiting. An X-ray of the abdomen may reveal a double-bubble sign, which suggests duodenal obstruction from an atresia or annular pancreas. Intestinal obstruction that presents after birth may result in marked abdominal distension, which will in turn elevate the diaphragm and compromise respiratory function.

Volvulus of the intestines can result in complete occlusion of the superior mesenteric artery. Because occlusion of this vessel can result in the necrosis of all bowel from the distal duodenum to transverse colon, volvulus can lead to a severe form of short-bowel syndrome with disastrous consequences. If volvulus is diagnosed, emergency laparotomy is indicated.

Implications for Aeromedical Evacuation

In the presence of suspected malrotation and/or signs of volvulus with ischemic bowel, urgent AE is indicated as this is a surgical emergency. An orogastric tube placed to suction should be placed as soon as possible to allow for bowel decompression, and maintenance IV fluids should be started. In the presence of respiratory compromise, elective intubation prior to AE should be considered. If there is a distal obstruction without signs of bowel ischemia or respiratory compromise, the infant can be placed on maintenance IV fluids, OG decompression achieved, and transport accomplished electively.

Omphalocele and Gastroschisis

Omphalocele and gastroschisis can be life-threatening if not recognized, stabilized, and treated promptly. Chromosomal disorders, heart disease, and other anomalies occur more commonly with omphalocele. Gastroschisis and ruptured omphalocele result in exposure of the bowel to the external environment. Significant heat and fluid loss can occur. Infection can be prevented with the use of sterile surgical-grade gauze soaked in warm saline, sterile bowel bags, and broad-spectrum antibiotic administration.

The circulation to the intestine should be assessed in a sterile manner. A well-perfused intestine should be pink and should not appear pale or dusky. Twisting of the superior mesenteric artery or cicatrix of the surrounding abdominal skin may compromise the circulation to the intestine. A compromised intestine may appear dark purple because of venous congestion. If the tight skin opening is causing ischemia, the local surgeon or transport team, in consultation with a pediatric surgeon, may need to widen the opening before transport.

Implications for Aeromedical Evacuation

These infants require urgent AE, and the stabilization and treatment during transport is similar for both conditions. Altitude effects upon gas volumes may compromise circulation to trapped segments. Prior to AE, an OG tube should be placed and connected to intermittent suction to allow for decompression.

These patients require strict attention to temperature control, fluid replacement, and cardiovascular support. They should be transported in an incubator that is kept at 36 ° C. The vehicle cabin should be kept as close as possible to 24 ° C (80 ° F).

It is not recommended that umbilical catheters be placed in these patients unless emergent and peripheral access is unable to be gained. Two peripheral IV lines should be established for transport. A peripherally inserted central catheter (PICC) can be placed at the receiving facility. IV maintenance fluids should be initiated and the infant should be closely monitored for adequate volume replacement. Tachycardia, poor capillary refill, metabolic acidosis, hypotension, and poor urine output are all indicative of inadequate volume repletion and should be managed with 10 mL/kg saline boluses and/or increase in the maintenance fluid rate.

To prevent torsion of the bowel blood supply, the infant should be placed on one side and the bowel supported with a donut-shaped roll of blankets or towels. Using warm, sterile saline maintains good moisture to the sterile surgical gauze covering the mass. Intestinal perfusion should be repeatedly reassessed and the findings documented with each set of vital signs.

Cyanotic Congenital Heart Disease

Cyanotic congenital heart disease (CHD) represents a group of conditions characterized by an alteration in blood flow that results in deoxygenated blood being delivered to the systemic circulation. This commonly occurs in one of three ways:

1. The presence of separate circulations and poor mixing of oxygenated and deoxygenated blood, e.g., transposition of the great arteries.
2. Restriction of pulmonary blood flow, e.g., tetralogy of Fallot, tricuspid atresia, and pulmonary atresia.
3. Complete mixing of oxygenated and deoxygenated blood, e.g., total anomalous pulmonary venous return or truncus arteriosus.

Cyanotic CHD should be suspected whenever a neonate remains cyanotic in the absence of respiratory distress. However, respiratory distress may be present and make it more challenging to pinpoint the etiology of the cyanosis. A neonate with a PaO_2 <200 mm Hg while receiving 100% inspired oxygen must be further evaluated for cyanotic CHD.

Acute nonsurgical therapy for most forms of cyanotic CHD is dependent upon maintenance of patency of the DA and control of pulmonary blood flow. Prostaglandin E1 (PGE1) is used to maintain ductal patency. Side effects of prostaglandin therapy include apnea, hypoventilation, and hyperthermia.

Proper ventilation techniques to control the partial pressure of oxygen and carbon dioxide and ensure optimal acid–base balance are critical. Management of the patient during transport should be discussed in advance with the cardiologist or critical care team to determine the best care plan for each specific cardiac defect. Commonly, prostaglandin therapy and SpO_2 values in the 80s are adequate.

Implications for Aeromedical Evacuation

Neonates with suspected cyanotic CHD should be transported by urgent AE. These patients require an altitude restriction to maximum cabin altitudes <2000 ft. or the altitude of the referring or accepting facility if higher. Oxygenation that has been maximized at sea level will often decrease at altitude. In-flight determination of arterial blood gases with portable laboratory equipment is useful for ensuring adequate acid–base balance in the presence of lower oxygenation. Close observation for apnea is warranted for any infant receiving PGE1. If there is concern for this, the transport team will often electively intubate the patient prior to transport.

Critical Coarctation of the Aorta

Infants with a critical coarctation may not present initially at birth due to a patent ductus arteriosus, allowing for systemic circulation beyond the obstruction. This should be found during screening in most nurseries as they will have a decreased SaO_2 in a lower extremity. These patients will typically present in the first couple weeks of life when the ductus closes. They are often in severe shock with significant metabolic acidosis. Key exam findings include decreased pulses/perfusion to the lower extremities with increased/normal pulses in the right upper extremity.

Implications for Aeromedical Evacuation

These neonates urgently require PGE1 at a dose of 0.1 μ(mu)g/kg per minute. They also often need significant resuscitation with fluids, bicarbonate, and potentially pressors. Hypoglycemia should also be treated. A definitive airway should be placed given their severity and use of Prostin.

Hypoplastic Left Heart Syndrome

Hypoplastic left heart syndrome (HLHS) is the most common cause of death from CHD during the first month of life and accounts for 9% of all newborn congenital heart defects. It accounts for more than one-third of pediatric cardiology cases transported by some critical care transport teams [51].

HLHS is characterized by underdevelopment of the left side of the heart in conjunction with mitral and aortic valve stenosis and narrowing of the ascending aorta. For HLHS to be compatible with life, both a right-to-left shunt and a left-to-right shunt must be present. These are usually in the form of ventricular and atrial septal defects or persistently patent foramen ovale and a patent ductus arteriosus.

Although newborns with HLHS often appear normal at birth, they usually display vague and nonspecific signs and symptoms, including increased respiratory effort and cyanosis when crying. If the foramen ovale or atrial septal defects restrict the delivery of oxygenated blood to the right atrium, the infant will appear cyanotic at birth.

The abrupt closing of the DA is a medical emergency for neonates who depend on it for blood flow to either the body (right-to-left shunting) or the lungs (left-to-right shunting). When the DA closes, cessation of blood flow to the body results in cyanosis, hypoxemia, and profound shock. Congestive heart failure and metabolic acidosis occur rapidly, with ensuing multiorgan failure. This condition can be reversed only by quickly reopening the DA.

Management centers on careful control of blood oxygen (PaO_2), carbon dioxide ($PaCO_2$), and pH. Ideally, the oxygen saturation should remain 60–80% and the blood slightly acidotic (pH 7.34–7.40). HLHS neonates should remain on room air because increased oxygen dilates the pulmonary bed, thus increasing blood flood to the lungs and decreasing blood flow to the body.

These infants should not be hyperventilated because accumulation of CO_2 and acidosis constrict pulmonary blood vessels, thus increasing blood flow to the body. Alternatively, high ventilator rates and large tidal volumes lower $PaCO_2$, resulting in alkalosis, dilated pulmonary beds, and increased blood flow to the lungs. An ideal $PaCO_2$ range is 40–50 mm Hg, titrated to maintain adequate systemic perfusion.

Infants with HLHS are routinely treated with PGE1 (0.01–0.05 μ[mu]g/kg per minute by IV infusion) to keep the DA patent, reduce pulmonary blood flow, and enhance systemic blood flow and coronary perfusion. PGE1 is titrated to the lowest effective dose to minimize side effects, including apnea, jitteriness, hypoglycemia, hyperthermia, and cutaneous vasodilatation. If the DA is suspected to have recently closed, a higher dose (~0.1 μ[mu]g/kg per minute) should first be utilized.

Implications for Aeromedical Evacuation

Although these neonates do better with relatively low O_2 saturations, an altitude restriction of <2000 ft. (or the altitude of the referring or accepting facility, if higher) will greatly simplify the in-flight management of HLHS. Otherwise, the most important aspects of air transport are the standard general principles of neonatal care, including maintenance of normothermia and prevention of hypoglycemia [51]. The neonate should have IV access before transport and an OG or NG tube for stomach decompression. Elective intubation before AE should be considered if the infant appears to be at risk for airway compromise or for apnea related to PGE1 infusion. Neuromuscular blockade with sedation helps minimize the oxygen consumption at the tissue level that often results from transport noise and vibration. Correct placement of all intravascular lines and tubes should be confirmed radiographically, then firmly secured with suture and/or tape. Arterial blood gas levels should be determined immediately before transport for comparison if the neonate should become hemodynamically unstable en route.

References

1. Bose CL. Neonatal transport. In: Avery GB, Fletcher MA, NG MD, editors. Neonatology, pathophysiology and management of the nwborn. 5th ed. Philadelphia, PA: Lippencott, Williams & Wilkins; 1999. p. 35–47.
2. Shepard KS. Air transportation of high risk infants utilizing a flying intensive care nursery. J Pediatr. 1970;77:148–9.
3. Pettett G, Merenstein GB, Battaglia FC, Butterfield LJ, Efird R. An analysis of air transport results in the sick newborn infant: part I. The transport team. Pediatrics. 1975;55:774–82.
4. American Academy of Pediatrics Section on Transport Medicine. Guidelines for air and ground transport of neonatal and pediatric atients. 4th ed. Elk Grove Village, IL: American Academy of Pediatrics; 2016.
5. US Department of the Air Force. Critical care air transport teams: air force tactics, C procedures 3-42.51. 2006. https://kx.afms.mil/doctrine.
6. US Department of the Air Force. Critical care air transport teams: air force tactics, techniques, and procedures 3-42.51. 2015. http://static.e-publishing.af.mil/production/1/af_sg/publication/afttp3-42.51/afttp3-42.51.pdf.
7. US Department of the Air Force. En route critical care: air force instruction 48-307, Volume 2. 2017. http://static.e-publishing.af.mil/production/1/af_sg/publication/afi48-307v2/afi48-307v2.pdf.
8. Commission on Accreditation of Medical Transport Systems. Tenth edition accreditation standards of the commission on accreditation of medical transport systems. 2015. https://www.camts.org.
9. Seidal JS, Knapp JF. Pediatric emergencies in the office, hospital and community: organizing systems of care. Pediatrics. 2000;106:337–8.
10. Air Force Research Laboratory. http://afmedl1.brooks.af.mil/aeromed/statusguide/.
11. United States Army Aeromedical Research Laboratory. http://www.usaarl.army.mil.
12. Extracorporeal Life Support Organization. ELSO guidelines for cardiopulmonary extracorporeal life support, version 1.4. 2017. http://www.elso.org.
13. Extracorporeal Life Support Organization. ELSO neonatal respiratory failure supplment to the ELSO general guidelines, version 1.4. 2017. http://www.elso.org.
14. Extracorporeal Life Support Organization. ECLS registry report international summary. 2018. http://www.elso.org.
15. Extracorporeal Life Support Organization. ELSO pediatric respiratory failure supplment to the ELSO general guidelines, version 1.3. 2013. http://www.elso.org.
16. Extracorporeal Life Support Organization. ELSO pediatric cardiac failure. 2017. http://www.elso.org.
17. Gleissner M, Jorch G, Avenarius S. Risk factors for intraventricular hemorrhage in a birth cohort of 3721 premature infants. J Perinat Med. 2000;28:104–10.
18. Shenai JP. Sound levels for neonates in transit. J Pediatr. 1977;90:811–2.
19. Children's Hospital Medical Center, Cincinatti, OH. Pediatric and neonatal transport diagnoses from July 1, 1999 through June 30, 2000. Unpublished data.
20. Meyer MT, Mikhailov TA, Kuhn EM, Collins MM, Scanlon MC. Pediatric specialty transport teams are

not associated with decreased 48-hour pediatric intensive care unit mortality: a propensity analysis of the VPS, LLC Database. Air Med J. 2016;35:73–8.
21. Ajizian SJ, Nakagawa TA. Interfacility transport of the critically ill pediatric patient. Chest. 2007;13:1361–7.
22. Centers for Disease Control and Prevention. Asthma: Data, Statistics, Surveillance. https://www.cdc.gov/asthma/most_recent_data.htm. Accessed 31 Aug 2018.
23. Centers for Disease Control and Prevention. Asthma mortality among persons aged 15–64 years, by industry and occupation – United States, 1999–2016. MMWR. 2018;67(2):60–5.
24. US Department of Health and Human Services: National Heart, Lung, and Blood Institute. National Asthma education and prevention program expert panel report 3: guidelines for the diagnosis and management of Asthma. 2007. https://www.nhlbi.nih.gov/files/docs/guidelines/asthsumm.pdf.
25. Rotta AT, Wiryawan B. Respiratory emergencies in children. Respir Care. 2003;48(3):248–58.
26. Mandal A, Kabra SK, Lodha R. Upper airway obstruction in children. Indian J Pediatr. 2015;82(8):737–44.
27. Mayo-Smith MF, Spinale JW, Donskey CJ, Yukawa M, Li RH, Schiffman FJ. Acute epiglottitis. An 18-year experience in Rhode Island. Chest. 1995;108:1640–7.
28. Brophy GM, Bell R, Claassen J, Alldredge B, Bleck TP, Glauser T, et al; Neurocritical Care Society Status Epilepticus Guideline Writing Committee. Guidelines for the evaluation and management of status epilepticus. Neurocrit Care. 2012;17(1):3–23.
29. Abend N, Loddenkemper T. Management of pediatric status epilepticus. Curr Treat Options Neurol. 2014;16(7):301.
30. Kaufman FR, Halvorson M, Kaufman ND. Evaluation of a snack bar containing uncooked cornstarch in subjects with diabetes. Diabetes Res Clin Pract. 1997;35:27–33.
31. Clarke WL, Gonder-Frederick L, Cox DJ. The frequency of severe hypoglycaemia in children with insulin-dependent diabetes mellitus. Hormone Res. 1996;45:48–52.
32. Wolfsdorf JI, Allgrove J, Craig ME, Edge J, Glaser N, Jain V, et al; International Society for Pediatric and Adolescent Diabetes. ISPAD Clinical Practice Consensus Guidelines 2014. Diabetic ketoacidosis and hyperglycemic hyperosmolar state. Pediatr Diabetes. 2014;15(Suppl. 20):154–79.
33. Buchanan BJ, Hoagland J, Fischer PR. Pseudoephedrine and air travel-associated ear pain in children. Arch Pediatr Adolesc Med. 1999;153:466–8.
34. Csortan E, Jones J, Haan M, Brown M. Efficacy of pseudoephedrine for the prevention of barotrauma during air travel. Ann Emerg Med. 1994;23:1324–7.
35. Centers for Disease Control and Prevention. Data and statistics on sickle cell disease. https://www.cdc.gov/ncbddd/sicklecell/data.html. Accessed 31 Aug 2018.
36. Platt OS, Brambilla DJ, Rosse WF, Milner PF, Castro O, Steinberg MH, Klug PP. Mortality in sickle cell disease: life expectancy and risk factors for early death. N Engl J Med. 1994;330:1639–44.
37. Lanzkron S, Carroll CP, Haywood C. Mortality rates and age at death from sickle cell disease: US, 1979–2005. Public Health Rep. 2013;128:110–28.
38. Green RL, Huntsman RG, Sergeant GR. Sickle-cell and altitude. Br Med J. 1972;1:803–4.
39. Ware M, Tyghter D, Staniforth S, Serjeant G. Airline travel in sickle-cell disease. Lancet. 1998;352(9128):652.
40. National Heart, Lung, and Blood Institute. Evidenced-based management of sickle cell disease: expert panel report, 2014. 2014. https://www.nhlbi.nih.gov/guidelines.
41. Centers for Disease Control and Prevention. Deaths: final data for 2015. National Vitals Statistics Report. 2017;66(6). https://www.cdc.gov/nchs/data/nvsr/nvsr66/nvsr66_06.pdf. Accessed 16 Sept 2018.
42. Ferguson NM, Sarnaik A, Miles D, Shafi N, Peters MJ, Truemper E, et al; Investigators of the Approaches and Decisions in Acute Pediatric Traumatic Brain Injury (ADAPT) Trial. Abusive head trauma and mortality – An analysis from an international comparative effectiveness study of children with severe traumatic brain injury. Crit Care Med. 2017; 45(8):1398–407.
43. American College of Surgeons Committee on Trauma. Advanced trauma life support student course manual. 9th ed. Chicago, IL: American College of Surgeons; 2013.
44. Nagler J, Krauss B. Intraosseous catheter placement in children. N Engl J Med. 2011;364:e14.
45. Riley AA, Arakawa Y, Worley S, Duncan BW, Fukamachi K. Circulating blood volumes: a review of measurement techniques and a meta-analysis in children. ASAIO J. 2010;56(3):260–4.
46. Harmsen AMK, Giannakopoulos GF, Moerbeek PR, Jansma EP, Bonjer HJ, Bloemers FW. The influence of prehospital time on trauma patient outcome: a systematic review. Injury. 2015;46:602–9.
47. Brain Trauma Foundation. Guidelines for the acute medical management of severe traumatic brain injury in infants, children, and adolescents: 2nd Ed. Pediatr Crit Care Med. 2012;13 Suppl 1:S1–S82.
48. Hansen G, McDonald PJ, Martin D, Vallance JK. Pre-trauma center management of intracranial pressure in severe pediatric brain injury. Pediatr Emer Care. 2018;34:330–3.
49. Martinon C, Duracher C, Blanot S, Escolano S, De Agostini M, Périé-Vintras AC, et al. Emergency tracheal intubation of severely head-injured children: changing daily practice after implementation of national guidelines. Pediatr Crit Care Med. 2011;12(1):65–70.
50. Cornblath M, Hawdon JM, Williams AF, Aynsley-Green A, Ward-Platt MP, Schwartz R, Kalhan SC. Controversies regarding definition of neonatal hypoglycemia: suggested operational thresholds. Pediatrics. 2000;105:1141–5.
51. Haselhuhn MR. Go blue: when blue is better for the neonate with hypoplastic left heart syndrome. J Emerg Nurs. 1999;25:392–6.

Aeromedical Evacuation of Psychiatric Casualties

23

Alan L. Peterson, Dhiya V. Shah, Jose M. Lara-Ruiz, and Elspeth Cameron Ritchie

Introduction

Evacuation of psychiatric casualties is a critical component of the military aeromedical evacuation (AE) process [1, 2]. The US military conflicts in Afghanistan, Iraq, and surrounding locations have resulted in significant psychiatric casualties. Psychiatric conditions were the fourth most common reason for US service members to be evacuated out of Afghanistan from 2001 to 2012 and out of Iraq from 2003 to 2010.

As battle injuries declined, mental disorders became the most common evacuation diagnostic category. Between 2013 and 2015, psychiatric disorders became the most common diagnostic category for US service members evacuated out of the US Central Command, which is responsible for Iraq and Afghanistan and other nearby countries. Psychiatric evacuation accounted for about 20% of all evacuations for male service members and more than 25% of female service members during this timeframe.

The majority of AE for psychiatric indications involves deployed military personnel and civilians working in military combat theaters [1–5]. Personnel deployed to combat theaters may be at a greater risk of developing psychiatric problems because of exposure to significant deployment-related stress. In some cases, service members with a history of psychiatric conditions are inadvertently deployed to combat environments and are exposed to additional stressors that may aggravate their pre-existing psychiatric conditions. This is why the military closely screens all military personnel prior to deployment. It is also why review and clearance by a military behavioral health provider is required for service members with a recent history of mental health treatment.

Psychiatric screening is also conducted for service members and their dependents prior to an overseas military permanent change of station assignment that is not part of the combat theater. Nonetheless, some military personnel and their dependents stationed at overseas locations (e.g., Pacific theater, Europe) require AE for psychiatric indications when local medical facilities do not have sufficient capabilities to treat or manage psychiatric patients. In civilian populations in developed countries, AE of psychiatric patients is

A. L. Peterson (✉)
Col, USAF (ret.), Department of Psychiatry, Division of Behavioral Medicine, The Military Health Institute, University of Texas Health Science Center, San Antonio, TX, USA
e-mail: petersona3@uthscsa.edu

D. V. Shah
Department of Psychiatry and Primary Care Center, Division of Behavioral Medicine, University of Texas Health Science Center, San Antonio, TX, USA

J. M. Lara-Ruiz
Department of Psychiatry, University of Texas Health Science Center, San Antonio, TX, USA

E. C. Ritchie
COL, MC, USA (ret.), Department of Psychiatry, Washington Hospital Center, Washington, DC, USA

W. W. Hurd, W. Beninati (eds.), *Aeromedical Evacuation*,
https://doi.org/10.1007/978-3-030-15903-0_23

a relatively rare event as there are hospitals that can care for them locally. The exception is after natural disasters, when there are insufficient local medical resources to care for these patients and ground transportation is not possible [6].

Psychiatric Disorders in Military Populations

In general, military populations are significantly healthier than civilian populations, in terms of both physical and psychological health. This is primarily because of the physical and mental fitness requirements for initial military enlistment and the additional fitness for duty requirements for continued service [7]. Most severe or chronic psychiatric conditions (e.g., psychotic disorders, bipolar disorder, etc.) are considered to be incompatible with military service [7].

Similar psychiatric fitness for duty requirements exist for active-duty military personnel as well as those serving in the National Guard and Reserves. However, community civilian providers often serve as the primary medical and psychiatric providers for National Guard and Reserve personnel when they are not activated into service. As a result, there is a greater likelihood of more severe medical and psychiatric conditions being present in National Guard and Reserve military personnel who are activated and deployed. In addition, during times of military conflict when these service members are most commonly active and deployed, the standard medical and psychiatric guidelines are sometimes modified to meet the needs of the military. For example, during the height of the US military operations in Afghanistan and Iraq when a significant increase in US military force strength was required, an increased number of waivers were approved for some medical and psychiatric conditions [8]. Starting in 2010, waivers for psychiatric conditions essentially were stopped being given.

The primary diagnostic guide for the diagnosis of mental disorders in military personnel is the fifth edition of the *Diagnostic and Statistical Manual of Mental Disorders* (*DSM-5*) [9]. One of the major revisions of the *DSM-5* included changes in the diagnostic criteria for post-traumatic stress disorder (PTSD), and some of these changes were to address the unique aspects of combat-related PTSD in military service members and veterans [10].

Deployment Psychiatry

Assessment and Treatment in Theater

Treatment in theater should be the first option for most patients who develop combat-related psychiatric symptoms during military deployments. However, this is not always successful and some psychiatric conditions, such as psychosis, are too severe and warrant immediate evacuation. Persistent suicidal or homicidal ideation are other examples. Psychiatric AE will likely have a significant negative career impact on most military service members. Therefore, the decision to evacuate should be given careful consideration.

During military deployments, behavioral health providers assess and treat a wide range of psychiatric health conditions including combat operational stress reactions. In order to maintain full operational capabilities in the combat theater, military behavioral health providers are tasked with trying to maintain the psychological fitness of all deployed military personnel and to limit AE whenever possible. However, under the significant stressors of combat deployments, some psychiatric conditions emerge that are so severe that immediate psychiatric AE is necessary. In other instances, providers may not be successful in treating patients sufficiently so they can remain in theater and fit for duty. In these cases, a decision may need to be made to evacuate patients.

Deployed military behavioral health providers should be aware that AE for a psychiatric diagnosis out of the combat theater may be a career-ending event for a military service member. A service member who deploys to perform the most important military duty assignment of his or her career and is subsequently AE out of theater for a psychiatric condition may ultimately be determined not to be fit for duty. Most psychiatric patients enter the AE system with a psychiatric inpatient classification code (i.e., 1A, 1B, 1C, or 3C; see Table 23.1).

Table 23.1 Psychiatric aeromedical evacuation patient classification codes

Code	Classification	Description
1A	Severe psychiatric inpatient	Psychiatric litter inpatient requiring the use of restraining apparatus, sedation, close supervision, and a medical attendant
		The medical attendant will be the same gender and preferably of equal or higher rank
		Patient must have standing and/or as needed (PRN) medication orders for agitation/anxiety/sleep
		Patients will have restraints on prior to boarding the aircraft, be sedated for flight, and have close supervision
		The referring physician, patient movement requirements center, medical attendant, or medical crew director may determine whether the patient's behavior is too high risk to flight safety, thus requiring further stabilization
		The patient will be stabilized prior to aeromedical evacuation movement with appropriate psychiatric medications that will effectively control symptoms of extreme agitation and/or anxiety
		Patients will travel in hospital garments, pajamas, or physical training (PT) gear. The PT gear should have all strings, laces, and belts removed
		Patients will only remain overnight at a bedded medical treatment facility
1B	Intermediate psychiatric inpatient	Psychiatric litter inpatient of intermediate severity
		Patient must have standing and/or as needed (PRN) medication orders for agitation/anxiety/sleep
		Patients should be transported on a litter. In coordination with the medical crew director/flight nurse/aeromedical evacuation technician, these patients may be allowed to sit up for comfort under close observation
		Psychiatric patients may require tranquilizing or sedating medications to prevent harm to self, aircrew members, or the aircraft
		Patients will have a restraint order for applying restraints or restraints immediately available at the litter
		Once available restraints are applied to the patient; the medical crew director will contact the validating flight surgeon for an applied restraint order
		They will not be seated near exits, flight deck, or where emergency equipment (i.e., oxygen, crash axes, or emergency oxygen shutoff valve) is kept
		All aircrew members will be informed of the patient's location
		Patients should travel in hospital garments, pajamas, or physical training (PT) gear. The PT gear should have all strings, laces, and belts removed
		Patients will only remain overnight at a bedded medical treatment facility
1C	Ambulatory psychiatric inpatient	Psychiatric patients who are cooperative and who have proved reliable under observation
		May or may not require an attendant for movement
		May be dressed in civilian or military clothing
		Will not be seated next to an emergency exit or oxygen shutoff valve
		May require a medical attendant if patient need dictates
		Patient will not self-medicate or carry their own medication
		Patients will only remain overnight at a bedded medical treatment facility
3C	Ambulatory substance abuse inpatient	Inpatient ambulatory, drug, alcohol, or substance abuse patient going for inpatient treatment or evaluation
		May be dressed in military or civilian clothing
		Individuals who have recent alcohol consumption may exhibit signs or symptoms of withdrawal
		Patient can be managed as an ambulatory psychiatric inpatient (1C) but may sit next to exits and oxygen shutoff valves, if determined to be competent by a flight nurse
		Patients may remain overnight at an En route patient staging system if determined by the flight surgeon and the senior nurse at the En route patient staging system to be stable and safe

(continued)

Table 23.1 (continued)

Code	Classification	Description
5B	Ambulatory substance abuse outpatient	Outpatient ambulatory, drug, alcohol, or substance abuse patient going for outpatient treatment or evaluation
		Patients may remain overnight at an En route patient staging system if determined by the flight surgeon and senior nurse at the En route patient staging system to be stable and safe
5C	Ambulatory psychiatric outpatient	Psychiatric outpatient going for treatment or evaluation
		Patients may remain overnight at an En route patient staging system if determined by the flight surgeon and senior nurse at the En route patient staging system to be stable and safe

Note: Adapted from Air Force Instruction 48–307, Volume 1, 9 January 2017. En Route Care and Aeromedical Evacuation Medical Operations [23]

One previous study evaluated the military career impact of a psychiatric inpatient hospitalization [11]. This study followed 1736 US Army soldiers who had an inpatient psychiatric hospitalization in 1998. The results indicated that within 6 months after their hospitalization, 45% of the soldiers had been separated from active duty compared with only 11% of those hospitalized for other, non-psychiatric medical illnesses. Two years after the psychiatric hospitalization, 67% of those who had an inpatient psychiatric hospitalization had been separated.

It is hypothesized that AE out of the combat theater resulting in an inpatient psychiatric hospitalization will have similar military career consequences. Therefore, deployed military behavioral health providers should do everything possible to assess and treat deployed military service members to keep them in theater and fit to perform their military duties. Additional research is needed to evaluate the long-term military career impact of AE for psychiatric indications from a combat theater.

Psychiatric Aeromedical Evacuation

Psychiatric Diagnoses

The most common diagnoses associated with psychiatric evacuations include adjustment disorders, mood disorders, anxiety disorders, trauma-related disorders, personality disorders, traumatic brain injury, and suicide ideation or attempts [12–19]. Several studies found that adjustment disorders were the most common diagnoses resulting in AE [4, 5, 12, 14, 20]. It is yet to be determined whether or not these adjustment disorders resolved after being evacuated or if they were later diagnosed with another mental disorder such as PTSD.

Recent changes in the publication of the *DSM-5* resulted in the development of a new diagnostic category called *trauma-related disorders* that include acute stress disorder (ASD) and PTSD, which previously were under the category of anxiety disorders in the *DSM-IV-TR*. In a sample of 195 military psychiatric patients who were surveyed at the Balad Contingency Aeromedical Staging Facility (CASF) prior to AE, 36% met criteria for an ASD diagnosis and 29% met criteria for PTSD [21]. In comparison, a study of 1336 deployed US military personnel seeking mental health treatment found that the most common psychiatric diagnosis was an anxiety disorder (31%, including 11% with PTSD) [20]. A larger study also found that PTSD accounted for 10.5% of diagnoses that subsequently resulted in approximately half of psychiatric evacuations. In this case, men were more frequently evacuated for PTSD (11.3%) compared to women (5.7%) [19]. Wilmoth and colleagues [22] also found a gender difference in post-concussion syndrome following a traumatic brain injury, with a prevalence of 6.0% in men compared to 1.4% in women. This is most likely due to the higher percentage of men serving in combat roles with a higher likelihood of exposure to blasts.

The majority of patients undergo AE for medical conditions other than mental disorders. However, many AE patients have comorbid mental disorders or significant psychological health symptoms. For example, chronic musculoskeletal pain is one of the most common diagnostic categories associated with AE [3–5], and there is a significant comorbidity of psychological health conditions with chronic pain. In most cases, these secondary psychiatric symptoms are not a primary focus of AE, unless they are significant enough to interfere with the AE process.

Psychiatric Patient Classification for Aeromedical Evacuation

Psychiatric patients entering the AE system are classified into three categories based on their specific needs and potential to cause problems during AE. A summary of the psychiatric AE patient classification codes is included in Table 23.1. The basic guidelines for patient classification codes for AE are included in Air Force Instruction 48-307, En Route Care and Aeromedical Evacuation Medical Operations [23].

The majority of psychiatric patients are evacuated with an inpatient classification code (1A, 1B, 1C, or 3C). In most cases, these patients require a medical escort or nonmedical attendant/escort. The attendant should be of the same gender and of equal or higher rank. The AE team should ensure that the attendant is aware of the duties and responsibilities of the attendant. In general, the attendant's duties are to monitor the psychiatric patient being transported at all times to help assure safe AE.

Psychiatric patients in the Severe Psychiatric Inpatient (Category 1A) and Intermediate Psychiatric Inpatient (Category 1B) require the closest monitoring by the attendant and AE team. Aeromedical evacuation checklists have been developed for Category 1A (Table 23.2) and 1B (Table 23.3) patients [23]. These checklists can be used to help ensure patients are properly screened and prepared prior to AE.

Prior to AE, patients in the 1A and 1B categories should be stabilized with tranquilizing or sedative medication to reduce agitation, anxiety, and sleep symptoms. These patients should be transported on a litter, and some may also need physical restraints. The ultimate goal is to help prevent injuries to the patient, attendant, flight crew, and other patients; help avoid damage to the aircraft; and avert an in-flight accident. Specific guidelines must be followed when using physical restraints [23].

Psychiatric Medications for Use in Aeromedical Evacuation

Patients with significant clinical symptoms should be treated medically for a long enough period to control their symptoms prior to undergoing AE [23]. This is especially true for patients who are actively psychotic, manic, or seriously suicidal, because it is potentially dangerous to put these patients on a flight. Most psychiatric symptoms—such as agitation, psychosis, and mania—will be adequately controlled after 3–5 days of treatment. Depressive symptoms may last much longer, but are less of a management problem aboard an aircraft.

Once a patient's symptoms have decreased enough to make AE safe, they should receive a 7-day supply of medications for the flight, plus extra medications for agitation or sedation in case they are needed. The following is a description of some of the most commonly prescribed psychiatric medications used prior to and during AE (see Table 23.4).

Agitation

All severely agitated patients should be sedated prior to AE regardless of their diagnoses. The most common medications used for sedation are the benzodiazepines because of their speed of onset and relative lack of side effects. Antipsychotics are also commonly used. Other antipsychotic, antimanic, and antidepressant medications may be used after the patient has

Table 23.2 Aeromedical evacuation (AE) checklist for Category 1A Severe Psychiatric Inpatients

Instructions: The following psychiatric evacuation requirement checklist should be completed prior to evacuation by the patients' medical attendant, the medical crew director, and/or the Patient Movement Requirements Center prior to and during psychiatric evacuation. A "Yes" response is required for every checklist item listed below

Category 1A: Severe psychiatric inpatient
Aeromedical evacuation requirement checklist

	Yes	No
1. Is the patient being transported on a litter?		
2. Is the patient dressed in a hospital garment or physical training (PT) gear?		
2.1. If PT gear is worn, have all strings, laces, and belts been removed?		
3. Has a medical attendant been assigned (preferably a mental health provider) for safety purposes for the duration of the psychiatric evacuation?		
3.1. Is the medical attendant of the same gender?		
3.2. Is the medical attendant of equal or higher rank as the patient?		
3.3. Is the medical attendant aware that the patient must be closely supervised for the duration of the flight and kept within line of sight at all times?		
4. Have restraints been applied prior to boarding the aircraft?		
4.1. Have four-point restraints been used?		
4.2. Have the short restraint belts, long restraint belts, wrist cuffs, and ankle cuffs been inspected for cuts, tears, or excessive wear?		
4.3. Has it been verified that the keys open the locking device on the restraints?		
4.4. Does medical attendant know the location of the restraints keys?		
4.5. Have steps been taken to ensure the restraints are not attached to or around the litter itself?		
5. Has the patient been sedated prior to flight to prevent harm to self, aircrew members, or the aircraft?		
5.1. Has respiratory status (including pulse oxygen) been continually monitored?		
5.2. Have signs of oversedation been continually monitored?		
6. Have standing and/or as needed (PRN) medication orders been written for agitation, anxiety, and sleep?		
7. Have arrangements been made to ensure that the patient will only remain overnight at a bedded medical treatment facility?		

Category 1A patients must be transported on a litter and require the use of restraining apparatus, sedation by medication, close supervision, and a medical attendant (preferably a mental health provider) for safety purposes during the entire duration of the psychiatric evacuation

Table 23.3 Aeromedical evacuation (AE) checklist for Category 1B Intermediate Psychiatric Inpatients

Instructions: The following psychiatric evacuation requirement checklist should be completed prior to evacuation by the medical crew director and/or the Patient Movement Requirements Center prior to and during psychiatric evacuation. A "Yes" response is required for every checklist item listed below

Category 1B: Intermediate psychiatric inpatient
Aeromedical evacuation requirement checklist

	Yes	No
1. Is the patient being transported on a litter? Note: In coordination with the medical crew director/flight nurse/aeromedical evacuation technician, these patients may be allowed to sit up for comfort under close observation		
2. Has patient been seated at a location that is not near exits, flight deck, or where emergency equipment (e.g., oxygen, crash axes, or emergency oxygen shutoff valve) is kept?		
3. Is the patient dressed in a hospital garment, pajamas, or physical training (PT) gear? Note: If PT gear is worn, all strings, laces, and belts should be removed		

Table 23.3 (continued)

Instructions: The following psychiatric evacuation requirement checklist should be completed prior to evacuation by the medical crew director and/or the Patient Movement Requirements Center prior to and during psychiatric evacuation. A "Yes" response is required for every checklist item listed below		
Category 1B: Intermediate psychiatric inpatient *Aeromedical evacuation requirement checklist*		
	Yes	No
4. Is there a restraint order for applying restraints or restraints immediately available at the litter? Note: Once available restraints are applied to the patient; the medical crew director will contact the validating flight surgeon for an applied restraint order		
5. Are tranquilizing or sedating medications available to prevent harm to self, aircrew members, or the aircraft?		
6. Have standing and/or as needed (PRN) medication orders been written for agitation, anxiety, and sleep?		
7. Have arrangements been made to ensure that the patient will only remain overnight at a bedded medical treatment facility?		
Category 1B patients must be transported on a litter, but restraints are not routinely applied for these patients and they are not routinely sedated. They may or may not require an attendant for movement. They may be allowed to sit up for comfort under close observation with approval of the AE medical crew director, flight nurse, or technician. These patients should travel in hospital garments, pajamas, or physical training (PT) gear. If PT gear is worn, all strings, laces, and belts should be removed. These patients cannot be seated near exits, flight deck, or where emergency equipment is kept, e.g., oxygen, crash axes, or emergency oxygen shutoff valve		

Table 23.4 Common psychiatric medications, doses, and side effects

Medications	Typical dose (mg)	Route	Interval	Side effect
Sedation				
Diazepam	5–10	PO	Every 4–12 h	Sedation, respiratory depression (rare)
Lorazepam	1–2	PO, IM, IV	Every 1–4 h	As above
Clonazepam	0.5–1	PO	Every 8–12 h	As above
Antipsychotic				
Haloperidol	5 1	PO, IM, IV	Every 4–6 h as needed	Extrapyramidal symptoms, akathisia, dystonias
Olanzapine	5–20	PO	At bedtime	Sedation, extrapyramidal symptoms (mild)
Risperidone	2–6	PO	At bedtime	Extrapyramidal symptoms
Anticholinergic				
Benztropine	1–2	PO, IM, IV	1–4 h as needed	Dry mouth, constipation
Diphenhydramine	25–50	PO, IM, IV	1–4 h as needed	As above
Mood stabilizer				
Lithium	300–600	PO	2–3/d	Polyuria, polydipsia, toxic at high doses
Valproic acid	500–750	PO	2/d	Sedation
Carbamazepine	200–400	PO	2/d	Ataxia, decreased white blood cell count
Antidepressant				
Fluoxetine	20–40	PO	Once daily	Sedation, nausea
Sertraline	50–200	PO	Once daily	As above
Paroxetine	20–40	PO	At bedtime	As above
Bupropion and bupropion SR	100–300	PO	2–3/d 1–2/d	
Nortriptyline	75–150	PO	At bedtime	Sedation, dry mouth, constipation
Amitriptyline	75–300	PO	At bedtime	As above
Doxepin	100–300	PO	At bedtime	As above

Abbreviations: PO orally, *IM* intramuscular, *IV* intravenous

been more completely evaluated, often when the patient is at a major medical center or back at their home station.

The most commonly used benzodiazepines are diazepam (Valium), lorazepam (Ativan), and clonazepam (Klonopin). Standard doses and time of administration vary depending on the agent used (see Table 23.4). However, doses significantly higher than standard may be required to calm an agitated patient prior to flight. One should begin with the standard dose and repeat in 1 hour if necessary. Benzodiazepines may be then repeated every 4–6 hours, if necessary, but the patient needs to be closely monitored.

Mania and Psychosis

Manic and psychotic patients should be stabilized for 3–5 days on antipsychotic agents before the flight, if at all possible. Some calming effect of these agents is usually evident within 1 or 2 hours, but the antipsychotic properties do not begin to take effect for 24–72 hours. It should be kept in mind that most antipsychotic agents work synergistically with benzodiazepines.

One of the most commonly used antipsychotic agents is still haloperidol (Haldol). Because this drug is associated with a high incidence of extrapyramidal symptoms (EPS) and dystonias, all patients on haloperidol should simultaneously be given an anticholinergic agent such as benztropine (Cogentin) or diphenhydramine (Benadryl). Some of the newer antipsychotic agents (e.g., olanzapine or risperidone) can significantly decreased risk of dystonias. However, these patients should still be provided with an anticholinergic agent to use, if needed, during the flight. The antipsychotic chlorpromazine (Thorazine) should be avoided because of the high incidence of anticholinergic symptoms.

Of the anticholinergic agents used to combat EPS, benztropine is more commonly used because it is less sedating than diphenhydramine. The side effects of both, especially at high doses, include dry mouth, constipation, inability to regulate heat, and confusion. All these medications may be given by the oral (PO), intramuscular (IM), or intravenous (IV) route.

Bipolar Mood Disorders

Bipolar (i.e., manic-depressive) mood disorders are most commonly treated with lithium, carbamazepine (Tegretol), or valproic acid (Depakote), although the latter two have not been approved for this purpose by the US Food and Drug Administration (FDA). These medications will normally have to be administered for 3–7 days before they will achieve a therapeutic effect. Because of their potential toxicity, all three must be monitored by following blood levels. Lithium has an especially narrow therapeutic window, with a therapeutic range between 0.6 and 1.2 mmol/L and toxicity >1.5 mmol/L. If a patient has been started on any of these drugs immediately prior to AE, they should be used only in the lowest effective dose because blood levels will be difficult or impossible to obtain while in transit.

Depression

The most commonly prescribed antidepressant medications are the selective serotonic reupdate inhibitors (SSRIs), both because of their relative effectiveness and because of the minimal risk of side effects. SSRIs in common use include sertraline (Zoloft), paroxetine (Paxil), and fluoxetine (Prozac). Bupropion (Wellbutrin) is also extensively used. The major drawback of all antidepressants is the 1- to 2-week delay between the start of administration and onset of therapeutic effects. Tricyclic agents are an older class of antidepressants less commonly prescribed because of anticholinergic side effects and the danger of overdose. They include nortriptyline (Pamelor), amitriptyline (Elavil), and doxepin (Sinequan).

Acute Management of Violent or Agitated Patients

Several medications, both oral and parenteral, are useful to treat violent or agitated patients acutely even if they are on other psychotropic medications (see Table 23.5). The ideal psychotropic for use in such a situation should have a quick calming effect with minimal risk of oversedation. An oversedated patient can have potentially life-threatening respiratory depression or depression of the normal gag reflexes.

Table 23.5 Medical management of the violent or agitated patient

Haloperidol	5 mg	Oral, IM, IV
Diphenhydramine	50 mg	As above
Lorazepam	2 mg	As above

Note: All three may be repeated in 30 minutes if the patient is not yet sedated
Abbreviations: IM intramuscular, *IV* intravenous

The most commonly used drugs for acute patient sedation include haloperidol (Haldol), diphenhydramine (Benadryl), and lorazepam (Ativan). These drugs have been chosen because they are often readily available and have a relatively fast onset of action and relatively broad safety margin. The combination of haloperidol, diphenhydramine, and lorazepam may also be mixed in the same syringe.

If the patient agrees, these medications should be given by mouth. If they are uncooperative, they may need to be restrained and the medications given by injection. It is not wise to attempt to restrain an agitated person without sufficient help—at least five people are needed to form the restraint team, one for each limb and one for the head. Indications for IM medications include severe disruption and danger to self, others, or property (see Table 23.5).

Restraints

Patients who are a danger to themselves or others and cannot be controlled medically are transported in restraints (see Table 23.1). The restraints most commonly used for AE are still the traditional 4-point leather restraints. They include two leather wrist cuffs and two larger ankle cuffs secured to the bed or litter by belts. There is also an optional waist belt. Because these restraints must be locked, the crew should verify prior to flight that they have the correct key to unlock the restraints in the event of an emergency. Hospitals accredited by Joint Commission on Accreditation of Health Care Organizations (JCAHO) are now required to use Velcro nonlocking cuffs. These do not require a key and are more comfortable for the patient.

The written orders for the use of restraints during AE must be detailed, specific, and written by the referring physician prior to flight [24]. The orders must specify the justification for placement, the date and time restraint will be used, the type of restraint, and the positions on the extremities. The orders should also outline other less restrictive means to control the patient, such as medication and family involvement. By regulation, the use of restraints must be time limited and cannot exceed 24 hours. Within those 24 hours, the restraints cannot be used for more than 4 hours for adults.

Restraint orders can authorize the medical attendant to continue restraints for an additional 24 hours at his or her discretion. However, even if no restraint orders have been given, the commanding officer of the AE crew may initiate the use of leather restraints in an emergency. If the commander is a flight nurse, as is often the case, a physician must be contacted for verbal authorization within 1 hour [24].

The use of restraints has certain risks to the patient. Most patients will be medicated. Some sedation (e.g., a benzodiazepine) is recommended to minimize the associated discomfort and humiliation. The patient will need to be carefully monitored by a dedicated attendant for signs of oversedation, resulting in hypoventilation or aspiration, or for evidence of circulatory problems related to the restraints themselves. Hydration and elimination needs must also be met. This intensive monitoring should be documented on a flow sheet at 15-minute intervals.

Procedures for Military Members and Dependents

Military members and their dependents may be treated at any military medical facility. However, medical and personnel records are usually best managed by the same branch of the military in which the patient serves. Patients returning from overseas should bring with them any important personnel documents and belongings, as it is unlikely that they will return to their unit.

Active-duty members should bring their uniforms as well because most military hospitals require that psychiatric patients wear them.

Both active-duty personnel and dependents should be encouraged to sign a voluntary admission form for the destination medical facility before AE. This will avoid the less-than-ideal situation in which a patient is transported great distances by AE only to refuse admission or to immediately sign out against medical advice. If a dependent declines to sign a voluntary admission form, it may be best to delay AE.

If an active-duty member disagrees with the plan for AE and voluntary admission, an involuntary admission can be ordered. This will require a command memorandum that details the need for continued psychiatric evaluation and/or treatment. The guidelines for command-directed mental health evaluations are covered in Mental Health Evaluations of Members of the Armed Forces (DODD 6490.1) and Requirements for Mental Health Evaluations of Members of the Armed Forces (DODI 6490.4) [25, 26].

Preparation for Aeromedical Evacuation

Patients with serious psychiatric conditions that cannot be effectively managed or treated locally must be prepared for AE. Patients should be thoroughly assessed, stabilized, classified, and cleared by a flight surgeon for AE. The first step in the evacuation of a psychiatric patient is communication and coordination between the referring physician and the accepting physician in a hospital facility. The referring physician should prepare a detailed evacuation summary, which includes the history of present illness and reason for continued psychiatric treatment. Often, the patient's mental status when they present to the receiving facility is vastly different from when they initially sought treatment. In many cases, this is related to the therapeutic effects of the psychotropic drugs they may be taking.

During Operation Iraqi Freedom and Operation New Dawn, a CASF was established at Joint Base Balad in Iraq. This was an ideal location for the CASF because it was adjacent to the 332nd Expeditionary Medical Group and the Air Force Theater Hospital at Balad [12, 21].

Patients from Iraq and surrounding locations who required psychiatric AE were transferred to Balad. Patients who required additional evaluation, stabilization, or classification were often first sent to the Air Force Theater Hospital prior to being transferred to the CASF. Other psychiatric patients who were already stable and classified were transferred directly to the CASF. The CASF was staffed with behavioral health providers, nurses, and technicians to further assess and manage psychiatric patients and to confirm the AE classification. If the psychiatric patient had a medical or nonmedical attendant, the CASF behavioral health staff would help ensure that the attendant was aware of the policies, procedures, and requirements to serve as an attendant.

For service members deployed to Afghanistan and surrounding locations in support of Operation Enduring Freedom and Operation Freedom's Sentinel, the CASF located adjacent to the Craig Joint Theater Hospital at Bagram Airfield (also known as Bagram Air Base) has served as the primary location for AE. The basic policies and procedures for the assessment, stabilization, classification, and clearance by a flight surgeon for AE at the Bagram CASF are similar to those described for Balad.

Indications for Return to Medical Facility Prior to Evacuation

Patients who have been transferred to a CASF are continuously assessed and monitored by the behavioral health staff members as well as by other CASF medical staff. If it is determined that a psychiatric patient is unstable and too high of a risk for flight safety and that further stabilization is required, he or she should be transferred back to the theater hospital or combat support hospital for additional treatment and stabilization. Once stabilized, the patient is transferred back to the CASF and prepared for psychiatric AE.

References

1. Ritchie EC. Aeromedical evacuation of psychiatric casualties. In: Hurd WW, Jernigan JG, editors. Aeromedical evacuation. New York, NY: Springer; 2003.
2. Peterson AL, McCarthy KR, Busheme DJ, Campise RL, Baker MT. The aeromedical evacuation. In: Ritchie EC, Bradley JC, Grammer GG, Forsten RD, Cozza SJ, Benedek DM, Schneider BJ, editors. Combat and operational mental health. San Antonio, TX: The Borden Institute; 2011. p. 191–207.
3. Armed Forces Health Surveillance Center. Medical evacuations from Operation Iraqi Freedom/ Operation New Dawn, active and reserve components, U.S. Armed Forces, 2003–2011. MSMR. 2012;19(2):18–21.
4. Armed Forces Health Surveillance Center. Medical evacuations from Afghanistan during Operation Enduring Freedom, active and reserve components, U.S. Armed Forces, 7 October 2001 to 31 December 2012. MSMR. 2013;20(6):2–8.
5. Williams VF, Stahlman S. Oh GT. Medical evacuations, active and reserve components, U.S. Armed Forces, 2013-2015. MSMR. 2017 Feb;24(2):15–21.
6. Lezama NG, Riddles LM, Pollan WA, Profenna LC. Disaster aeromedical evacuation. Mil Med. 2011 Oct;176(10):1128–32.
7. National Research Council, Division of Behavioral and Social Sciences and Education; Board on Behavioral, Cognitive, and Sensory Sciences, Committee on the Youth Population and Military Recruitment: Physical, Medical, and Mental Health Standards. In: Sackett PR, Mavor AS, editors. Assessing fitness for military enlistment: physical, medical, and mental health standards. Washington, DC: The National Academies Press; 2006.
8. Bollinger MJ, Schmidt S, Pugh JA, Parsons HM, Copeland LA, Pugh MJ. Erosion of the healthy soldier effect in veterans of US military service in Iraq and Afghanistan. Popul Health Metrics. 2015;13:8.
9. American Psychiatric Association. Diagnostic and statistical manual of mental disorders. 5th ed. Arlington, VA: The American Psychiatric Association; 2013.
10. Pai A, Suris AM, North CS. Posttraumatic stress disorder in the DSM-5: controversy, change, and conceptual considerations. Behav Sci. 2017;7(1):7.
11. Hoge CW, Toboni HE, Messer SC, Bell N, Amoroso P, Orman DT. The occupational burden of mental disorders in the U.S. military: psychiatric hospitalizations, involuntary separations, and disability. Am J Psychiatry. 2005;162(3):585–91.
12. Peterson AL, Baker MT, McCarthy KR. Combat stress casualties in Iraq. Part 2: Psychiatric screening prior to aeromedical evacuation. Perspect Psychiatr Care. 2008;44(3):159–68.
13. Cohen SP, Brown C, Kurihara C, Plunkett A, Nguyen C, Strassels SA. Diagnoses and factors associated with medical evacuation and return to duty for service members participating in Operation Iraqi Freedom or Operation Enduring Freedom: a prospective cohort study. Lancet. 2010;375(9711):301–9.
14. Rundell JR. Demographics of and diagnoses in Operation Enduring Freedom and Operation Iraqi Freedom personnel who were psychiatrically evacuated from the theater of operations. Gen Hosp Psychiatry. 2006;28(4):352–6.
15. Goodman GP, DeZee KJ, Burks R, Waterman BR, Belmont PJ. Epidemiology of psychiatric disorders sustained by a US Army brigade combat team during the Iraq War. Gen Hosp Psychiatry. 2011;33(1):51–7.
16. Hauret KG, Taylor BJ, Clemmons NS, Block SR, Jones BH. Frequency and causes of nonbattle injuries air evacuated from operations Iraqi freedom and enduring freedom, US Army, 2001–2006. Am J Prev Med. 2010;38(1):S94–107.
17. Jones N, Fear NT, Wessely S, Thandi G, Greenberg N. Forward psychiatry–early intervention for mental health problems among UK armed forces in Afghanistan. Eur Psychiatry. 2017;39:66–72.
18. Stetz MC, McDonald JJ, Lukey BJ, Gifford RK. Psychiatric diagnoses as a cause of medical evacuation. Aviat Space Environ Med. 2005;76(7):C15–20.
19. Turner MA, Kiernan MD, McKechanie AG, Finch PJ, McManus FB, Neal LA. Acute military psychiatric casualties from the war in Iraq. Br J Psychiatry. 2005;186(6):476–9.
20. Schmitz KJ, Schmied EA, Galarneau MR, Edwards NK. Psychiatric diagnoses and treatment of US military personnel while deployed to Iraq. Mil Med. 2012;177(4):380–9.
21. Peterson AL, Baker MT, McCarthy KR. Combat stress casualties in Iraq. Part 1: behavioral health consultation at an expeditionary medical group. Perspect Psychiatr Care. 2008s;44(3):146–58.
22. Wilmoth MC, Linton A, Gromadzki R, Larson MJ, Williams TV, Woodson J. Factors associated with psychiatric evacuation among service members deployed to Operation Enduring Freedom and Operation Iraqi Freedom, January 2004 to September 2010. Mil Med. 2015;180(1):53–60.
23. US Department of the Air Force. En route care and aeromedical evacuation medical operations. Air Force Instruction 48-307, Vol. 1. 2017. http://static.e-publishing.af.mil/production/1/af_sg/publication/afi48-307v1/afi48-307v1.pdf. Accessed 31 Oct 2018.
24. Department of the Air Force. Aeromedical evacuation patient considerations and standards of care. Washington, DC: US Government Printing Office; 1997. AFI 41-307
25. Department of Defense. Requirements of mental health evaluations of members of the armed forces. Washington, DC: US Government Printing Office; 1997. Directive 6490.1.
26. Department of Defense. Requirements of mental health evaluations of members of the armed forces. Washington, DC: US Government Printing Office; 1997. Instruction 6490.4

Index

W. W. Hurd, W. Beninati (eds.), *Aeromedical Evacuation*,
https://doi.org/10.1007/978-3-030-15903-0

N

P